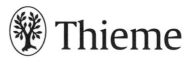

Anatomy

An Essential Textbook

Latin Nomenclature
Second Edition

Anne M. Gilroy, MA
Professor Emeritus
Department of Radiology
University of Massachusetts Medical School
Worcester, Massachusetts

Consulting Editor
Hugo Zeberg, MD
Department of Neuroscience
Karolinska Institute, Stockholm, Sweden

Illustrations by
Markus Voll
Karl Wesker

735 illustrations

Thieme
New York • Stuttgart • Delhi • Rio de Janeiro

Illustrations by Voll M and Wesker K. From: Schuenke M, Schulte E, Schumacher U, *THIEME Atlas of Anatomy*.
Compositor: DiTech

Library of Congress Cataloging-in-Publication Data

Names: Gilroy, Anne M., author. | Zeberg, Hugo, editor. | Voll, Markus M., illustrator. | Wesker, Karl, illustrator.

Title: Anatomy : an essential textbook : Latin nomenclature / Anne M. Gilroy, MA, Professor Emeritus, Department of Radiology, University of Massachusetts Medical School, Worcester, Massachusetts ; consulting editor, Hugo Zeberg, MD, Department of Neuroscience, Karolinska Institute, Stockholm, Sweden ; illustrations by Markus Voll, Karl Wesker.

Description: Second edition. | New York : Thieme, 2022. | Includes index. | Summary: "Building on the tradition of the highly acclaimed prior editions, Anatomy: An Essential Textbook, Latin Nomenclature, Second Edition by Anne M. Gilroy features new learning components that leverage the Thieme companion, Atlas of Anatomy, Fourth Edition, Latin Nomenclature. Concise, bulleted text paired with large, detailed anatomic figures enhance visual learning and retention of knowledge, using Latin nomenclature. Organized by eight units, the book starts with basic concepts and a general overview of anatomic systems. Subsequent units focused on regional anatomy cover the Back, Thorax, Abdominal Wall and Inguinal Region, Pelvis and Perineum, Upper Limb, Lower Limb, and Head and Neck. Each unit includes a chapter on the practical application of regional imaging and extensive question sets with detailed explanations. A new ordering of chapters now mirrors the revised organization of the Atlas and sequence of dissections in most gross anatomy programs. This is the quintessential resource for medical students to build anatomy knowledge and confidence as they progress in their medical careers"-- Provided by publisher.

Identifiers: LCCN 2022024299 (print) | LCCN 2022024300 (ebook) | ISBN 9781684205134 (paperback) | ISBN 9781684205158 (pdf) | ISBN 9781684205141 (epub)

Subjects: LCSH: Human anatomy. | Human anatomy-Nomenclature.

Classification: LCC QM23.2 .G56 2022 (print) | LCC QM23.2 (ebook) | DDC 611-dc23/eng/20220729

LC record available at https://lccn.loc.gov/2022024299

LC ebook record available at https://lccn.loc.gov/2022024300

©2023. Thieme. All rights reserved.

Thieme Medical Publishers, Inc.
333 Seventh Avenue, 18th Floor
New York, NY 10001, USA
www.thieme.com
+1 800 782 3488, customerservice@thieme.com

Cover design: Thieme Publishing Group

Printed in Germany by Appl   5 4 3 2 1

ISBN 978-1-68420-513-4

Also available as an e-book:
eISBN (PDF): 978-1-68420-515-8
eISBN (ePub): 978-1-68420-514-1

Important note: Medicine is an ever-changing science undergoing continual development. Research and clinical experience are continually expanding our knowledge, in particular our knowledge of proper treatment and drug therapy. Insofar as this book mentions any dosage or application, readers may rest assured that the authors, editors, and publishers have made every effort to ensure that such references are in accordance with **the state of knowledge at the time of production of the book.**

Nevertheless, this does not involve, imply, or express any guarantee or responsibility on the part of the publishers in respect to any dosage instructions and forms of applications stated in the book. **Every user is requested to examine carefully** the manufacturers' leaflets accompanying each drug and to check, if necessary in consultation with a physician or specialist, whether the dosage schedules mentioned therein or the contraindications stated by the manufacturers differ from the statements made in the present book. Such examination is particularly important with drugs that are either rarely used or have been newly released on the market. Every dosage schedule or every form of application used is entirely at the user's own risk and responsibility. The authors and publishers request every user to report to the publishers any discrepancies or inaccuracies noticed. If errors in this work are found after publication, errata will be posted at www.thieme.com on the product description page.

Some of the product names, patents, and registered designs referred to in this book are in fact registered trademarks or proprietary names even though specific reference to this fact is not always made in the text. Therefore, the appearance of a name without designation as proprietary is not to be construed as a representation by the publisher that it is in the public domain.

MIX
Paper | Supporting responsible forestry
FSC® C004592
www.fsc.org

To my mother, Mary Gilroy, a woman of courage and love;
To Colin and Bryan, my strength and sanity;
And once more, to my Dad.

Contents

I Introduction to Anatomic Systems and Terminology

II Back

III Thorax

IV Abdomen

V Pelvis and Perineum

VI Upper Limb

VII Lower Limb

VIII Head and Neck

Acknowledgments

Special thanks to authors Michael Schuenke, Erik Schulte, and Udo Schumacher of the award-winning three-volume *Thieme Atlas of Anatomy* and illustrators Markus Voll and Karl Wesker for their work over the course of many years

For their careful and thoughtful review of the manuscript, thanks to

William J. Swartz, PhD
Department of Cell Biology and Anatomy
LSU Health Sciences Center
New Orleans, Louisiana

For their contributions to the problems sets, thanks to

Frank J. Daly, PhD
Department of Biomedical Sciences
University of New England
School of Osteopathic Medicine
Biddeford, Maine

Geoffrey Guttman, PhD
Department of Cell Biology and Anatomy
University of North Texas Health Science Center
Texas College of Osteopathic Medicine
Fort Worth, Texas

Contributor: Clinical Imaging Basics
Joseph Makris, MD
Department of Radiology
Baystate Medical Center
Springfield, Massachusetts

Krista S. Johansen, MD
Department of Medical Education
Tufts University School of Medicine
Boston, Massachusetts

Michelle Lazarus, PhD
Center for Human Anatomy Education
Monash University
Melbourne, Victoria, Australia

Preface to the Second Edition

Since publication of the original version of the *Anatomy – An Essential Textbook,* the intent has been to offer an accurate, current and user-friendly resource for students of anatomy. But beyond those basic considerations, the inclusion of clinical content, the exquisite illustrations, and the carefully planned organization are designed to inspire students to fully appreciate the intrinsic role that anatomy will play throughout their medical careers. The relevance of anatomy to medical diagnosis and treatment continually evolves and it is my hope that this text will equip students with a fundamental knowledge that will be instrumental not only in today's medical environment but in the medical world of the future.

This book follows the general scheme of the original text. Basic concepts and a general overview of anatomic systems are covered in the first unit while subsequent units focus on regional anatomy. These include an overview of systems followed by chapters that focus more closely on the form and function of individual systems. Each unit includes a chapter on the practical application of regional imaging and an extensive question set.

In this second edition some helpful organizational changes have been included. A Table of Contents has been added at the beginning of each unit, listing chapters and sections as well as the tables and clinical boxes that appear within them. An effort has been made to coordinate with Thieme's fourth edition of the *Atlas of Anatomy*, often used as a companion resource. In this regard, readers will notice matching colored side tabs that allow quick access to similar units in both books. Note also that the chapter on the neck has been moved forward to immediately follow the introductory chapter in the Head and Neck unit. This new order follows the revised organization of the Atlas and mirrors the sequence of dissections in most gross anatomy programs.

Although the previous edition was rich with illustrations, over 100 new figures have been added with many others updated, including revised versions of all autonomic schematics. New topics in clinical and developmental anatomy, such as clinically important vascular anastomoses, spinal cord development, and common anatomic anomalies, are addressed throughout the text and an additional 50 clinical and developmental correlations are now illustrated with descriptive images, radiographs or schematics.

New content in several areas, such as defecation and fecal continence, structure of urethral sphincters, and the ulnocarpal complex of the wrist, expands, clarifies and updates existing text. The Clinical Imaging Basics chapters, first introduced in the second edition, proved to be popular with students and instructors and have been revised and enhanced with new images here. The self-testing sections in each unit have also been expanded with over 40 new USMLE-style question sets with detailed explanations.

As with each of the previous texts, this new edition came together through the work of a talented and dedicated team. I am exceedingly grateful to the steadfast support, patience and professional perspectives of Judith Tomat, Developmental Editor, Barbara Chernow, PhD, Production Editor, and Torsten Scheihagen, Senior Content Service Manager. Their guidance was unquestionably the most valuable asset throughout the project. Also, thanks to my colleague Joseph Makris, MD, who lent his experience as an educator and clinician to create the Clinical Imaging Basics chapters in the previous edition and further developed them for this edition.

A special acknowledgement goes to authors Michael Schuenke, Erik Schulte, and Udo Schumacher of the three-volume *Thieme Atlas of Anatomy* and illustrators Markus Voll and Karl Wesker whose work is seen throughout this text.

Finally, the design for each new edition has been motivated largely by user input. I deeply appreciate the many students and instructors who offered their comments, corrections and suggestions, with a particular thanks to William Swartz, PhD, for his very thorough and meticulous review. I look forward to their responses to this newest edition.

Anne M Gilroy
Worcester, Massachusetts

A Note on the Use of Latin Terminology

To introduce the Latin nomenclature into an English textbook is a delicate task, particularly because the many Latin loanwords have passed into general use. Some loanwords are so common that fluency of the text would be disturbed if they were to be translated back into Latin. The Latin loanwords have typically undergone several adaptations before becoming part of the English language. A term such as *sympathetic trunk* (lat. *truncus sympaticus*) has undergone morphological adaptation (through the loss of masculine suffix -*us*), orthographical adaptation (through the substitution of a 'Germanic' *k* for a Latin *c*), and phonological adaptation (*th* and *e* instead of *t* and *i*).

In addition, the word order has been reversed. The Latin term *sympaticus* is in fact borrowed from late Greek *sympathetikos* (from *sympathes* 'having a fellow feeling, affected by like feelings'), thereby illustrating that terms move between languages when cultures meet. Other anatomical terms are so colloquial (e.g., *hand*), that a Latin term (e.g., *manus*) would be inappropriate to use at all occasions. Clearly, the text would easily become unreadable if a strict translation of all English terms into Latin were imposed.

As a result, Latin has been used as long as it does not disrupt the flow of the text and whenever possible in figures and tables. In some cases, dual terminology has been used, with either the English or Latin word in parentheses. As much as possible, the terminology of *Terminologia Anatomica* (1998) has been followed.

For their assistance in reviewing the Latin nomenclature of this edition, I would like to express my gratitude to my talented assistant teachers — Miklós Szabó, Anna Thoss, John Bairoh, Adonis Sotoodeh, Eslem Nur Söğütlü, Julia Lichtenstein, Jacob Torakai, Zabih Aurfan, Tyra Hasselrot, David Freiholtz, Ville Hasselberg, Ida Norberg, Jenny Wang, Erica Rauhala, Milou Gamage, and Megan Gjordeni.

Hugo Zeberg
Stockholm, Sweden

Unit I   Introduction to Anatomic Systems and Terminology

1 Introduction to Anatomic Systems and Terminology

Anatomy of the human body can be studied by inspection of all the systems that occupy a specific region or by considering the global aspects of a particular system throughout the entire body. The first approach tends to focus on anatomic relationships while the second is better suited to studying physiologic influences. Most systems, however, are conveniently confined to one or two regions, and in this text are discussed in the units devoted to those regions. Some systems, however, (those included in this chapter) are more pervasive throughout the body, and a fundamental understanding of their basic organization is important before undertaking the study of the systems they support.

1.1 Structural Design of the Human Body

The most preliminary inspection of the human body reveals that it is structurally divided into a head and neck region, a trunk, and paired upper and lower extremities (limbs). Each is further divided into smaller regions (**Fig. 1.1; Table 1.1**). These house the structures that make up the functional organ systems that perform the basic bodily functions (**Table 1.2**). Although the primary organ of a system is often confined to a single anatomic region (e.g., the brain resides in the head), systems extend beyond regional borders, both anatomically and physiologically, to integrate their influences on normal function and growth.

Table 1.1 Regional Subdivisions of the Body

Head (Caput)

Neck (Collum)

Trunk (Truncus)
- Thorax (chest)
- Abdomen
- Pelvis

Upper limb (Membrum superius)
- Shoulder girdle (Cingulum membri superioris)
- Free upper limb (Pars libera membri superioris)

Lower limb (Membrum inferius)
- Pelvic girdle (Cingulum membri inferioris)
- Free lower limb (Pars libera membri inferioris)

Table 1.2 Functional Subdivisions by Organ Systems

Locomotor system (musculoskeletal system)
- Skeleton and skeletal connections (passive part)
- Striated skeletal musculature (active part)

Viscera
- Cardiovascular system
- Hemolymphatic system
- Endocrine system
- Respiratory system
- Digestive system
- Urinary system
- Male and female reproductive system

Nervous system
- Central and peripheral nervous system
- Sensory organs

The skin and its appendages

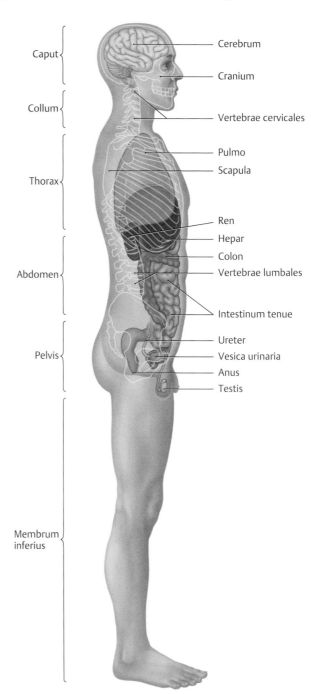

Fig. 1.1 Structural design of the human body: location of the internal organs
(From Schuenke M, Schulte E, Schumacher U. THIEME Atlas of Anatomy, Vol 1. Illustrations by Voll M and Wesker K. 3rd ed. New York: Thieme Publishers; 2020.)

1.2 Terms of Location and Direction, Cardinal Planes, and Axes

— All locational and directional terms used in anatomy, and in medical practice, refer to the human body in the **anatomic position,** in which the body is upright, arms at the side, with the eyes, palms of the hands, and feet directed forward (**Fig. 1.2, Table 1.3**).
— Three perpendicular cardinal planes and three axes based on the three spatial coordinates can be drawn through the body (**Fig. 1.3**).
  • The **plana sagittalia** passes through the body from front to back, dividing it into right and left sides.

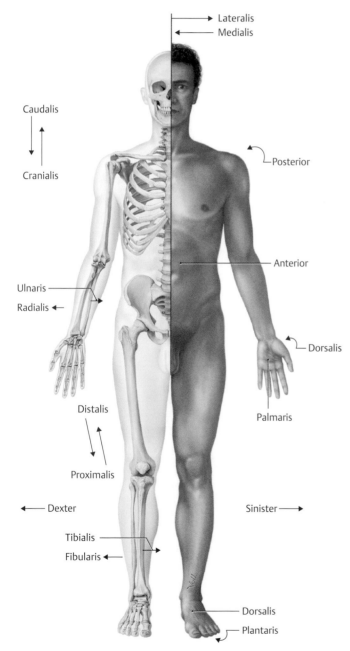

Fig. 1.2 Anatomic position
Anterior view. (From Schuenke M, Schulte E, Schumacher U. THIEME Atlas of Anatomy, Vol 1. Illustrations by Voll M and Wesker K. 3rd ed. New York: Thieme Publishers; 2020.)

Table 1.3 General Terms of Location and Direction

Term	Explanation
Upper Body (Caput, Collum, and Truncus)	
Cranialis	Pertaining to, or located toward, the head
Caudalis	Pertaining to, or located toward, the tail
Anterior	Pertaining to, or located toward, the front; synonym: ventralis (used for all animals)
Posterior	Pertaining to, or located toward, the back; synonym: dorsalis (used for all animals)
Superior	Upper or above
Inferior	Lower or below
Axialis	Pertaining to the axis of a structure
Transversus	Situated at right angles to the long axis of a structure
Longitudinalis	Parallel to the long axis of a structure
Horizontalis	Parallel to the plane of the horizon
Verticalis	Perpendicular to the plane of the horizon
Medialis	Toward the median plane
Lateralis	Away from the median plane (toward the side)
Medianus	Situated in the median plane or midline
Peripheralis	Situated away from the center
Superficialis	Situated near the surface
Profundus	Situated deep beneath the surface
Externus	Outer or lateral
Internus	Inner or medial
Apicalis	Pertaining to the top or apex
Basalis	Pertaining to the bottom or base
Sagittalis	Situated parallel to the sutura sagittalis
Coronalis	Situated parallel to the sutura coronalis (pertaining to the crown of the head)
Limbs	
Proximalis	Close to, or toward, the truncus, or toward the point of origin
Distalis	Away from the truncus (toward the end of the limb), or away from the point of origin
Radialis	Pertaining to the radius or the lateral side of the antebrachium
Ulnaris	Pertaining to the ulna or the medial side of the antebrachium
Tibialis	Pertaining to the tibia or the medial side of the crus
Fibularis	Pertaining to the fibula or the lateral side of the crus
Palmaris (volaris)	Pertaining to the palma
Plantaris	Pertaining to the planta
Dorsalis	Pertaining to the dorsum manus or dorsum pedis

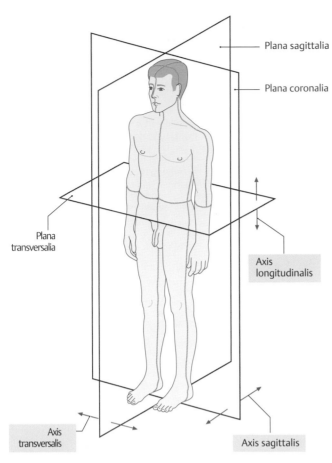

Fig. 1.3 Cardinal planes and axes
Neutral position, left anterolateral view. (From Schuenke M, Schulte E, Schumacher U. THIEME Atlas of Anatomy, Vol 1. Illustrations by Voll M and Wesker K. 3rd ed. New York: Thieme Publishers; 2020.)

- The **plana coronalia** passes through the body from side to side, dividing it into front (anterior) and back (posterior) parts.
- The **plana transversalia** (axial, horizontal, cross-sectional planes) divides the body into upper and lower parts. A particular transverse section is often given the designation of the corresponding vertebral level, such as *T IV*, which passes through vertebra thoracica T IV.
- The **axis longitudinalis** passes along the height of the body in a craniocaudal direction.
- The **axis sagittalis** passes from the front to the back (or the back to the front) of the body in an anteroposterior direction.
- The **axis transversalis** (horizontal axis) passes through the body from side to side.

1.3   Landmarks and Reference Lines

— In surface anatomy, palpable structures or visible markings on the surface of the body are used to identify the location of underlying structures. **Reference lines** are vertical or transverse planes that connect palpable structures or markings (**Tables 1.4, 1.5,** and **1.6;** see also **Fig. 1.5**).

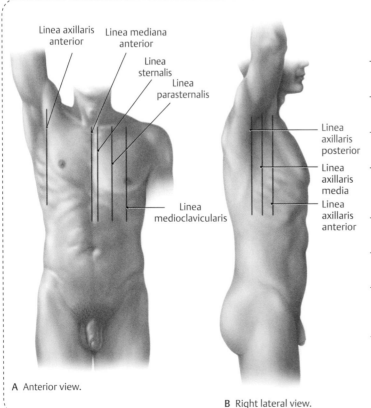

A Anterior view.

B Right lateral view.

Table 1.4 Anterior and Lateral Reference Lines on the Trunk
(From Schuenke M, Schulte E, Schumacher U. THIEME Atlas of Anatomy, Vol 1. Illustrations by Voll M and Wesker K. 3rd ed. New York: Thieme Publishers; 2020.)

Linea mediana anterior	Passes through the center of the sternum
Linea sternalis	Passes along the lateral border of the sternum
Linea medioclavicularis	Passes through the midpoint of the clavicula
Linea parasternalis	Passes through a point midway between the linea sternalis and linea medioclavicularis
Linea axillaris anterior	Marks the anterior axillary fold formed by the m. pectoralis major
Linea axillaris posterior	Marks the posterior axillary fold formed by the m. teres major
Linea axillaris media	Marks the midpoint between the linea axillaris anterior and linea axillaris posterior

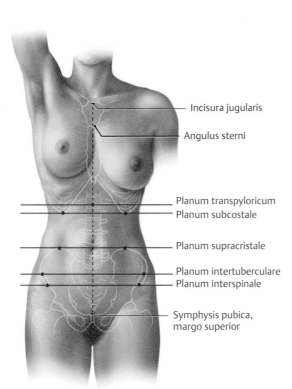

Incisura jugularis
Angulus sterni
Planum transpyloricum
Planum subcostale
Planum supracristale
Planum intertuberculare
Planum interspinale
Symphysis pubica, margo superior

Table 1.5 Landmarks and Transverse Planes on the Anterior Trunk
(From Schuenke M, Schulte E, Schumacher U. THIEME Atlas of Anatomy, Vol 1. Illustrations by Voll M and Wesker K. 3rd ed. New York: Thieme Publishers; 2020.)

Incisura jugularis	Marks the superior border of the manubrium sterni
Angulus sterni	Marks the junction of manubrium and corpus sterni
Planum transpyloricum	Passes through the midpoint between the incisura jugularis and symphysis pubica
Planum subcostale	Marks the lowest level of the cavea thoracis, cartilago costalis X
Planum supracristale	Connects the top of the cristae iliacae
Planum intertuberculare	Passes through the tubercula iliaca
Planum interspinale	Connects the cristae iliacae anterior superior

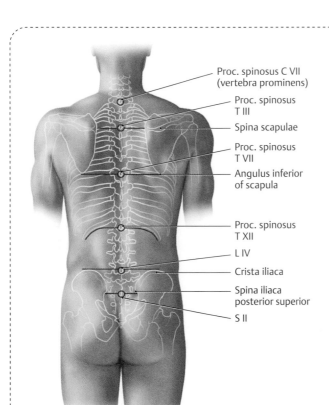

Proc. spinosus C VII (vertebra prominens)
Proc. spinosus T III
Spina scapulae
Proc. spinosus T VII
Angulus inferior of scapula
Proc. spinosus T XII
L IV
Crista iliaca
Spina iliaca posterior superior
S II

Table 1.6 Vertebral Spinous Processes and Posterior Landmarks
(From Schuenke M, Schulte E, Schumacher U. THIEME Atlas of Anatomy, Vol 1. Illustrations by Voll M and Wesker K. 3rd ed. New York: Thieme Publishers; 2020.)

C VII	Vertebra prominens
T III	Level of the medial edge of spinae scapulae
T VII	Level of the anguli inferiores scapulae
T XII	Level of the lower limit of cavitas thoracis
L IV	Level of the cristae iliacae
S II	Level of the spinae iliacae posteriores superiores

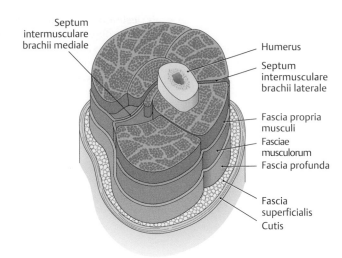

Fig. 1.4 Fascia
Cross section through the brachium dexter, proximal view. (From Schuenke M, Schulte E, Schumacher U. THIEME Atlas of Anatomy, Vol 1. Illustrations by Voll M and Wesker K. 3rd ed. New York: Thieme Publishers; 2020.)

1.4   Connective and Supporting Tissues

— Connective tissue comprises a variety of forms that are found throughout the body. Its common characteristic is a predominance of extracellular material made up largely of fibrous proteins and an amorphous ground substance and widely spaced cells that may include adipocytes, fibroblasts, and mesenchymal stem cells as well as macrophages and lymphocytes. Bone and cartilage are specialized types of connective tissue.

— The classification of connective tissue types is based on the degree to which the fibrous components are organized.
  • Irregular types include
    ◦ Loose, or areolar, connective tissue, which is widely distributed around vessels and nerves and within organs, where it binds lobes and groups of muscle fascicles. It provides support while allowing movement of structures.
    ◦ Dense connective tissue, which supports structures under mechanical stress. It ensheathes muscles and nerves and forms the capsules of organs such as the testis.
    ◦ Adipose tissue, or fat, which is found in specialized areas such as the subcutaneous tissue of the skin, the female breast (mamma), and padding on the soles of the feet and in the renal bed surrounding the kidneys (renes).
  • Regular connective tissue, which is largely fibrous but may also contain elastin fibers, makes up the tendons, ligaments, and aponeuroses as well as fascial layers that enclose muscles and underlie the skin.

— Fascia is a general term that has been redefined in recent years to describe any easily discernable connective tissue sheet or sheath. The most common usages pertain to the connective tissue layers between the skin and muscle, formerly known as the fasciae superficialis and fasciae profunda. New terminology refers to these layers as the **subcutaneous connective tissue** with two layers **(Fig. 1.4)**:
  • A **fatty layer** of varying thickness that lies deep to the skin, composed of loose connective tissue and fat, traversed by superficial nerves and vessels.
  • A **membranous layer** of dense connective tissue layer that lies under (deep to) the fatty layer and is devoid of fat. It forms an investing layer, which envelops neurovascular structures and muscles of the limbs, trunk wall, head, and neck. Invaginations of this layer form intermuscular septa that compartmentalize limb musculature into functional groups.

1.5   The Integumentary System

The skin (integument), the largest organ of the body, protects underlying tissue from biologic, mechanical, and chemical injury; regulates body temperature; and participates in metabolic processes, such as the synthesis of vitamin D.

— The skin is composed of
  • an outer waterproof avascular layer, the **epidermis,** which has a superficial layer of keratinized cells that shed continuously and a deep basal layer of regenerating cells, and
  • an inner richly vascularized and innervated layer, the **dermis,** which supports the epidermis and contains hair follicles.

1.6   The Skeletal System

The bones and cartilages of the body, which make up the skeletal system, provide leverage for muscles and protect the internal organs. Bone is also the site for calcium storage and blood cell production.

— There are two anatomic divisions of the skeleton **(Fig. 1.5)**:
  • The **axial skeleton,** which consists of the skull, vertebrae, os sacrum, os coccygis, ribs (costae), and sternum
  • The **appendicular skeleton,** which includes the clavicle and scapula of the pectoral girdle, the coxal bones of the pelvic girdle, and the bones of the upper and lower limbs

— **Periosteum** is a thin layer of fibrous connective tissue that coats the outer surface of each bone **(Fig. 1.6)**. **Perichondrium** forms a similar layer around cartilaginous structures. These tissues nourish and assist in the healing of the underlying bone.
— All bones have a superficial layer of dense **compact** (cortical) **bone** that surrounds a less dense **cancellous** (spongy) **bone.** In some areas of the bone, a **medullary cavity** contains yellow (fatty) or red (blood cell or platelet-forming) **bone marrow.**
— Bones develop from **mesenchyme** (embryonic connective tissue) through two processes of ossification (bone formation).

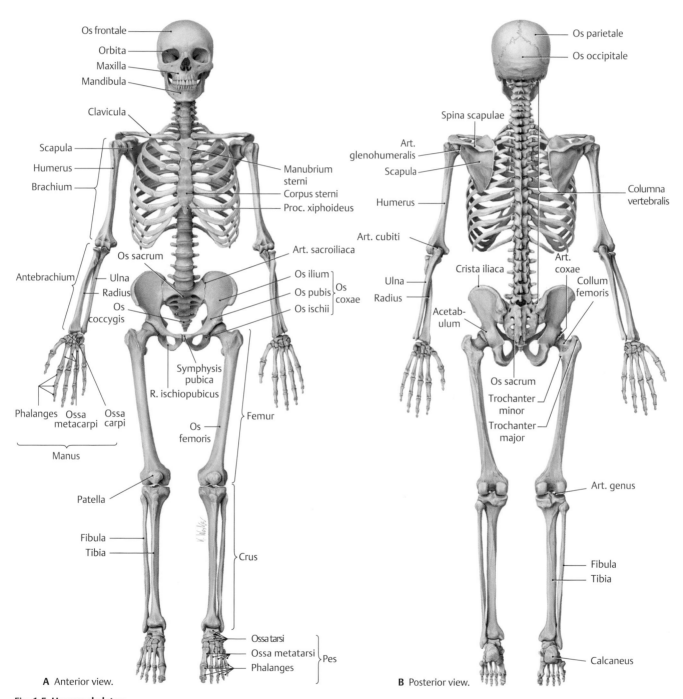

A Anterior view.   **B** Posterior view.

Fig. 1.5 **Human skeleton**
Left forearm is pronated, and both feet are in plantarflexion. (From Schuenke M, Schulte E, Schumacher U. THIEME Atlas of Anatomy, Vol 1. Illustrations by Voll M and Wesker K. 3rd ed. New York: Thieme Publishers; 2020.)

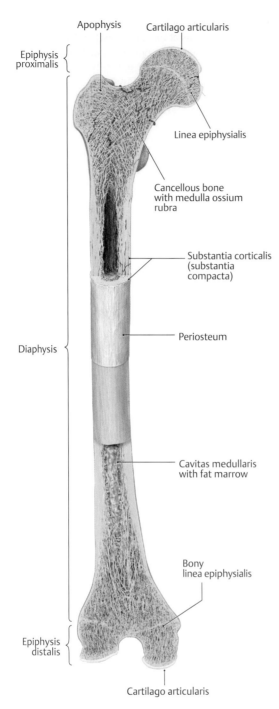

Fig. 1.6 **Structure of a typical long bone**
Illustrated for the femur. Coronal cuts through the proximal and distal parts of an adult femur. (From Schuenke M, Schulte E, Schumacher U. THIEME Atlas of Anatomy, Vol 1. Illustrations by Voll M and Wesker K. 3rd ed. New York: Thieme Publishers; 2020.)

- The clavicle and some bones of the skull develop by **membranous ossification,** in which the bones form through direct ossification of mesenchymal templates that are set down during the embryonic period.
- Most bones, including the long bones of the limbs, develop by **endochondral ossification,** in which a cartilaginous template, formed from mesenchyme, is laid down during the fetal period. Over the first and second decades of life, bone replaces most of the cartilage.
  - Within each bone undergoing endochondral ossification, bone formation occurs first at a **primary ossification center,** which is in the **diaphysis** (shaft) of the long bones. **Secondary ossification centers** appear later at the **epiphyses** (growing ends) of the bones.
— Long bones of the skeleton increase in length through growth of the epiphyses and diaphysis on either side of the **lamina epiphysialis,** an intervening cartilaginous area. During childhood and adolescence the laminae epiphysiales gradually shorten as they are replaced by bone. In the adult these areas are completely ossified, and only thin **linea epiphysialis** remain.
— **Apophyses,** bony outgrowths that lack their own growth center, serve as attachment sites for ligaments or tendons. Specific apophyses are referred to as condyles, tubercles, spines, crests, trochanters, or processes.
— **Ligaments** are connective tissue bands that connect bones to each other or to cartilage. (Within the body cavities, the term *ligament* refers to folds or condensations of a serous or fibrous membrane that support visceral structures.)
— Joints are classified according to the type of tissue that connects the bones.
  - **Syndesmoses** (fibrous joints), such as those found in the sutures of the skull and interosseous membrane of the forearm, are united by fibrous tissue and allow minimal movement (**Fig. 1.7**).
  - **Synchondroses** (cartilaginous joints) are united either by fibrocartilaginous segments, such as the cartilago costalis of costae, disci intervertebrales, and symphysis pubica (**Fig. 1.8A,B**), or by cartilago articularis, often found in

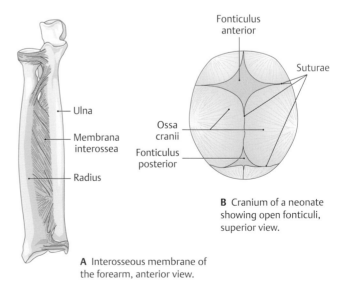

A Interosseous membrane of the forearm, anterior view.

B Cranium of a neonate showing open fonticuli, superior view.

Fig. 1.7 **Syndesmoses**
(From Schuenke M, Schulte E, Schumacher U. THIEME Atlas of Anatomy, Vol 1. Illustrations by Voll M and Wesker K. 3rd ed. New York: Thieme Publishers; 2020.)

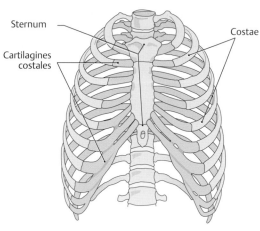

A Cartilago costalis.

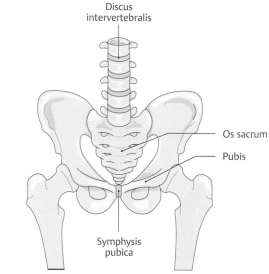

B Symphysis pubica and disci intervertebrales.

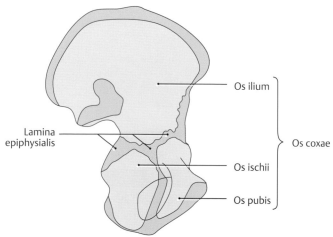

C Os coxae before closure of laminae epiphysiales.

Fig. 1.8 Synchondroses
(From Schuenke M, Schulte E, Schumacher U. THIEME Atlas of Anatomy, Vol 1. Illustrations by Voll M and Wesker K. 3rd ed. New York: Thieme Publishers; 2020.)

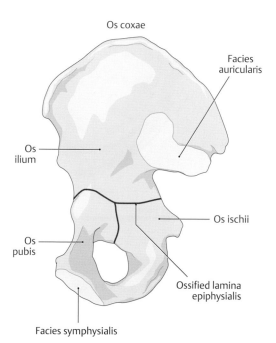

Fig. 1.9 Synostoses
Os coxae (fusion of ischium, ilium, and pubis). (From Schuenke M, Schulte E, Schumacher U. THIEME Atlas of Anatomy, Vol 1. Illustrations by Voll M and Wesker K. 3rd ed. New York: Thieme Publishers; 2020.)

temporary joints, such as those that join the ilium, ischium, and pubis of the hip bone **(Fig. 1.8C)**. Subsequent fusion of these temporary joints creates **synostoses** (sites of bony fusion) **(Fig. 1.9)**.

- **Synovial joints,** the most common type of joint, allow free movement **(Fig. 1.10)** and typically have
    - a **cavitas articularis** that is enclosed by a fibrous **capsula articularis** and lined by a **synovial membrane,** which secretes a thin film of lubricating **synovial fluid;**
    - articulating ends of the bones that are covered by cartilago epiphysialis; and
    - extrinsic ligaments on the outer surface, which reinforce the joints.
    - Some synovial joints also contain intrinsic ligaments and intra-articular fibrocartilaginous structures.
- **Bursae** are closed sacs that contain a thin film of fluid and are lined with a synovial membrane. Commonly found around joints of the limbs, bursae cushion prominent bony processes from external pressure and prevent friction where tendons cross bony surfaces.

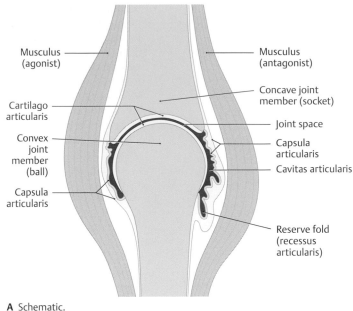

A Schematic.

B Intracapsular structures of the art. genus.

Fig. 1.10 Structure of a synovial joint
(From Schuenke M, Schulte E, Schumacher U. THIEME Atlas of Anatomy, Vol 1. Illustrations by Voll M and Wesker K. 3rd ed. New York: Thieme Publishers; 2020.)

BOX 1.1: ANATOMIC NOTES

EXTRA-ARTICULAR AND INTRA-ARTICULAR STRUCTURES OF SYNOVIAL JOINTS (SEE FIG. 1.10)

The joint capsule of a synovial joint is composed of an outer fibrous membrane and an inner synovial membrane. The intima (innermost lining) of the synovial membrane produces the synovial fluid, which lubricates and nourishes intra-articular structures.

— Ligaments of synovial joints act as primary joint stabilizers. They may be:
  • Extra-capsular (e.g., lig. collaterale fibulare of the knee), which lie outside the fibrous capsule.
  • Intra-capsular, which run either within the fibrous membrane (e.g., lig. collaterale tibiale of the art. genus) or

between the fibrous and synovial membranes (e.g., ligg. cruciata).

— Menisci, articular disks, and articular labra are intra-articular structures composed of connective tissue and fibrocartilage:
  • Menisci are crescent-shaped structures found in the art. genus. They act as shock absorbers and modify the incongruity of the articulating surfaces.
  • Articular disks divide joints into separate chambers and are found in the artt. sternoclavicularis and radiocarpea.
  • Articular labra are wedge-shaped structures that line the glenoid of the scapula and acetabulum of the os coxae, thus enlarging the articular surfaces of the shoulder and hip joints.

1.7 The Muscular System

The muscular system is composed of muscles and their tendons, which produce movement through contraction of muscle cells.

— **Muscle cells** are the structural units of the muscular system. Connective tissue binds muscle cells (fibers) together to form bundles, which in turn are bound together to form muscles (**Fig. 1.11**).

— A **motor unit** is the functional unit of muscles and describes the group of muscle fibers innervated by a single motor neuron. Motor units are relatively small in muscles that perform fine movements but larger in muscles that are responsible for maintaining posture or performing gross movements.

— Muscles function through tensing and contraction of the muscle fibers, which provide movement and stability
  • **Phasic contractions** can change the length of the muscle through shortening (**concentric contractions**), or lengthening (**eccentric contractions**), or simply increasing the muscle tension (**isometric contractions**).
  • **Tonic contractions** contribute to stability of joints and position but do not provide any movements.
  • **Reflexive contractions** are involuntary and are responsive to muscle stretch.

— Muscle tissue is classified by location (somatic or visceral), appearance (striated or nonstriated), and innervation (voluntary or involuntary).

— **Somatic**, or **skeletal muscles**, the most prevalent type, are found in the neck, trunk wall, and limbs, where they move and support the skeleton (**Fig. 1.12**). They are multinucleated, striated, and voluntary.

• Somatic muscle fibers are interwoven with three sheaths of connective tissue including the **endomysium**, the innermost sheath, which surrounds and condenses muscle fibers into primary bundles; the **perimysium,** which surrounds and condenses primary bundles into secondary bundles; and the **epimysium**, a loose connective tissue layer that surrounds the muscle and lies deep to the muscle fascia.

• **Muscle fascia** is the tough connective tissue sheath that encloses the muscle, maintains its shape, and allows frictionless movement between muscles and muscle groups.

• **Tendons**, dense fibrous bands, connect muscles to their bony attachments. **Aponeuroses** are tendons that form flat sheets, which attach the muscle to the skeleton, other muscles, or organs.

• Muscles shapes are described according to the arrangement of the muscle fibers as pennate (uni-, bi-, multi-), fusiform, circular, convergent, or parallel.

• **Tendon (synovial) sheaths**, such as those found in the wrist and ankle, facilitate the movement of tendons over bone. Similar to a capsula articularis, they are composed of an outer vagina fibrosa lined with a two-layered synovial membrane. The space between the synovial layers is filled with synovial fluid.

— **Visceral muscles,** considered involuntary**,** alter the shape of internal structures, such as the heart (cor) and gastrointestinal tract. There are two types:
  • **Cardiac muscle**, which makes up the thick muscular layer (myocardium) of the heart, is striated.
  • **Smooth muscle,** which is found in the walls of blood vessels and hollow internal organs, is nonstriated.

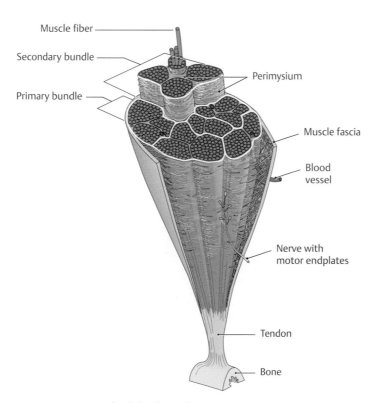

Muscle fiber
Secondary bundle
Primary bundle
Perimysium
Muscle fascia
Blood vessel
Nerve with motor endplates
Tendon
Bone

Fig. 1.11 Structure of a skeletal muscle
Cross section through a skeletal muscle. (From Schuenke M, Schulte E, Schumacher U. THIEME Atlas of Anatomy, Vol 1. Illustrations by Voll M and Wesker K. 3rd ed. New York: Thieme Publishers; 2020.)

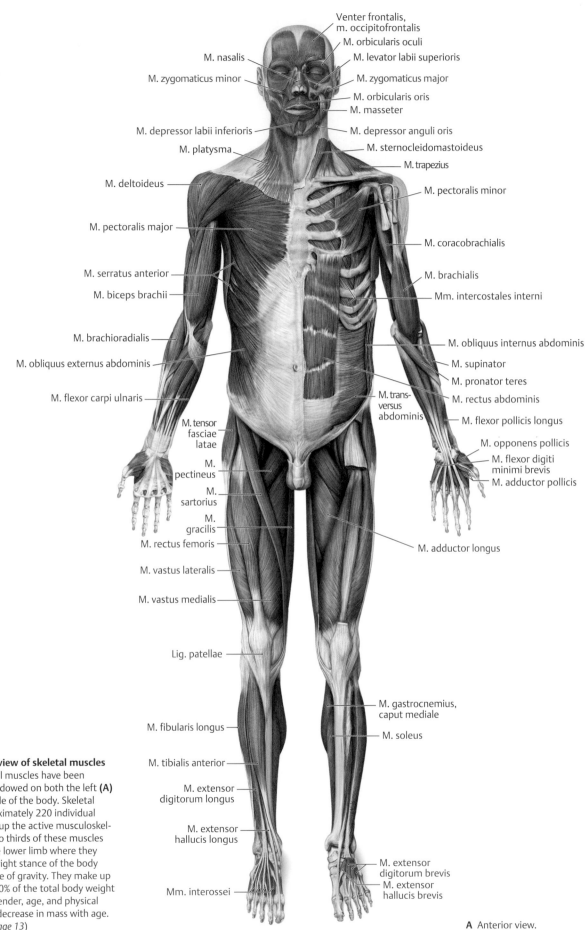

Venter frontalis,
m. occipitofrontalis

M. orbicularis oculi

M. nasalis

M. levator labii superioris

M. zygomaticus minor

M. zygomaticus major

M. orbicularis oris

M. masseter

M. depressor labii inferioris

M. depressor anguli oris

M. platysma

M. sternocleidomastoideus

M. trapezius

M. deltoideus

M. pectoralis minor

M. pectoralis major

M. coracobrachialis

M. serratus anterior

M. brachialis

M. biceps brachii

Mm. intercostales interni

M. brachioradialis

M. obliquus internus abdominis

M. obliquus externus abdominis

M. supinator

M. pronator teres

M. flexor carpi ulnaris

M. rectus abdominis

M. trans-
versus
abdominis

M. flexor pollicis longus

M. tensor
fasciae
latae

M. opponens pollicis

M. flexor digiti
minimi brevis

M.
pectineus

M. adductor pollicis

M.
sartorius

M.
gracilis

M. rectus femoris

M. adductor longus

M. vastus lateralis

M. vastus medialis

Lig. patellae

M. gastrocnemius,
caput mediale

M. fibularis longus

M. soleus

M. tibialis anterior

M. extensor
digitorum longus

M. extensor
hallucis longus

M. extensor
digitorum brevis

M. extensor
hallucis brevis

Mm. interossei

Fig. 1.12 Overview of skeletal muscles
Some superficial muscles have been removed or windowed on both the left **(A)** and right **(B)** side of the body. Skeletal muscles (approximately 220 individual muscles) make up the active musculoskeletal system. Two thirds of these muscles are found in the lower limb where they support the upright stance of the body against the force of gravity. They make up an average of 40% of the total body weight (varying with gender, age, and physical condition) but decrease in mass with age. (continued on page 13)

A Anterior view.

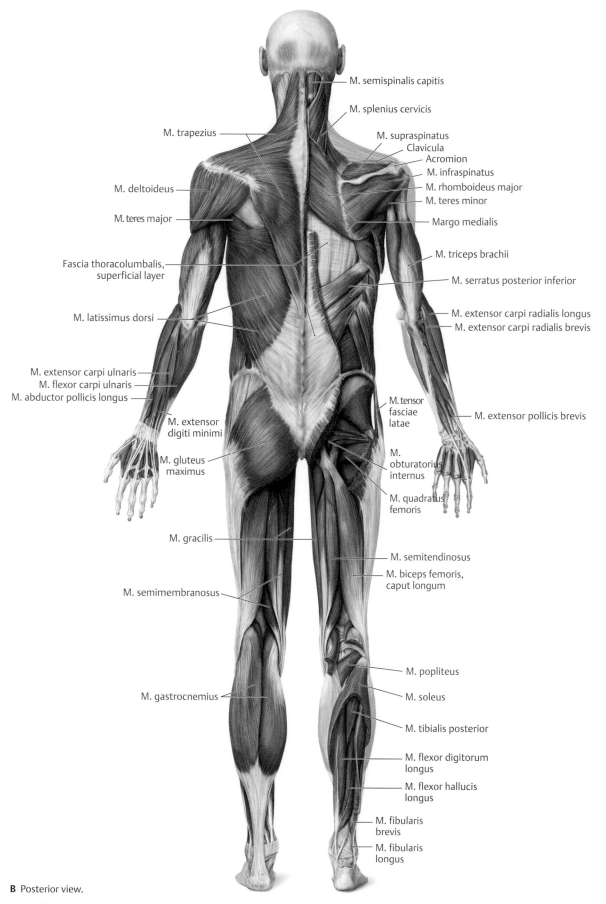

M. semispinalis capitis

M. splenius cervicis

M. trapezius

M. supraspinatus
Clavicula
Acromion
M. infraspinatus
M. deltoideus
M. rhomboideus major
M. teres minor
M. teres major
Margo medialis

Fascia thoracolumbalis,
superficial layer

M. triceps brachii

M. serratus posterior inferior

M. latissimus dorsi

M. extensor carpi radialis longus
M. extensor carpi radialis brevis

M. extensor carpi ulnaris
M. flexor carpi ulnaris
M. abductor pollicis longus

M. tensor
fasciae
latae

M. extensor pollicis brevis

M. extensor
digiti minimi

M.
obturatorius
internus

M. gluteus
maximus

M. quadratus
femoris

M. gracilis

M. semitendinosus

M. biceps femoris,
caput longum

M. semimembranosus

M. popliteus

M. gastrocnemius

M. soleus

M. tibialis posterior

M. flexor digitorum
longus

M. flexor hallucis
longus

M. fibularis
brevis

M. fibularis
longus

B Posterior view.

Fig. 1.12 (continued) **Overview of skeletal muscles**
(From Schuenke M, Schulte E, Schumacher U. THIEME Atlas of Anatomy, Vol 1. Illustrations by Voll M and Wesker K. 3rd ed. New York: Thieme Publishers; 2020.)

1.8   The Circulatory System

The heart and blood vessels, which make up the circulatory system (**Figs. 1.13** and **1.14**), transport blood to tissues of the body for the exchange of gases, waste products, and nutrients.

— The muscular heart provides the pumping action that maintains the flow of blood through the vessels.

— The blood vessels of the circulatory system (**Fig. 1.15**) are classified as follows:

- **Arteries,** which transport blood away from the heart and branch into many smaller **arterioles**
- **Veins,** which carry blood toward the heart and are formed by the convergence of many small **venules**

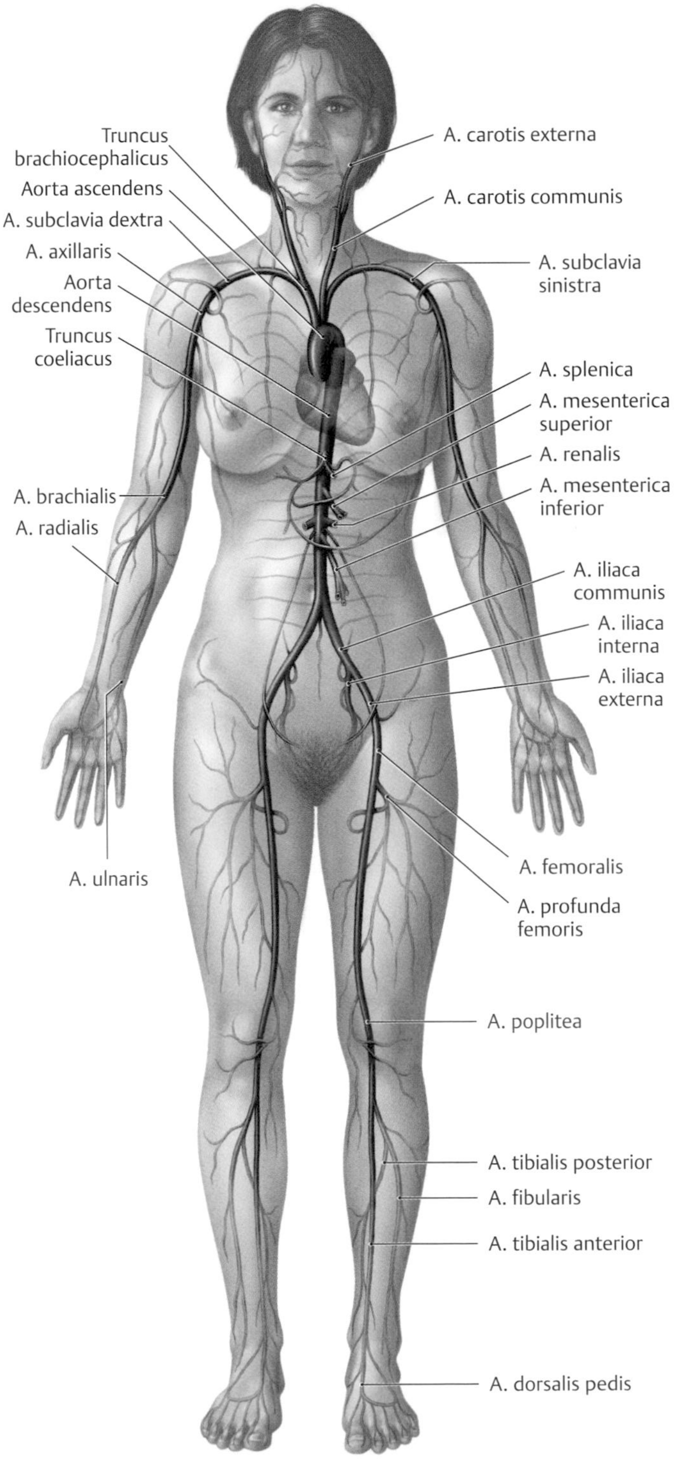

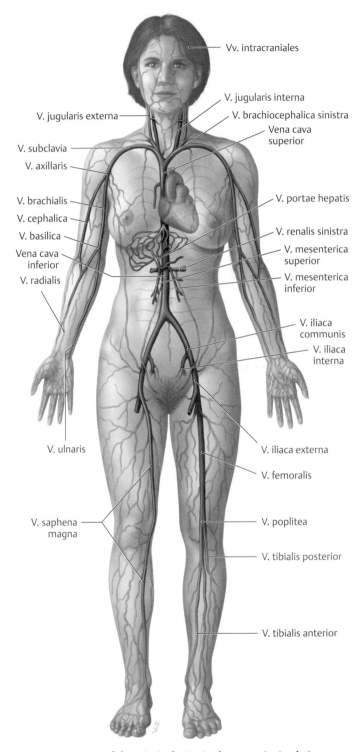

Fig. 1.13 Overview of the principal arteries in the systemic circulation
Anterior view. (From Schuenke M, Schulte E, Schumacher U. THIEME Atlas of Anatomy, Vol 2. Illustrations by Voll M and Wesker K. 3rd ed. New York: Thieme Publishers; 2020.)

Fig. 1.14 Overview of the principal veins in the systemic circulation
Anterior view. The portal circulation of the hepar is shown in purple. Deep veins shown on the left limb, superficial veins shown on the right limb. (From Schuenke M, Schulte E, Schumacher U. THIEME Atlas of Anatomy, Vol 2. Illustrations by Voll M and Wesker K. 3rd ed. New York: Thieme Publishers; 2020.)

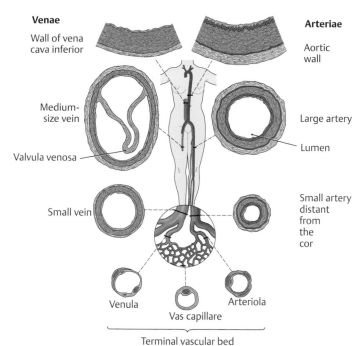

Venae

Wall of vena
cava inferior

Medium-
size vein

Valvula venosa

Small vein

Venula

Vas capillare

Arteriola

Terminal vascular bed

Arteriae

Aortic
wall

Large artery

Lumen

Small artery
distant
from
the
cor

Fig. 1.15 Structure of blood vessels
Blood vessels in different regions of the systemic circulation, shown in
cross section. (From Schuenke M, Schulte E, Schumacher U. THIEME Atlas
of Anatomy, Vol 1. Illustrations by Voll M and Wesker K. 3rd ed. New York:
Thieme Publishers; 2020.)

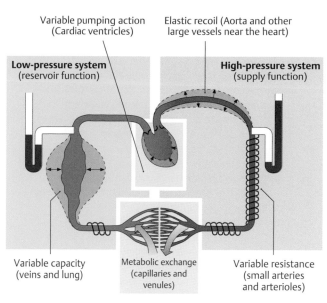

Variable pumping action
(Cardiac ventricles)

Elastic recoil (Aorta and other
large vessels near the heart)

Low-pressure system
(reservoir function)

High-pressure system
(supply function)

Variable capacity
(veins and lung)

Metabolic exchange
(capillaries and
venules)

Variable resistance
(small arteries
and arterioles)

Fig. 1.16 Pressure gradients in the cardiovascular system
(*Note:* No distinction is made between the systemic and pulmonary
systems in the diagram; Klinke R, Sibernagel S. Lehbuch der Phyiologic.
3rd ed. Stuttgart: Thieme; 2001.)

BOX 1.2: ANATOMIC NOTES

FUNCTIONAL ASPECTS OF THE CIRCULATORY SYSTEM
Blood is transported through the circulatory system along a pressure gradient that is influenced by the size, number, and structure
of the vessels through which it flows **(Fig. 1.16)**. Relatively high
pressure is maintained in the arterial system. Large elastic type
arteries can accommodate the intermittent volume ejected from
the heart while more distal muscular arteries, through vasodilation (expansion) and vasoconstriction (contraction), can control
vascular resistance and regulate local blood flow.

The venous system maintains a much lower pressure, and
veins have comparatively thinner walls and larger diameters. They
can accommodate up to 80% of the total blood volume and therefore serve an important reservoir function. Return of venous
blood to the heart is aided by factors such as (a) venous valves
that prevent backflow, (b) arteriovenous coupling that transmits
the arterial pulse to accompanying veins, and (c) the pumping
action of surrounding muscles **(Fig. 1.17)**.

Terminal vascular beds, formed by the extensive branching
of capillaries, connect the arterial and venous circulations. These
vascular networks are characterized by a large increase in cross-
sectional area and a corresponding decrease in the flow velocity,
which is necessary for the exchange process between the blood
and interstitial fluid. Flow through these vascular beds can be regulated locally by contraction and relaxation of precapillary
sphincters. Only one fourth to one third of capillary networks are
perfused under normal resting conditions.

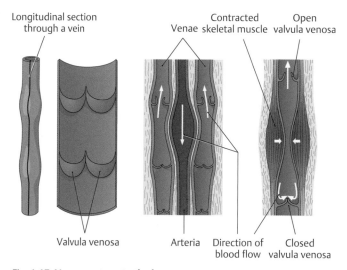

Longitudinal section
through a vein

Contracted
Venae skeletal muscle

Open
valvula venosa

Valvula venosa

Arteria

Direction of
blood flow

Closed
valvula venosa

Fig. 1.17 Venous return to the heart
(From Schuenke M, Schulte E, Schumacher U. THIEME Atlas of Anatomy,
Vol 1. Illustrations by Voll M and Wesker K. 3rd ed. New York: Thieme
Publishers; 2020.)

- ◦ Many veins, particularly in the limbs, have multiple valves along their length to prevent backward flow due to gravity.
  - ◦ The veins are divided into **venae superficiales** that travel in the fascia superficialis and **venae profundae** that accompany the arteries. **Venae perforantes** connect the superficial and deep venous circulations.
  - ◦ Veins are more numerous and more variable than arteries and often form plexi venosi (networks), which are named for the structure they surround (e.g., plexus venosus uterinus).
- • **Capillaries,** which form networks that intervene between the arteries and veins at the **terminal vascular beds,** where gas, nutrient, and waste exchange occurs
- • **Sinusoids,** which are wide, thin-walled vessels that replace capillaries in some organs, such as the liver (hepar)
— The circulatory system has two circuits **(Fig. 1.18)**:
  1. The **pulmonary circulation** transports oxygen-poor blood from the right side of the heart to the lungs (pulmones) through **arteriae pulmonales.** Oxygen-rich blood from the lungs flows back to the left side of the heart through **venae pulmonales.**
  2. The **systemic circulation** distributes oxygen-rich blood from the left side of the heart to body tissues through the systemic arteries (the **aorta** and its branches). Oxygen-poor blood returns to the heart through the systemic veins (the **venae cavae superior** and **inferior** and their tributaries—sometimes referred to as the **caval system—** and the sinus coronarius).
— A **portal circulation** is a route within the systemic circulation that diverts blood to a second capillary network before returning it to the systemic veins. The largest of these, the hepatic **portal system,** diverts blood from the gastrointestinal tract to the capillaries (sinusoids) in the liver before returning it to the systemic veins. A similar portal system is found in the glandula pituitaria.
— An **anastomosis,** a communication between blood vessels, allows blood to bypass its normal route and flow through an alternate, or collateral, route. Although blood volume through the anastomosis is usually minimal, it increases when the lumen of vessels along the normal route is obstructed.
— **End arteries** are vessels that lack anastomoses, such as the a. centralis retinae and aa. renales. Gradual narrowing of end arteries stimulates the formation of new vessels, but an abrupt obstruction of an end artery can cause necrosis (death) of the target tissue.

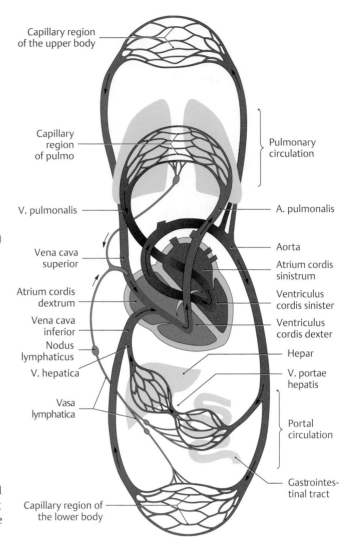

Fig. 1.18 Circulation
Schematic showing the pulmonary and systemic circulations. The portal circulation through the hepar is part of the systemic circulation. Arteries are shown in red, veins in blue, and lymphatic vessels in green. (From Schuenke M, Schulte E, Schumacher U. THIEME Atlas of Anatomy, Vol 1. Illustrations by Voll M and Wesker K. 3rd ed. New York: Thieme Publishers; 2020.)

1.9 The Lymphatic System

The lymphatic system, which runs parallel to the circulatory system, consists of lymph, lymphatic vessels, and lymphoid organs.

— The lymphatic system performs the following functions:
  - Drains excess extracellular fluid from body tissues and returns it to veins of the systemic circulation
  - Mounts an immune response in the body
  - Transports fat and large protein molecules that cannot be taken up by venous capillaries

— Lymphoid organs and tissues that are part of the body's immune system include
  - primary lymphatic organs: the thymus and medulla ossium
  - secondary lymphatic organs: the spleen (splen), nodi lymphoidei, mucosa-associated lymphatic tissue (MALT), pharyngeal lymphatic (Waldeyer's) ring, bronchus-associated lymphatic tissue (BALT) in the airway, and gut-associated lymphatic tissue (GALT)—such as Peyer's patches and appendix vermiformis—in the gastrointestinal tract (**Fig. 1.19**).

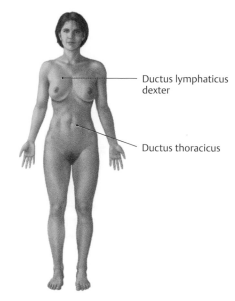

Fig. 1.20 Lymphatic drainage by body quadrants
(From Gilroy AM et al. Atlas of Anatomy. 4th ed. 2020. Based on: Schuenke M, Schulte E, Schumacher U. THIEME Atlas of Anatomy. Internal Organs. Illustrations by Voll M and Wesker K. 3rd ed. New York: Thieme Medical Publishers; 2020.)

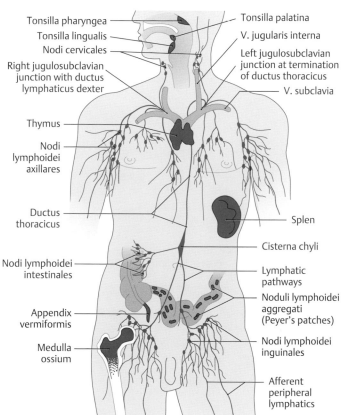

Fig. 1.19 Lymphatic system
The lymphatic system parallels the veins of the circulatory system and includes lymph nodes, lymphatic vessels, and lymphatic organs. (From Schuenke M, Schulte E, Schumacher U. THIEME Atlas of Anatomy, Vol 1. Illustrations by Voll M and Wesker K. 3rd ed. New York: Thieme Publishers; 2020.)

— **Lymph,** extracellular fluid that is extracted by lymph capillaries and transported by lymphatic vessels, is a clear, watery substance similar to blood plasma.

— The conducting vessels of the lymphatic system include
  - blind-ended **vasa lymphocapillares** that begin in the tissues and drain to lymphatic vessels;
  - **vasa lymphatica,** which are interposed with lymph nodes along their length and drain to lymphatic trunks; and
  - two major **trunci lymphatici,** the ductus thoracicus (ductus lymphaticus sinister) and ductus lymphaticus dexter, which drain into large veins of the neck.

— The ductus lymphaticus sinister, or **ductus thoracicus** (~ 40 cm long), is the larger of the two major lymphatic trunks. It originates from the **cisterna chyli**, a dilated lymphatic vessel in the abdomen, and drains lymph from the right and left lower quadrants and left upper quadrant of the body. The smaller **ductus lymphaticus dexter** (~ 1 cm long) drains only the right upper quadrant of the body (**Fig. 1.20**).

— Lymph carried by the ductus thoracicus and ductus lymphaticus dexter returns to the systemic venous circulation at the **left** and **right venous angles** (junction of the vena jugularis interna and vena subclavia), also known as the **jugulosubclavian junction**, in the neck (**Fig. 1.21**).

— Tributaries of the ductus thoracicus (ductus lymphaticus sinister) include the:
  - truncus jugularis sinister, which drains the left half of the head and neck

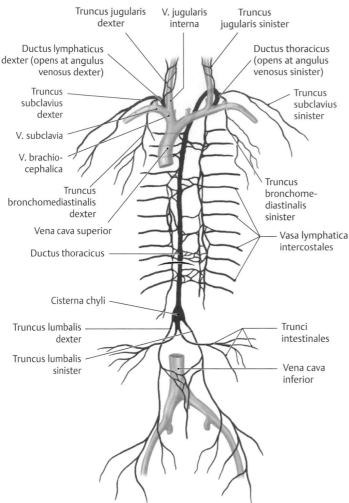

Truncus jugularis dexter
V. jugularis interna
Truncus jugularis sinister
Ductus lymphaticus dexter (opens at angulus venosus dexter)
Ductus thoracicus (opens at angulus venosus sinister)
Truncus subclavius dexter
Truncus subclavius sinister
V. subclavia
V. brachio-cephalica
Truncus bronchomediastinalis dexter
Truncus bronchome-diastinalis sinister
Vena cava superior
Vasa lymphatica intercostales
Ductus thoracicus
Cisterna chyli
Truncus lumbalis dexter
Trunci intestinales
Truncus lumbalis sinister
Vena cava inferior

Fig. 1.21 Lymphatic pathways
Anterior view. (From Schuenke M, Schulte E, Schumacher U. THIEME Atlas of Anatomy, Vol 1. Illustrations by Voll M and Wesker K. 3rd ed. New York: Thieme Publishers; 2020.)

- truncus subclavius sinister, which drains the left upper limb, left sides of the chest, and back wall
- truncus bronchomediastinalis sinister, which drains viscera of the left thoracic cavity (except from the lower lobe of the left lung, which can drain to the ductus lymphaticus dexter). This trunk commonly empties directly into the vena subclavia sinistra.
- intestinal trunks from the abdominal organs
- truncus lumbalis dexter and sinister, which drain both lower limbs, all of the pelvic viscera, and walls of the pelvis and abdomen
— Tributaries of the ductus lymphaticus dexter include the:
  - truncus jugularis dexter, which drains the right half of the head and neck
  - truncus subclavius dexter, which drains the right upper limb and right sides of the chest and back walls
  - truncus bronchomediastinalis dexter, which drains the viscera of the right thoracic cavity. This trunk commonly empties directly into the vena subclavia dextra.

1.10   The Nervous System

The nervous system receives, transmits, and integrates information throughout the body through the conduction of nerve impulses. This complex system can be classified according to many different criteria. Although these classifications are somewhat artificial, they are useful for understanding the numerous interconnections within the nervous systems (**Fig. 1.22**).
— The nervous system has two major structural, or anatomic, divisions (**Fig. 1.23**):
  - **central nervous system,** or **systema nervosum centrale** (CNS), which consists of the brain and spinal cord (medulla spinalis), where information about the body's internal and external environment is processed
  - A **peripheral nervous system** (PNS), which consists of 12 pairs of nervi craniales, 31 pairs of nervi spinales, and autonomic (visceral) nerves; peripheral nerves transmit information between the CNS and target organs and tissues in the rest of the body.
— The nervous system can also be divided into functional divisions (**Fig. 1.24**). Both the CNS and PNS contain components of each functional division.
  - The **somatic nervous system** controls voluntary functions such as contraction of skeletal muscles.
  - The **autonomic** (visceral) **nervous system** controls involuntary functions such as gland secretion.
— **Nerve cells** or **neurons,** the functional unit of the nervous system found in the CNS and PNS, are specialized for conducting nerve impulses. They generate electrical signals, the

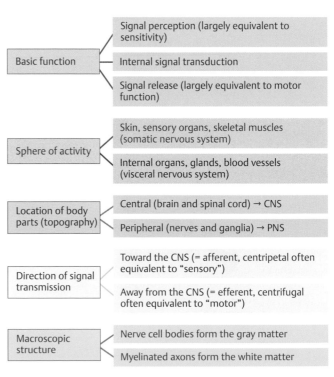

Basic function	Signal perception (largely equivalent to sensitivity)
	Internal signal transduction
	Signal release (largely equivalent to motor function)

| Sphere of activity | Skin, sensory organs, skeletal muscles (somatic nervous system) |
| | Internal organs, glands, blood vessels (visceral nervous system) |

| Location of body parts (topography) | Central (brain and spinal cord) → CNS |
| | Peripheral (nerves and ganglia) → PNS |

| Direction of signal transmission | Toward the CNS (= afferent, centripetal often equivalent to "sensory") |
| | Away from the CNS (= efferent, centrifugal often equivalent to "motor") |

| Macroscopic structure | Nerve cell bodies form the gray matter |
| | Myelinated axons form the white matter |

Fig. 1.22 Classification of systema nervosum—overview (From Schuenke M, Schulte E, Schumacher U. THIEME Atlas of Anatomy, Vol 3. Illustrations by Voll M and Wesker K. 3rd ed. New York: Thieme Publishers; 2020.)

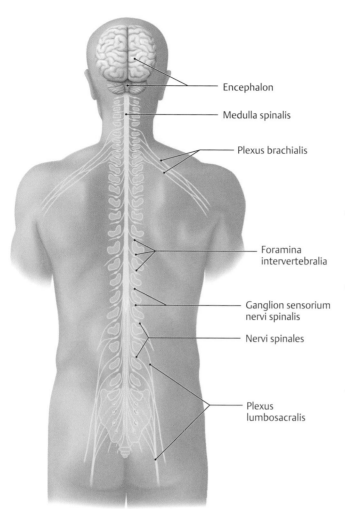

— Encephalon

— Medulla spinalis

— Plexus brachialis

— Foramina intervertebralia

— Ganglion sensorium nervi spinalis

— Nervi spinales

— Plexus lumbosacralis

Fig. 1.23 Topography of the nervous system
Posterior view. (From Schuenke M, Schulte E, Schumacher U. THIEME Atlas of Anatomy, Vol 1. Illustrations by Voll M and Wesker K. 3rd ed. New York: Thieme Publishers; 2020.)

action potential, and pass them on to other nerve or muscle cells. A variety of neurons can be described based on their appearance but the basic structure remains similar. The typical **neuron (Fig. 1.25A)** has

- a **cell body** (soma). An aggregate of cell bodies in the CNS is called a **nucleus;** an aggregate of cell bodies in the PNS is called a **ganglion.**
- multiple short branching **dendrites**, which receive information from other neurons and transmit impulses toward the cell body.
- a single long **axon** or nerve fiber, which transmits impulses away from the cell body. Bundles of axons in the CNS form **tracts;** bundles of axons in the PNS form **nerves.**

— Neurons transmit electrical signals from cell to cell across junctions called **synapses**. At the synapse the electrical impulse of the **presynaptic** nerve fiber initiates the release of a chemical signal, or transmitter, which generates an electrical impulse in the receptor, or **postsynaptic** nerve cell (**Fig 1.25B**).

— Neurons are classified by function as

- **sensory** (afferent) **nerves**, which carry information regarding pain, temperature, and pressure to the CNS from peripheral structures.
- **motor** (efferent) **nerves**, which transmit impulses from the CNS that elicit responses from peripheral target organs.

— **Neuroglia,** or **glial** cells, the non-neuronal cellular components of the nervous system, act as supporting cells and perform a variety of metabolic functions. Glial cells are responsible for producing the **myelin sheath**, a lipid-rich layer that surrounds axons and increases the speed of impulse conduction (**Fig. 1.26**). The myelin-producing cells in the PNS are called **Schwann cells** and in the CNS are called **oligodendrocytes**.

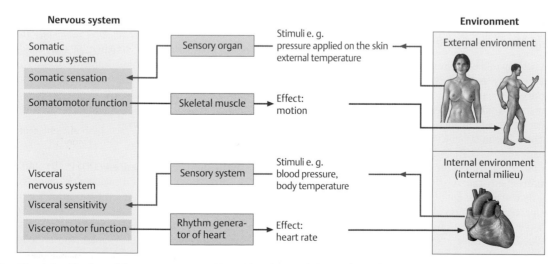

Fig. 1.24 Functional classification of the nervous system (From Schuenke M, Schulte E, Schumacher U. THIEME Atlas of Anatomy, Vol 3. Illustrations by Voll M and Wesker K. 3rd ed. New York: Thieme Publishers; 2020.)

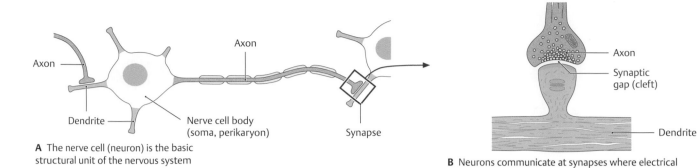

A The nerve cell (neuron) is the basic structural unit of the nervous system

B Neurons communicate at synapses where electrical signals initiate the release of neurotransmitters (chemical transmitters), which create an excitatory or inhibitory response at the target (postsynaptic) neuron.

Fig. 1.25 Nerve cell and synapse (From Schuenke M, Schulte E, Schumacher U. THIEME Atlas of Anatomy, Vol 3. Illustrations by Voll M and Wesker K. 3rd ed. New York: Thieme Publishers; 2020.)

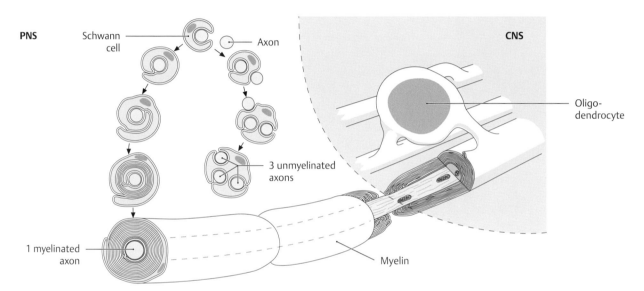

Fig. 1.26 Glial cells in the CNS and PNS
Glial cells form myelin sheaths around axons. This increases the speed with which impulses travel in the nervous system. In myelinated axons, multiple layers of glial membrane surround a single axon forming a distinct myelin sheath. In unmyelinated axons, a glial cell surrounds and supports multiple axons without forming a myelin sheath. (From Schuenke M, Schulte E, Schumacher U. THIEME Atlas of Anatomy, Vol 3. Illustrations by Voll M and Wesker K. 3rd ed. New York: Thieme Publishers; 2020.)

The Central Nervous System

The detailed anatomy of the CNS is most appropriately described in texts on neuroanatomy, and therefore is not included in this text. However, because an appreciation of its structure is essential to understanding the functioning of peripheral structures, a brief overview is included here, with further discussions to follow in Section 2.2 (spinal cord [medulla spinalis]) and Section 18.2 (brain [encephalon]).

— The brain and spinal cord of the CNS **(Fig. 1.27)** consist of
  • **gray matter (substantia grisea),** which contains the cell bodies, dendrites, and unmyelinated axons of neurons;
  • **white matter (substantia alba),** which contains the myelinated axons of neurons; and
  • neuroglial cells, which are abundant in both white and gray matter.
— The brain resides in the cranial cavity of the skull. The tissue of the brain consists of an outer **cortex cerebri** of gray

matter, an inner core of white matter, and islands of gray matter deep within the brain known as **basal ganglia**. Axonal tracts of the white matter link regions of the brain with each other and with the spinal cord.
— The brain **(Fig. 1.28)** is subdivided into
  • **cerebral hemispheres**
  • **diencephalon**
  • **cerebellum**
  • **brainstem (truncus encephali)**
— The bony vertebral column encloses the spinal cord. Gray matter in the spinal cord is located centrally and is surrounded by white matter tracts. The gray matter forms an H-shaped area that consists of bilateral
  • **cornua anteriora,** which contain motor neurons;
  • **cornua posteriora,** which contain sensory neurons;
  • **cornua lateralia** in the thoracic and upper lumbar region, which contain visceromotor neurons.

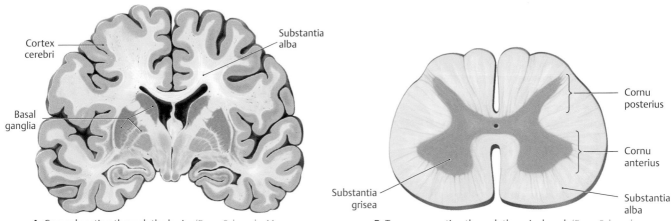

A Coronal section through the brain. (From Schuenke M, Schulte E, Schumacher U. THIEME Atlas of Anatomy, Vol 3. Illustrations by Voll M and Wesker K. 3rd ed. New York: Thieme Publishers; 2020.)

B Transverse section through the spinal cord. (From Schuenke M, Schulte E, Schumacher U. THIEME Atlas of Anatomy, Vol 3. Illustrations by Voll M and Wesker K. 3rd ed. New York: Thieme Publishers; 2020.)

Fig. 1.27 Gray and white matter in the central nervous system
Nerve cell bodies appear gray in gross inspection, whereas nerve cell processes (axons) and their insulating myelin sheaths appear white.

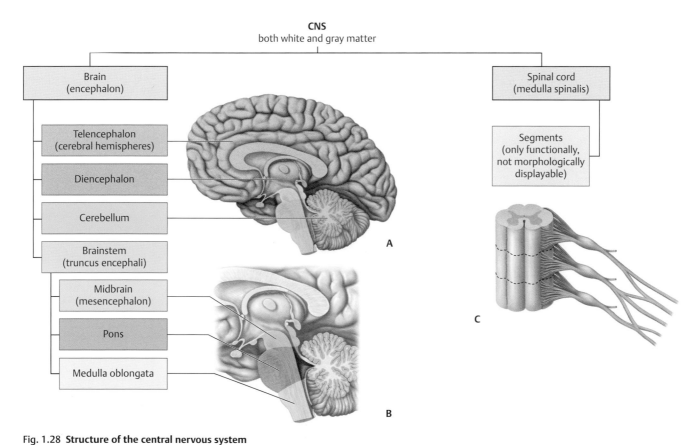

Fig. 1.28 Structure of the central nervous system
(A, B) Right side of brain, medial view. **(C)** Anterior view of a section of the spinal cord. (From Gilroy AM, MacPherson BR, Wikenheiser JC. Atlas of Anatomy. Illustrations by Voll M and Wesker K. 4th Edition. New York: Thieme Publishers; 2020.)

The Peripheral Nervous System

— The peripheral nervous system includes the peripheral parts of the autonomic and somatic divisions. Components of each system (**Fig. 1.29**) are found in
  - 12 pairs of **cranial nerves (nervi craniales)** (traditionally designated, in order from cranial to caudal, by Roman numeral) that arise from the brain and primarily innervate structures of the head and neck. The **nervus vagus** (n. cranialis X) also innervates viscera of the thorax and abdomen.
  - 31 pairs of **spinal nerves (nervi spinales)** that arise from the spinal cord and exit the vertebral column through **foramina intervertebralia** (openings between vertebrae). Spinal nerves are named for the section of the spinal cord from which they arise (e.g., T4 is the fourth segment of the thoracic part of the spinal cord).
— Most nerves of the peripheral nervous system are mixed nerves that contain both motor and sensory fibers (**Fig. 1.30**).
  - The somatic nervous system contains a combination of fiber types:
    - **somatic sensory** (somatosensory) **fibers**, which transmit the information from skin and skeletal muscles
    - **somatic motor** (somatomotor) **fibers**, which innervate skeletal muscles
  - The autonomic nervous system contains only **visceral motor** (visceromotor) **fibers**, which innervate smooth muscle, cardiac muscle, and glands.
  - **Visceral sensory** (viscerosensory) **fibers** transmit information from smooth muscle, cardiac muscle, and internal organs. Although these often accompany the visceral motor fibers, they are generally not considered part of the autonomic system.
  - In addition to those named above, cranial nerves may also contain special fiber types that are associated with structures in the head:
    - **Special somatic sensory** (somatomotor) **fibers**, which conduct information from the retina of the eye, and auditory and vestibular apparatus of the ear
    - **Special visceral sensory** (viscerosensory) **fibers,** which transmit information from the taste buds of the tongue and olfactory mucosa
    - **Special visceral motor fibers** (visceromotor, branchio-motor), which innervate skeletal muscles that originate from the pharyngeal arches (arcus pharyngei)
— The somatic component of the nervous system transmits the motor output to, and sensory input from, structures over which we have voluntary and conscious control. (Consider a simple activity like walking, in which we have control over the movement of our legs and are aware of the pain elicited by an arthritic art. genus or a splinter in the sole of the foot.)
— The autonomic component transmits the motor output to structures that function without conscious control. Its two divisions work to excite (**sympathetic**) or relax (**parasympathetic**) visceral responses based on internal and external stimuli. Together they work to maintain a stable (homeostatic) internal environment. (Consider the increase in heart rate when you have won the lottery and the crucial corresponding slowing of the heart rate when you need to sleep.)

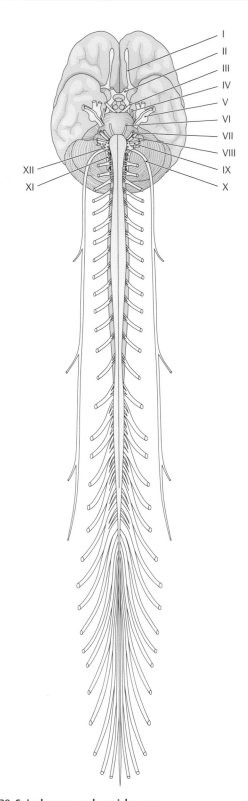

Fig. 1.29 Spinal nerves and cranial nerves
Anterior view. Thirty-one pairs of nn. spinales arise from the medulla spinalis in the peripheral nervous system, compared with 12 pairs of cranial nerves that arise from the brain. The nn. craniales pairs are traditionally designated by Roman numerals. (From Gilroy AM, MacPherson BR, Wikenheiser JC. Atlas of Anatomy. Illustrations by Voll M and Wesker K. 4th Edition. New York: Thieme Publishers; 2020.)

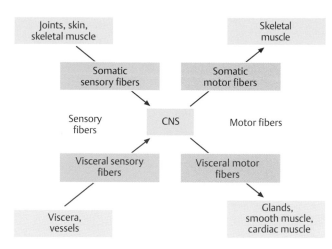

Fig. 1.30 Information flow in the systema nervosum
Fibers that carry information to the central nervous system (CNS) are called sensory or afferent fibers; fibers that carry signals away from the CNS are called motor or efferent fibers. (From Schuenke M, Schulte E, Schumacher U. THIEME Atlas of Anatomy, Vol 1. Illustrations by Voll M and Wesker K. 3rd ed. New York: Thieme Publishers; 2020.)

— The somatic and autonomic nervous systems each have their own network of nerves that transmit information between the CNS and PNS. Although somatic and autonomic nerves may travel together, the nerve fibers remain anatomically and functionally distinct.
— Most cranial nerves and all spinal nerves carry somatic nerve fibers; some also carry autonomic fibers:
  • parasympathetic fibers are carried by nn. craniales III, VII, IX, and X and nn. spinales S2–S4
  • sympathetic fibers originate at medulla spinalis levels T1–L2 but, via the truncus sympathicus, are distributed to, and travel with, nn. spinales at all levels.
— Nerves from each system typically form nerve plexuses (i.e., somatic nerve plexus, autonomic nerve plexus). Each contains nerves arising from multiple levels of the spinal cord.
  • Somatic plexuses are made up of large, distinct, easily identifiable nerve roots and give rise to nerves that are given descriptive names (n. medianus, n. femoralis).
  • Autonomic plexuses appear as dense mats of thin hair-like nerves that frequently extend peripherally along major arteries.
— Both somatic and autonomic nerves carry motor information from the CNS to a peripheral structure, but the type of target organ they innervate and the response they elicit is very different.
  • Somatic nerves initiate voluntary responses (such as contraction of the m. biceps brachii).
  • Autonomic nerves initiate visceral responses (such as secretion of pancreatic juices).

— Somatic sensory and visceral sensory nerves carry sensory information from target organs to the CNS.
  • Sensations carried by visceral sensory fibers are vague and poorly localized (such as nausea).
  • Sensations carried by somatic sensory fibers are sharp and localized (such as a paper cut).
  • In all cases, the cell bodies of peripheral sensory neurons lie in sensory (spinal/dorsal root) ganglia that lie outside the CNS.
— **Splanchnic nerves (nn. splanchnici)** are nerves of the autonomic nervous system that innervate visceral structures (splanchnic refers to internal organs or viscera). They may carry either sympathetic or parasympathetic fibers (never both) and contain no somatic fibers. All splanchnic nerves contain visceral sensory and visceral motor fibers.

1.11 Body Cavities and Internal Organ Systems

The large organs of the endocrine, respiratory, digestive, urinary, and reproductive systems are housed in the cavitas thoracis, cavitas abdominis, and cavitas pelvis. These large spaces are divided into serous cavities and connective tissue spaces.
— A serous cavity is a fully enclosed potential space that is lined by a serous (fluid secreting) membrane. The outer, or **parietal,** layer of this membrane lines the inner wall of the cavity. It is continuous with the inner, or **visceral,** layer that reflects from the wall to cover or enclose the viscera within the cavity. The large serous cavities include:
  • In the thorax
    ◦ paired **cavitates pleurales**, which contain the lungs
    ◦ a **cavitas pericardiaca**, which contains the heart
  • In the abdomen and pelvis
    ◦ a **cavitas peritonealis**, which contains the gastrointestinal tract and its accessory structures
— Connective tissue spaces are potential spaces that lie outside the serous cavities. They are often defined by adjacent layers of fascia or may lie between opposing serous cavities. Major examples include:
  • The **deep cervical space** between fascial layers of the neck
  • The **mediastinum**, which lies between the pleural cavities in the thorax
  • The **spatium retroperitoneale**, which lies posterior to the cavitas peritoneales in the abdomen, and its continuation into the pelvis below the peritoneum, where it is known as the **spatium infraperitoneale**. Urinary and reproductive organs, as well as the major vascular structures, reside within these extraperitoneal spaces.

2 Clinical Imaging Basics Introduction

Imaging is the primary diagnostic method used by physicians in nearly all medical specialties. All physicians should have a basic understanding of radiology concepts and how imaging can be optimally utilized in the care of their patients. The clinical imaging basics covered in this text are meant to be a brief introduction to the extraordinary diagnostic and therapeutic capabilities of radiology. Although imaging can be quite daunting to the first year medical student who has yet to master anatomy, you are encouraged to become familiar with the basics outlined here and in other introductory works. It is upon these basic fundamentals that you will build your foundation to better understand anatomy and physiology, and also to achieve the ultimate goal of using imaging to take the best care of your patients, regardless of which career path you choose.

The four most commonly used imaging modalities are
1. Radiographs (x-rays)
2. CT (computed tomography)
3. MRI (magnetic resonance imaging)
4. Ultrasound

X-Rays

— X-rays are a form of electromagnetic energy and are ionizing radiation. An x-ray tube generates energy in the form of photons, which are directed toward the patient. An electronic detector is positioned behind the patient, which detects the photons (x-ray energy) that pass through the patient to produce an image (**Fig. 2.1**). The degree to which that energy is able to pass through different tissues of the body produces the light, dark, and intermediate grays that are seen on the image. Tissues are rendered as
  • white when the energy is blocked (metal)
  • black when the energy is not blocked (air)
  • gray when the energy is partially blocked (soft tissues)
— The amount of x-ray energy passing through the body depends on the type of tissue encountered by the x-ray beam and the thickness of the tissues. Based on these principles, five densities can be identified on a radiograph (**Table 2.1**).

Table 2.1 Radiographic Densities

Tissue	Radiographic Density
Air	Dark black
Fat	Light black
Water and soft tissue	Shades of gray
Bone (calcium)	White
Metal	Bright white

— Additional descriptive terms are "opacity," "density," and "shadow," which indicate a whiter area on the x-ray; "lucency" indicates a blacker area.
— The image created is a summation of shadows based on the type and thickness of tissues the x-ray photons encounter (**Fig. 2.2**). This summation of shadows creates a two-dimensional representation of the three-dimensional structure of the body. Because it is frequently difficult to determine the depth of a structure in a two-dimensional image, an additional orthogonal (right angle) projection may be required to mentally "construct" a three-dimensional visualization (**Fig. 2.3**).
— The position of the patient and direction of the x-ray beam are manipulated to optimize image quality and produce different physical and physiological effects such as fluid moving to the most inferior (dependent) part of the patient due to gravity. The resulting image is described in terms of both patient position and x-ray beam direction, for example, upright frontal view (**Fig. 2.4**) or supine lateral view. Standard patient positions include
  • Upright (standing or sitting up)
  • Supine (lying on back)

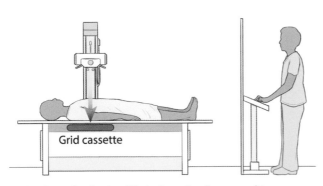

Fig. 2.1 Example of a simplified schematic of x-ray machine
(From Gunderman R. Essential Radiology, 3rd ed. New York: Thieme; 2014.)

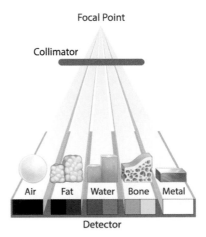

Fig. 2.2 The effects of density (tissue type) and thickness of tissue on the exposure of an x-ray image using the five basic x-ray densities
Note that air virtually blocks none of the beam (all energy passes through), whereas metal virtually blocks all of the x-ray energy.

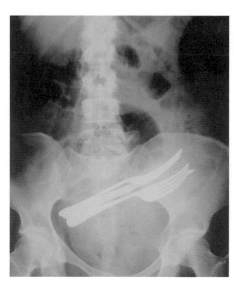

Fig. 2.3 Abdominal radiograph in a patient who swallowed multiple foreign objects The objects are two forks, one plastic hairbrush with partially metallic bristles, and one plastic pen with a metallic tip. As the image is a summation of the shadows produced by the objects and the tissue, it is impossible to know based on this single x-ray if the objects are in front of or behind the patient, or if they are indeed inside the abdomen. Given the patient's history of swallowing foreign objects, however, we deduce that they are inside the gastrointestinal tract. A lateral view (orthogonal to the frontal view) could confirm this. Using the frontal and lateral view can help triangulate the position of the objects and visualize the abdomen in three dimensions. (From Gunderman R. Essential Radiology, 3rd ed. New York: Thieme; 2014.)

- Prone
- Decubitus (lying on the side)
- Oblique
Standard direction of x-ray beams include
- Frontal (either PA or AP.) Note that the distinction between posterior anterior (PA) or anterior posterior (AP) x-ray beams is beyond the scope of this text, and we will refer to them collectively as a frontal view.
- Lateral

— Radiographs are oriented in a standard fashion for viewing.
  - Frontal images are viewed with the patient in the anatomic position (always facing the observer). The patient's right side is seen on the observer's left and vice versa, and each side is labeled as R or L.
  - The lateral projection can be viewed with the patient facing either right or left, but you should be consistent with your viewing patterns. The lateral view is best used in conjunction with the frontal view to convey the 3-dimensional nature of the structure. The lateral view is also helpful in seeing "hidden" areas on the frontal view such as behind the sternum and heart.
— When evaluating radiographs, a systematic approach is important and should include a checklist of major anatomic structures, which are discussed in the appropriate units.

CT (Computed Tomography)

— CT scans are created by rotating an x-ray beam around the patient. The computer reconstructs these data into image sets of consecutive sections or "slices" (think of a loaf of bread cut into slices). **(Fig. 2.5;** see also **Fig. 2.7).** Because the CT scan is made up of a large number of individual x-rays, the radiation dose is considerably higher. For this reason CT scanning is used judiciously.
— The images produced are based on the computer calculation of the x-ray attenuation of each pixel on each slice and expressed in Hounsfield units (Hounsfield was one of the discoverers of CT). Water is arbitrarily set to 0 Hounsfield units; more dense structures are more white (bone), and less dense structures are darker (air). However, CT can discriminate more subtle shades of gray, black, and white than radiographs, which improves soft tissue detail. For example, CT can distinguish between fluid and organs and between blood and other types of fluids. When IV contrast is used, soft tissue detail/contrast is improved significantly.
— Individual CT slices are oriented in the transverse (axial) plane and, by convention, are viewed from the inferior perspective (looking from the feet toward the head) **(Fig. 2.6).**

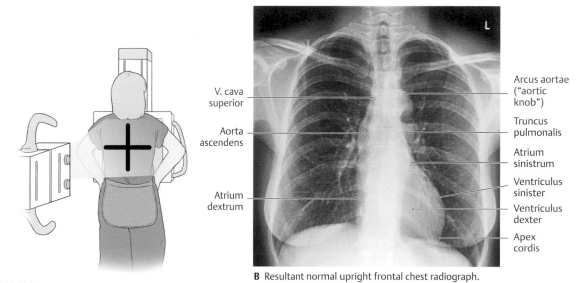

A Standing (upright) posteroanterior (PA) radiograph being produced in an x-ray room.

V. cava superior
Aorta ascendens
Atrium dextrum

Arcus aortae ("aortic knob")
Truncus pulmonalis
Atrium sinistrum
Ventriculus sinister
Ventriculus dexter
Apex cordis

B Resultant normal upright frontal chest radiograph.

Fig. 2.4 Positioning of patient and direction of x-ray beam
(From Gilroy AM, MacPherson BR, Wikenheiser JC. Atlas of Anatomy. 2nd Edition. New York: Thieme Publishers; 2012.)

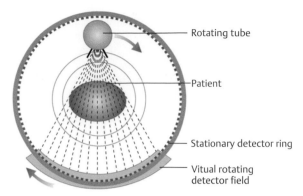

Rotating tube

Patient

Stationary detector ring

Vitual rotating detector field

Fig. 2.5 How computed tomography (CT) scanners work
The x-ray tube rotates continuously around the patient, as the patient, lying on the table, slides through the machine. The curved x-ray detector is opposite to the x-ray tube and registers the amount of x-ray energy that passes through the body. Taking into account the tube position and patient position at each time point of measurement, the computer constructs a data matrix and ultimately a set of images. (From Eastman G, et al. Getting Started in Radiology. Stuttgart: Thieme; 2005.)

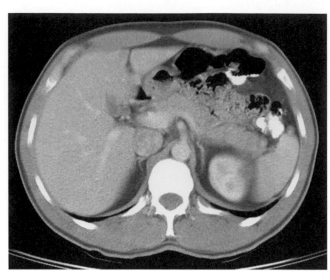

Fig. 2.6 Example of single axial slice from a normal abdominal CT
This image is shown in soft tissue windows to highlight the solid organs and blood vessels. (From Moeller TB, Reif E. Pocket Atlas of Sectional Anatomy, Vol 2, 3rd ed. New York: Thieme; 2007.)

However, CT scanners can also generate a volume of data that can be viewed in any plane, including three dimensions (3D reconstruction). Additionally, individual images can be "windowed," which involves changing the brightness or the contrast, to optimize the appearance of structures with specific densities, such as a bone or soft tissue "window."

MRI (Magnetic Resonance Imaging)

— A magnetic resonance image is produced by the interactions of a strong magnetic field on the protons within cells and a radiofrequency energy pulse that disturbs the protons. These spinning protons produce a "signal" that is picked up by a receiver and converted via computerized mathematical manipulation into images.
— MRIs are especially useful because they lack ionizing radiation, produce superb soft tissue contrast, and can be oriented in any plane (**Fig. 2.7**). The soft tissue contrast of MRI is far superior to other imaging modalities and is a key feature that makes MRI so powerful. Disadvantages include the high cost, long study acquisition time, and small confined space that patients must tolerate. MRI machines look similar to CT machines, but the tube that the patient slides into is smaller in diameter and longer.
— MRI images are traditionally viewed in the axial, sagittal, and coronal planes, but these can be skewed to optimize "out of plane" structures such as the heart (cor). As in CT, axial images are viewed as if the patient is supine and the observer is looking superiorly from the feet (i.e., inferior view).
— An MRI exam consists of multiple sequences with each sequence highlighting different types of tissue. The same tissues can look different on different sequences. The two basic MRI sequences are T1 and T2 (T represents time constant).
  • T1 sequence: fluid appears dark (black).
  • T2 sequence: fluid appears bright (white).
  • Cortical bone usually appears black on all sequences.

Ultrasound

— Ultrasound images are created by using a transducer, which emits high-frequency sound waves that penetrate the body. It then "listens" for the return echo, similar to the way sonar operates in a submarine (**Fig. 2.8**). Because tissues of different densities attenuate the sound wave to different degrees, the returning echo produces an image of varying shades of gray (**Fig. 2.9**).
— Ultrasound travels most easily through water, which appears black on the image, but it travels poorly through air and bone, which block the sound energy and appear white on the image. Common terms used to describe ultrasound images include *hypoechoic*, meaning blacker, and *hyperechoic* or *echogenic*, meaning gray or white.
— Ultrasound is relatively inexpensive and is radiation free, so it is used whenever possible and is the primary imaging modality in pediatrics, obstetrics, and when imaging both male and female gonads.
— Ultrasound images are displayed as a single slice, usually as a longitudinal or transverse section through the target organ, but also in any plane necessary to identify certain features or pathology.
— Note that the images are oriented to the organ itself, not the whole body.
— Ultrasound can also make use of the Doppler effect to identify and characterize motion. In medical imaging, Doppler is primarily used to characterize flow in blood vessels and to assess heart physiology. Color Doppler encodes direction and velocity into colors. By convention, blood flowing toward the ultrasound transducer is red and blood flowing away from the transducer is blue (regardless of vessel type). Spectral Doppler gives a graphical representation of the speed of flow with respect to time and thus can demonstrate characteristics of arterial vs. venous flow and identify abnormal flow patterns.

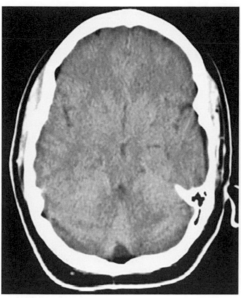
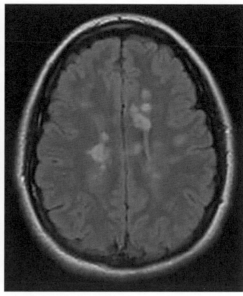

Fig. 2.7 Example of the improved soft tissue contrast and sensitivity of magnetic resonance imaging (MRI)
(From Gunderman R. Essential Radiology, 2nd ed. New York: Thieme; 2000)

A Axial slice of CT scan of the brain in a young woman with blurry vision. This scan is normal.

B Axial slice from an MRI at the same location in the same patient, showing bright spots in the substantia alba, indicating multiple sclerosis.

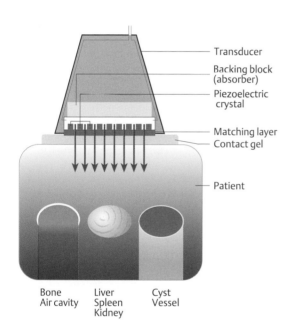

Transducer

Backing block (absorber)

Piezoelectric crystal

Matching layer
Contact gel

Patient

Bone   Liver   Cyst
Air cavity Spleen   Vessel
           Kidney

Fig. 2.8 Schematic of ultrasound probe held against patient's skin
Gel is used to acoustically couple the probe to the patient. Sound waves travel into the patient and are absorbed, reflected, or scattered based on type of tissue and tissue interfaces. The probe listens for the return echoes and the computer reconstructs the echoes into a two-dimensional image slice. (From Eastman G, et al. Getting Started in Radiology. Stuttgart: Thieme; 2005.)

Abdominal wall

Fig. 2.9 Example ultrasound image of a normal left kidney
The probe was positioned on the abdomen such that the kidney could be seen oriented longitudinally. The image is through the mid-kidney. Ultrasound differentiates the pyramides renales, which are blacker because of higher relative water content. The renal sinus fat is shown to be whiter. Note the liver tissue anterior and superior to the kidney. (From Gunderman R. Essential Radiology, 3rd ed. New York: Thieme; 2014.)

Cranial

Caudal

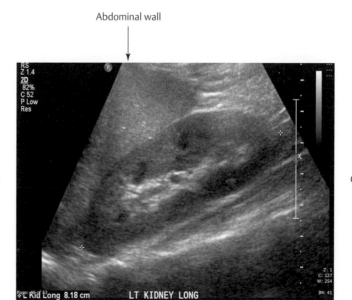

Unit I   Review Questions: Introduction

1. Which of the following is associated with membranous bone formation?
   A. Primary ossification centers
   B. Epiphyses
   C. Direct ossification of mesenchymal templates
   D. Long bones of the limbs
   E. Diaphyses

2. A portal system is associated with
   A. venous shunts that divert blood toward the heart (cor)
   B. the pulmonary circulation
   C. arterial-venous anastomoses
   D. capillary beds in the liver (hepar)
   E. lymphatic capillaries

3. In the anatomic position the
   A. eyes are directed forward
   B. palms are directed forward
   C. body is erect with arms at the sides
   D. feet are directed forward
   E. All of the above

4. Which of the following is true of nn. splanchnici?
   A. They synapse in ganglia near their target organ.
   B. They innervate viscera of the abdomen.
   C. They may carry sympathetic fibers.
   D. They may carry parasympathetic fibers.
   E. All of the above

5. A 43-year-old high school teacher complained to her physician of abdominal bloating and pelvic pain. Radiographic studies showed a large tumor involving her right ovary. Although the patient was scheduled for surgery to remove the tumor, the physician was concerned about the spread of the cancer along lymphatic channels. What is the lymphatic drainage pattern of pelvic viscera?
   A. Ipsilateral drainage to the ductus lymphaticus dexter and ductus thoracicus
   B. Contralateral drainage to the ductus lymphaticus dexter and ductus thoracicus
   C. Bilateral drainage to the ductus lymphaticus dexter and ductus thoracicus
   D. All pelvic viscera drain to the ductus lymphaticus dexter.
   E. All pelvic viscera drain to the ductus thoracicus.

6. As an inexperienced medical student, you volunteer at an outpatient clinic where you're asked to assist in administering vaccines to its large homeless population. As you deliver these percutaneous (through the skin) injections, you recall your knowledge of subcutaneous connective tissue and understand that deep to the skin the needle will first pass through
   A. a fatty layer of regular connective tissue
   B. a fatty layer of areolar and adipose connective tissue
   C. a membranous layer of dense connective tissue
   D. two layers of dense connective tissue
   E. a layer of fascia that is devoid of all superficial vessels and nerves

7. As a junior orthopedic resident, you are tasked with delivering a lecture to first-year medical students on the anatomy of joints. Which of the following statements might you include as a take-away point on your final summary slide?
   A. Most synovial joints are stabilized by intrinsic ligaments and intra-articular structures such as menisci.
   B. Synchondroses are defined as temporary cartilaginous joints that subsequently form synostoses, sites of bony fusion.
   C. Synovial joints typically contain a joint space lined by a synovial membrane.
   D. The complementary articulating surfaces of bones within a joint provide the greatest stability.
   E. Syndesmoses are fibrous joints found only in the sutures of the neonate skull.

8. Which of the following pertains to visceral muscles?
   A. The most prevalent type of muscle in the body
   B. Tendons connect them to bony attachments
   C. Tendon sheaths facilitate movement across joints
   D. They include a striated type of muscle found in the heart
   E. Aponeuroses attach them to other muscles or organs

9. After experiencing sudden unexplained weight loss and severe abdominal pain, your uncle sought advice from his primary physician. A CT scan revealed a 3-cm pancreatic tumor in the center of his abdomen. The physician explained that the pain resulted from pressure of the tumor on nearby nerves and ganglia associated with his sympathetic nervous system. The nerves transmitting the pain contain which type of fibers?
   A. Special visceral sensory
   B. Special somatic sensory
   C. Visceral sensory
   D. Somatic sensory
   E. Special visceral motor

10. Which of the following imaging methods do not use ionizing radiation as its energy source?
    A. Ultrasound
    B. Radiographs
    C. CT scan
    D. MRI

11. Which of the following structures would be the darkest as seen on an x-ray?
    A. Liver (hepar)
    B. Spleen (splen)
    C. Heart (cor)
    D. Gas-filled bowel loop
    E. Fluid-filled bowel loop

Answers and Explanations

1.   **C.** In the process of membranous ossification, embryonic mesenchymal templates are replaced by bone (Section 1.6).

    A. A primary ossification center, usually in the shaft of the long bones, is the site at which endochondral ossification begins.

    B. Epiphyses, located on either end of the long bones, are the secondary ossification centers for endochondral ossification.

    D. Long bones of the limbs undergo endochondral bone formation, in which a cartilaginous template forms from the embryonic mesenchyme before being replaced by bone.

    E. A diaphysis is the shaft of a long bone, which undergoes endochondral ossification.

2.   **D.** The body's largest portal system diverts blood from capillary beds in the gastrointestinal tract to secondary capillary beds in the liver before returning it to systemic veins (Section 1.8).

    A. A portal system diverts venous blood from one capillary network to another, instead of allowing it to flow directly into systemic veins toward the heart.

    B. A portal system is a venous system within the systemic (general body) circulation, but not within the pulmonary circulation.

    C. A portal system diverts blood from one capillary network to another, unlike arterial-venous anastomoses, which divert blood away from capillary beds.

    E. Lymphatic capillaries are restricted to the lymphatic system and are not involved with portal venous systems.

3.   **E.** The anatomic position is the standard position of the body used in medical references. The body is upright, facing the observer, with arms at the side and the head, eyes, palms, and feet directed forward (Section 1.1).

    A. Eyes are directed forward, and other positions are correct as well (E).

    B. Palms are directed forward, and other positions are correct as well (E).

    C. Body is erect with arms at side, and other positions are correct as well (E).

    D. Feet are directed forward, and other positions are correct as well (E).

4.   **E.** All of the above (Section 1.10).

    A. Nn. splanchnici synapse near their target organ either in prevertebral ganglia or in small ganglia on the viscera. B through D are correct also (E).

    B. Nn. splanchnici are autonomic nerves that innervate viscera in the thorax, abdomen, and pelvis. A, C, and D are correct also (E).

    C. Sympathetic fibers arise from the T1–L2 medulla spinalis to form thoracic, lumbar, and sacral splanchnic nerves. A, B, and D are correct also (E).

    D. Parasympathetic fibers arise from the S2–S4 medulla spinalis and form nn. splanchnici pelvici. A through C are correct also (E).

5.   **E.** The ductus thoracicus receives lymph from the entire body below the diaphragm, as well as from the left side of the thorax, head, and neck and the left upper limb. The right lymphatic duct receives lymph only from the right side of the thorax, head, and neck and the right upper limb (Section 1.9).

    A. Viscera from the right and left sides of the pelvis drain to the ductus thoracicus.

    B. All pelvic viscera drain to the ductus thoracicus.

    C. All pelvic viscera drain to the ductus thoracicus.

    D. Only the right upper quadrant of the body drains to the ductus lymphaticus dexter.

6.   **B.** The needle would first pass through the most superficial layer of the subcutaneous connective tissue, which is composed of areolar and adipose tissues (Section 1.4).

    A. Both areolar and adipose connective tissues, which make up the fatty layer, are irregular types of connective tissue.

    C. The needle would pierce the membranous layer after first passing through the more superficial fatty layer.

    D. Subcutaneous connective tissue is composed of a superficial fatty layer and deeper membranous layer.

    E. The fatty layer is traversed by the superficial vessels and nerves.

7.   **C.** Synovial joints typically have a joint space enclosed by a fibrous capsule lined by a synovial membrane (Section 1.6).

    A. Most synovial joints are stabilized by extrinsic ligaments, although some also have intrinsic ligaments. Intra-articular structures are found in only certain joints, like the knee or shoulder.

    B. While some synchondroses subsequently become fully fused (synostoses) many remain as cartilaginous joints.

    D. Extrinsic ligaments are the primary stabilizers of most joints.

    E. Syndesmoses are also found in the adult skull as well in the interosseous membranes that join bones of the forearm and leg.

8.   **D.** The heart is made of cardiac muscle, one of two types of visceral muscles (Section 1.8).

    A. Somatic, or skeletal muscle, is the most prevalent type of muscle.

    B. Visceral muscles do not have tendons and are not attached to bones.

    C. Tendon sheaths surround the tendons of somatic muscles to facilitate movement as they cross joints.

    E. Aponeuroses are tendons that form flat sheets and are associated with somatic muscles.

9.   **C.** Visceral sensory fibers transmit sensation from internal organs (Section 1.10).

   A. Special visceral sensory fibers transmit only taste from the tongue (lingua) and smell from the olfactory mucosa.

   B. Special somatic sensory fibers transmit information only from the retina of the eye and auditory and vestibular apparatus of the ear.

   D. Somatic sensory fibers conduct information from somatic structures, the skin, and skeletal muscles.

   E. Special visceral motor fibers innervate only specific muscles that are derived from the branchial arches.

10.   **A** and **D.** Ultrasound utilizes acoustic energy (high-frequency sound waves), and MRI uses radiofrequency energy within a high-strength magnetic field (Chapter 2).

   B. Radiographs (or x-rays) utilize ionizing radiation in the form of high-energy electromagnetic waves.

   C. CT scans utilize the same type of electromagnetic energy as x-rays.

11.   **D.** The gas (air) in a gas-filled bowel loop does not attenuate the x-ray energy as much as soft tissues, so therefore will be rendered as darker gray (Chapter 2).

   A, B, C, and **E.** The liver, spleen, heart, and fluid-filled bowel would all be similar densities on an x-ray. These are all "soft tissue densities," which cannot be reliably differentiated by conventional radiography. Remember that CT has much higher soft tissue contrast than regular x-rays.

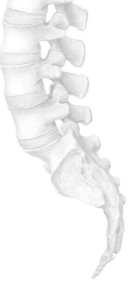

Unit II   Back

3 Back

3.1 The Vertebral Column (Columna Vertebralis)

The back includes the columna vertebralis, medulla spinalis, and nn. spinales, and the overlying muscles and skin.

General Features

— The vertebral column (columna vertebralis)
  • encloses and protects the spinal cord (medulla spinalis),
  • supports the head and trunk,
  • provides an attachment for the limbs, and
  • transfers the weight of the body to the lower limbs.
— The vertebral column, which extends from its articulation with the skull to the coccyx, comprises 33 vertebrae and the intervening disci intervertebrales, which are divided among five regions (**Fig. 3.1**):
  • 7 cervical vertebrae
  • 12 thoracic vertebrae
  • 5 lumbar vertebrae
  • 5 fused sacral vertebrae
  • 4 (3–5) fused coccygeal vertebrae
— Within each region, individual vertebrae are identified by number, a designation often referred to as a **vertebral level** (such as T8 vertebral level).
— Vertebrae increase in size from the cervical to the lumbar regions and decrease in size from the top of os sacrum to os coccygis.
— When the vertebral column is viewed laterally, two types of curvatures are evident (**Fig. 3.2**):
  • The **kyphtoic curvatures** (**kyphosis thoracica** and **kyphosis sacralis**), known as primary curvatures, are curved posteriorly and are present before birth.
  • The **lordotic curvatures** (**lordosis cervicis** and **lordosis lumbalis**), curved anteriorly, are secondary curvatures that develop postnatally.
— A **canalis vertebralis** passes through the center of the vertebral column and encloses the spinal cord, the spinal meninges (membranes surrounding the spinal cord), and the roots of the spinal nerves, and associated vasculature (see Section 3.2).
— **Foramina intervertebralia**, openings between vertebrae, allow the passage of nn. spinales.
— Strong vertebral ligaments support the joints of the vertebral column while allowing flexibility of the trunk.
— Fibrocartilaginous intervertebral discs (disci intervertebrales) lie between the vertebral bodies (corpora vertebrarum) of all vertebrae, except between C I and C II. They act as shock absorbers for the spine and allow flexibility between vertebrae. With the vertebral bodies, they form the anterior wall of the canalis vertebralis.

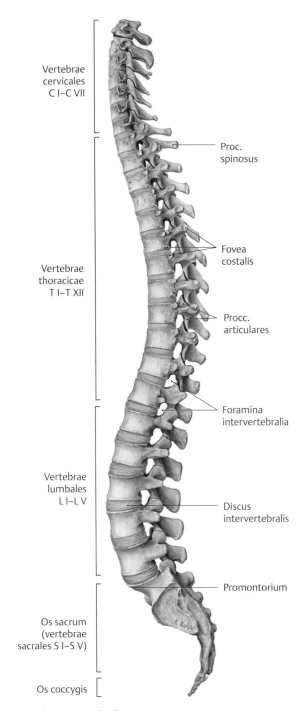

Fig. 3.1 Columna vertebralis
Left lateral view. (From Schuenke M, Schulte E, Schumacher U. THIEME Atlas of Anatomy, Vol 1. Illustrations by Voll M and Wesker K. 3rd ed. New York: Thieme Publishers; 2020.)

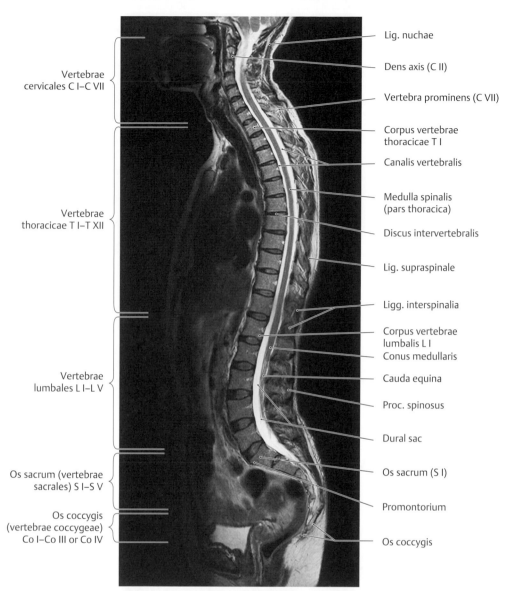

Vertebrae
cervicales C I–C VII

Vertebrae
thoracicae T I–T XII

Vertebrae
lumbales L I–L V

Os sacrum (vertebrae
sacrales) S I–S V

Os coccygis
(vertebrae coccygeae)
Co I–Co III or Co IV

Lig. nuchae

Dens axis (C II)

Vertebra prominens (C VII)

Corpus vertebrae
thoracicae T I

Canalis vertebralis

Medulla spinalis
(pars thoracica)

Discus intervertebralis

Lig. supraspinale

Ligg. interspinalia

Corpus vertebrae
lumbalis L I
Conus medullaris

Cauda equina

Proc. spinosus

Dural sac

Os sacrum (S I)

Promontorium

Os coccygis

Fig. 3.2 MRI of the spine
Sagittal view. (From Moeller TB,
Reif E. Pocket Atlas of Sectional
Anatomy: The Musculoskeletal
System. New York: Thieme
Publishers; 2009.)

BOX 3.1: DEVELOPMENTAL CORRELATION

SPINAL DEVELOPMENT
The characteristic curvatures of the adult spine appear over the course of postnatal development, being only partially present in a newborn. The newborn has a "kyphotic" spinal curvature (**A**); lumbar lordosis develops later and becomes stable at puberty (**C**).

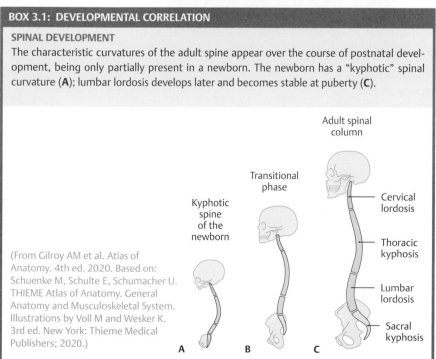

Kyphotic
spine
of the
newborn

Transitional
phase

Adult spinal
column

Cervical
lordosis

Thoracic
kyphosis

Lumbar
lordosis

Sacral
kyphosis

(From Gilroy AM et al. Atlas of
Anatomy. 4th ed. 2020. Based on:
Schuenke M, Schulte E, Schumacher U.
THIEME Atlas of Anatomy. General
Anatomy and Musculoskeletal System.
Illustrations by Voll M and Wesker K.
3rd ed. New York: Thieme Medical
Publishers; 2020.)

A   B   C

BOX 3.2: CLINICAL CORRELATION

ABNORMAL CURVATURES OF THE VERTEBRAL COLUMN: KYPHOSIS, LORDOSIS, AND SCOLIOSIS

Kyphosis ("hunchback"), an excessive anterior curvature of the thoracic spine, is often seen in elderly women. Although it may be congenital or posture related, it is usually secondary to degenerative changes (collapse) of the vertebral bodies. Lordosis ("swayback"), an excessive posterior curvature of the lumbar spine, frequently develops as a temporary side effect during pregnancy, but in nonpregnant individuals it may have pathologic or even weight-related causes. Scoliosis is a lateral curvature of the spine and may be congenital or neuromuscular, caused by diseases such as cerebral palsy and muscular dystrophy.

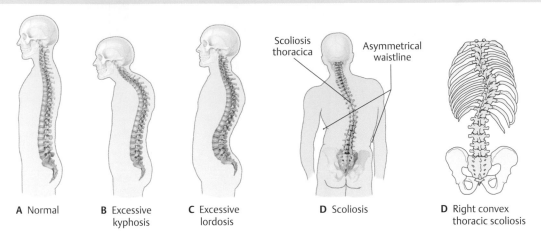

A Normal   **B** Excessive kyphosis   **C** Excessive lordosis   **D** Scoliosis   **D** Right convex thoracic scoliosis

(From Gilroy AM et al. Atlas of Anatomy. 4th ed. 2020. Based on: Schuenke M, Schulte E, Schumacher U. THIEME Atlas of Anatomy. General Anatomy and Musculoskeletal System. Illustrations by Voll M and Wesker K. 3rd ed. New York: Thieme Medical Publishers; 2020.)

BOX 3.3: CLINICAL CORRELATION

OSTEOPOROSIS

The spine is the primary target for degenerative diseases of the skeleton, such as osteoporosis, in which the rate of reabsorption by osteoclasts exceeds that of bone formation by osteoblasts. The resulting loss of bone mass predisposes the individual to compression fractures of the spine.

Regional Characteristics of Vertebrae

Most vertebrae share a typical form **(Fig. 3.3)**, although specific features vary by region.

— Most vertebrae have the following:
  • An anterior corpus vertebrae
  • A posterior arcus vertebrae formed by paired pediculi and paired laminae (the pediculi attach to the corpus vertebrae, and the paired laminae join to form a proc. spinosus)
  • Paired procc. transversi that project laterally from the arcus vertebrae
  • Proc. articularis superior and proc. articularis inferior that articulate with the adjacent vertebrae
  • A foramen vertebrale encircled by the corpus vertebrae and arcus vertebrae (the combined foramina vertebrales form the canalis vertebralis)

— Vertebrae cervicales, the smallest of all of the vertebrae, support the head and form the posterior skeleton of the neck **(Fig. 3.4)**. The seven vertebrae cervicales are characterized as typical or atypical.
  • Typical vertebrae cervicales **(Fig. 3.5A)**
    ○ C III–C VI have a small body, a large foramen vertebrale, and often bifid (two-pronged) procc. spinosi.

• Atypical vertebrae cervicales
  ○ C I, the **atlas**, lacks a corpus vertebrae and proc. spinosus **(Fig. 3.5B)**. It has arcus anterior atlantis and arcus posterior atlantis that are connected on each side by **lateral masses.** C I articulates superiorly with the os occipitale of the skull and inferiorly with C II.
  ○ C II, the axis, has a peglike **dens** projecting superiorly from its body that articulates with arcus anterior atlantis of C I **(Fig. 3.5C)**.
  ○ C VII, the **vertebra prominens**, has a long, palpable proc. spinosus.

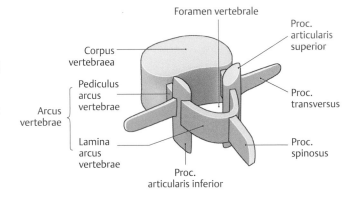

Fig. 3.3 Structural elements of a vertebra

Left posterosuperior view. With the exception of the atlas (C I) and axis (C II), all vertebrae consist of the same structural elements. (From Schuenke M, Schulte E, Schumacher U. THIEME Atlas of Anatomy, Vol 1. Illustrations by Voll M and Wesker K. 3rd ed. New York: Thieme Publishers; 2020.)

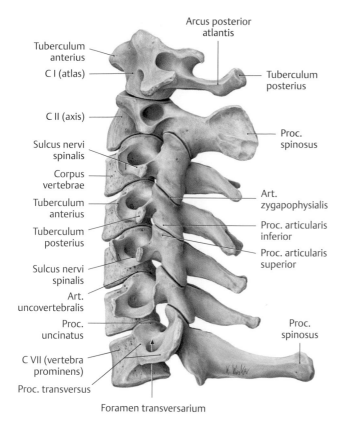

Fig. 3.4 **Vertebrae cervicales**
Bones of the vertebrae cervicales, left lateral view. (From Gilroy AM et al. Atlas of Anatomy. 4th ed. 2020. Based on: Schuenke M, Schulte E, Schumacher U. THIEME Atlas of Anatomy. General Anatomy and Musculoskeletal System. Illustrations by Voll M and Wesker K. 3rd ed. New York: Thieme Medical Publishers; 2020.)

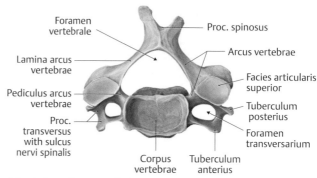

A Typical vertebra cervicalis (C IV), superior view.

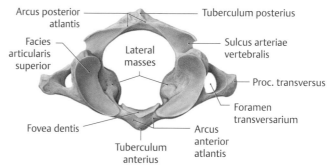

B Atlas (C I), superior view.

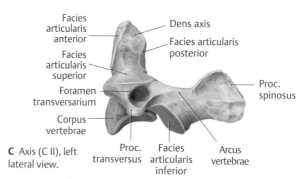

C Axis (C II), left lateral view.

Fig. 3.5 **Vertebrae cervicales**
(From Schuenke M, Schulte E, Schumacher U. THIEME Atlas of Anatomy, Vol 1. Illustrations by Voll M and Wesker K. 3rd ed. New York: Thieme Publishers; 2020.)

- • All vertebrae cervicales have paired **foramina transversaria,** openings formed by the tuberculum anterior and posterior of each proc. transversus.
- — Paired **aa. vertebrales** ascend in the neck through the foramina transversaria of C I–C VI, pass through a groove on the posterior arch of C1, and enter the base of the skull through a large opening, the **foramen magnum.**
- — Thoracic vertebrae **(Fig. 3.6)** have
  - • long procc. spinosi that project inferiorly,
  - • heart-shaped vertebral bodies,
  - • **facies articularis superior** and **facies articularis inferior** that are oriented in the coronal plane, and
  - • **foveae costales** that articulate with the ribs (costae).
- — Lumbar vertebrae **(Fig. 3.7),** the largest vertebrae, have
  - • large bodies;
  - • short, broad procc. spinosi; and
  - • an **interarticular part** (pars interarticularis), part of the lamina between the facies articulares superior and inferior, that forms the neck of the "Scottie dog" seen on oblique views of lumbar spine radiographs. It is a common site of vertebral fractures.
- — The five vertebrae sacrales are fused into a single bone, the **os sacrum (Fig. 3.8),** which forms the posterosuperior wall of the pelvis and articulates laterally with the ossa coxae. The os sacrum contains

- • the **canalis sacralis,** a continuation of the canalis vertebralis, which is open inferiorly at the **hiatus sacralis;**
- • the **crista sacralis mediana,** the fused procc. spinosi of the vertebrae sacrales;
- • paired **cristae sacrales mediales** that end inferiorly as the **cornua sacralia** on either side of the hiatus sacralis;
- • four pairs of **foramina sacralia anteriora** and **posteriora** for the passage of the branches of nn. spinales; and
- • the **promontorium,** formed by the anterior lip of the corpus vertebrae of vertebra S I.
- — The small vertebrae coccygeae, usually four (but this can vary from three to five), fuse into a single triangularly shaped bone, the **os coccygis,** which articulates with the os sacrum at the **art. sacrococcygea.**

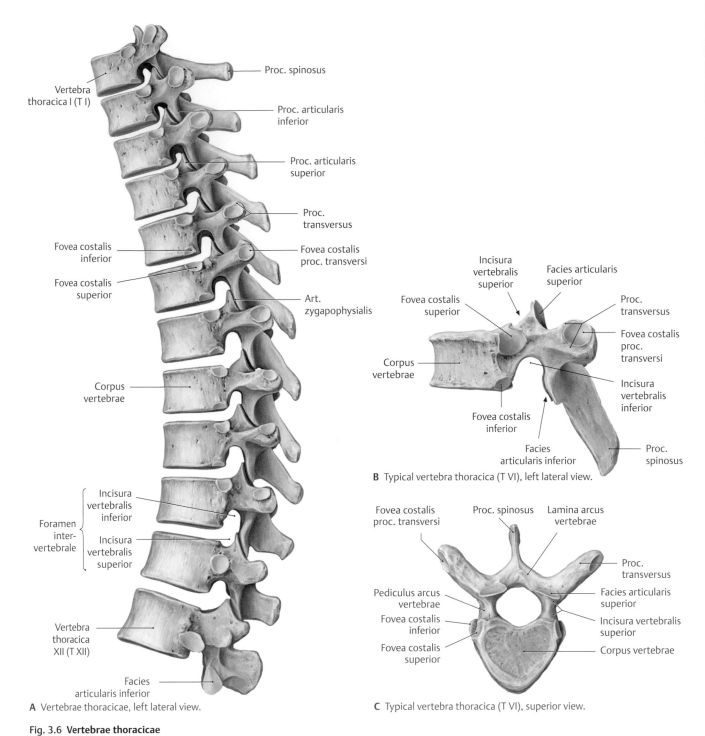

A Vertebrae thoracicae, left lateral view.

B Typical vertebra thoracica (T VI), left lateral view.

C Typical vertebra thoracica (T VI), superior view.

Fig. 3.6 Vertebrae thoracicae
(From Schuenke M, Schulte E, Schumacher U. THIEME Atlas of Anatomy, Vol 1. Illustrations by Voll M and Wesker K. 3rd ed. New York: Thieme Publishers; 2020.)

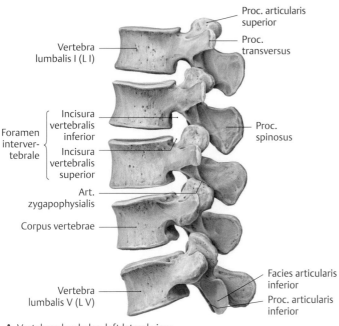

A Vertebrae lumbales, left lateral view.

Vertebra lumbalis I (L I)

Proc. articularis superior

Proc. transversus

Foramen intervertebrale

Incisura vertebralis inferior

Incisura vertebralis superior

Art. zygapophysialis

Corpus vertebrae

Proc. spinosus

Vertebra lumbalis V (L V)

Facies articularis inferior

Proc. articularis inferior

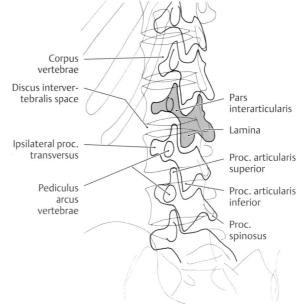

B Schematic. Oblique view of the vertebrae lumbales, showing the "Scottie dog" as seen on vertebrae lumbales radiographs.

Corpus vertebrae

Discus intervertebralis space

Ipsilateral proc. transversus

Pediculus arcus vertebrae

Pars interarticularis

Lamina

Proc. articularis superior

Proc. articularis inferior

Proc. spinosus

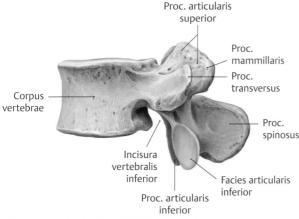

C Typical vertebra lumbalis (L4), left lateral view.

Proc. articularis superior

Proc. mammillaris

Proc. transversus

Corpus vertebrae

Proc. spinosus

Incisura vertebralis inferior

Facies articularis inferior

Proc. articularis inferior

D Typical vertebra lumbalis (L IV), superior view.

Proc. spinosus

Facies articularis superior

Proc. mammillaris

Proc. costalis

Arcus vertebrae

Foramen vertebrale

Corpus vertebrae

Proc. articularis superior

Incisura vertebralis superior

Fig. 3.7 Vertebrae lumbales
(From Gilroy AM et al. Atlas of Anatomy. 4th ed. 2020. Based on: Schuenke M, Schulte E, Schumacher U. THIEME Atlas of Anatomy. General Anatomy and Musculoskeletal System. Illustrations by Voll M and Wesker K. 3rd ed. New York: Thieme Medical Publishers; 2020.)

Box 3.4: CLINICAL CORRELATION

SPONDYLOLYSIS AND SPONDYLOLISTHESIS

Spondylolysis is a fracture across the interarticular part of the lamina, usually at L V, and appears as a collar on the "Scottie dog" seen on lumbar radiographs. When the defect is bilateral, the corpus vertebrae may separate from its arcus vertebrae and shift anteriorly relative to the vertebra below it, a condition known as *spondylolisthesis*. Mild cases can be asymptomatic, but more severe cases compress the nn. spinales and cause pain in the lower limbs and back. Note: Spondylosis, a similar-sounding name but unrelated condition, refers to age-related degeneration and the formation of osteophytes (see Box 3.7 Age-Related Changes in Vertebrae).

A 50% anterolisthesis of one corpus vertebrae on another, with the facies articularis inferior of the upper vertebra locked in front of the facies articularis superior of the lower vertebra. Naturally, this anterolisthesis tends to compromise the canalis vertebralis and threatens the cord. (From Gunderman R. Essential Radiology, 3rd ed. New York: Thieme; 2014)

Spondylolisthesis with locked facets

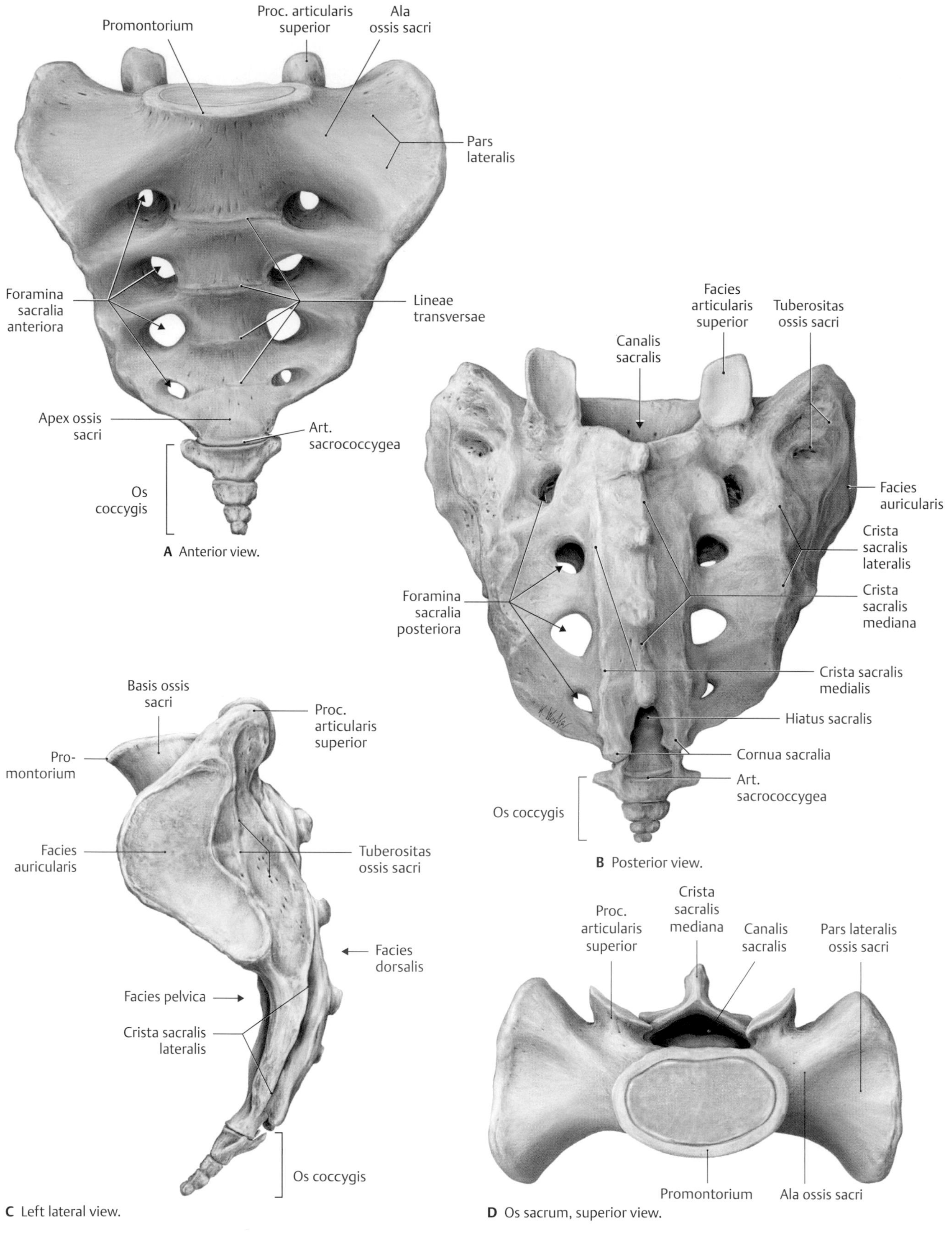

Promontorium

Proc. articularis superior

Ala ossis sacri

Pars lateralis

Foramina sacralia anteriora

Lineae transversae

Apex ossis sacri

Art. sacrococcygea

Os coccygis

A Anterior view.

Canalis sacralis

Facies articularis superior

Tuberositas ossis sacri

Foramina sacralia posteriora

Facies auricularis

Crista sacralis lateralis

Crista sacralis mediana

Crista sacralis medialis

Hiatus sacralis

Cornua sacralia

Art. sacrococcygea

Os coccygis

B Posterior view.

Basis ossis sacri

Proc. articularis superior

Pro-montorium

Facies auricularis

Tuberositas ossis sacri

Facies dorsalis

Facies pelvica

Crista sacralis lateralis

Os coccygis

C Left lateral view.

Proc. articularis superior

Crista sacralis mediana

Canalis sacralis

Pars lateralis ossis sacri

Promontorium

Ala ossis sacri

D Os sacrum, superior view.

Fig. 3.8 Os sacrum and os coccygis
(From Schuenke M, Schulte E, Schumacher U. THIEME Atlas of Anatomy, Vol 1. Illustrations by Voll M and Wesker K. 3rd ed. New York: Thieme Publishers; 2020.)

Joints of the Vertebral Column

Joints of the vertebral column include articulations between adjacent vertebral bodies and articulations between adjacent vertebral arches. Joints also form between the vertebral column and the skull (**Table 3.1**). Individual vertebral joints allow small local movements, but the combination of these movements over multiple vertebral levels accounts for the considerable flexibility of the vertebral column.

— **Craniovertebral joints (Fig. 3.9)** are synovial joints between the skull and C I, and between C I and C II:

- Paired **atlanto-occipital joints** between the os occipitale of the skull and the atlas (C I) allow flexion and extension of the head (as when nodding "yes").
- **Atlantoaxial joints,** which include one median and two lateral articulations between the atlas and axis (C I and C II), allow rotation of the head from side to side (as when saying "no").

BOX 3.5: CLINICAL CORRELATION

INJURIES OF THE VERTEBRAE CERVICALES
The laxity of the vertebrae cervicales makes it prone to hyperextension injuries, such as "whiplash," the excessive and often violent backward movement of the head, resulting in fractures of the dens axis and traumatic spondylolisthesis (see Box 3.4 Spondylolysis and Spondylolisthesis). Patient prognosis is largely dependent on the spinal level of the injuries.

— **Uncovertebral joints** form between the **proc. uncinatus** (lateral lips on the superior edges of the vertebral bodies) of C III–C VII vertebrae and the vertebral bodies immediately superior to them.

- These joints, which are not present at birth, form during childhood, probably as a result of a fissure in the cartilage of the discus intervertebralis that then assumes a joint-like character.

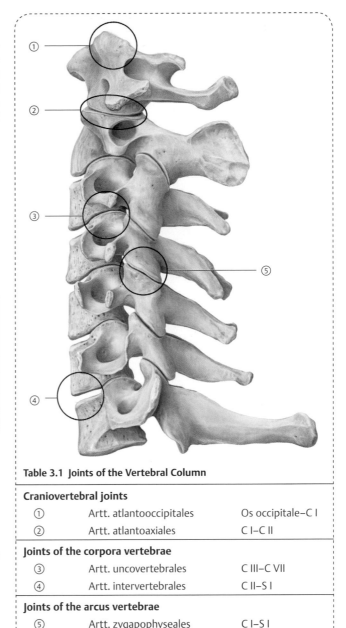

Table 3.1 Joints of the Vertebral Column

Craniovertebral joints		
①	Artt. atlantooccipitales	Os occipitale–C I
②	Artt. atlantoaxiales	C I–C II
Joints of the corpora vertebrae		
③	Artt. uncovertebrales	C III–C VII
④	Artt. intervertebrales	C II–S I
Joints of the arcus vertebrae		
⑤	Artt. zygapophyseales	C I–S I

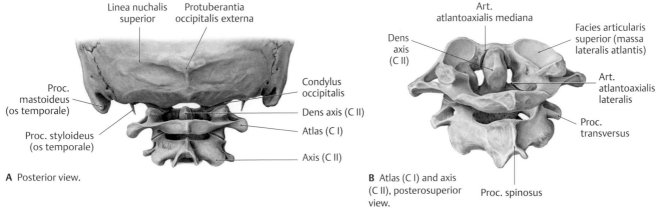

A Posterior view.

Linea nuchalis superior
Protuberantia occipitalis externa
Proc. mastoideus (os temporale)
Proc. styloideus (os temporale)
Condylus occipitalis
Dens axis (C II)
Atlas (C I)
Axis (C II)

B Atlas (C I) and axis (C II), posterosuperior view.

Art. atlantoaxialis mediana
Dens axis (C II)
Facies articularis superior (massa lateralis atlantis)
Art. atlantoaxialis lateralis
Proc. transversus
Proc. spinosus

Fig. 3.9 Craniovertebral joints

(From Gilroy AM et al. Atlas of Anatomy. 4th ed. 2020. Based on: Schuenke M, Schulte E, Schumacher U. THIEME Atlas of Anatomy. General Anatomy and Musculoskeletal System. Illustrations by Voll M and Wesker K. 3rd ed. New York: Thieme Medical Publishers; 2020.)

BOX 3.6: CLINICAL CORRELATION

HERNIATION OF DISCUS INTERVERTEBRALIS

As elasticity of the anulus fibrosus declines with age, compressive forces can cause the nucleus pulposus to protrude through weakened areas. If the fibrous ring of the anulus ruptures posteriorly, the herniated material may compress the contents of the dural sac, but posterolateral herniations that compress nn. spinales are most common, particularly at the L4–L5 or L5–S1 level. In the lumbar region, where nn. spinales exit the canalis vertebralis above the discus intervertebralis, the hernia is likely to compress the n. spinalis inferior to that level (e.g., a herniation of the discus intervertebralis L IV–L V will impact the n. spinalis L5), and pain is felt along the corresponding dermatome.

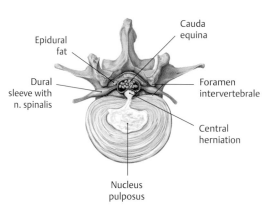

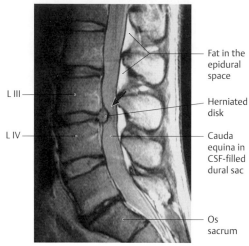

A Superior view. (From Schuenke M, Schulte E, Schumacher U. THIEME Atlas of Anatomy, Vol 1. Illustrations by Voll M and Wesker K. 3rd ed. New York: Thieme Publishers; 2020.)

B Midsagittal T2-weighted MRI. (From Jallo J and Vaccaro AR. Neurotrama and Critical Care of the Spine, 2nd ed. New York: Thieme Publishers; 2018.)

Posterior herniation (A,B). In the MRI a conspicuously herniated disk at the level of L III–L IV protrudes posteriorly. The dural sac is deeply indented at that level. CSF, cerebrospinal fluid.

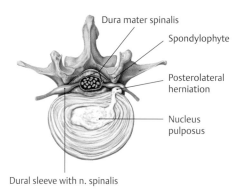

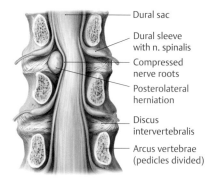

C Superior view. (From Schuenke M, Schulte E, Schumacher U. THIEME Atlas of Anatomy, Vol 1. Illustrations by Voll M and Wesker K. 3rd ed. New York: Thieme Publishers; 2020.)

D Posterior view, vertebral arches removed. (From Schuenke M, Schulte E, Schumacher U. THIEME Atlas of Anatomy, Vol 1. Illustrations by Voll M and Wesker K. 3rd ed. New York: Thieme Publishers; 2020.)

Posterolateral herniation (C,D). A posterolateral herniation may compress the n. spinalis as it passes through the foramen intervertebrale. If more medially positioned, the herniation may spare the nerve at that level but impact nerves at inferior levels.

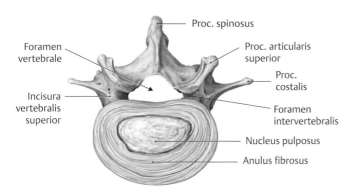

Fig. 3.10 Discus intervertebralis
Vertebra lumbalis IV, superior view. (From Schuenke M, Schulte E, Schumacher U. THIEME Atlas of Anatomy, Vol 1. Illustrations by Voll M and Wesker K. 3rd ed. New York: Thieme Publishers; 2020.)

— **Intervertebral joints** form between **disci intervertebrales** and the articular surfaces of vertebral bodies. There is no discus intervertebralis between C I and C II, and those between sacral and coccygeal vertebrae are rudimentary.
- The disci intervertebrales act as shock absorbers and are composed of an outer fibrous ring, the **anulus fibrosus,** and a gelatinous core, the **nucleus pulposus (Fig. 3.10)**.
- The height of the discus intervertebralis relative to the height of the corpus vertebrae determines the degree of

mobility of the joint; mobility is greatest in the cervical and lumbar regions.
- The differences between anterior and posterior heights of the cervical and lumbar disks contribute to the lordotic curvatures.
— **Artt. zygapophysiales,** also known as **facet joints,** are synovial joints that join the facies articularis superior and facies articularis inferior of adjacent vertebrae. The orientation of these joints differs among regions and influences the degree and direction of movement of the vertebral column.
- In the cervical region, the joints are mostly in the horizontal plane and allow movement in most directions.
- In the thorax, the joints largely lie in the coronal plane, limiting movement to lateral flexion.
- In the lumbar region, the joints are in the sagittal plane, facilitating flexion and extension.

Vertebral Ligaments

Vertebral ligaments support the joints of the vertebral column.
— Ligaments that support the cranial vertebral joints (**Fig. 3.11**) include
- the **atlanto-occipital membranes,** which connect the os occipitale to the arcus anterior atlantis and arcus posterior atlantis (C I);
- the **ligg. alaria,** which secure the dens of C II to the skull; and

---

BOX 3.7: CLINICAL CORRELATION

AGE-RELATED CHANGES IN VERTEBRAE
With advancing age, a decrease in bone density and aging of the disci intervertebrales can lead to an increase in compressive forces on the vertebral joints. Subsequent degenerative changes can include the depletion of articular cartilage and the formation of osteophytes (bony spurs). Osteophyte formation at the periphery of the vertebral bodies where they join the disci intervertebrales is known as **spondylosis**. Similar degenerative changes of the artt. zygapophysiales indicate osteoarthritis, common in the vertebrae cervicalis and vertebrae lumbales but also manifested in the joints of the hand, hip, and knee.

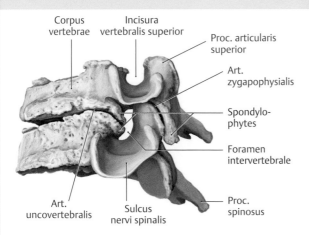

Advanced uncovertebral arthrosis of the vertebrae cervicales. (Drawing based on specimen from the Anatomical Collection at Kiel University.) (From Schuenke M, Schulte E, Schumacher U. THIEME Atlas of Anatomy, Vol 1. Illustrations by Voll M and Wesker K. 3rd ed. New York: Thieme Publishers; 2020.)

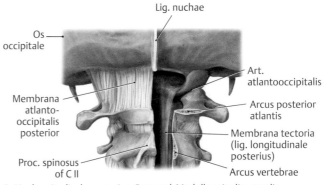

A Lig. longitudinale posterius. *Removed:* Medulla spinalis; canalis vertebralis windowed.

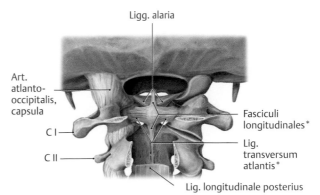

B Lig. cruciforme atlantis (*). *Removed:* Membrana tectoria.

Fig. 3.11 Dissection of the craniovertebral joint ligaments
Posterior view. (From Gilroy AM et al. Atlas of Anatomy. 4th ed. 2020. Based on: Schuenke M, Schulte E, Schumacher U. THIEME Atlas of Anatomy. General Anatomy and Musculoskeletal System. Illustrations by Voll M and Wesker K. 3rd ed. New York: Thieme Medical Publishers; 2020.)

- the **lig. cruciforme atlantis,** formed by longitudinal fascicles (fibers) and a transverse ligament, which secures the dens against the arcus anterior atlantis.

— Two longitudinal ligaments **(Figs. 3.12** and **3.13)** join all of the vertebral bodies:
1. The **lig. longitudinale anterius,** a broad fibrous band extending from the os occipitale of the skull to the os sacrum, attaches to the anterior and lateral surfaces of the vertebral bodies and disci intervertebrales and prevents hyperextension.
2. The **lig. longitudinale posterius,** a thin fibrous band extending from C II to the os sacrum along the anterior aspect of the canalis vertebralis, attaches primarily to the disci intervertebrales and offers weak resistance to hyperflexion. Superiorly, this ligament extends into the skull as the **membrana tectoria** (see **Fig. 2.15A**).

— Ligaments that join the arcus vertebrae of adjacent vertebrae include the following:
- the paired **ligg. flava,** which join the laminae of adjacent vertebrae on the posterior wall of the canalis vertebralis. They limit flexion and provide postural support of the vertebral column **(Fig. 3.14).**
- the **lig. supraspinale**, which connects the posterior ridge of the procc. spinosi **(Fig. 3.15)**
- the **lig. nuchae,** a finlike expansion of the lig. supraspinale in the neck that extends from the os occipitale to the proc. spinosus of C VII **(Fig. 3.15)**

— Additional vertebral ligaments connect elements of the arcus vertebrae and procc. spinosi (see **Fig. 3.12**).

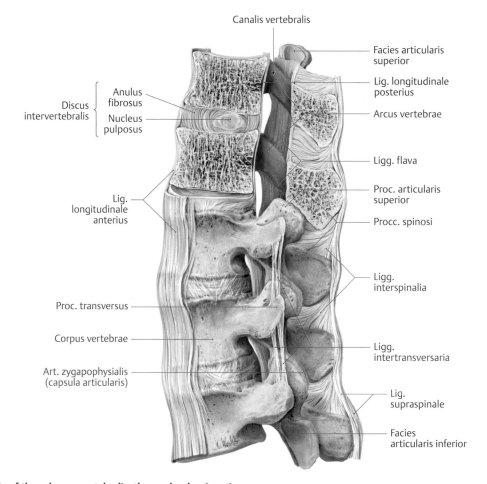

Fig. 3.12 Ligaments of the columna vertebralis: thoracolumbar junction
Left lateral view of T XI–L III, with T XI–T XII sectioned in the midsagittal plane. (From Gilroy AM et al. Atlas of Anatomy. 4th ed. 2020. Based on: Schuenke M, Schulte E, Schumacher U. THIEME Atlas of Anatomy. General Anatomy and Musculoskeletal System. Illustrations by Voll M and Wesker K. 3rd ed. New York: Thieme Medical Publishers; 2020.)

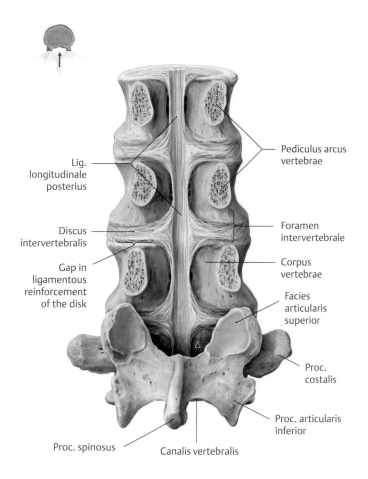

Lig. longitudinale posterius

Discus intervertebralis

Gap in ligamentous reinforcement of the disk

Proc. spinosus

Canalis vertebralis

Pediculus arcus vertebrae

Foramen intervertebrale

Corpus vertebrae

Facies articularis superior

Proc. costalis

Proc. articularis inferior

Fig. 3.13 Lig. longitudinale posterius
Posterior view of opened canalis vertebralis at level of L II–L V.
Removed: L II–L IV arcus vertebrae. (From Gilroy AM et al. Atlas of Anatomy. 4th ed. 2020. Based on: Schuenke M, Schulte E, Schumacher U. THIEME Atlas of Anatomy. General Anatomy and Musculoskeletal System. Illustrations by Voll M and Wesker K. 3rd ed. New York: Thieme Medical Publishers; 2020.)

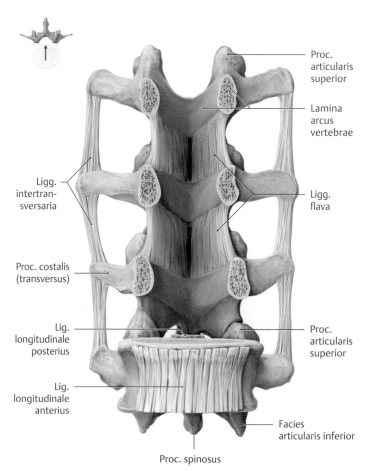

Proc. articularis superior

Lamina arcus vertebrae

Ligg. flava

Proc. articularis superior

Facies articularis inferior

Proc. spinosus

Ligg. intertransversaria

Proc. costalis (transversus)

Lig. longitudinale posterius

Lig. longitudinale anterius

Fig. 3.14 Ligg. flava and ligg. intertransversaria
Anterior view of opened canalis vertebralis at level of L II–L V.
Removed: L II–L IV corpora vertebrae. (From Gilroy AM et al. Atlas of Anatomy. 4th ed. 2020. Based on: Schuenke M, Schulte E, Schumacher U. THIEME Atlas of Anatomy. General Anatomy and Musculoskeletal System. Illustrations by Voll M and Wesker K. 3rd ed. New York: Thieme Medical Publishers; 2020.)

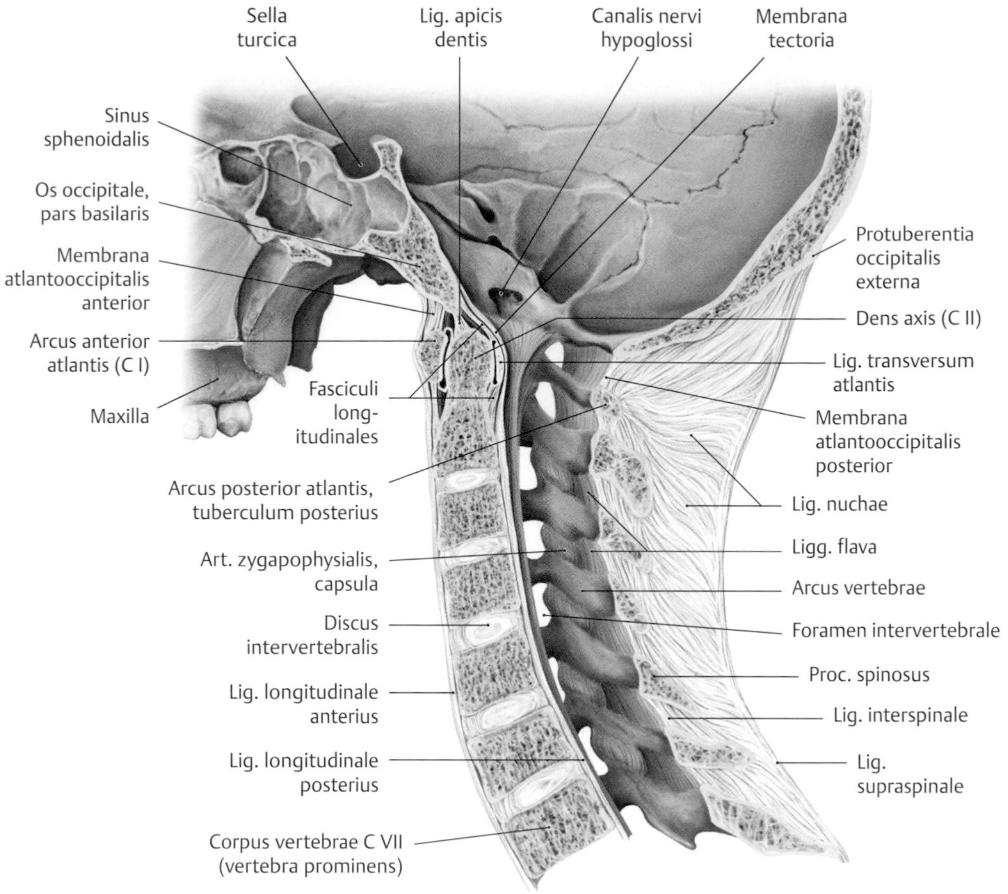

Fig. 3.15 Ligaments of the cervical spine
Midsagittal section, left lateral view. Lig. nuchae is the broadened, sagittally oriented part of the lig. supraspinale that extends from the vertebra prominens (C VII) to the protuberentia occipitalis externa. (From Gilroy AM et al. Atlas of Anatomy. 4th ed. 2020. Based on: Schuenke M, Schulte E, Schumacher U. THIEME Atlas of Anatomy. General Anatomy and Musculoskeletal System. Illustrations by Voll M and Wesker K. 3rd ed. New York: Thieme Medical Publishers; 2020.)

Neurovasculature of the Vertebral Column

— The following arteries (**Fig. 3.16**) supply the vertebrae, vertebral ligaments, meninges, and spinal cord:
  - The segmental arteries, paired branches of the aorta descendens such as the **aa. intercostales posteriores and aa. lumbales,** that arise in the thoracic and lumbar regions
  - Branches of the **a. subclavia** in the neck, including the a. intercostalis suprema (which supplies the first and second intercostal arteries), and the a. vertebralis and **a. cervicalis ascendens**
  - The **a. sacralis mediana**, arising near the aortic bifurcation, and the **a. iliolumbalis** and **aa. sacrales lateralis**, branches of the **a. iliaca interna** in the pelvis
— The **plexus venosus vertebralis** (Batson plexus) surrounds the vertebral bodies and drains the spinal cord, meninges, and vertebrae (**Fig. 3.17**).
  - **Plexus venosus vertebralis externus anterior** and **posterior** surround the vertebrae, and **plexus venosus vertebralis internus anterior** and **posterior** lie within the spatium epidurale in the canalis vertebralis.
  - Both the internal and external plexuses drain into **vv. intervertebrales**, which in turn drain to **vv. vertebrales** of

the cervical region and segmental veins (paired tributaries of the v. cava inferior and azygos system) in the thoracic, lumbar, and sacral regions.
  - The veins of the plexus venosus vertebralis have few valves; thus, there is free venous communication between the skull, neck, thorax, abdomen, and pelvis.
— Lymphatic drainage from the vertebrae and vertebral ligaments generally follows the arteries that supply each region and end in nodi lymphoidei cervicales, thoracis, lumbales, and sacrales.
— Posterior rami, and meningeal branches of anterior rami, of nn. spinales innervate the vertebrae, vertebral ligaments, and spinal meninges.

BOX 3.8: CLINICAL CORRELATION

METASTASIS AND THE PLEXUS VENOSUS VERTEBRALIS
The plexus venosus vertebralis links the venous drainages of viscera in the thorax, abdomen, and pelvis and the venous sinuses of the brain. These communications have been identified as a likely route of metastases of carcinoma of the prostata (commonly), breast, and lung (less commonly) to the central nervous system (systema nervosum centrale) and bone.

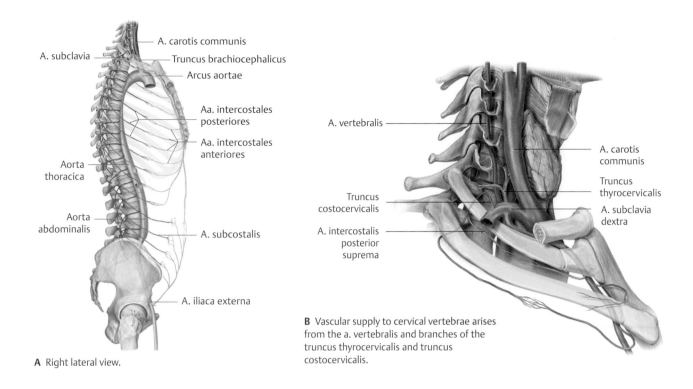

A. subclavia

A. carotis communis

Truncus brachiocephalicus

Arcus aortae

Aa. intercostales posteriores

Aa. intercostales anteriores

Aorta thoracica

Aorta abdominalis

A. subcostalis

A. iliaca externa

A Right lateral view.

A. vertebralis

A. carotis communis

Truncus thyrocervicalis

Truncus costocervicalis

A. subclavia dextra

A. intercostalis posterior suprema

B Vascular supply to cervical vertebrae arises from the a. vertebralis and branches of the truncus thyrocervicalis and truncus costocervicalis.

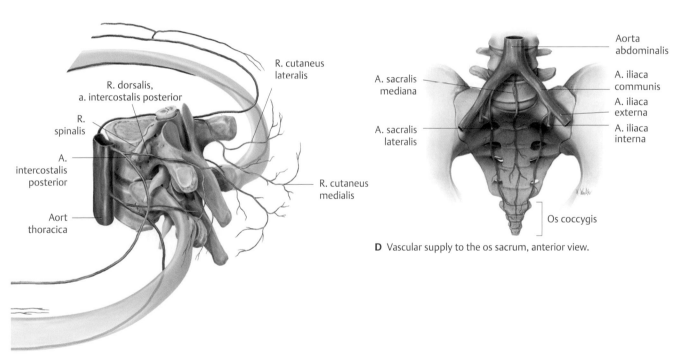

R. cutaneus lateralis

R. dorsalis, a. intercostalis posterior

R. spinalis

A. intercostalis posterior

Aort thoracica

R. cutaneus medialis

Aorta abdominalis

A. sacralis mediana

A. iliaca communis

A. iliaca externa

A. sacralis lateralis

A. iliaca interna

Os coccygis

D Vascular supply to the os sacrum, anterior view.

C Aa. intercostales posteriores, oblique posterosuperior view. The aa. intercostales posteriores give rise to cutaneous and muscular branches, as well as spinal branches that supply the medulla spinalis.

Fig. 3.16 Arteries of the trunk
(From Gilroy AM et al. Atlas of Anatomy. 4th ed. 2020. Based on: Schuenke M, Schulte E, Schumacher U. THIEME Atlas of Anatomy. General Anatomy and Musculoskeletal System. Illustrations by Voll M and Wesker K. 3rd ed. New York: Thieme Medical Publishers; 2020.)

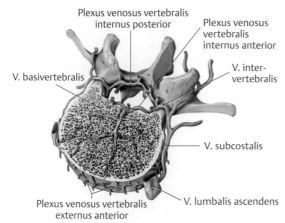

A Vertebral venous plexuses, superior view.

- Plexus venosus vertebralis internus posterior
- Plexus venosus vertebralis internus anterior
- V. basivertebralis
- V. intervertebralis
- V. subcostalis
- Plexus venosus vertebralis externus anterior
- V. lumbalis ascendens

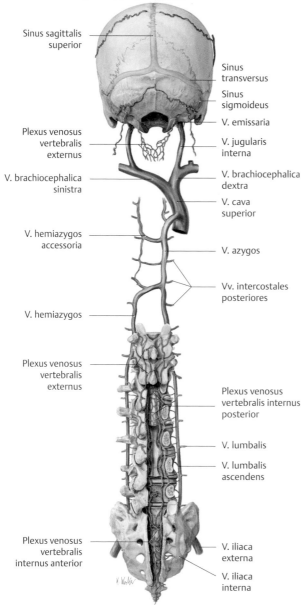

B Plexus venosus vertebralis, posterior view with canalis vertebralis windowed in the lumbar and sacral spine.

- Sinus sagittalis superior
- Sinus transversus
- Sinus sigmoideus
- V. emissaria
- Plexus venosus vertebralis externus
- V. jugularis interna
- V. brachiocephalica sinistra
- V. brachiocephalica dextra
- V. cava superior
- V. hemiazygos accessoria
- V. azygos
- Vv. intercostales posteriores
- V. hemiazygos
- Plexus venosus vertebralis externus
- Plexus venosus vertebralis internus posterior
- V. lumbalis
- V. lumbalis ascendens
- Plexus venosus vertebralis internus anterior
- V. iliaca externa
- V. iliaca interna

Fig. 3.17 Plexus venosus vertebralis
The vv. intervertebrales and vv. basivertebrales connect the plexus venosus vertebrales interni and plexus venosus vertebralis externus, which drain into the azygos system. (From Gilroy AM et al. Atlas of Anatomy. 4th ed. 2020. Based on: Schuenke M, Schulte E, Schumacher U. THIEME Atlas of Anatomy. Head, Neck, and Neuroanatomy. Illustrations by Voll M and Wesker K. 3rd ed. New York: Thieme Medical Publishers; 2020.)

3.2   The Spinal Cord (Medulla Spinalis)

The spinal cord is the part of the central nervous system (systema nervosum centrale) that relays information between the brain and the body. The spinal cord, along with its nn. spinales, surrounding membranes (the **meninges**), and associated vasculature, is enclosed within the canalis vertebralis.

Structure of the Spinal Cord

— The spinal cord, a slightly flattened cylindrical structure, is continuous with the brainstem. Within the canalis vertebralis, it extends from the skull base to a tapered end, the **conus medullaris**, at the level of L I or L II vertebra (**Fig. 3.18**).

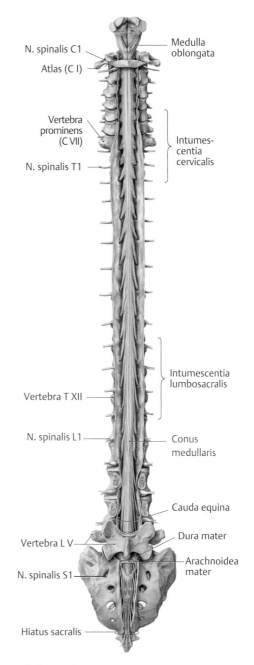

- N. spinalis C1
- Medulla oblongata
- Atlas (C I)
- Vertebra prominens (C VII)
- Intumescentia cervicalis
- N. spinalis T1
- Intumescentia lumbosacralis
- Vertebra T XII
- N. spinalis L1
- Conus medullaris
- Cauda equina
- Vertebra L V
- Dura mater
- N. spinalis S1
- Arachnoidea mater
- Hiatus sacralis

Fig. 3.18 Medulla spinalis in situ
Posterior view with canalis vertebralis windowed. (From Gilroy AM et al. Atlas of Anatomy. 4th ed. 2020. Based on: Schuenke M, Schulte E, Schumacher U. THIEME Atlas of Anatomy. Head, Neck, and Neuroanatomy. Illustrations by Voll M and Wesker K. 3rd ed. New York: Thieme Medical Publishers; 2020.)

— Along its length, two swellings occur in the regions of the spinal cord that innervate the limbs:
  • The **cervical enlargement** at C IV–T I is related to the plexus brachialis, a plexus of nerves that innervate the upper limb.
  • The **lumbosacral enlargement** at T XI–S I is related to the plexus lumbosacralis, nerve plexuses that innervate the abdominal wall and lower limb.
— The spinal cord consists of 31 segments (8 cervical, 12 thoracic, 5 lumbar, 5 sacral, and 1 coccygeal), each of which innervates a specific area of the trunk or limbs. Each spinal cord segment is associated with a pair of **nn. spinales** that pass to and from the canalis vertebralis through the foramina intervertebralia at the corresponding vertebral level. Both spinal cord segments and nn. spinales are identified by region and number (e.g., T IV).
— The adult spinal cord is considerably shorter than the vertebral column, occupying only the superior two thirds of the canalis vertebralis. As a result, most spinal cord segments do not lie adjacent to the vertebral level of the same number although the nn. spinales arising from those segments still exit through the corresponding foramina intervertebralia (**Fig. 3.19**).
— The spinal cord is surrounded by three layers, or **meninges**, and is suspended within cerebrospinal fluid (liquor cerebrospinalis).

Meninges of the Spinal Cord

The **spinal meninges** are membranes that surround the spinal cord and nerve roots and that contain the **cerebrospinal fluid** (liquor cerebrospinalis, a fluid that cushions and nourishes the brain and spinal cord) (**Fig. 3.20**; see also Section 26.2).
— The three layers of spinal meninges are continuous with the meninges that surround the brain:
  1. **Dura mater,** a tough outer layer that forms the **dural sac** enclosing the spinal cord and extending along the nerve roots to the foramina intervertebralia. The dural sac begins at the foramen magnum of the skull and ends at the level of S II.
  2. **Arachnoidea,** a delicate middle layer that lines the dural sac and is connected to the underlying membrane by **trabeculae arachnoideae** (strands of connective tissue).
  3. **Pia mater,** a thin layer that adheres to the surface of the spinal cord. **Ligg. denticulata,** transverse extensions of the pia mater, attach to the dura mater and suspend the spinal cord within the dural sac.
— The **filum terminale,** a thin cord of connective tissue invested by pia mater, extends from the conus medullaris to the apex of the dural sac. There it is surrounded by dura mater spinalis and extends to the end of the canalis vertebralis, where it anchors both membranes to the os coccygis.
— Three spaces separate the layers of meninges (**Fig. 3.21**):
  • The **spatium epidurale** lies between the bony wall of the canalis vertebralis and the dura mater. It contains fat and the plexus venosus vertebralis.
  • The **spatium subdurale,** a potential space between the dura and arachnoid layers, contains a thin film of lubricating fluid.
  • The **spatium subarachnoideum** lies deep to the arachnoid layer and contains the cerebrospinal fluid which bathes the spinal cord and roots of the nn. spinales. This space expands inferiorly as the **cisterna lumbalis** between the end of the spinal cord at the L I/L II vertebra, and the end of the arachnoid-lined dural sac at the S II vertebra.

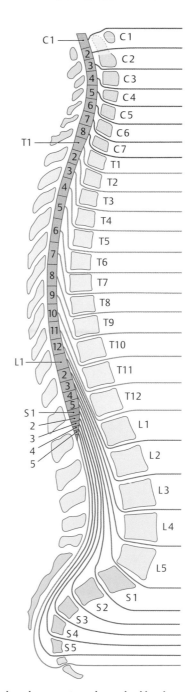

Fig. 3.19 Spinal cord segments and vertebral levels
Medulla spinalis is divided into four major regions: cervical, thoracic, lumbar, and sacral. Spinal cord segments are numbered by the exit points of their associated nn. spinales. (From Schuenke M, Schulte E, Schumacher U. THIEME Atlas of Anatomy, Vol 1. Illustrations by Voll M and Wesker K. 3rd ed. New York: Thieme Publishers; 2020.)

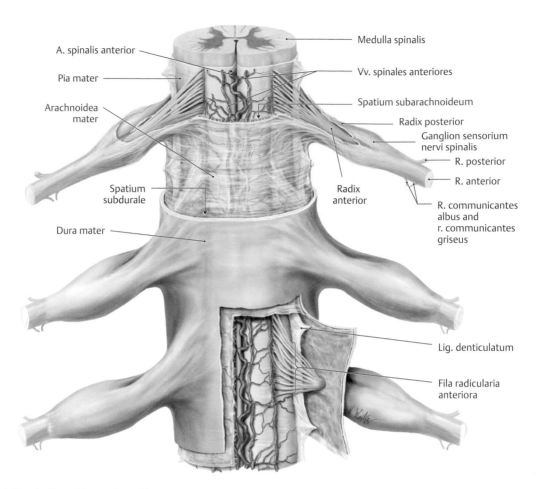

Fig. 3.20 Medulla spinalis and its meningeal layers
Anterior view. The dura mater is opened, and the arachnoidea is sectioned. (From Gilroy AM et al. Atlas of Anatomy. 4th ed. 2020. Based on: Schuenke M, Schulte E, Schumacher U. THIEME Atlas of Anatomy. Head, Neck, and Neuroanatomy. Illustrations by Voll M and Wesker K. 3rd ed. New York: Thieme Medical Publishers; 2020.)

BOX 3.9: CLINICAL CORRELATION

LUMBAR PUNCTURE, SPINAL ANESTHESIA, AND EPIDURAL ANESTHESIA

A lumbar puncture, used to extract cerebrospinal fluid from the spinal subarachnoid space, is administered by inserting a needle between the proc. spinosus of L III and L IV (sometimes between L IV and L V). The needle pierces the lig. flavum and wall of the dural sac before entering the cisterna lumbalis (2). The injection of a local anesthetic for spinal anesthesia is also administered in this manner. A similar approach may be used for epidural anesthesia (1), to anesthetize emerging nn. spinales, but the anesthetic is injected into the spatium epidurale without entering the dural sac. A caudal approach through the hiatus sacralis also allows access to the spatium epidurale (3).

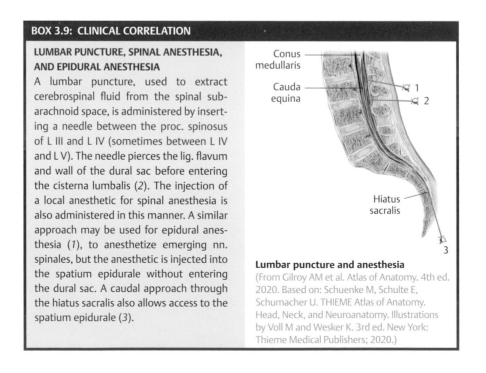

Lumbar puncture and anesthesia
(From Gilroy AM et al. Atlas of Anatomy. 4th ed. 2020. Based on: Schuenke M, Schulte E, Schumacher U. THIEME Atlas of Anatomy. Head, Neck, and Neuroanatomy. Illustrations by Voll M and Wesker K. 3rd ed. New York: Thieme Medical Publishers; 2020.)

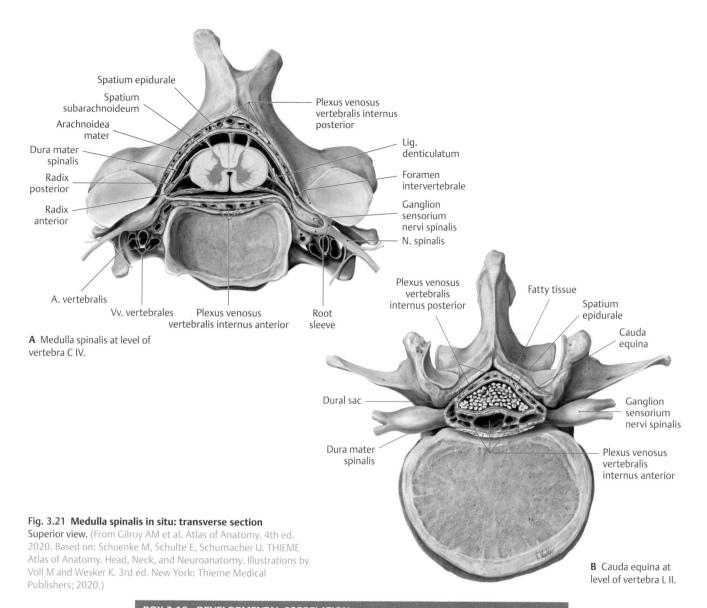

A Medulla spinalis at level of vertebra C IV.

B Cauda equina at level of vertebra L II.

Fig. 3.21 Medulla spinalis in situ: transverse section
Superior view. (From Gilroy AM et al. Atlas of Anatomy. 4th ed. 2020. Based on: Schuenke M, Schulte E, Schumacher U. THIEME Atlas of Anatomy. Head, Neck, and Neuroanatomy. Illustrations by Voll M and Wesker K. 3rd ed. New York: Thieme Medical Publishers; 2020.)

BOX 3.10: DEVELOPMENTAL CORRELATION

DEVELOPMENTAL CHANGES OF THE SPINAL CORD, DURAL SAC, AND VERTEBRAL COLUMN
During postnatal development, the longitudinal growth of the vertebral column exceeds that of the spinal cord. At birth, the conus medullaris is at the level of the L III vertebra, but in the average adult it lies at the level of the L I or L II vertebra. At all ages, the cisterna lumbalis of the dural sac extends into the canalis sacralis.

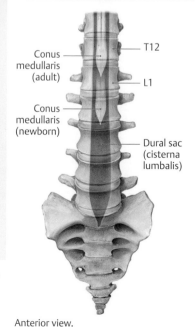

(From Gilroy AM et al. Atlas of Anatomy. 4th ed. 2020. Based on: Schuenke M, Schulte E, Schumacher U. THIEME Atlas of Anatomy. Head, Neck, and Neuroanatomy. Illustrations by Voll M and Wesker K. 3rd ed. New York: Thieme Medical Publishers; 2020.)

Anterior view.

Blood Supply to the Spinal Cord

Arterial blood supply to the spinal cord arises from the aa. verte-brales as well as from branches of the aa. subclaviae and aorta descendens **(Fig. 3.22)**.

— Longitudinal aa. spinales supply the superior part of the spinal cord.
- A single **a. spinalis anterior** arises from the two aa. vertebrales (branches of the aa. subclaviae) and supplies the anterior two thirds of the spinal cord.
- Paired **aa. spinales posteriores** arise from the aa. vertebrales (or one of their branches, the posterior cerebellar artery) and supply the posterior third of the spinal cord.
— **A. medullaris segmentalis anterior** and **a. medullaris segmentalis posterior** are large, irregularly spaced vessels that communicate with the aa. spinales.
- They arise from branches of the a. subclavia and segmental arteries in the thoracic and lumbar regions.
- The aa. medullares enter the canalis vertebralis through the foramina intervertebralia and are found mainly at the cervical and lumbar enlargements.
— The **a. radicularis magna** (Adamkiewicz), a single large, usually left-sided vessel, can provide an important contribu-tion to the circulation of the lower two thirds of the spinal cord.
- It arises as a branch of a lower thoracic or lumbar segmental artery.
- It enters the canalis vertebralis through a foramen interver-tebrale in the lower thorax or upper lumbar region.
— The **a. radicularis anterior** and **a. radicularis posterior** are small arteries that supply the roots of the nn. spinales and the superficial **substantia grisea** of the spinal cord. They do not communicate with the aa. spinales.

Veins of the spinal cord, which are more numerous than the arter-ies, have the same distribution, anastomose freely with one another, and drain into the plexus venosus vertebralis internus **(Fig. 3.23)**.

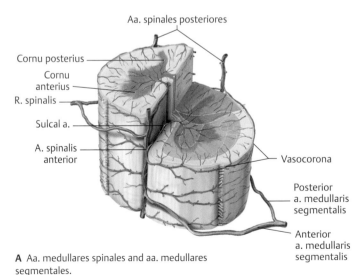

A Aa. medullares spinales and aa. medullares segmentales.

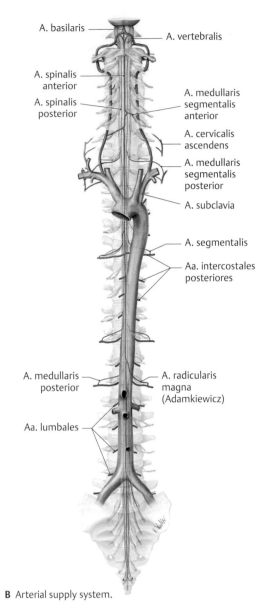

B Arterial supply system.

Fig. 3.22 Arteries of the medulla spinalis
The unpaired aa. spinales anteriores and paired aa. spinales posteriores typically arise from the aa. vertebrales. As they descend within the canalis vertebralis, the aa. spinales are reinforced by a. medullaris anterior and a. medullaris posterior. Depending on the spinal level, these reinforcing branches may arise from the a. vertebralis, a. cervicalis ascendens, a. cervicalis profunda, a. intercostalis posterior, aa. lumbales, or aa. sacrales laterales. (From Gilroy AM et al. Atlas of Anatomy. 4th ed. 2020. Based on: Schuenke M, Schulte E, Schumacher U. THIEME Atlas of Anatomy. Head, Neck, and Neuroanatomy. Illustrations by Voll M and Wesker K. 3rd ed. New York: Thieme Medical Publishers; 2020.)

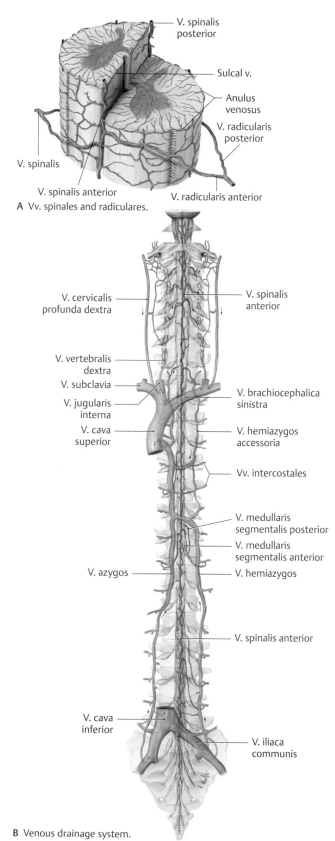

A Vv. spinales and radiculares.

- V. spinalis posterior
- Sulcal v.
- Anulus venosus
- V. radicularis posterior
- V. radicularis anterior
- V. spinalis anterior
- V. spinalis

B Venous drainage system.

- V. cervicalis profunda dextra
- V. spinalis anterior
- V. vertebralis dextra
- V. subclavia
- V. jugularis interna
- V. brachiocephalica sinistra
- V. cava superior
- V. hemiazygos accessoria
- Vv. intercostales
- V. medullaris segmentalis posterior
- V. medullaris segmentalis anterior
- V. azygos
- V. hemiazygos
- V. spinalis anterior
- V. cava inferior
- V. iliaca communis

Fig. 3.23 Veins of the medulla spinalis
The interior of medulla spinalis drains via venous plexuses into vv. spinales anterior and posterior. The vv. medullares and spinales connect the veins of the medulla spinalis with the plexus venosus vertebralis internus. The vv. intervertebrales and basivertebrales connect the plexus venosus vertebralis internus and externus, which drain into the azygos system. (From Gilroy AM et al. Atlas of Anatomy. 4th ed. 2020. Based on: Schuenke M, Schulte E, Schumacher U. THIEME Atlas of Anatomy. Head, Neck, and Neuroanatomy. Illustrations by Voll M and Wesker K. 3rd ed. New York: Thieme Medical Publishers; 2020.)

3.3 Spinal Nerves (Nn. Spinales)

Nn. spinales transmit information between peripheral body tissues and the spinal cord. A single pair of nn. spinales arises from each segment of the spinal cord.

- There are 31 pairs of nn. spinales: 8 cervical, 12 thoracic, 5 lumbar, 5 sacral, and 1 coccygeal. Each pair is named for the spinal cord segment from which it arises.
- Nn. spinales are formed by the merging of (**Fig. 3.24**)
  - a **radix anterior** carrying motor (efferent) fibers whose cell bodies are located in the cornu anterius of the spinal cord, and
  - a **radix posterior** carrying sensory (afferent) fibers whose cell bodies are located in a ganglion sensorium nervi spinalis located outside the spinal cord.
- Nn. spinales pass through the foramina intervertebralia at the corresponding vertebral level.
  - Nn. cervicales C1–C7 exit the canalis vertebralis superior to the vertebra of the same number (e.g., n. spinalis C4 exits between vertebrae C VII and T I).
  - N. spinalis C8 exits below vertebra C VII (between vertebrae C III and C IV).
  - Nn. spinales T1–Co1 exit the canal inferior to the corresponding vertebra.
- Because the spinal cord is shorter than the vertebral column, nerve roots from the lower spinal cord (L2–Co1) must descend below the conus medullaris within the cisterna lumbalis of the dural sac before exiting through the respective foramina intervertebralia. This loose group of nerve roots within the dural sac is called the **cauda equina** (see **Figs. 3.19** and **3.21**).

Peripheral Nerve Pathways of the Somatic Nervous System

The somatic nervous system innervates structures under conscious control including the skin and skeletal muscles.

- As nn. spinales emerge from the foramina intervertebralia, they split to form rami (branches) that contain both sensory

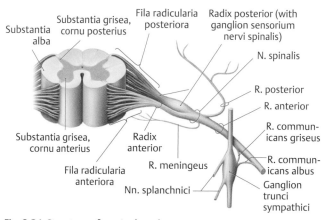

- Substantia alba
- Substantia grisea, cornu posterius
- Fila radicularia posteriora
- Radix posterior (with ganglion sensorium nervi spinalis)
- N. spinalis
- R. posterior
- R. anterior
- R. communicans griseus
- R. communicans albus
- Ganglion trunci sympathici
- Nn. splanchnici
- R. meningeus
- Radix anterior
- Substantia grisea, cornu anterius
- Fila radicularia anteriora

Fig. 3.24 Structure of a spinal cord segment
Anterior view. Spinal cord segments are defined as a section of medulla spinalis that is associated with a single pair of nn. spinales. The nerves arise as anterior (motor) and posterior (sensory) rootlets that combine to form anterior and posterior roots, respectively. The two roots fuse within the foramen intervertebrale to form a mixed n. spinalis. Subsequent branches of the n. spinalis contain both motor and sensory fibers (except the meningeal branch, which is only sensory). (From Gilroy AM et al. Atlas of Anatomy. 4th ed. 2020. Based on: Schuenke M, Schulte E, Schumacher U. THIEME Atlas of Anatomy. Head, Neck, and Neuroanatomy. Illustrations by Voll M and Wesker K. 3rd ed. New York: Thieme Medical Publishers; 2020.)

and motor fibers (except C1, which contains only motor fibers) **(Fig. 3.24)**.
- **Rami posteriores** innervate skin and muscles of the posterior trunk, head, and neck.
- **Rami anteriores** form peripheral nerves and plexuses that innervate the rest of the body.
— Rr. posteriores do not form plexuses, and most are referred to by the spinal cord segment from which they originate (e.g., r. posterior T4). The n. suboccipitalis (C1), n. occipitalis major (C2), and n. occipitalis tertius (C3) that innervate the scalp are the only individually named rr. posteriores **(Fig. 3.25A)**.
— Rr. anteriores have a larger distribution than rr. posteriores, and most have a more complex course **(Fig. 3.25)**.
- Rr. anteriores of thoracic nn. spinales do not form plexuses but become **nn. intercostales,** which run in the spaces between ribs to innervate the thoracic and anterolateral abdominal walls.

- Rr. anteriores of the cervical, lumbar, and sacral regions form plexuses that give rise to multi-segmental nerves that may carry only sensory or only motor fibers, or they may be mixed nerves, carrying both sensory and motor fibers. These nerves are usually given specific names (e.g., n. radialis, n. femoralis). These somatic plexuses include:
  - Plexus cervicalis (C1–C4) innervates muscles of the neck and skin over the neck and scalp.
  - Plexus brachialis (C5–T1) innervates the pectoral girdle and upper limb.
  - Plexus lumbalis (L1–L4) innervates the lower anterior abdominal wall and anterior thigh.
  - Plexus sacralis (L4–S3) innervates the gluteal region, posterior thigh, and leg.
— In somatic nerve plexuses, sensory nerve fibers associated with a single spinal cord segment are distributed among several peripheral nerves. Traveling from the periphery toward the

Medulla Spinalis Segment	Anterior Branches (rami anteriores)	Posterior Branches (rami posteriores)
C1		N. suboccipitalis
C2	Plexus cervicalis	N. occipitalis major
C3		N. occipitalis tertius
C4		
C5	Plexus brachialis	
C6		
C7		
C8		
T1		
T2		
T3		
T4		
T5		
T6		
T7	Nn. intercostales	
T8		
T9		
T10		Rami posteriores
T11		
T12		
L1	Plexus lumbalis	
L2		
L3		
L4		
L5	Plexus sacralis	
S1		
S2		
S3		
S4		
S5	Plexus coccygeus	
Co1		
Co2		

A Anterior and posterior branches of the nn. spinales.

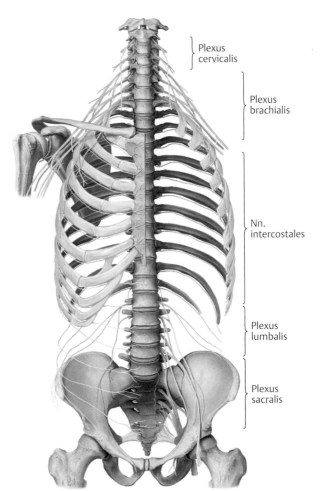

B Nerves of the trunk wall, anterior view. *Removed:* Anterior part of the left half of cavea thoracis.

Fig. 3.25 Nerves of the trunk wall
(From Schuenke M, Schulte E, Schumacher U. THIEME Atlas of Anatomy, Vol 1. Illustrations by Voll M and Wesker K. 3rd ed. New York: Thieme Publishers; 2020.)

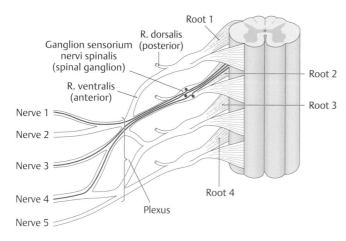

Fig. 3.26 Principles of plexus formation: sensory nerves (nervi sensorii)
The axons, which form the afferents from a dermatome, extend
from that dermatome to a single root in medulla spinalis. (From Gilroy AM
et al. Atlas of Anatomy. 4th ed. 2020. Based on: Schuenke M, Schulte E,
Schumacher U. THIEME Atlas of Anatomy. General Anatomy and
Musculoskeletal System. Illustrations by Voll M and Wesker K. 3rd ed. New
York: Thieme Medical Publishers; 2020.)

spinal cord, the sensory fibers converge to enter the
spinal cord via the radix posterior. There they synapse
with sensory neurons in the cornu posterius of the spinal cord
(**Fig. 3.26**).

— Sensory roots from each spinal cord segment correspond to
the sensory (cutaneous) innervation of a particular area of
skin, known as a **dermatome** (**Fig. 3.27**). Because sensory
fibers from each segment are distributed among multiple
peripheral nerves, there is a large area of overlap between
adjacent dermatomes. Thus, the lesion of a single sensory
nerve root (such as by the impingement of a herniated disk)
would have a minimal effect.

— Typically peripheral sensory nerves carry fibers from several
spinal cord levels. Lesions of a sensory nerve, therefore, would
affect a larger cutaneous territory covering multiple dermatomes (**Fig. 3.28**).

— Cutaneous sensations transmitted by somatic sensory nerves
include those of pain, pressure (touch), and temperature.
Sensory nerves also transmit a sense of position, or **proprio-
ception,** that provides information about the spatial position
of the limbs.

— Similar to the distribution of sensory fibers in a plexus,
motor fibers from multiple spinal cord levels may combine in
a peripheral nerve to innervate a single skeletal muscle. In
other cases, muscles may be innervated by a single spinal
cord segment. Muscles are divided into two groups based
on their innervation patterns (**Fig. 3.29**):

- **Monosegmentally** innervated muscles are innervated
by motor neurons from a single spinal cord
segment.

- **Polysegmentally** innervated muscles are innervated by
neurons whose nuclei extend over several spinal cord
segments.

— **Myotomes** represent the muscle mass that is innervated
by a single spinal cord segment. For example, although
the n. femoralis and the n. obturatorius both contain rr.
anteriores of L2–L4, they innervate different muscles. The L2
myotome would comprise all of the muscle fibers innervated
by the L2 spinal segment, whether carried in the n. femoralis
or n. obturatorius.

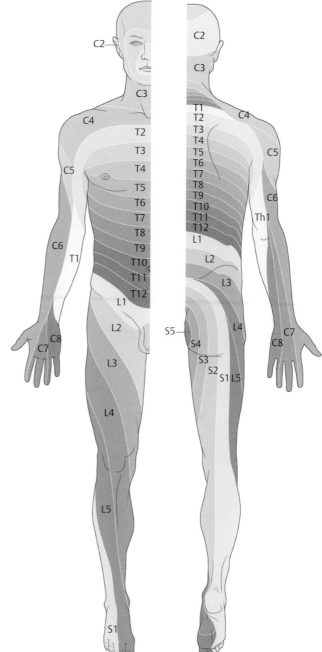

Fig. 3.27 Dermatomes of the head, trunk, and limbs
Each spinal cord segment innervates a particular skin area (dermatome).
Dermatomes are band-like areas of skin innervated by a pair of nn.
spinales arising from a single spinal cord segment. Since n. spinalis C1
carries only motor fibers, there is no corresponding dermatome. (From
Schuenke M, Schulte E, Schumacher U. THIEME Atlas of Anatomy, Vol 1.
Illustrations by Voll M and Wesker K. 3rd ed. New York: Thieme Publishers;
2020.)

— Muscles that are innervated by a single segment of the spinal
cord (monosegmental) can be evaluated clinically by testing a
corresponding **reflex**. Reflexes, such as the patellar tendon
reflex, are mediated by motor (efferent limb) and sensory
(afferent limb) neurons that are located within a single segment of the spinal cord.

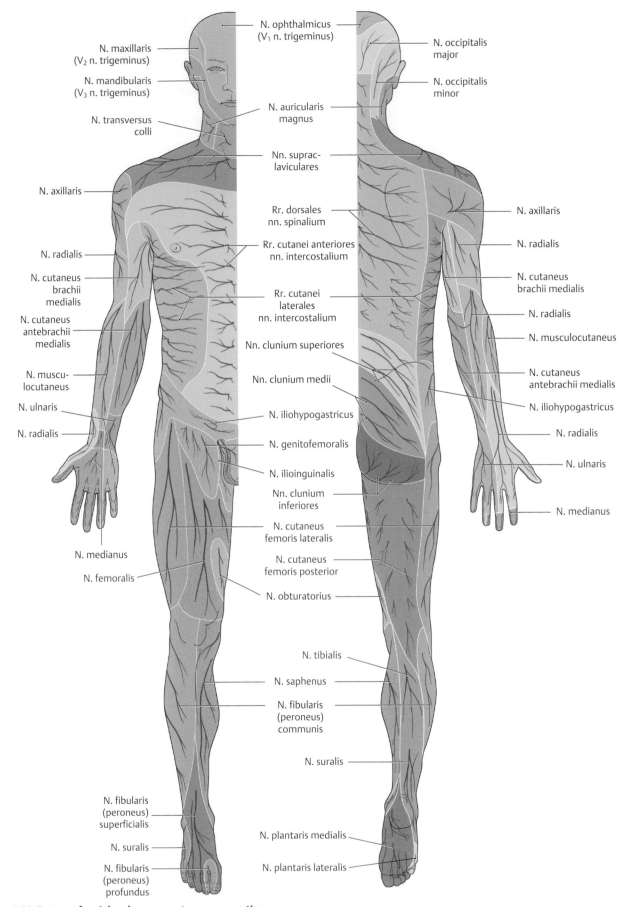

Fig. 3.28 Pattern of peripheral sensory cutaneous sensation
Sensory loss patterns that are associated with a peripheral nerve lesion overlap multiple dermatomes. (From Schuenke M, Schulte E, Schumacher U. THIEME Atlas of Anatomy, Vol 1. Illustrations by Voll M and Wesker K. 3rd ed. New York: Thieme Publishers; 2020.)

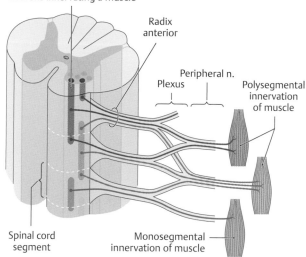

Fig. 3.29 Monosegmental and polysegmental innervation
(From Gilroy AM et al. Atlas of Anatomy. 4th ed. 2020. Based on: Schuenke M, Schulte E, Schumacher U. THIEME Atlas of Anatomy. General Anatomy and Musculoskeletal System. Illustrations by Voll M and Wesker K. 3rd ed. New York: Thieme Medical Publishers; 2020.)

Peripheral Nerve Pathways of the Autonomic Nervous System

The autonomic nervous system, the visceral part of the peripheral nervous system regulates the internal environment in response to both internal and external stimuli.

— Its two divisions often have antagonistic effects on the same organ and coordinate these responses to maintain a homeostatic internal environment (**Fig. 3.30; Table 3.2**):
  • The **sympathetic division** allows the body to respond to stress ("fight or flight").
  • The **parasympathetic division** allows the body to maintain, or return to, a state of homeostasis ("rest and digest").
— Nerve pathways of both the sympathetic and parasympathetic systems consist of a two-neuron chain between the central nervous system (systema nervosum centrale) and the target organ: a proximal preganglionic (presynaptic) neuron and distal postganglionic (postsynaptic) neuron that synapse with each other in an intervening ganglion (**Fig. 3.31**).
— Autonomic nerves often form dense plexuses, which travel to their target organs along arterial routes. Plexuses are named for the organs they innervate, such as cardiac or hepatic, or for the artery they follow, such as internal carotid, celiac, or renal.
— The sympathetic division is known as the thoracolumbar component because its nerves arise from the cornu laterale of the spinal cord in the thoracic and lumbar regions (T1–L2). They exit through the foramina intervertebralia with the motor fibers of the corresponding nn. spinales.
— In addition to sympathetic nerves, the sympathetic system includes paired **trunci sympathici**, chains of **paravertebral ganglia** that contain the cell bodies of postganglionic sympathetic nerves. The trunks run along each side of the vertebral bodies from C1 to S5. The paravertebral ganglia are connected to nn. spinales via
  • **rr. communicantes grisei,** which connect paravertebral ganglia at all levels (C1–S5) to the corresponding nn. spinales; and
  • **rr. communicantes albi**, which connect only paravertebral ganglia between T1 and L2 to the corresponding nn. spinales.

— Shortly after emerging from the vertebral column, the preganglionic sympathetic fibers leave the n. spinalis via the r. communicans albus to enter the paravertebral ganglion. From this point the sympathetic fibers can take three different routes:
  • They can synapse with the postganglionic neuron in the paravertebral ganglia at that level and return to the n. spinalis via the r. communicans griseus. As part of the n. spinalis, these fibers will follow the sensory and motor fibers of the anterior and posterior rami to innervate structures in the dermatome.
  • They can course up or down within the trunk to synapse with ganglia at other levels. The postganglionic fibers then join the nn. spinales at those levels. This route allows sympathetic fibers to be distributed to nn. spinales along the entire length of the spinal cord, and thus to all regions of the body, even though they originate only from the thoracolumbar segment.
  • They can pass through the paravertebral ganglia without synapsing to form **nn. splanchnici thoracici, nn. splanchnici lumbales,** or **nn. splanchnici sacrales**. These synapse in **prevertebral ganglia**, such as the celiac ganglion (see Section 11.2). Postganglionic fibers contribute to autonomic plexuses in the thorax, abdomen, and pelvis that travel along periarterial routes to innervate viscera in those regions.
— The parasympathetic division is known as the **craniosacral** component because its nerves arise from the brain and the S2–S4 segments of the sacral medulla spinalis.
  • Preganglionic parasympathetic fibers that arise from the brain travel with nn. craniales III, VII, IX, and X and synapse in parasympathetic ganglia of the head or, in the case of the n. vagus, ganglia near the target organ. The neural pathways involved are discussed in detail in Section 26.3.
    ○ The n. vagus is the only n. cranialis that extends inferior to the neck. Its parasympathetic fibers reach as far as the colon transversum in the abdomen. Thus, it provides parasympathetic innervation to all thoracic viscera and most of the abdominal viscera.
  • Similar to sympathetic fibers in the thoracolumbar region, sacral nn. parasympathici leave the medulla spinalis with the motor nerves of the corresponding somatic nn. spinales (S2–S4). These preganglionic parasympathetic fibers are known as **nn. splanchnici pelvici.** They contribute to autonomic plexuses in the pelvis and abdomen and synapse in small ganglia located close to, or within, their target organ.
— Smooth muscle in the skin and body wall (important for vasoconstriction, piloerection, gland secretion) does not receive any parasympathetic innervation. Sympathetic innervation is responsible for constriction of blood vessels; vasodilation results when sympathetic stimulation ceases.
— Visceral sensory fibers convey sensations from physiologic processes, such as distension of the bladder (vesicula urinaria). Nociceptive (pain) fibers have been shown to accompany both sympathetic and parasympathetic nerves.
  • Nociceptive fibers from viscera travel in the nn. splanchnici to ganglia sympathica and reach the n. spinalis by way of the r. communicans albus. Like somatic sensory neurons, their cell bodies are located in ganglia spinalia. They enter the cornu posterius of the spinal cord through the posterior roots.
  • Nociceptive fibers traveling with cranial parasympathetic fibers have their cell bodies in the inferior or superior ganglia of the n. vagus (n. cranialis X). Those traveling with sacral parasympathetic nerves have their cell bodies in the sacral ganglia spinalia of S2–S4.

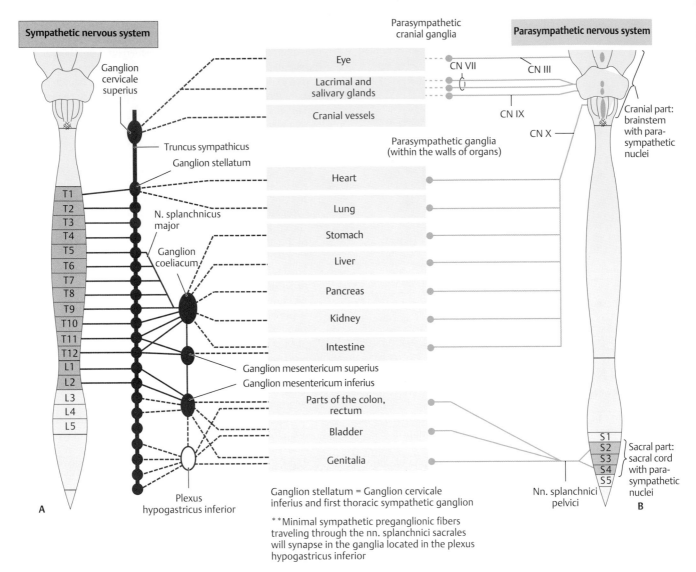

Fig. 3.30 Autonomic nervous system
The autonomic nervous system is subdivided into **(A)** sympathetic (thoracolumbar) and **(B)** parasympathetic (craniosacral) divisions. Each utilizes a two-neuron pathway in which preganglionic neurons synapse with postganglionic neurons in peripheral autonomic ganglia. (From Gilroy AM et al. Atlas of Anatomy. 4th ed. 2020. Based on: Schuenke M, Schulte E, Schumacher U. THIEME Atlas of Anatomy. General Anatomy and Musculoskeletal System. Illustrations by Voll M and Wesker K. 3rd ed. New York: Thieme Medical Publishers; 2020.)

Table 3.2 Effects of the Sympathetic and Parasympathetic Nervous Systems

Organ	Sympathetic Nervous System	Parasympathetic Nervous System
Eye	Pupillary dilation	Pupillary constriction and increased curvature of the lens
Salivary glands	Decreased salivation (scant, viscous)	Increased salivation (copious, watery)
Heart	Elevation of the heart rate	Slowing of the heart rate
Lungs	Decreased bronchial secretions; bronchial dilation	Increased bronchial secretions; bronchial constriction
Gastrointestinal tract	Decreased secretions and motor activity	Increased secretions and motor activity
Pancreas	Decreased secretion from the endocrine part of the gland	Increased secretion
Male sex organs	Ejaculation	Erection
Skin	Vasoconstriction, sweat, secretion, piloerection	No parasympathetic innervation

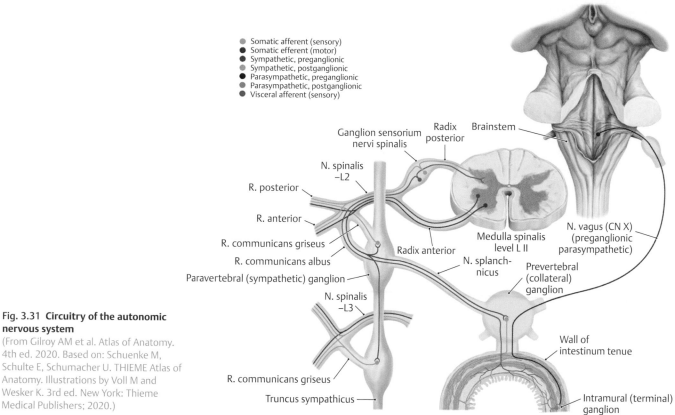

- ● Somatic afferent (sensory)
- ● Somatic efferent (motor)
- ● Sympathetic, preganglionic
- ● Sympathetic, postganglionic
- ● Parasympathetic, preganglionic
- ● Parasympathetic, postganglionic
- ● Visceral afferent (sensory)

Fig. 3.31 Circuitry of the autonomic nervous system
(From Gilroy AM et al. Atlas of Anatomy. 4th ed. 2020. Based on: Schuenke M, Schulte E, Schumacher U. THIEME Atlas of Anatomy. Illustrations by Voll M and Wesker K. 3rd ed. New York: Thieme Medical Publishers; 2020.)

BOX 3.11: CLINICAL CORRELATION

REFERRED PAIN
Referred pain is a sensation that originates from viscera but is perceived as if coming from an overlying or nearby somatic structure. It occurs because the somatic and visceral sensory fibers converge onto the same spinal cord segment. Diaphragmatic irritation from a splenic abscess, for example, is typically referred to the shoulder because both the diaphragma and the skin over the shoulder convey sensory information to C3–C5 segments of the spinal cord **(Fig. 3.32)**.

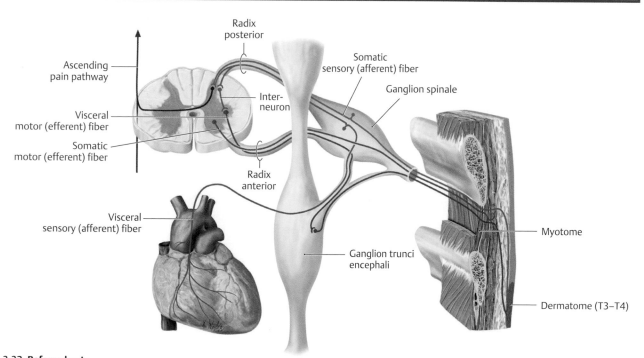

Fig. 3.32 Referred pain
It is believed that nociceptive sensory fibers from dermatomes (somatic pain) and internal organs (visceral pain) terminate on the same relay neurons in the medulla spinalis. The convergence of somatic and visceral sensory fibers confuses the relationship between the perceived and actual sites of pain, a phenomenon known as referred pain. The pain is typically perceived at the somatic site given that somatic pain is well localized while visceral pain is not. (From Gilroy AM et al. Atlas of Anatomy. 4th ed. 2020. Based on: Schuenke M, Schulte E, Schumacher U. THIEME Atlas of Anatomy. Head, Neck, and Neuroanatomy. Illustrations by Voll M and Wesker K. 3rd ed. New York: Thieme Medical Publishers; 2020.)

3.4   Muscles of the Back and Suboccipital Region

— **Extrinsic muscles,** the most superficial muscles that overlie the back, stabilize and move the upper limb. (See Chapter 19 for a discussion of the muscles of the upper limb.)
  • Extrinsic muscles include the m. trapezius, m. latissimus dorsi, m. levator scapulae, and m. rhomboideus major and m. rhomboideus minor.
— **Intrinsic muscles,** which attach to vertebrae or ribs, move and support the vertebral column **(Table 3.3)**.
  • They are arranged in superficial, intermediate, and deep layers **(Figs. 3.33** and **3.34)**.
  • The superficial layer includes the **splenius** muscle group that covers the deeper neck muscles laterally and posteriorly. These muscles extend and rotate the head and neck. They extend superolaterally from the procc. spinosi of vertebrae cervicales and upper thoracic vertebrae to the os occipitale and procc. transversi of C I and C II.
  • The intermediate layer includes the **erector spinae** muscle group that extends from the midline of the back to the angle of the ribs laterally. These large muscles are the main extensors and stabilizers of the thoracic and lumbar vertebral column. They include:
    ◦ the **m. iliocostalis,** the most lateral column that arises from the **fascia thoracolumbalis,** the os sacrum, crista iliaca, and ribs and extends superolaterally to the ribs and to cervical and lumbar vertebrae.
    ◦ the **m. longissimus,** the middle column that arises from the os sacrum, crista iliaca, procc. spinosi of lumbar vertebrae, and procc. transversi of thoracic and cervical vertebrae. It inserts superiorly on the temporal

bone of the skull, to cervical, thoracic and lumbar vertebrae and to the ribs.
  ◦ the **m. spinalis,** the most medial column that extends between the procc. spinosi of cervical and thoracic vertebrae.
  • The deep layer includes short muscles at multiple vertebral levels that produce small movements along the entire vertebral column. They are divided into a **transversospinalis** muscle group and a **deep segmental** muscle group. The mm. transversospinales extend between the procc. transversi and spinosi of the vertebrae. They include:
    ◦ the **mm. semispinales,** the most superficial group
    ◦ the **m. multifidus,** most prominent in the lumbar region
    ◦ the **mm. rotatores,** the deepest muscles of the transversospinalis group, best developed in the thoracic region
  • The deep segmental muscles are minor muscles of the back. They include the **mm. interspinales** and **intertransversarii** that connect adjacent vertebrae, and the **mm. levatores costarum** that connect vertebrae to ribs.

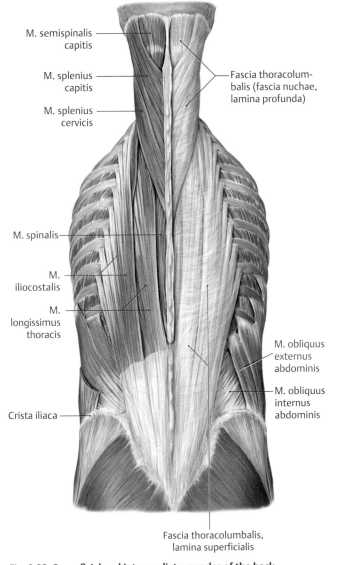

Fig. 3.33 Superficial and intermediate muscles of the back
Posterior view. *Removed:* Fascia thoracolumbalis *(left)*. (From Gilroy AM et al. Atlas of Anatomy. 4th ed. 2020. Based on: Schuenke M, Schulte E, Schumacher U. THIEME Atlas of Anatomy. General Anatomy and Musculoskeletal System. Illustrations by Voll M and Wesker K. 3rd ed. New York: Thieme Medical Publishers; 2020.)

Table 3.3 Muscles of the Back and Suboccipital Region

Muscle Group	Innervation	Action
Intrinsic muscles of the back		
Superficial layer M. splenius capitis M. splenius cervicis	Rami posteriores of nn. spinales cervicales	Extend, rotate, and laterally flex the head and vertebrae cervicales
Intermediate layer (erector spinae) M. spinalis M. longissimus thoracis M. iliocostalis	Rami posteriores of nn. spinales	Extend and laterally flex the columna vertebralis

Deep layer
Mm. transversospinales
  Mm. rotatores (brevis and longus)
  M. multifidus
  M. semispinalis
Deep segmental group
  Mm. interspinales
  Mm. intertransversarii
  Mm. levatores costarum
	Rami posteriores of nn. spinales	Extend, rotate, and laterally flex the head and columna vertebralis

Muscles of the suboccipital region		
M. rectus capiti posterior major M. rectus capitis posterior minor M. obliquus capitis superior M. obliquus capitis inferior	N. suboccipitalis (C1)	Extend and rotate the head

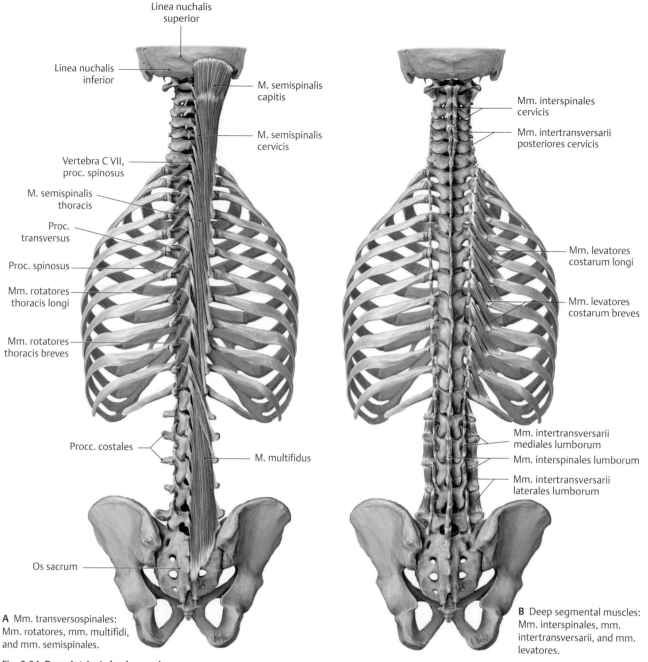

A Mm. transversospinales: Mm. rotatores, mm. multifidi, and mm. semispinales.

B Deep segmental muscles: Mm. interspinales, mm. intertransversarii, and mm. levatores.

Fig. 3.34 Deep intrinsic back muscles
Posterior view. (From Gilroy AM et al. Atlas of Anatomy. 4th ed. 2020. Based on: Schuenke M, Schulte E, Schumacher U. THIEME Atlas of Anatomy. General Anatomy and Musculoskeletal System. Illustrations by Voll M and Wesker K. 3rd ed. New York: Thieme Medical Publishers; 2020.)

- A deep fascia that encloses the intrinsic muscles runs laterally from the posterior midline to the cervical and lumbar transverse processes and to the ribs. This **fascia thoracolumbalis** continues into the neck as the deep layer of the **fascia nuchae**, the posterior extension of the **fascia cervicalis** (see Section 25.2).
- Muscles of the posterior neck occupy the small **suboccipital compartment (Fig. 3.35)** that is inferior to the base of the skull and deep to the m. trapezius and intrinsic back muscles that extend into the neck. The mm. suboccipitales arise from C I or C II and extend upward to insert on the os occipitale or proc. transversus of C I. All assist in the positioning of the head and are innervated by the n. suboccipitalis, the posterior

ramus of C1. They include the **m. rectus capitis posterior major, m. rectus capitis posterior minor, m. obliquus capitis inferior,** and **m. obliquus capitis superior.**
- Aa. intercostales posteriores and aa. lumbales (branches of the aorta descendens and a. subclavia) supply the skin and muscles of the back.
- Vv. intercostales posteriores and vv. lumbales accompany the corresponding arteries to drain muscles of the back. These veins are tributaries of the azygos system, which communicates with both the vertebral venous plexus and the vena cava.
- Rami posteriores of nn. intercostales and nn. lumbales supply the skin and intrinsic muscles of the back **(Figs. 3.36** and **3.37).**

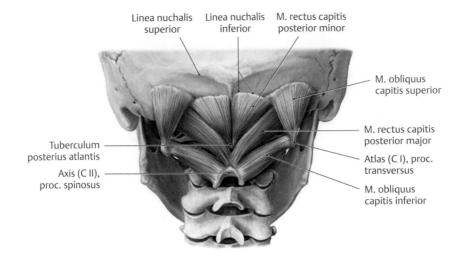

Linea nuchalis superior

Linea nuchalis inferior

M. rectus capitis posterior minor

M. obliquus capitis superior

M. rectus capitis posterior major

Atlas (C I), proc. transversus

M. obliquus capitis inferior

Tuberculum posterius atlantis

Axis (C II), proc. spinosus

Fig. 3.35 Short nuchal and craniovertebral joint muscles
Mm. suboccipitales, posterior view. (From Schuenke M, Schulte E, Schumacher U. THIEME Atlas of Anatomy, Vol 1. Illustrations by Voll M and Wesker K. 3rd ed. New York: Thieme Publishers; 2020.)

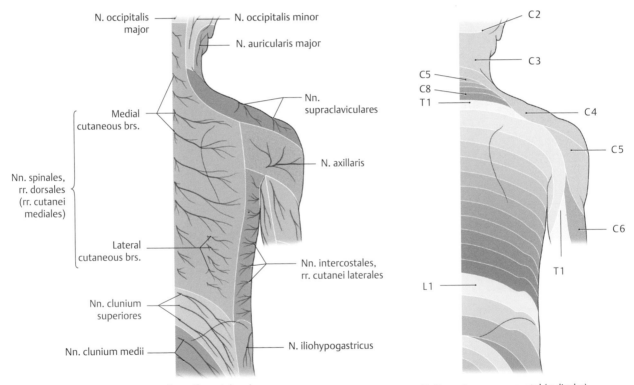

N. occipitalis major

N. occipitalis minor

N. auricularis major

Nn. supraclaviculares

Medial cutaneous brs.

Nn. spinales, rr. dorsales (rr. cutanei mediales)

N. axillaris

Lateral cutaneous brs.

Nn. intercostales, rr. cutanei laterales

Nn. clunium superiores

Nn. clunium medii

N. iliohypogastricus

C2

C3

C5

C8

T1

C4

C5

C6

T1

L1

A Cutaneous innervation patterns of specific peripheral nerves.

B Dermatomes: segmental (radicular) cutaneous innervation of the back. *Note:* Ramus posterior of C1 is purely motor; there is consequently no C1 dermatome.

Fig. 3.36 Cutaneous innervation of the back
(From Gilroy AM et al. Atlas of Anatomy. 4th ed. 2020. Based on: Schuenke M, Schulte E, Schumacher U. THIEME Atlas of Anatomy. General Anatomy and Musculoskeletal System. Illustrations by Voll M and Wesker K. 3rd ed. New York: Thieme Medical Publishers; 2020.)

Oesophagus   Aorta

Ganglion trunci
sympathici

R. communicantes
albus and
r. communicantes
griseus

R. meningeus

R. cutaneus medialis

R. cutaneus
lateralis

Outer layer,
dura mater

Inner layer,
arachnoidea

Radix anterior

Ganglion
sensorium
nervi spinalis

Radix posterior

N. spinalis

R. anterior

R. posterior

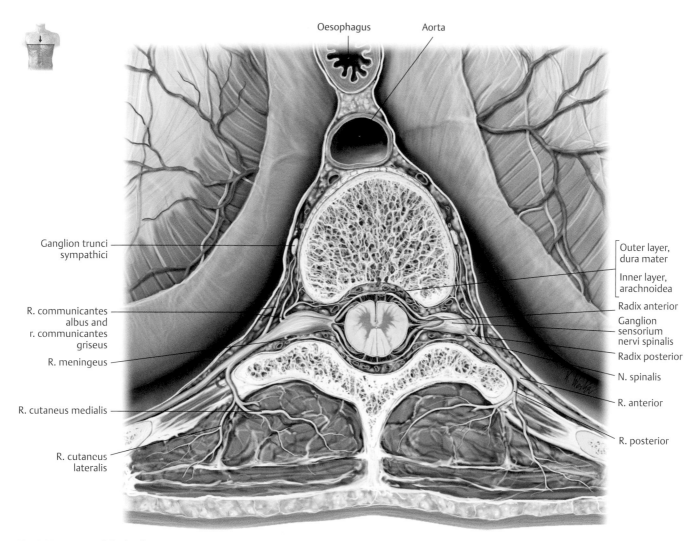

Fig. 3.37 Nerves of the back
Cross section through the columna vertebralis and medulla spinalis with surrounding musculature, superior view. (From Gilroy AM et al. Atlas of
Anatomy. 4th ed. 2020. Based on: Schuenke M, Schulte E, Schumacher U. THIEME Atlas of Anatomy. General Anatomy and Musculoskeletal System.
Illustrations by Voll M and Wesker K. 3rd ed. New York: Thieme Medical Publishers; 2020.)

4 Clinical Imaging Basics of the Spine

Radiographs provide a fast initial assessment of overall alignment of the spine and are often the first imaging study obtained in trauma patients. However, nondisplaced fractures may be invisible on x-ray and only detected with the high resolution and detail of computed tomography (CT). Because x-ray and CT do not show soft tissues well, magnetic resonance imaging (MRI) is used for optimal evaluation of the spinal cord (medulla spinalis), nerve roots, ligaments, and disci intervertebrales (**Table 4.1**). The fully developed adult spine is not suitable for ultrasound analysis as the bones of the vertebrae block the sound waves. In infants, the posterior aspect of the vertebral bodies (corpora vertebrarum) are not yet ossified, allowing for sound transmission into the canalis spinalis from the infant's back (**Fig. 4.1**). This anatomic

consideration, the infant's small size, and the lack of radiation make ultrasound ideal for evaluation of the spinal cord and canalis spinalis in infants in the evaluation of developmental spinal anomalies, such as a tethered cord.

Radiographic examination of the spine should include both frontal and lateral views. This is especially important for assessing alignment. Note that in both views the vertebral bodies appear as rectangles, the result of the "summation shadow" (**Figs. 4.2** and **4.3**). The procc. spinosi and the pedicles of each vertebra, superimposed on the vertebral bodies, are easily seen on the frontal radiographs because of the brightness of the cortical edges. The artt. zygapophysiales are best assessed on the lateral view. CT provides superior details of the bony anatomy and columna vertebralis. Additionally, images can be reconstructed into multiple planes and into three-dimensional images to optimize the evaluation of pathologic conditions (**Fig. 4.4**). MRI is extremely valuable in spine/back imaging. The superior soft tissue detail and contrast are invaluable for evaluation of the spinal cord, nerve roots, intervertebral discs, bone marrow of the vertebral bodies, and surrounding soft tissues (**Figs. 4.5** and **4.6**).

Table 4.1 Suitability of Imaging Modalities for the Back and Spine

Modality	Clinical Notes
Radiographs (x-rays)	Excellent for first-line evaluation of alignment of the columna vertebralis and assessment for fractures in trauma patients; vertebral anatomy is well depicted
CT (computed tomography)	Although important soft structures are not well seen, other anatomic relationships are seen with exceptional detail; more sensitive than radiographs for the evaluation of fractures (especially nondisplaced fractures) and injuries to the posterior structures
MRI (magnetic resonance imaging)	Best for evaluation of the disci intervertebrales, radices nervorum, medulla spinalis, ligaments, and other soft tissues
Ultrasound	Used only in young infants whose columna vertebralis is not fully ossified, allowing for excellent imaging of the infant medulla spinalis

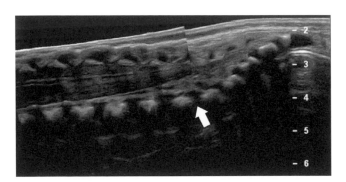

Fig. 4.1 Infant spinal ultrasound
Longitudinal view of a normal lower spine/canalis spinalis in an infant. Note the two successive images are "stitched" together at the L V–S I level (*arrow*) to create this panoramic view. The probe is placed on the lower back of the infant and oriented as to center the canalis spinalis. (From Beek E, Van Rijn R, ed. Diagnostic Pediatric Ultrasound. 1st ed. New York: Thieme; 2015)

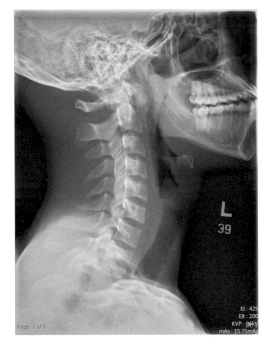

Fig. 4.2 Radiograph of the cervical spine
Left lateral view.
In a normal radiograph of the spine, the vertebral bodies (corpora vertebrarum) appear roughly rectangular in shape and the corners of each vertebral body line up with the corners of the vertebral body above and below it. The spaces of disci intervertebrales are uniform from level to level and the proc. spinosus of each vertebra is easily identified. (Courtesy of Joseph Makris, MD, Baystate Medical Center.)

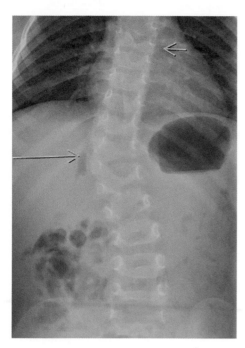

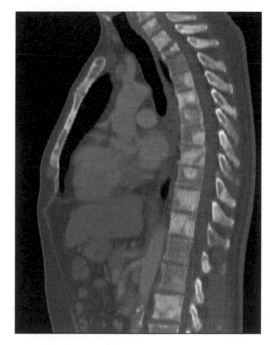

Fig. 4.3   Frontal view of the lower thoracic and lumbar spine in an infant
The inferior ribs can be seen articulating with lower vertebrae thoracicae; the lower-most vertebral body (corpus vertebrae) with an adjacent rib is T XII. Note the abnormal shape of the corpus vertebrae T XII and that there are two pedicles on its right side (*long arrow*). Also note the abnormal shape of the corpus vertebrae T VII (*short arrow*) with a central vertical cleft—this a "butterfly" vertebra. Vertebral bodies should be rectangular, and each should have a small rounded pedicle visible on each side (small white circles due to the cortical bone). (Courtesy of Joseph Makris, MD, Baystate Medical Center.)

Fig. 4.4   CT reconstruction of the spine
Midsagittal section.
This midsagittal section represents a single slice of a digitally reconstructed CT scan. This image is a single slice of the midline that was digitally "reconstructed" in the sagittal plane from the original CT images. The spine is easier to evaluate in this plane because the relationships between vertebrae are better depicted. This image is presented in the "bone window," which is best for evaluating the osseous structures. The multiple densities (whiter spots) throughout many of the vertebral bodies (corpora vertebrarum) are metastatic lesions from prostate cancer, referred to as sclerotic or blastic lesions because there is increased bone at the metastatic focus. Although these may be visible on an x-ray of the spine, they are more obvious with CT. As with radiographs, the edges of each vertebral body should line up with the edges of the vertebral body above and below. (From Gunderman R. Essential Radiology, 3rd ed. New York: Thieme; 2014.)

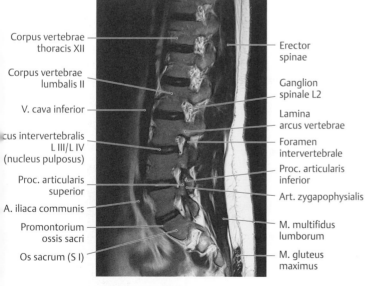

Corpus vertebrae thoracis XII
Corpus vertebrae lumbalis II
V. cava inferior
cus intervertebralis L III/L IV (nucleus pulposus)
Proc. articularis superior
A. iliaca communis
Promontorium ossis sacri
Os sacrum (S I)

Erector spinae
Ganglion spinale L2
Lamina arcus vertebrae
Foramen intervertebrale
Proc. articularis inferior
Art. zygapophysialis
M. multifidus lumborum
M. gluteus maximus

Fig. 4.5   MRI of the lumbar spine
Parasagittal section through the lateral edges of the vertebral bodies (corpora vertebrarum) and the foramina intervertebralia. Left lateral view. (*Fat = white, muscles = black, nerve roots = light gray, bone = dark gray.*) This image demonstrates MRI's superior ability to show soft tissues, an advantage over radiographs and CT. The foramina intervertebralia are clearly visualized with the dark nerve roots surrounded by fat within the foramina intervertebralia. If this patient had a disk herniation, the disk tissue would be clearly visible intruding into the canalis spinalis. Note the white nucleus pulposus in the middle of the disci intervertebrales. (From Moeller TB, Reif E. Pocket Atlas of Sectional Anatomy, Vol 3, 2nd ed. New York: Thieme; 2017.)

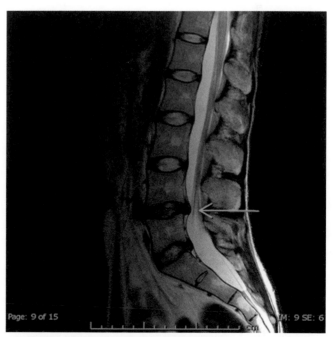

Fig. 4.6   MRI of the lumbar spine, herniated disc
Sagittal section through the mid-lumbar spine showing protrusion of the disci intervertebrales into the canalis spinalis, most pronounced at the L IV/L V level. (Courtesy of Joseph Makris, MD, Baystate Medical Center.)

Unit II Review Questions: Back

1. During the surgical repair of an aortic aneurysm in a 62-year-old patient, the left T10 intercostal artery that supplied the a. radicularis magna (of Adamkiewicz) was inadvertently ligated. A likely consequence of this would be a disruption of the blood supply to
   A. the cervical enlargement of the spinal cord (medulla spinalis)
   B. the lumbosacral enlargement of the spinal cord
   C. the lower vertebrae thoracicae
   D. the deep intrinsic muscles of the back
   E. the posterior one third of the spinal cord

2. A 57-year-old woman who runs a 4-mile route three times a week complained to her primary care physician of low back pain and an irritating paresthesia (tingling) along the inner aspect of her right leg. Electromyographic studies identified a lesion of her n. spinalis L4 on the right side.
   The n. spinalis L4
   A. carries only sensory fibers
   B. contributes to both the plexus lumbalis and plexus sacralis
   C. contains sympathetic nerve fibers that innervate pelvic viscera
   D. exits the foramen intervertebrale between the L III and L IV vertebrae
   E. innervates intrinsic muscles and skin of the back via its r. anterior

3. The filum terminale is best described as
   A. an extension of the arachnoidea that connects to the pia mater
   B. a transverse ligament that suspends the spinal cord within the dural sac
   C. an extension of the pia mater that descends within the cisterna lumbalis
   D. a ligament that connects the procc. spinosi of the vertebrae
   E. an extension of the pia mater that anchors the conus medullaris to the L II vertebra

4. The nerves that descend within the cisterna lumbalis of the dural sac are called
   A. plexus lumbalis
   B. plexus sacralis
   C. cauda equina
   D. rr. posteriores
   E. sacral spinal nerves

5. An 87-year-old man sees his primary care physician with a complaint of mental confusion and back pain. Although the physician considers that these symptoms may be a normal consequence of the patient's age, examination reveals that the patient has advanced prostate cancer that has spread to his brain and columna vertebralis. The probable route of metastasis is identified as the vertebral venous plexus, which
   A. drains the vertebrae and disci intervertebrales but does not drain the spinal cord
   B. lies within the spatium subarachnoidale
   C. consists of veins with multiple valves along their length
   D. consists of paired longitudinal veins within the canalis vertebralis
   E. is a valveless system of veins

6. A 47-year-old construction worker presented to his physician with debilitating pain in his lower back and lower limb. Radiographic studies showed a herniated discus intervertebralis at the L IV–L V vertebral level. Which of the following is true?
   A. The herniated disk most likely signals a weakness of the lig. longitudinale anterius.
   B. A posterior herniation of this disk could result in compression of the adjacent spinal cord.
   C. Pain from this hernia would most likely be felt along the L4 dermatome.
   D. The herniation is the result of a loss of elasticity of the anulus fibrosus, which allowed protrusion of the nucleus pulposus.
   E. None of the above

7. The splenius muscle group
   A. lies deep to the m. trapezius
   B. is enclosed by the fascia thoracolumbalis
   C. extends the cervical spine and head
   D. is innervated by rr. posteriores of cervical nn. spinales
   E. All of the above

8. A 92-year-old woman remains mentally alert and physically active but has lost several inches in height, and her posture is stooped forward. Her geriatrician explains that this exaggerated curvature is due to degeneration of the bodies of two of her vertebrae thoracicae that often occurs in older women as a result of decreased bone density. The curvature exhibited by this patient is known as
   A. scoliosis
   B. spondylolysis
   C. lordosis
   D. kyphosis
   E. spondylosis

9. The spinal cord terminates caudally as the
   A. lig. denticulatum
   B. filum terminale
   C. conus medullaris
   D. cisterna lumbalis
   E. hiatus sacralis

10. Which of the following ligaments would prevent hyperextension of the vertebral column?
    A. Lig. longitudinale anterius
    B. Lig. longitudinale posterius
    C. Ligamentum flavum
    D. Lig. alare
    E. Lig. cruciforme

11. Which of the following vertebral characteristics is paired with the correct vertebral region?
    A. Promontorium—sacral
    B. Vertebra prominens—thoracic
    C. Dens—thoracic
    D. Foramen transversarium—lumbar
    E. Fovea costalis—cervical

12. Parasympathetic stimulation is responsible for responses such as contraction of the pupil of the eye, slowing of the heart rate, and erection of the penis in the male. Which of the following statements accurately describes characteristics of the parasympathetic system?
    A. Preganglionic fibers synapse in large sacral ganglia spinalia.
    B. Nn. splanchnici pelvici are parasympathetic nerves that arise from levels S2–S4 to innervate viscera of the pelvis.
    C. Preganglionic fibers that arise from the brain travel with nn. craniales III, IV, V, and X.
    D. Parasympathetic nerves in the skin innervate smooth muscle responsible for constriction of blood vessels.
    E. Nociceptive (pain) fibers travel only with nerves of the sacral component of the parasympathetic system.

13. During the last month of her pregnancy, Janice confided to her obstetrician that she was very anxious about motherhood and was particularly concerned about the pain that she knew accompanied the delivery. Her physician suggested she undergo a procedure that would provide a degree of anesthesia to lessen the discomfort. Her recommendation most likely involved
    A. an injection of anesthetic into the spatium epidurale
    B. a lumbar puncture
    C. an injection for spinal anesthesia at the T XII–L I level
    D. an extraction of liquor cerebrospinalis from the spatium subarachnoidale
    E. an extraction of liquor cerebrospinalis from the cisterna lumbalis

14. The evaluation of reflexes is part of most standard physical exams. It measures the integrity of the nerve supply to muscles. A reflex, such as the patellar reflex, involves all of the following except:
    A. primarily autonomic nerves that arise from the truncus sympathicus
    B. a sensory (afferent) and a motor (efferent) limb that are located within a single spinal cord segment
    C. only monosegmentally innervated muscles
    D. only skeletal muscles
    E. nerves that likely arise from a somatic nerve plexus

15. Valerie is an active 55-year-old executive who has recently experienced some pain and "cracking" in her neck. Although she can relieve the pain with ibuprofen, she's noticed that the rotation of her head from side to side is a bit more limited than previously. During her yearly physical, an x-ray of her cervical spine showed a slight loss of bone density and the formation of osteophytes. Her physician explained that this was a common result of aging and recommended continued use of mild pain relievers and regular exercise. Which of the following best describes her condition?
    A. a fracture of the dens of her vertebra cervicalis II
    B. spondylolisthesis
    C. spondylosis
    D. spondylolysis
    E. increased laxity of the cervical spine

16. Which statement correctly distinguishes between a dermatome and a myotome?
    A. A dermatome carries only sensory fibers; a myotome carries only motor fibers.
    B. Dermatomes are composed of somatic muscle fibers; myotomes are composed of smooth muscle.
    C. Sensory nerves of dermatomes transmit sensation of pain, pressure, and temperature; sensory nerves of myotomes carry sensation of proprioception (sense of position).
    D. Each dermatome is innervated by a pair of nn. spinales from a single spinal cord segment; each myotome is innervated by a pair of nn. spinales from multiple spinal cord segments.
    E. Lesions of a single spinal root would have a major impact on the corresponding dermatome; it would have minimal effect on the corresponding myotome.

17. A 45-year-old man has severe back pain and pain radiating down his left leg (sciatica). Your physical exam reveals relative weakness and decreased sensation on the left side. Which imaging modality would be best suited for evaluating your suspicion that the patient has a herniated discus intervertebralis?
    A. MRI
    B. CT
    C. Ultrasound
    D. Radiography (x-ray)

18. A teenager is complaining of neck pain after being in a motor vehicle accident. He is otherwise doing well. The cervical spine has been stabilized by a collar by the EMTs on the scene. Which imaging modality would you choose as a first-line assessment of the cervical spine?
    A. MRI
    B. CT
    C. Ultrasound
    D. Radiography (x-ray)

Answers and Explanations

1. **B.** The a. radicularis magna (of Adamkiewicz) supplies the inferior two thirds of the spinal cord, which includes the region of the lumbosacral enlargement (T11–S1) (Section 3.2).

    A. The a. radicularis magna (of Adamkiewicz) supplies the inferior two thirds of the spinal cord, which does not include the region of the cervical enlargement (C4–T1).

    C. Vertebrae are supplied by segmental arteries of the aorta descendens, as well as by branches of the a. subclavia and arteries of the pelvis.

    D. Intrinsic muscles of the back get their blood supply from posterior branches of the aa. intercostales and aa. lumbales.

    E. The aa. spinales posteriores that usually arise from the aa. vertebrales in the neck supply the posterior third of the spinal cord.

2. **B.** The plexus lumbalis includes rr. anteriores of nn. spinales L1–L4, and the plexus sacralis includes rr. anteriores of nn. spinales L4–S4 (Section 3.3).
   A. All nn. spinales carry both sensory and motor fibers
   C. Sympathetic fibers are carried only in nn. spinales between T1 and L2.
   D. Except for nerves in the cervical region, nn. spinales exit below the vertebra of the corresponding number; thus, L4 exits between the L IV and L V vertebrae.
   E. Intrinsic muscles and skin of the back are innervated by rr. posteriores of nn. spinales.

3. **C.** The filum terminale is a filament of pia mater that runs within the cisterna lumbalis with the cauda equina, from the conus medullaris to the end of the dural sac. Inferior to the dural sac, it is surrounded by spinal dura mater and extends to the os coccygis (Section 3.2).
   A. The trabeculae arachnoideae connect the arachnoidea to the pia mater.
   B. Ligg. denticulata suspend the spinal cord within the dural sac.
   D. The lig. supraspinale connects the procc. spinosi of all thoracic, lumbar, and sacral vertebrae. In the cervical region it expands as the lig. nuchae, a finlike ligament that attaches superiorly to the os occipitale.
   E. The end of the spinal cord, the conus medullaris, lies adjacent to the L II vertebra but is not attached to it.

4. **C.** Because the spinal cord is shorter than the columna vertebralis, nn. spinales L2–Co1 descend as a group (cauda equina) within the dural sac before exiting at the appropriate foramen intervertebrale (Section 3.3).
   A. The plexus lumbalis forms outside the canalis vertebralis on the posterior abdominal wall and contains only rr. anteriores of lumbar nn. spinales (L1–L4).
   B. The plexus sacralis forms outside the canalis vertebralis on the posterior wall of the pelvis and contains only rr. anteriores of nn. spinales L4–S4.
   D. The nerves of the cauda equina are nn. spinales, which contain both rr. anteriores and rr. posteriores.
   E. The cauda equina contains both lumbar and sacral nn. spinales.

5. **E.** The vertebral venous plexus is a valveless system that allows communication between the caval and azygos systems, which drain the trunk, and the venous sinuses of the brain (Section 3.1).
   A. The vertebral venous plexus drains the vertebrae, meninges, and spinal cord.
   B. The internal vertebral venous plexus lies in the spatium epidurale. The external plexus surrounds the outside of the vertebral column.
   C. The vertebral venous plexus is a valveless system that allows communication between the caval and azygos systems, which drain the trunk, and the venous sinuses of the brain.
   D. The venous plexus consists of interconnecting veins that form an internal plexus within the canalis vertebralis and an external plexus that surrounds the vertebrae.

6. **D.** Loss in elasticity of the anulus fibrosus, which may occur with aging, allows herniation of the nucleus pulposus (Section 3.1).

A. The lig. longitudinale anterius supports the vertebral bodies and disks anteriorly. The lig. longitudinale posterius supports the disks posteriorly where herniation normally occurs.
   B. The spinal cord ends at L II and is not present in this part of the canalis vertebralis.
   C. The n. spinalis L4 exits the foramen intervertebrale superior to the discus intervertebralis and is usually unaffected by the herniation. The hernia would compress the next inferior n. spinalis, L5, and pain would be felt along that dermatome.
   E. Not applicable

7. **E.** All of the above (Section 3.4)
   A. The mm. splenii are superficial intrinsic back muscles that lie deep to the m. trapezius, an extrinsic muscle of the upper back. B through D are also correct (E).
   B. All intrinsic back muscles, including the splenius group, are enclosed by the deep fascia of the back, the fascia thoracolumbalis. A, C, and D are also correct (E).
   C. Mm. splenii extend the cervical spine and head when working bilaterally. Unilaterally, they flex and rotate the head to the same side. A, B, and D are also correct (E).
   D. The mm. splenii are innervated by the rr. posteriores of nn. spinales C1–C6. A through C are also correct (E).

8. **D.** Kyphosis is an abnormal posterior curvature of the thoracic spine often seen in older women (Section 3.1).
   A. Scoliosis is a lateral curvature of the spine.
   B. Spondylolysis refers to a fracture or defect across the interarticular part of the lamina of the lumbar vertebrae.
   C. Lordosis is an exaggerated anterior curvature of the lumbar spine often seen in pregnant women.
   E. Spondylosis is a degeneration of the discus intervertebralis and corresponding vertebral body that results in osteophyte formation.

9. **C.** The spinal cord terminates caudally as the conus medullaris. This usually corresponds to the L I–L II vertebral level in an adult (Section 3.2).
   A. Ligg. denticulata are transverse extensions of the pia mater that attach to dura mater and suspend the spinal cord within the dural sac.
   B. Pia mater terminates caudally as the filum terminale.
   D. The cisterna lumbalis is part of the spatium subarachnoidale that lies between the conus medullaris and the inferior end of the dural sac.
   E. The hiatus sacralis is the inferior opening of the canalis sacralis, which is a continuation of the canalis vertebralis.

10. **A.** The lig. longitudinale anterius attaches the anterior and lateral surfaces of the vertebral bodies and disci intervertebrales and prevents hyperextension (Section 3.1).
   B. The lig. longitudinale posterius attaches primarily to the disci intervertebrales and produces weak resistance to hyperflexion.
   C. The ligg. flava join the laminae of adjacent vertebrae. They limit flexion and provide postural support of the columna vertebralis.
   D. The ligg. alaria secure the dens of C II to the skull.
   E. The lig. cruciforme, formed by longitudinal fibers and a lig. transversum, secure the dens against the arcus anterior atlantis.

11. **A.** The anterior lip of S1 forms the promontorium of the os sacrum (Section 3.1).
     B. The vertebral prominens is the vertebra C VII, named for its long palpable proc. spinosus.
     C. Only the vertebra C II has a dens, the peg-like process that articulates with C I.
     D. Only vertebrae cervicales have foramina transversaria.
     E. Only vertebrae thoracicae have foveae costales where they articulate with the ribs.

12. **B.** Nn. splanchnici pelvici (S2–S4) form the parasympathetic component of the autonomic plexuses that innervate pelvic viscera (Section 3.3).
     A. Preganglionic nerves synapse in small ganglia near, or within, their target organ.
     C. Only nn. craniales III, VII, IX, and X carry parasympathetic nerves.
     D. Vasoconstriction occurs through sympathetic stimulation. Blood vessels receive no parasympathetic innervation.
     E. Nociceptive fibers travel with both cranial and sacral parts of the parasympathetic system, as well as with sympathetic nn. splanchnici.

13. **A.** Epidural anesthesia, often used during delivery, involves an injection of anesthetic into the spatium epidurale (Section 3.2).
     B. Lumbar puncture is used to extract liquor cerebrospinalis and does not involve injection of anesthetic.
     C. Injections into the canalis spinalis should be performed inferior to L II, below the level of the conus medullaris in order to avoid damage to the spinal cord.
     D and **E.** Anesthesia of the relevant nn. spinales requires an injection of anesthetic, not the extraction of liquor cerebrospinalis.

14. **A.** Autonomic nerves innervate only involuntary muscle and are not involved in reflexes (Section 3.3).
     B. An intact reflex involves both sensory and motor limbs that are mediated at the spinal cord level.
     C. Both the sensory and motor limbs of the reflex are located within a single segment of the spinal cord.
     D. Only skeletal muscles are involved in reflexes. Smooth or cardiac muscles are innervated by autonomic nerves and not involved in reflexes.
     E. Reflexes are conducted by somatic nerves, which most often (except nn. intercostales) form somatic nerve plexuses.

15. **C.** Spondylosis is an age-related condition characterized by loss of bone density and the formation of osteophytes (Section 3.1).
     A. Only a traumatic incident, such the violent "whiplash" resulting from a car accident, normally results in the fracture of the dens.
     B. Spondylolisthesis describes a condition in which a vertebral body is displaced anteriorly relative to the vertebral body below it.
     C. Spondylolysis describes a fracture of one or both lamina of the vertebra. When bilateral, it may result in spondylolisthesis.

     E. Increased laxity of the cervical spine makes the spine more prone to injury but is not a result of aging or cause of bone loss and osteocyte formation.

16. **A.** A dermatome is a band of skin, which is innervated by a sensory nerve from a single spinal cord segment. A myotome refers to the muscle mass that's innervated by a motor nerve from a single spinal cord segment (Section 3.3).
     B. Dermatomes are bands of skin; myotomes refer to a group of skeletal (somatic) muscle fibers.
     C. Sensory nerves of dermatomes transmit sensations of pain, pressure, temperature, and proprioception; myotomes are groups of muscle fibers innervated by motor nerves, which do not transmit sensory information.
     D. Both dermatomes and myotomes are innervated by nerves from a single spinal cord segment.
     E. Because of the considerable overlap among dermatomes, the loss of a single spinal nerve root would have minimal impact on sensation in that dermatome.

17. **A.** MRI is best for evaluation of the disci intervertebrales, radices nervorum, canalis spinalis, and surrounding soft tissues. In this case, MRI would show the herniated portion of the discus intervertebralis extending into the foramen intervertebrale and impinging on the exiting radix nervi.
     B. CT is highly sensitive for fractures and malalignment of the spine but does not have sufficient soft tissue contrast to reliably diagnose nerve root, spinal cord, and disk pathology.
     C. Ultrasound has no role in the evaluation of the adult spine. Unlike in infants, the adult trunk is too large and the adult columna vertebralis is too ossified to allow for an adequate sonographic window.
     D. Radiography is best for evaluating overall spinal alignment and for displaced fractures but would not be helpful in identifying disk or other soft tissue pathology.

18. **D.** Radiographs would be the best choice here as they provide excellent evaluation of spinal alignment, are good for screening for fractures, and can be obtained quickly. If the x-ray is normal, you could then "clear" the cervical spine by a thorough physical examination of the neck after removing the collar.
     A. MRI would be reserved for evaluating a patient with an abnormal physical exam or if the pain is persistent, or if physical exam cannot be reliably performed (unconscious).
     B. Although CT is more sensitive for fractures and subtle malalignment, its use would be reserved for cases where the radiographs are abnormal or suboptimal in quality (e.g., very large patients), especially in children to reduce overall radiation exposure. CT is also often used in unconscious patients who cannot have a reliable physical examination.
     C. Ultrasound has no role in the evaluation of spinal trauma.

Unit III   Thorax

5 Overview of the Thorax

The thorax is the region of the trunk between the neck and abdomen. The throacic cavity (cavitas thoracis), surrounded by a bony cage that protects the thoracic contents, is open to the neck through the superior thoracic aperture (apertura thoracis superior) but separated from the abdomen at the inferior thoracic aperture (apertura thoracis inferior) by a muscular diaphragma. The viscera of the thorax include the primary organs of the respiratory and cardiovascular systems, as well as components of the gastrointestinal, endocrine, and lymphatic systems.

5.1 General Features

— The thorax is divided into two lateral compartments, the **cavitas pleuralis dextra** and **sinistra**, which contain the lungs and pleural sac, and a central compartment, the **mediastinum**, which contains the heart (cor), pericardial sac, trachea and bronchi, oesophagus, thymus, and neurovasculature **(Fig. 5.1; Table 5.1)**.
— **A pericardial sac** surrounds the heart, and a **pleural sac** surrounds each lung (pulmo). These closed membranous sacs contain a thin layer of serous fluid that ensures frictionless movement, which is crucial to the function of these organs.

— The lungs (pulmones) are the organs of respiration. They communicate with the **tracheobronchial tree** (the passages for air between the lungs and outside environment) and the heart through the **hilum pulmonis,** an indentation on the medial surface of each lung.
— The heart is a four-chambered muscular organ that functions as a dual pump that propels blood through the body. Each pump is made up of two chambers: a thin-walled **atrium** and a thick-walled **ventriculus.**
— During a cardiac cycle, the right pump receives deoxygenated blood from the **systemic circulation** (circulation of blood through all regions of the body except the lungs) and directs it to the **pulmonary circulation** in the lungs. The left pump receives oxygenated blood from the pulmonary circulation and returns it to the systemic circulation for the distribution of oxygen and nutrients **(Fig. 5.2)**.
— Coordinated contraction of atria and ventriculi, known as the **cardiac cycle,** is self-moderated by specialized tissue within the cardiac muscle that makes up the cardiac **conduction system.**

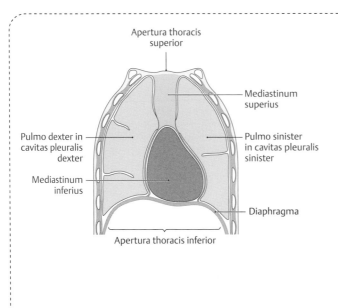

Table 5.1 Major Structures of the Cavitas Thoracis
(From Gilroy AM, MacPherson BR, Wikenheiser JC. Atlas of Anatomy. Illustrations by Voll M and Wesker K. 4th ed. New York: Thieme Publishers; 2020.)

Mediastinum	Mediastinum superius		Thymus, great vessels, trachea, oesophagus, and ductus thoracicus
	Mediastinum inferius	Mediastinum anterius	Thymus
		Mediastinum medium	Cor, pericardium, and roots of great vessels
		Mediastinum posterius	Aorta thoracica, ductus thoracicus, oesophagus, and azygos venous system
Cavitates pleurales	Cavitas pleuralis dexter		Pulmo dexter, pleura
	Cavitas pleuralis sinister		Pulmo sinister, pleura

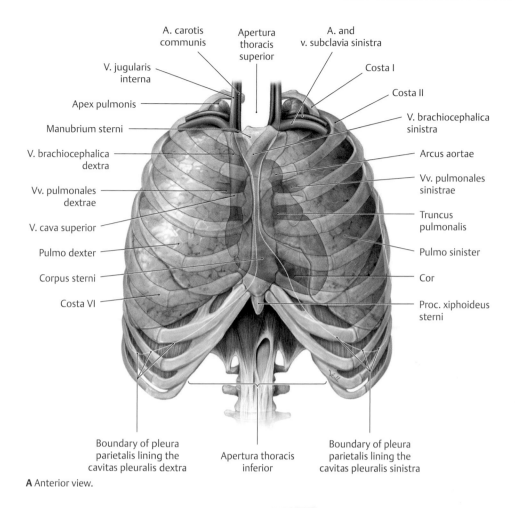

A Anterior view.

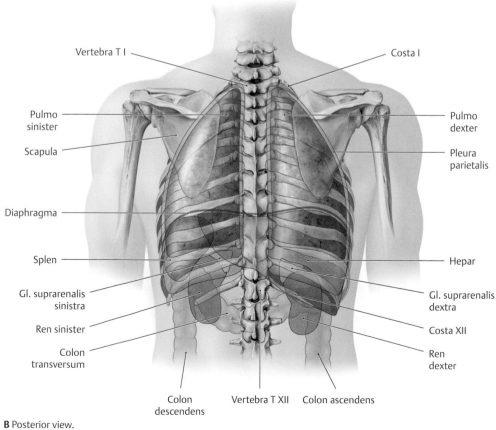

B Posterior view.

Fig. 5.1 Overview of the thorax
(From Schuenke M, Schulte E, Schumacher U. THIEME Atlas of Anatomy, Vol 2. Illustrations by Voll M and Wesker K. 3rd ed. New York: Thieme Publishers; 2020.)

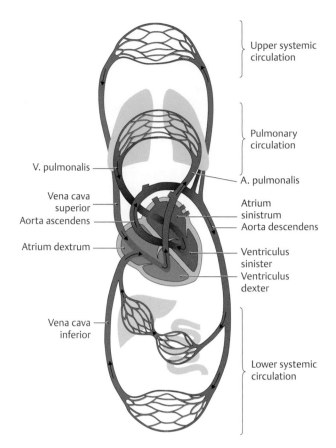

Upper systemic circulation

Pulmonary circulation

V. pulmonalis

A. pulmonalis

Vena cava superior

Aorta ascendens

Atrium dextrum

Atrium sinistrum

Aorta descendens

Ventriculus sinister

Ventriculus dexter

Vena cava inferior

Lower systemic circulation

Fig. 5.2 Systemic and pulmonary circulation
Red, oxygenated blood; *blue,* deoxygenated blood. (From Schuenke M, Schulte E, Schumacher U. THIEME Atlas of Anatomy, Vol 1. Illustrations by Voll M and Wesker K. 3rd ed. New York: Thieme Publishers; 2020.)

5.2   Neurovasculature of the Thorax

The "great vessels," which include the aa. pulmonales, the vv. pulmonales, the aorta, the v. cava superior, and the v. cava inferior, direct blood into and out of the heart and lungs. Their branches and further details of their anatomy, along with more detailed descriptions of lymphatic drainage and nerves of the thorax, are discussed in Chapters 7 and 8 on the mediastinum and pulmonary cavities.

Arteries of the Thorax

— The **truncus pulmonalis** directs deoxygenated blood from the right side of the heart into the pulmonary circulation. It arises from the ventriculus dexter on the anterior surface of the heart, passes superiorly and posteriorly, and, under the arcus aortae, divides into **a. pulmonalis dextra** and **a. pulmonalis sinistra (Fig. 5.3).**
— One a. pulmonalis enters each lung, where it branches into generations of smaller vessels that accompany the respi-

ratory passages. The aa. pulmonales transport deoxygenated blood to the small respiratory units in the lungs.
— The **aorta thoracica** arises from the left side of the heart and carries oxygenated blood that is distributed to the systemic circulation. It is divided into three sections **(Fig. 5.4):**
  • The **aorta ascendens** arises from the ventriculus sinister of the heart and ascends to the level of the vertebra T IV. The a. coronaria dextra and a. coronaria sinistra are its only branches.
  • The **arcus aortae** (radiographically, the "aortic knob") ascends anterior to the a. pulmonis dextra and the bifurcatio tracheae (where the trachea splits into the bronchus dexter and bronchus sinister). It courses posteriorly and to the left, arching over the structures entering the left lung, and then turns inferiorly to descend to the left of the trachea and oesophagus. It terminates on the left side of the corpus vertebrae T IV. Three large branches arise from the arch:
    ○ The **truncus brachiocephalicus,** which ascends posterior to the art. sternoclavicularis dextra, where it bifurcates into the **a. carotis communis dextra** and **a. subclavia dextra.**
    ○ The **a. carotis communis sinistra,** which enters the neck posterior to the art. sternoclavicularis sinistra.
    ○ The **a. subclavian sinistra,** which arises from the distal segment of the arch and enters the neck posterior to the art. sternoclavicularis sinistra.
  • The **aorta descendens,** a continuation of the arcus aortae, descends within the mediastinum posterius, where it passes posterior to the root of the left lung and anterior and to the left of the thoracic vertebral bodies. It passes into the abdomen through the diaphragma at T XII. Its thoracic branches **(Fig. 5.5; Table 5.2)** are
    ○ the 3rd through 11th **aa. intercostales posteriores** (the 1st and 2nd arise from a. subclavia), which run anteriorly within the corresponding intercostal spaces (between the ribs), where they anastomose with the rr. intercostales anteriores; and
    ○ the visceral branches to the oesophagus, trachea, bronchi, and pericardium.
— The **aa. thoracicae internae** arise from the aa. subclavia in the neck and descend deep to the ribs on either side of the sternum. Their branches, which supply the thoracic and abdominal walls include **(Fig. 5.6):**
  • the **rr. intercostales anteriores,** which run within the spatia intercostalia;
  • the **aa. musculophrenicae,** terminal branches of the aa. thoracicae internae, which arise at the level of the sixth cartilago costalis and follows the lower margin of the rib cage laterally; and
  • the **aa. epigastricae superiores,** terminal branches of the aa. thoracicae internae, which run inferiorly to supply muscles of the anterior abdominal wall.

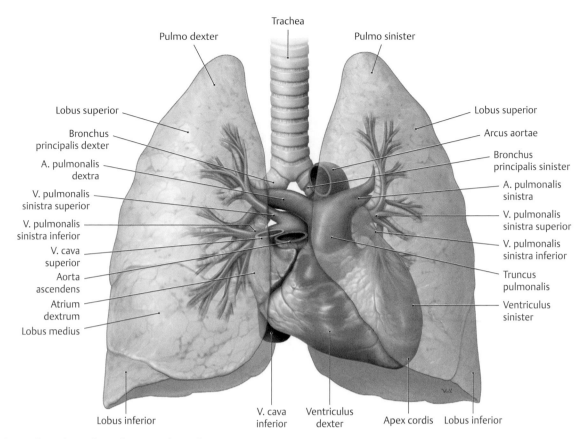

Fig. 5.3 **Arteriae pulmonales and venae pulmonales**
Distribution of the a. pulmonales and v. pulmonales, anterior view. (From Schuenke M, Schulte E, Schumacher U. THIEME Atlas of Anatomy, Vol 2. Illustrations by Voll M and Wesker K. 3rd ed. New York: Thieme Publishers; 2020.)

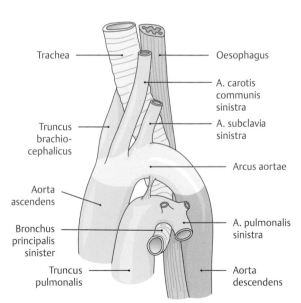

A Parts of the arcus aortae, left lateral view. *Note:* The arcus aortae begins and ends at the level of the angulus sterni (T4–T5). (From Gilroy AM et al. Atlas of Anatomy. 4th ed. 2020. Based on: Schuenke M, Schulte E, Schumacher U. THIEME Atlas of Anatomy. Internal Organs. Illustrations by Voll M and Wesker K. 3rd ed. New York: Thieme Medical Publishers; 2020.)

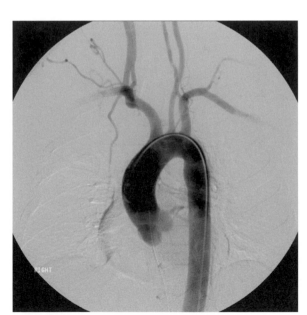

B Digital subtraction angiogram of the arcus aortae. (From Gunderman R. Essential Radiology, 3rd ed. New York: Thieme; 2014)

Fig. 5.4 **Aorta thoracica**

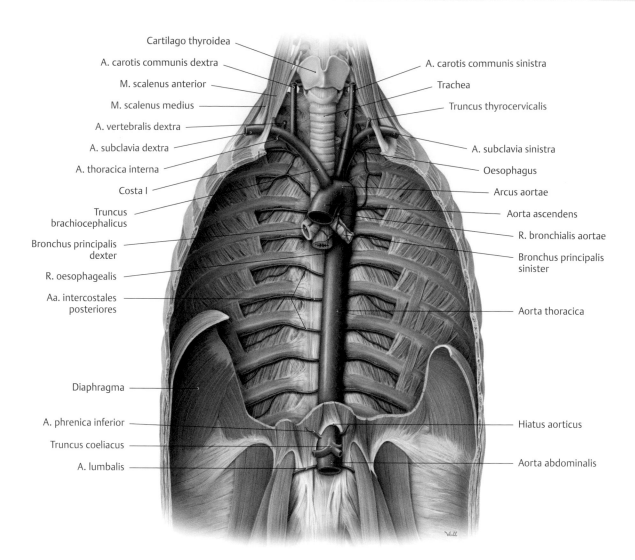

Fig. 5.5 Aorta thoracica in situ, anterior view
Removed: Cor, pulmones, and portions of the diaphragma. (From Gilroy AM et al. Atlas of Anatomy. 4th ed. 2020. Based on: Schuenke M, Schulte E, Schumacher U. THIEME Atlas of Anatomy. Internal Organs. Illustrations by Voll M and Wesker K. 3rd ed. New York: Thieme Medical Publishers; 2020.)

Table 5.2 Branches of the Aorta Thoracica

The thoracic organs are supplied by direct branches from the aorta thoracica, as well as indirect branches from the aa. subclaviae.

Part of aorta	Branches			Region supplied
Aorta ascendens	A. coronaria dextra, a. coronaria sinistra			Cor, bronchi, trachea, oesophagus
Arcus aortae	Truncus brachiocephalicus	A. subclavia dextra	(See a. subclavia sinistra for complementary branches and regions supplied)	
		A. carotis communis dextra		Cor and neck
	A. carotis communis sinistra			
	A. subclavia sinistra	A. vertebralis		
		A. thoracica interna	Rr. intercostales anteriores	Anterior chest wall
			Rr. thymici	Thymus
			Rr. mediastinales	Mediastinum posterior
			A. pericardiacophrenica	Pericardium, diaphragma
		Truncus thyrocervicalis	A. thyroidea inferior	Oesophagus, trachea, gl. thyroidea
		Truncus costocervicalis	A. intercostalis superior	Chest wall
Aorta descendens	Visceral brs.			Bronchi, trachea, oesophagus
	Parietal brs.		Aa. intercostales posteriores	Posterior chest wall
			Aa. phrenicae superiores	Diaphragma

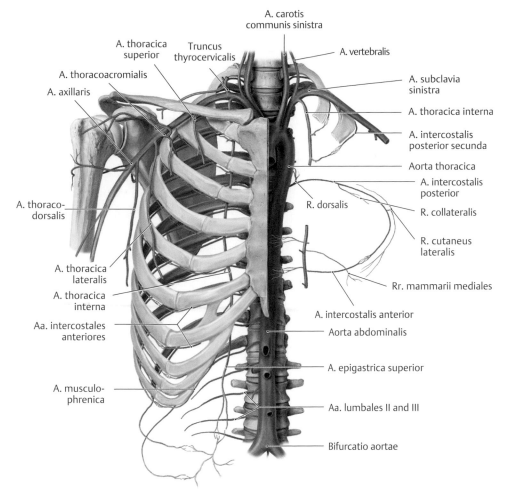

Fig. 5.6 Arteries of the thoracic wall
Anterior view. (From Gilroy AM et al. Atlas of Anatomy. 4th ed. 2020. Based on: Schuenke M, Schulte E, Schumacher U. THIEME Atlas of Anatomy. General Anatomy and Musculoskeletal System. Illustrations by Voll M and Wesker K. 3rd ed. New York: Thieme Medical Publishers; 2020.)

Veins of the Thorax (Fig. 5.7)

— **Vv. thoracicae internae,** which receive the vv. intercostales anteriores, accompany the aa. thoracicae internae and drain into the vv. brachiocephalicae of the mediastinum superius.
— The **vv. brachiocephalica dextra** and **sinistra,** which drain the head, neck, and upper limb, form behind the clavicula by the convergence of the v. jugularis interna and v. subclavia. The v. brachiocephalica sinistra, which is longer than the v. brachiocephalica dextra, crosses the midline just anterior to the branches of the arcus aortae and converges with the v. brachiocephalica dextra to form the v. cava superior.
— The **v. cava superior,** which returns deoxygenated blood from the upper body to the heart, forms on the right side, posterior to the cartilago costalis of the first rib by the junction of the vv. brachiocephalicae. It descends behind and to the right side of the aorta and drains into the superior pole of the atrium dextrum.
— The **v. cava inferior,** which returns deoxygenated blood to the heart from the abdomen, pelvis, and lower limbs, enters the atrium dextrum after passing through the diaphragma from the abdomen. Only a small portion, therefore, is located within the thorax.

— The **vv. pulmonales,** two on each side (often three on the left side), carry oxygenated blood from the lungs to the left side of the heart (see **Fig. 5.3**).
— The **azygos system** drains veins of the thoracic and antero-lateral abdominal walls (**Figs. 5.7** and **5.8**).
  • The **v. azygos** ascends along the right side of the thoracic vertebral bodies as it drains the **vv. intercostales posteriores** of the thoracic wall on that side. It arches over the root of the right lung to empty into the v. cava superior.
  • The **v. hemiazygos accessoria** and **v. hemiazygos** run along the left side of the vertebrae thoracicae and drain the thoracic wall on the left side. They cross the midline independently (or they may join to form a single vessel) to drain into the v. azygos on the right side.
  • The vv. azygos and hemiazygos are the continuations of the **vv. lumbales ascendentes** in the abdomen, which communicate with the v. cava inferior. Thus the azygos system links the drainages of the vv. cavae superior and inferior and provides a collateral (alternate) pathway for blood back to the heart.
  • **Vv. mediastinales, vv. oesophageales,** and **vv. bronchiales** in the thorax, and the plexus venosus vertebralis (see Section 3.2) are also tributaries of the azygos system.

Fig. 5.7 Veins of the thoracic wall
Anterior view with rib cage (cavea thoracis) opened.
Removed: Clavicula. (From Gilroy AM et al. Atlas of Anatomy. 4th ed. 2020. Based on: Schuenke M, Schulte E, Schumacher U. THIEME Atlas of Anatomy. General Anatomy and Musculoskeletal System. Illustrations by Voll M and Wesker K. 3rd ed. New York: Thieme Medical Publishers; 2020.)

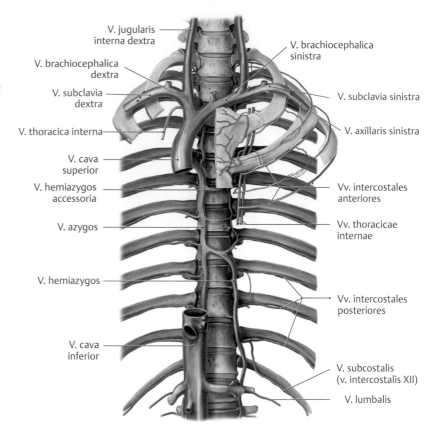

Fig. 5.8 Azygos system
Anterior view. (From Schuenke M, Schulte E, Schumacher U. THIEME Atlas of Anatomy, Vol 2. Illustrations by Voll M and Wesker K. 3rd ed. New York: Thieme Publishers; 2020.)

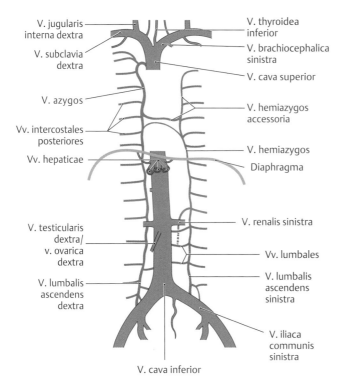

BOX 5.1: CLINICAL CORRELATION

SUPERIOR VENA CAVA SYNDROME

The superior vena cava syndrome is an obstruction of the v. cava superior, which in the majority of cases is caused by mediastinal tumors such as metastatic lung carcinoma (the lobus superior of the pulmo dexter lies next to the v. cava superior), lymphoma, breast cancer, or thyroid cancer. Noncancerous causes include thromboses (blood clots) that obstruct the lumen and infections that produce scarring. The onset of symptoms is usually gradual and includes dyspnea (shortness of breath) and swelling of the face, neck, and arms.

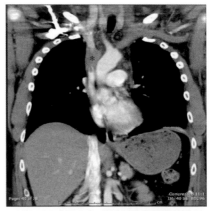

A coronal computed tomography (CT) scan image with intravenous (IV) contrast demonstrates a hypodense mass (*) occluding the v. cava superior, causing a swelling of the face and upper limbs.
(From Gunderman R. Essential Radiology, 3rd ed. New York: Thieme Publishers; 2014)

Lymphatics of the Thorax (see Section 1.9)

— The **ductus thoracicus,** the main lymphatic vessel of the body,
  • drains the abdomen, pelvis, and lower limbs, and the left side of the thorax, head, neck, and left upper limb (except the lower lobe of the left lung; see Section 8.5);
  • enters the thorax from its origin in the abdomen and passes superiorly in the midline of the mediastinum posterius; and
  • terminates at the junction of the v. subclavia sinistra and v. jugularis interna sinistra (jugulosubclavian junction or "venous angle") in the neck.
— The **ductus lymphaticus dexter,** which has a variable form,
  • drains lymph from the right side of the thorax, the lower lobe of the left lung, the head, and neck, and the right upper limb; and

  • usually terminates at the junction of the v. subclavia dextra and right v. jugularis interna (the jugulosubclavian junction).
— Lymph from most thoracic structures drains through chains of lymph nodes that empty into **trunci bronchomediastinales** in the mediastinum (**Figs. 5.9** and **5.10**). This includes
  • nll. parasternales and intercostales of the thoracic wall and superior surface of the diaphragma;
  • nll. bronchopulmonales and nll. intrapulmonales of the lungs and bronchi; and
  • nll. tracheobronchiales, nll. paratracheales, and nll. juxtaoesophageales of the heart, pericardium, trachea, and oesophagus.
— The trunci bronchomediastinales may empty into the ductus thoracicus and ductus lymphaticus dexter, but, more commonly, they empty directly into the vv. subclaviae in the neck.

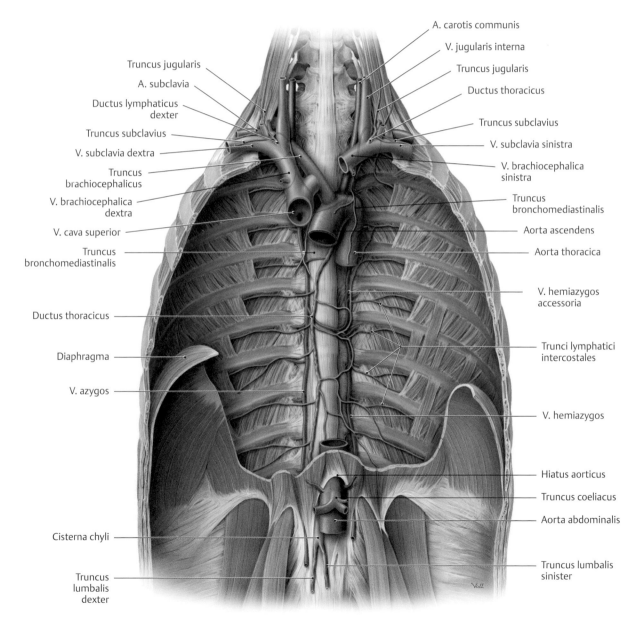

Fig. 5.9 Lymphatic trunks in the thorax
Anterior view of opened thorax. (From Schuenke M, Schulte E, Schumacher U. THIEME Atlas of Anatomy, Vol 2. Illustrations by Voll M and Wesker K. 3rd ed. New York: Thieme Publishers; 2020.)

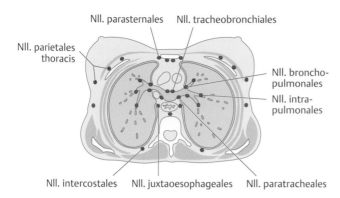

Fig. 5.10 Nodi lymphoidei thoracis
Transverse section at the level of the bifurcatio tracheae (at approximately T IV), viewed from below. Topographically, the nodi lymphoidei thoracis can be divided into three broad groups:
— Nodi lymphoidei in the thoracic wall (*pink*)
— Nodi lymphoidei in the pulmones and at the divisions of the arbor bronchialis (*blue*)
— Nodi lymphoidei associated with the trachea, oesophagus, and pericardium (*green*)
(From Schuenke M, Schulte E, Schumacher U. THIEME Atlas of Anatomy, Vol 2. Illustrations by Voll M and Wesker K. 3rd ed. New York: Thieme Publishers; 2020.)

Nerves of the Thorax (Figs. 5.11, 5.12, 5.13, 5.14)

— Pairs of **nn. intercostales posteriores** arise from the anterior rami of T1–T11 and pass along the inferior edge of the ribs on their deep surface.
  • The nerves innervate the muscles between the ribs, overlying muscles and skin of the thoracic wall and the breast (mamma).
— **Nn. phrenici** arise in the neck from anterior rami of C3, C4, and C5 ("to keep the diaphragm alive") and descend into the thorax.
  • On the right, the n. phrenicus runs along the v. cava superior; on the left, it crosses lateral to the arcus aortae.
  • Both nerves pass anterior to the hilum pulmonis as they descend to the diaphragma between the pericardial and pleural sacs.
  • The nn. phrenici provide motor innervation to the diaphragma and transmit sensory input from the mediastinum, mediastinal and diaphragmatic pleura, and peritoneum on the inferior diaphragmatic surface.
— The **trunci sympathici** run along either side of the thoracic vertebral column.

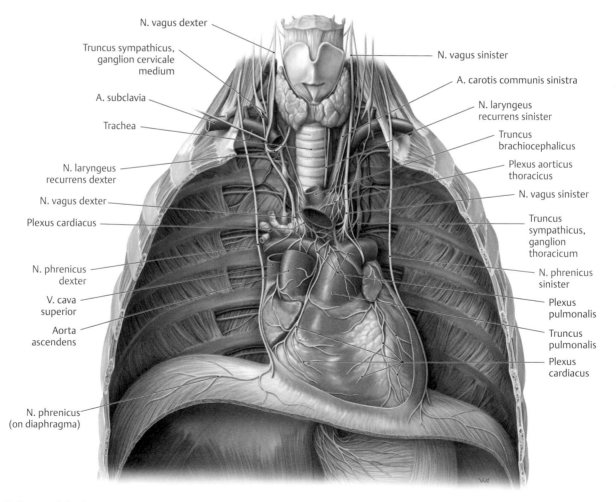

Fig. 5.11 Nerves of the thorax
Anterior view of opened thorax. (From Schuenke M, Schulte E, Schumacher U. THIEME Atlas of Anatomy, Vol 2. Illustrations by Voll M and Wesker K. 3rd ed. New York: Thieme Publishers; 2020.)

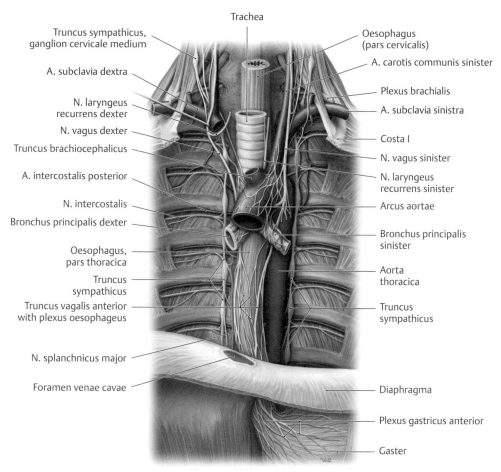

Trachea

Truncus sympathicus, ganglion cervicale medium

A. subclavia dextra

N. laryngeus recurrens dexter

N. vagus dexter

Truncus brachiocephalicus

A. intercostalis posterior

N. intercostalis

Bronchus principalis dexter

Oesophagus, pars thoracica

Truncus sympathicus

Truncus vagalis anterior with plexus oesophageus

N. splanchnicus major

Foramen venae cavae

Oesophagus (pars cervicalis)

A. carotis communis sinister

Plexus brachialis

A. subclavia sinistra

Costa I

N. vagus sinister

N. laryngeus recurrens sinister

Arcus aortae

Bronchus principalis sinister

Aorta thoracica

Truncus sympathicus

Diaphragma

Plexus gastricus anterior

Gaster

Fig. 5.12 Nerves of the mediastinum posterius
Anterior view. (From Gilroy AM et al. Atlas of Anatomy. 4th ed. 2020. Based on: Schuenke M, Schulte E, Schumacher U. THIEME Atlas of Anatomy. Internal Organs. Illustrations by Voll M and Wesker K. 3rd ed. New York: Thieme Medical Publishers; 2020.)

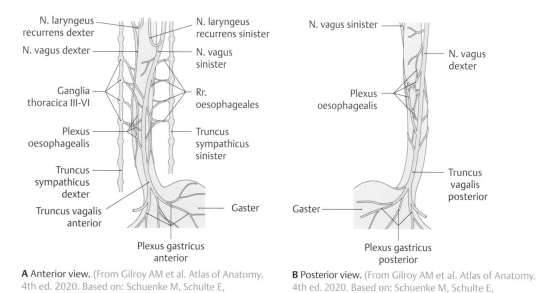

N. laryngeus recurrens dexter

N. vagus dexter

Ganglia thoracica III-VI

Plexus oesophagealis

Truncus sympathicus dexter

Truncus vagalis anterior

N. laryngeus recurrens sinister

N. vagus sinister

Rr. oesophageales

Truncus sympathicus sinister

Gaster

Plexus gastricus anterior

A Anterior view. (From Gilroy AM et al. Atlas of Anatomy. 4th ed. 2020. Based on: Schuenke M, Schulte E, Schumacher U. THIEME Atlas of Anatomy. Internal Organs. Illustrations by Voll M and Wesker K. 3rd ed. New York: Thieme Medical Publishers; 2020.)

N. vagus sinister

N. vagus dexter

Plexus oesophagealis

Truncus vagalis posterior

Gaster

Plexus gastricus posterior

B Posterior view. (From Gilroy AM et al. Atlas of Anatomy. 4th ed. 2020. Based on: Schuenke M, Schulte E, Schumacher U. THIEME Atlas of Anatomy. Internal Organs. Illustrations by Voll M and Wesker K. 3rd ed. New York: Thieme Medical Publishers; 2020.)

Fig. 5.13 Plexus oesophagealis

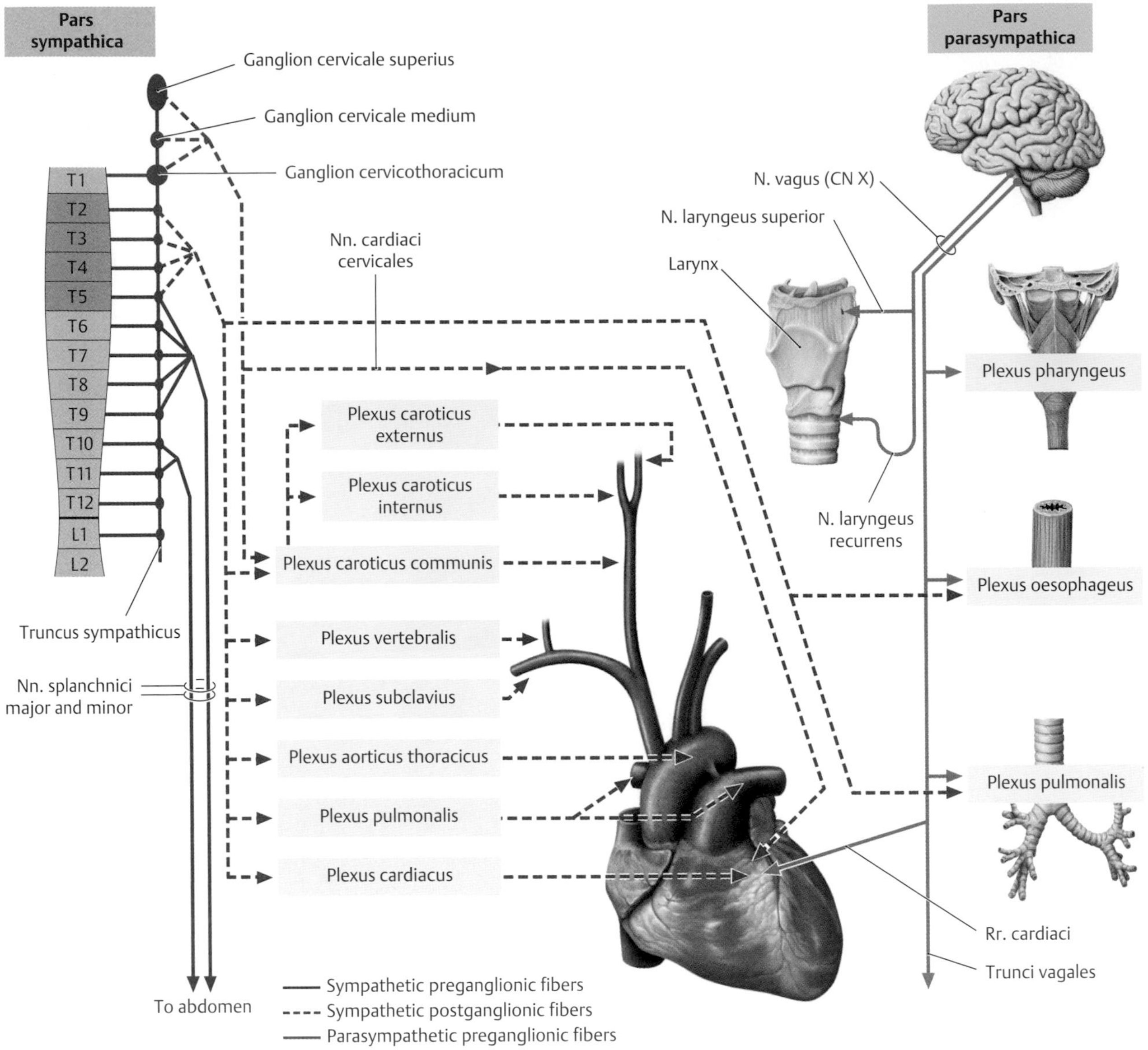

Fig. 5.14 Sympathetic and parasympathetic nervous systems in the thorax
Schematic. (From Gilroy AM et al. Atlas of Anatomy. 4th ed. 2020. Based on: Schuenke M, Schulte E, Schumacher U. THIEME Atlas of Anatomy. Internal Organs. Illustrations by Voll M and Wesker K. 3rd ed. New York: Thieme Medical Publishers; 2020.)

- Ganglia sympathica (paravertebral ganglia) at each spinal level communicate with nn. spinales through rami communicantes albus and griseus.
  - The T1 ganglion may combine with the ganglion at C8 to form a large star-shaped ganglion stellatum.
  - Small nn. splanchnici course medially from the truncus sympathicus to contribute to the autonomic plexuses of the thorax, which innervate thoracic viscera.
- Three large additional nn. splanchnici arise from the truncus sympathicus thoracis on each side, the **n. splanchnicus major** (T5–T9 or T10), **n. splanchnicus minor** (T10–T11), and **n. splanchnicus imus** (T12), and course inferomedially along the thoracic vertebral bodies into the abdomen. They contain preganglionic fibers that synapse in prevertebral ganglia of abdominal autonomic nerve plexuses (**Table 5.3**).

- The **nn. vagi** (CN X) descend from the neck into the thorax.
  - The n. vagus dexter courses behind the v. cava superior, medial to the arcus venae azygos; the n. vagus sinister runs lateral to the arcus aortae.
  - Both nn. vagi pass posterior to the hilum pulmonis before merging on the wall of the oesophagus.
  - The nn. vagi contribute parasympathetic fibers to the plexus cardiacus, pulmonalis, and oesophageus (**Table 5.4**).
- The **n. laryngeus recurrens sinister,** a branch of the n. vagus sinister, passes under the arcus aortae, posterior to the **lig. arteriosum** (see Section 5.6), and turns superiorly to ascend in the neck in the groove between the trachea and oesophagus.

Table 5.3 Peripheral Sympathetic Nervous System

Origin of Preganglionic Fibers*	Ganglion Cells	Course of Postganglionic Fibers	Target
Medulla spinalis	Sympathetic trunk	Follow nn. intercostalis	Blood vessels and glands in chest wall
		Accompany intrathoracic aa.	Visceral targets
		Gather in n. splanchnicus major and n. splanchnicus minor	Abdomen

*The axons of preganglionic neurons exit the medulla spinalis via the anterior roots and synapse with postganglionic neurons in the sympathetic ganglia.

Table 5.4 Peripheral Parasympathetic Nervous System

Origin of Preganglionic Fibers	Course of Postganglionic Motor Axons		Target
Brainstem	N. vagus (CN X)	Rr. cardiaca	Plexus cardiacus
		Rr. oesophagei	Plexus oesophageus
		Rr. tracheales	Trachea
		Rr. bronchiales	Plexus pulmonalis (bronchi, pulmonary vessels)

*The ganglion cells of the parasympathetic nervous system are scattered in microscopic groups in their target organs. The n. vagus thus carries the preganglionic motor axons to these targets.
CN, n. cranialis

- • The n. laryngeus recurrens dexter, a branch of the n. vagus dexter, recurs around the a. subclavia in the neck and is not a thoracic structure.
- — The **plexus oesophageus** surrounds the lower oesophagus.
  - • It is composed of preganglionic parasympathetic fibers from the n. vagus dexter and sinister and postganglionic fibers from the truncus sympathicus thoracis
  - • The **truncus vagalis anterior** and **truncus vagalis posterior** arise from the plexus and pass into the abdomen, anterior and posterior to the oesophagus.
- — The **plexus cardiacus (Fig. 5.13)**, which is located above the heart in the concavity of the arcus aortae, continues along the aa. coronariae. It innervates the conducting system of the heart and contains
  - • preganglionic sympathetic fibers from T1 to T5 and postganglionic sympathetic fibers from cardiopulmonary branches of the truncus sympathicus cervicalis and thoracis;

- • preganglionic parasympathetic fibers from cardiac branches of the n. vagus that arise in the cervical region and contributions from the nn. laryngei recurrentes; and
- • visceral sensory fibers that travel with sympathetic and parasympathetic nerves.
- — The **plexus pulmonalis** is a continuation of the plexus cardiacus onto the bifurcatio tracheae and the bronchi that penetrate the hilum pulmonis.
  - • It regulates the constriction and dilation of the pulmonary vessels and respiratory passages.
  - • It transmits sensation from the lung and visceral, or inner, layer of the pleural sac that is adherent to the surface of the lung.

6 Thoracic Wall

A bony and muscular cage, which communicates superiorly with the neck and inferiorly with the abdomen, encloses and protects the thoracic contents. A superficial layer of extrinsic muscles overlies the thoracic cage (cavea thoracis), although these muscles act primarily on the upper limb. The breast (mamma), a derivative of the epidermis (outermost layer of skin), is a prominent superficial structure of the thoracic wall.

6.1 The Breast (Mamma)

General Features

The breast (mamma) is made up of the **mammary gland (gl. mammaria),** a modified sweat gland, and its supporting fat and fibrous tissue **(Figs. 6.1** and **6.2).** Breasts remain rudimentary in males but are prominent structures of the female pectoral region.

- Female breasts extend from the lateral border of the sternum to the midaxillary line and overlie the 2nd through 6th ribs.
- The breast is embedded in the subcutaneous layer of the skin overlying the deep fascia of the m. pectoralis major and m. serratus anterior.
- The **retromammary space** is a plane of loose connective tissue that separates the breast from underlying fascia of the m. pectoralis major and allows movement of the breasts on the thoracic wall.
- The highest prominence of the breast, the **nipple (papilla mammaria),** is located at the center of the areola (areola mammae). Circularly arranged smooth muscle fibers cause erection of the nipple in response to cold or tactile stimulation. In men and young women, the nipple is at the T IV vertebral level, but in older women this location varies considerably.
- The **areola,** the pigmented skin surrounding the nipple, contains sebaceous glands (glandulae areolares) whose oily secretions lubricate the area during nursing.
- An **axillary tail,** or small finger of glandular tissue, may extend into the axilla (armpit) along the lower edge of the m. pectoralis.
- The volume of fat, not the volume of glandular tissue, largely determines the differences in breast size among women.

Mammary Gland (Glandula Mammaria)

The mammary gland (gl. mammaria) has two components:
- The **parenchyma,** or milk-producing part of the gland (see **Fig. 6.2)**
  - The parenchyma consists of lobes divided into 15 to 20 lobules, which contain grapelike clusters of **alveoli,** hollow balls lined by secretory cells.
  - **Lactiferous ducts (ductus lactiferi)** in the parenchyma drain each lobule and open at the nipple. Deep to the areola, each duct has a small, dilated portion called the **lactiferous sinus (sinus lactifer)** where, in lactating females, a small amount of milk is stored.
- The **stroma,** or fibrous framework, of the gland that separates the lobules and supports the lobes
  - Stroma is attached to the overlying dermis of the skin by **suspensory (Cooper) ligaments (ligg. suspensoria mammaria),** which are particularly strong on the superior surface of the breast.

Neurovasculature of the Breast

- Rr. intercostales anteriores and rr. mammarii medialis (from perforating branches) of the a. thoracica interna, **rr. thoracici laterales** and **rr. thoracodorsales** of the a. axillaris, and the 2nd, 3rd, and 4th aa. intercostales posteriores supply the breast (see Sections 5.2 and 6.4).
- Venous blood drains primarily to the v. axillaris but also to the v. thoracica interna.
- Most lymph (> 75%) from the breast drains (particularly from the lateral quadrant) to axillary lymph nodes **(Fig. 6.3)**; from there it travels to nodes around the clavicle and the ipsilateral lymphatic duct.
  - Some lymph may drain to deep pectoral nodes, where it joins the bronchomediastinal drainage in the mediastinum.
  - Medial portions of the breast may drain to nll. parasternales and to the contralateral breast; inferior segments may drain to abdominal nodes.
- The rr. cutaneus anteriores and laterales of the 4th, 5th, and 6th nn. intercostales innervate the breast.

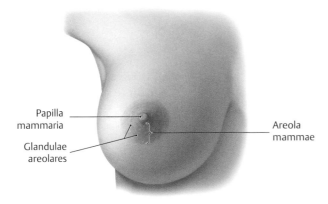

Papilla mammaria

Glandulae areolares

Areola mammae

Fig. 6.1 Surface anatomy of the breast
Mamma dextra, anterior view. (From Schuenke M, Schulte E, Schumacher U. THIEME Atlas of Anatomy, Vol 1. Illustrations by Voll M and Wesker K. 3rd ed. New York: Thieme Publishers; 2020.)

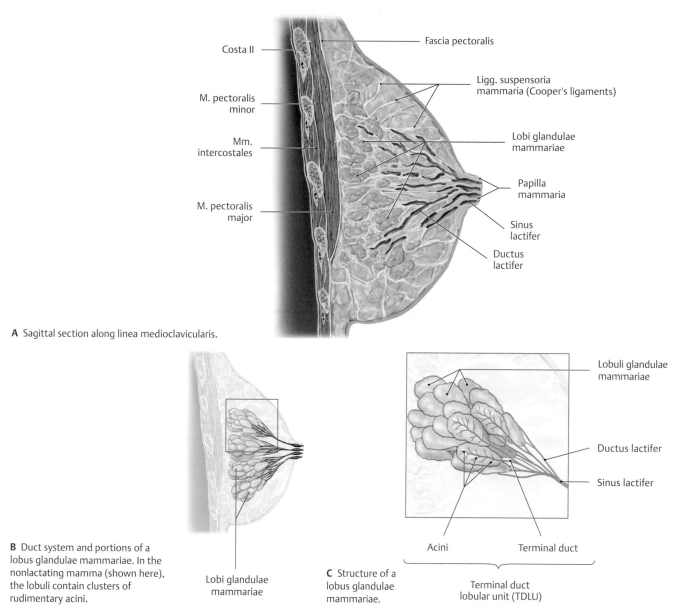

Costa II

M. pectoralis minor

Mm. intercostales

M. pectoralis major

Fascia pectoralis

Ligg. suspensoria mammaria (Cooper's ligaments)

Lobi glandulae mammariae

Papilla mammaria

Sinus lactifer

Ductus lactifer

A Sagittal section along linea medioclavicularis.

Lobuli glandulae mammariae

Ductus lactifer

Sinus lactifer

Acini

Terminal duct

B Duct system and portions of a lobus glandulae mammariae. In the nonlactating mamma (shown here), the lobuli contain clusters of rudimentary acini.

Lobi glandulae mammariae

C Structure of a lobus glandulae mammariae.

Terminal duct lobular unit (TDLU)

Fig. 6.2 Structure of the breast
(From Gilroy AM et al. Atlas of Anatomy. 4th ed. 2020. Based on: Schuenke M, Schulte E, Schumacher U. THIEME Atlas of Anatomy. General Anatomy and Musculoskeletal System. Illustrations by Voll M and Wesker K. 3rd ed. New York: Thieme Medical Publishers; 2020.)

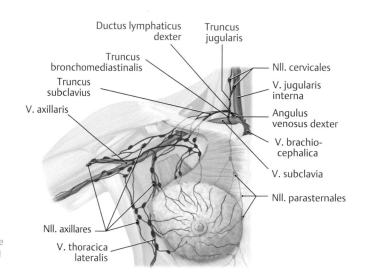

Ductus lymphaticus dexter

Truncus jugularis

Truncus bronchomediastinalis

Truncus subclavius

V. axillaris

Nll. cervicales

V. jugularis interna

Angulus venosus dexter

V. brachio-cephalica

V. subclavia

Nll. parasternales

Nll. axillares

V. thoracica lateralis

Fig. 6.3 Lymphatic drainage of the female breast
Nll. axillares, parasternales, and cervicales. Right thoracic and axillary region with the arm abducted, anterior view. (From Schuenke M, Schulte E, Schumacher U. THIEME Atlas of Anatomy, Vol 1. Illustrations by Voll M and Wesker K. 1st ed. New York: Thieme Publishers; 2007.)

BOX 6.1: CLINICAL CORRELATION

CARCINOMA OF THE BREAST
The most common type of breast cancer, invasive ductal carcinoma, arises from the lining of the ductus lactiferi. Typically, it metastasizes through lymphatic channels, most abundantly to axillary nodes from the supralateral quadrant but it may also travel to supraclavicular nodes, the contralateral breast, and the abdomen. Obstruction of the lymphatic drainage causes edema, and fibrosis (shortening) of the ligg. suspensoria can cause a pitted appearance of the skin. Through venous communication with the azygos system and vertebral venous plexus, breast cancer can metastasize to the vertebrae, cranium, and brain. Elevation of the breast with contraction of the m. pectoralis major suggests invasion of the fascia pectoralis and retromammary space.

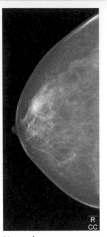

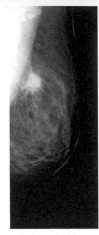

Normal mammogram. (From Gunderman R. Essential Radiology, 3rd ed. New York: Thieme; 2014.)

This mediolateral-oblique mammogram demonstrates a spiculated mass in the upper outer quadrant, an infiltrating ductal carcinoma, in this 63-year-old woman. (From Gunderman R. Essential Radiology, 3rd ed. New York: Thieme Publishers; 2014.)

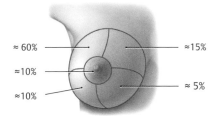

≈ 60%   ≈15%
≈10%
≈10%   ≈ 5%

Origin of malignant breast tumors by quadrant
Right breast. (From Schuenke M, Schulte E, Schumacher U. THIEME Atlas of Anatomy, Vol 1. Illustrations by Voll M and Wesker K. 3rd ed. New York: Thieme Publishers; 2020.)

6.2   The Thoracic Skeleton

The thoracic skeleton protects the thoracic viscera and provides attachment for the upper limb. The thoracic cage includes the sternum, 12 pairs of ribs, and the 12 thoracic vertebrae **(Fig. 6.4)**.

The Sternum

The **sternum** is a flat, elongated bone that has three parts:
1. The **manubrium,** which articulates laterally with the costal cartilages (cartilagines costales, cartilage that attaches the ribs to the sternum) of the 1st and 2nd ribs. A deep **jugular notch (incisura jugularis)** separates the right and left artt. sternoclaviculares, where the manubrium articulates with the clavicles.
2. The **body of the sternum (corpus sterni),** which is fused superiorly with the manubrium at the **manubriosternal joint (symphysis manubriosternalis).** Laterally, the body articulates with costal cartilages of the 2nd to 7th ribs.
3. The **proc. xiphoideus,** the lowest part of the sternum, which joins superiorly with the body of the sternum at the xiphisternal joint (synchondrosis xiphosternalis).
   - The **angulus sterni** is an important surface landmark on the anterior thoracic wall that provides orientation to the internal anatomy of the thorax. It is a palpable ridge that marks the fusion of the manubrium and body of the sternum. A horizontal plane through the angulus sterni intersects
     - the articulation between the sternum and the costal cartilages of the 2nd ribs,
     - the division of the mediastinum into superior and inferior regions,

- the origin and termination of the arcus aortae,
- the bifurcation of the trachea, and
- the T IV–T V disci intervertebrales.

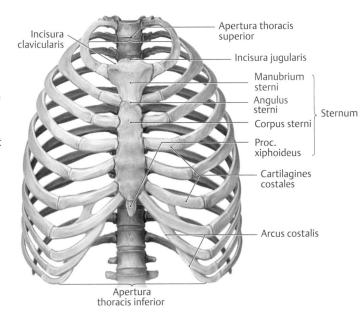

Incisura clavicularis
Apertura thoracis superior
Incisura jugularis
Manubrium sterni
Angulus sterni
Sternum
Corpus sterni
Proc. xiphoideus
Cartilagines costales
Arcus costalis
Apertura thoracis inferior

Fig. 6.4 Thoracic skeleton
Anterior view. (From Schuenke M, Schulte E, Schumacher U. THIEME Atlas of Anatomy, Vol 1. Illustrations by Voll M and Wesker K. 3rd ed. New York: Thieme Publishers; 2020.)

The Ribs (Costae)

— The ribs (costae) are numbered 1 to 12 (costae I–XII) from superior to inferior, and each rib articulates with a thoracic vertebra of the same number.
— The ribs hang obliquely downward from their articulation with the columna vertebralis. Their anterior ends may be two to five vertebral levels lower than their posterior attachment.
— Ribs 1 to 10 articulate anteriorly with a cartilaginous segment called the **costal cartilage (cartilago costalis).**
— The ribs are classified according to their articulation of their costal cartilage with the sternum **(Fig. 6.5)**:
  • **True ribs (costae verae, costae I–VII)** articulate directly with the sternum via individual costal cartilages.
  • **False ribs (costae spuriae, costae VIII–X)** articulate indirectly with the sternum through costal cartilages that are connected to the cartilage superior to it.
  • **Floating ribs (costae fluctuantes, costae XI -XII)** have no connection to the sternum.
— Most ribs articulate at three joints **(Fig. 6.6)**:
  1. **Costochondral joints (artt. costochondrales)** between the bony segments of ribs 1 to 10 and their respective **costal cartilages**
  2. **Sternochondral joints (artt. sternochondrales)** between the sternum and costal cartilages of ribs 1 to 7 on each side
  3. **Costovertebral joints (artt. costovertebrales)** between the ribs and vertebrae. These joints may contain multiple articulations.
     ◦ The **costal tubercle (tuberculum costae)** of each rib articulates with the fovea costalis on its accompanying thoracic vertebra (see **Fig. 3.6**).
     ◦ The **heads** of ribs 2 to 10 articulate with the vertebra of the same number and with the vertebra superior to them. Ribs 1, 11, and 12 articulate only with their own vertebra.

Thoracic Apertures

— The thoracic cage has superior and inferior openings (see **Fig. 6.4**):

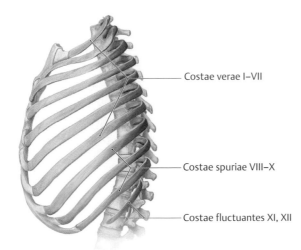

Fig. 6.5 Types of ribs (costae)
Left lateral view. (From Schuenke M, Schulte E, Schumacher U. THIEME Atlas of Anatomy, Vol 1. Illustrations by Voll M and Wesker K. 3rd ed. New York: Thieme Publishers; 2020.)

Costae verae I–VII

Costae spuriae VIII–X

Costae fluctuantes XI, XII

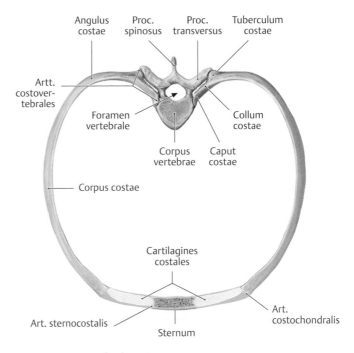

Fig. 6.6 Structure of a thoracic segment
Superior view of 6th costal pair. (From Schuenke M, Schulte E, Schumacher U. THIEME Atlas of Anatomy, Vol 1. Illustrations by Voll M and Wesker K. 3rd ed. New York: Thieme Publishers; 2020.)

Angulus costae

Proc. spinosus

Proc. transversus

Tuberculum costae

Artt. costovertebrales

Foramen vertebrale

Collum costae

Corpus vertebrae

Caput costae

Corpus costae

Cartilagines costales

Art. sternocostalis

Sternum

Art. costochondralis

• The **apertura thoracis superior (thoracic inlet)**, which is bounded by the T1 vertebra, the 1st ribs, and the manubrium of the sternum. The thorax communicates with the neck through this opening.
• The **apertura thoracis inferior (thoracic outlet)**, which is bounded by the T12 vertebra, the 11th and 12th ribs, the **arcus costalis** (lower border of the thoracic cage), and the proc. xiphoideus. A muscular diaphragma closes this aperture, separating the cavitas thoracis from the cavitas abdominis.

6.3 Muscles of the Thorax

Muscles of the Thoracic Wall (Fig. 6.7; Table 6.1)

— Extrinsic muscles of the upper limb, including the **m. pectoralis major, m. pectoralis minor,** and **m. serratus anterior,** cover the thorax. Although they mainly move or stabilize the upper limb, these muscles also assist in movements of the ribs during deep inspiration. (See Chapter 18, Overview of the Upper Limb.)
— The **m. scalenus anterior, m. scalenus medius,** and **m. scalenus posterior** originate on the procc. transversi of the vertebrae cervicales and insert onto the 1st and 2nd ribs. They assist the intrinsic thoracic muscles during inspiration and are considered extrinsic muscles of respiration.
— Intrinsic muscles of the thoracic wall are the chief muscles that move the ribs during respiration.
  • The **mm. intercostales** occupy the intercostal spaces between the ribs. They extend from the inferior border of one rib to the superior border of the next inferior rib. The mm. intercostales move the ribs primarily during forced respiration. During quiet respiration, they stabilize the thoracic wall. They include

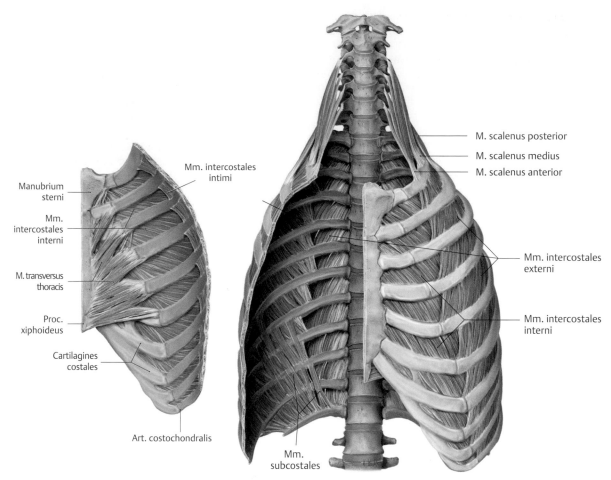

Fig. 6.7 Transversus thoracis
Anterior view with cavea thoracis opened to expose posterior surface of anterior wall. The external and internal intercostal membranes have been removed. (From Gilroy AM et al. Atlas of Anatomy. 4th ed. 2020. Based on: Schuenke M, Schulte E, Schumacher U. THIEME Atlas of Anatomy. General Anatomy and Musculoskeletal System. Illustrations by Voll M and Wesker K. 3rd ed. New York: Thieme Medical Publishers; 2020.)

Table 6.1 Muscles of the Thoracic Wall

Muscle		Origin	Insertion	Innervation	Action
Mm. scaleni	M. scalenus anterior	Vertebrae C III–C VI (proc. transversus, tuberculum anterius)	Costa I (tuberculum m. scaleni anterioris)	C4–C6	Raise the upper costae during inspiration
	M. scalenus medius	Vertebrae C I–C II (proc. transversus) Vertebrae C III–C VII (proc. transversus, tuberculum posterius)	Costa I (posterior to sulcus arteriae subclaviae)	C3–C8	
	M. scalenus posterior	Vertebrae C V–C VII (proc. transversus, tuberculum posterius)	Costa II (outer surface)	C6–C8	
Mm. intercostales	Mm. intercostales externi	Lower margin of costa to upper margin of next lower costa (courses obliquely forward and downward from tuberculum costae to junctura costochondralis)		Nn. intercostales I–XI	Raise the costae during inspiration
	Mm. intercostales interni	Lower margin of costa to upper margin of next lower costa (courses obliquely forward and upward from angulus costae to sternum)			Lower the costae during expiration
	Mm. intercostales intimi				
Mm. subcostales		Lower margin of lower costae to inner surface of costae two to three costae below		Adjacent lower nn. intercostales	Lower the costae during expiration
M. transversus thoracis		Sternum and proc. xiphoideus (inner surface)	Costae II–VI (cartilago costalis, inner surface)	Nn. intercostales II–VI	Weakly lower the costae during expiration

- ◦ the **mm. intercostales externi,** with fibers directed inferoanteriorly, which make up the most superficial layer
- ◦ the **mm. intercostales interni** and **mm. intercostales intimi,** which occupy the middle and deepest layers of the thoracic wall, respectively, with their fibers directed inferoposteriorly
- The **mm. subcostales** are most prominent along the lower thoracic wall, where they cross the inner surface of one or two intercostal spaces.
- The **mm. transversi thoracis** consist of four of five thin slips that extend superiorly and laterally from the posterior surface of the sternum to the ribs.

The Thoracic Diaphragm

The **thoracic diaphragm** (or simply, the **diaphragma**), a musculo-tendinous sheet that separates the thorax from the abdomen, is the principal muscle of respiration. The diaphragma forms the floor of the thorax, the roof of the abdomen, and a portion of the posterior abdominal wall (**Fig. 6.8**).

— The skeletal muscle fibers of the diaphragma originate along the costal margin, the corpora vertebrae L I–L III, the **lig. arcuatum medianum** and **lig. arcuatum laterale**, and the proc. xiphoideus. They insert on the diaphragma's **centrum tendineum.**

— **Crura dextrum and sinistrum,** extensions of the posterior diaphragma, attach to the bodies of the lumbar vertebrae, with the right crus extending slightly lower than the left crus.

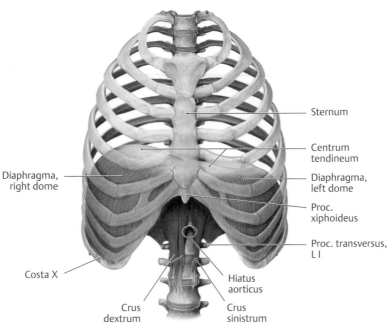

A Anterior view.

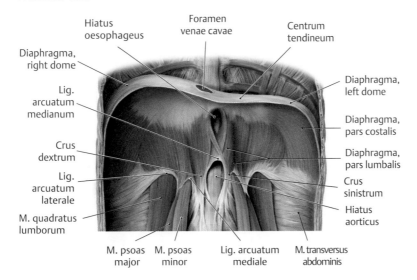

B Coronal section with diaphragma in intermediate position.

Fig. 6.8 Diaphragma
The diaphragma, which separates the thorax from the abdomen, has two asymmetric domes (hemidiaphragmata) and three apertures (for the aorta, vena cava, and oesophagus). (From Gilroy AM et al. Atlas of Anatomy. 4th ed. 2020. Based on: Schuenke M, Schulte E, Schumacher U. THIEME Atlas of Anatomy. General Anatomy and Musculoskeletal System. Illustrations by Voll M and Wesker K. 3rd ed. New York: Thieme Medical Publishers; 2020.)

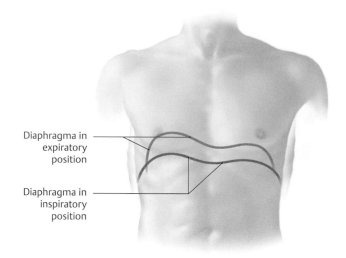

Fig. 6.9 Projection of the diaphragma onto the trunk
Anterior view. Position of the diaphragma in inspiration and expiration. (From Schuenke M, Schulte E, Schumacher U. THIEME Atlas of Anatomy, Vol 2. Illustrations by Voll M and Wesker K. 3rd ed. New York: Thieme Publishers; 2020.)

— The domes on the right and left sides of the diaphragma are asymmetric; the right hemidiaphragm is generally higher than the left.

— During full expiration the diaphragma is 4 to 6 cm higher than during full inspiration. During expiration it ascends to the level of the 4th or 5th rib on the right and slightly lower on the left, although this varies with respiration, posture, and body type (**Fig. 6.9**).

— The diaphragma has three openings to allow the passage of structures between the thorax and abdomen (**Fig. 6.10**):

1. The **caval opening (foramen venae cavae)**, which is a passage for the v. cava inferior through the centrum tendineum at the T VIII vertebral level.

2. The **hiatus oesophageus**, which is an opening at the T X vertebral level for the oesophagus, the truncus vagalis anterior and truncus vagalis posterior, and a. and v. gastrica sinistra. It is usually formed by the crus dextrum of the diaphragma (occasionally by the crus dextrum and crus sinistrum) that, when contracted, forms a sphincter around the oesophagus.

3. The **hiatus aorticus**, which is a passageway for the aorta between the crus dextrum and crus sinistrum as it passes behind the diaphragm at T12. The ductus thoracicus, and often the vv. azygos and hemiazygos, also passes through this aperture.

— The aa. phrenicae inferiores, branches of the aorta abdominalis (or truncus coeliacus) are the primary blood supply to the diaphragma. aa. phrenicae superiores, aa. pericardiophrenica, and aa. musculophrenica make additional contributions (**Fig. 6.11**).

— Venous blood drains to the azygos system through vv. intercostales posteriores and vv. phrenicae superiores.

— The n. phrenicus (C3–C5) provides all of the motor and most of the sensory innervation to the diaphragma. The nn. subcostales and nn. intercostales supply sensory innervation to the periphery of the diaphragma (**Fig. 6.12**).

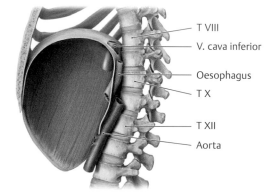

A Left lateral view of opened thorax. (From Gilroy AM et al. Atlas of Anatomy. 4th ed. 2020. Based on: Schuenke M, Schulte E, Schumacher U. THIEME Atlas of Anatomy. General Anatomy and Musculoskeletal System. Illustrations by Voll M and Wesker K. 3rd ed. New York: Thieme Medical Publishers; 2020.)

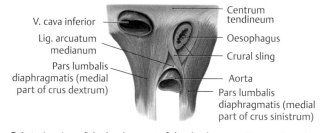

B Anterior view of the lumbar part of the diaphragma. (From Schuenke M, Schulte E, Schumacher U. THIEME Atlas of Anatomy, Vol 2. Illustrations by Voll M and Wesker K. 3rd ed. New York: Thieme Publishers; 2020.)

Fig. 6.10 Diaphragmatic apertures

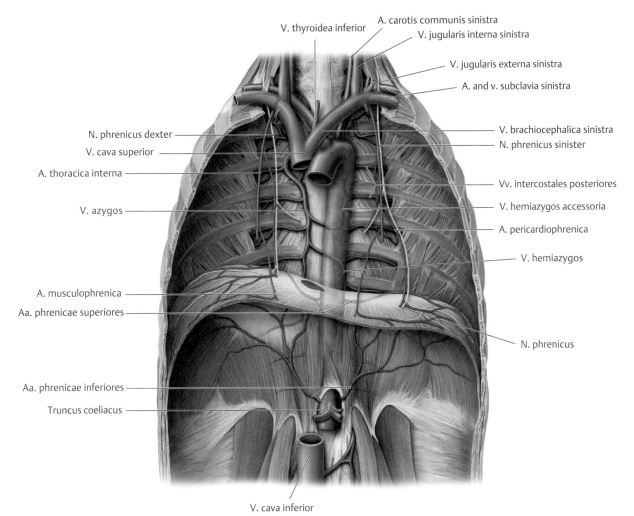

V. thyroidea inferior
A. carotis communis sinistra
V. jugularis interna sinistra
V. jugularis externa sinistra
A. and v. subclavia sinistra
V. brachiocephalica sinistra
N. phrenicus sinister
Vv. intercostales posteriores
V. hemiazygos accessoria
A. pericardiophrenica
V. hemiazygos
N. phrenicus
N. phrenicus dexter
V. cava superior
A. thoracica interna
V. azygos
A. musculophrenica
Aa. phrenicae superiores
Aa. phrenicae inferiores
Truncus coeliacus
V. cava inferior

A Anterior view of open cavea thoracis. (From Gilroy AM et al. Atlas of Anatomy. 4th ed. 2020. Based on: Schuenke M, Schulte E, Schumacher U. THIEME Atlas of Anatomy. Internal Organs. Illustrations by Voll M and Wesker K. 3rd ed. New York: Thieme Medical Publishers; 2020.)

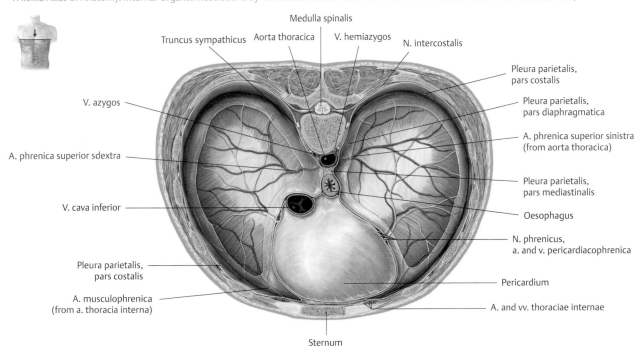

Medulla spinalis
Truncus sympathicus
Aorta thoracica
V. hemiazygos
N. intercostalis
Pleura parietalis, pars costalis
Pleura parietalis, pars diaphragmatica
A. phrenica superior sinistra (from aorta thoracica)
Pleura parietalis, pars mediastinalis
Oesophagus
N. phrenicus, a. and v. pericardiacophrenica
Pericardium
A. and vv. thoraciae internae
V. azygos
A. phrenica superior sdextra
V. cava inferior
Pleura parietalis, pars costalis
A. musculophrenica (from a. thoracica interna)
Sternum

B Superior view of diaphragma. (From Schuenke M, Schulte E, Schumacher U. THIEME Atlas of Anatomy, Vol 2. Illustrations by Voll M and Wesker K. 3rd ed. New York: Thieme Publishers; 2020.)

Fig. 6.11 Neurovasculature of the diaphragma

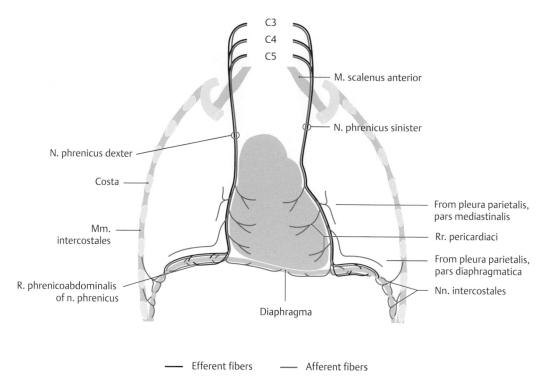

Fig. 6.12 Innervation of the diaphragma
Anterior view. The n. phrenicus lies on the lateral surface of the pericardium fibrosum together with the a. pericardiophrenica and v. pericardiophrenica. *Note:* The n. phrenicus also innervates the pericardium. (From Gilroy AM et al. Atlas of Anatomy. 4th ed. 2020. Based on: Schuenke M, Schulte E, Schumacher U. THIEME Atlas of Anatomy. Internal Organs. Illustrations by Voll M and Wesker K. 3rd ed. New York: Thieme Medical Publishers; 2020.)

6.4   Neurovasculature of the Thoracic Wall

— Intercostal neurovascular bundles course along the inferior surface of the ribs within the sulcus costae (**Figs. 6.13, 6.14, 6.15, 6.16**).
  • Rr. intercostales anteriores (branches of the a. thoracica interna) and aa. intercostales posteriores (branches of the aorta thoracica and a. subclavia) supply the muscles and skin of the thoracic wall (**Fig. 6.14**).
  • Vv. intercostales drain primarily to the azygos system but also into the v. brachiocephalica and vv. thoracicae internae, which join the vena cava superior (**Fig. 6.15**).
— The **v. thoracoepigastrica** is a superficial vein that drains the subcutaneous tissue of the anterolateral thoracic and abdominal walls. It drains superiorly to the v. axillaris of the upper limb and inferiorly to the v. epigastrica superficialis (**Fig. 6.16**).

— The thoracic wall is drained by three major groups of lymph nodes:
  • The **nll. parasternales,** which are scattered along the a. thoracica interna. They receive lymph from the breast, anterior thoracic wall, liver, and upper deep surface of the anterior abdominal wall.
  • The **nll. intercostales,** which are located in the intercostal spaces near the heads and necks of the ribs. They drain the posterolateral part of the chest and gll. mammariae.
  • The **nll. phrenici superiores,** which are located on the superior surface of the diaphragma. They drain the centrum tendineum of the diaphragma, the pericardium fibrosum, and the superior surface of the liver.
— Nn. intercostales T1–T11 innervate the muscles of the thoracic wall. In the linea axillaris media these nerves give off a r. cutaneus lateralis that supplies the superficial muscles and skin of the thorax (**Figs. 6.17** and **6.18**).

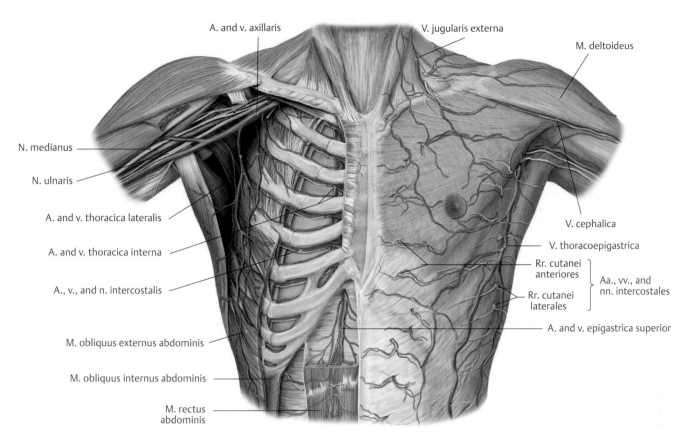

Fig. 6.13 Neurovascular topography of the thoracic wall
(From Gilroy AM et al. Atlas of Anatomy. 4th ed. 2020. Based on: Schuenke M, Schulte E, Schumacher U. THIEME Atlas of Anatomy. General Anatomy and Musculoskeletal System. Illustrations by Voll M and Wesker K. 3rd ed. New York: Thieme Medical Publishers; 2020.)

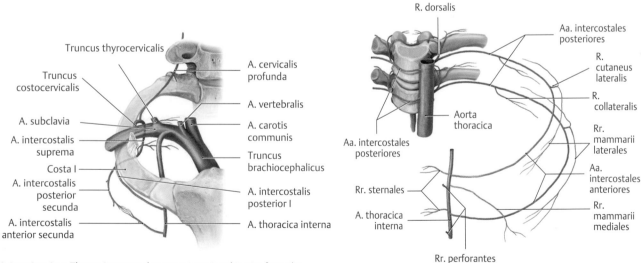

A Anterior view. The aa. intercostales posteriores I and II arise from the a. intercostalis suprema, an indirect branch of the a. subclavia.

B Anterior view. Aa. intercostales posteriores III–XI are segmental branches of the aorta thoracica.

Fig. 6.14 Course and branches of the arteriae intercostales
(From Schuenke M, Schulte E, Schumacher U. THIEME Atlas of Anatomy, Vol 1. Illustrations by Voll M and Wesker K. 3rd ed. New York: Thieme Publishers; 2020.)

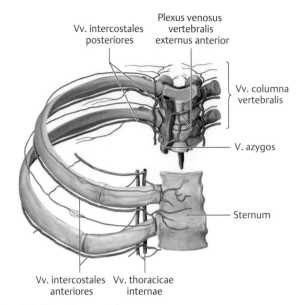

Fig. 6.15 Venae intercostales
Anteriosuperior view. Vertebral column and rib segment. (From Schuenke M, Schulte E, Schumacher U. THIEME Atlas of Anatomy, Vol 1. Illustrations by Voll M and Wesker K. 3rd ed. New York: Thieme Publishers; 2020.)

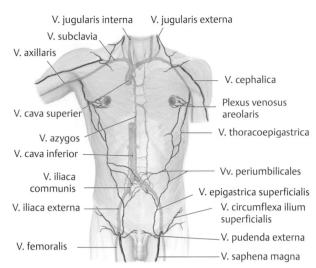

Fig. 6.16 Superficial veins
Anterior view. The vv. thoracoepigastricae are a potential superficial collateral venous drainage route in the event of obstruction of the v. cava superior or v. cava inferior. (From Schuenke M, Schulte E, Schumacher U. THIEME Atlas of Anatomy, Vol 1. Illustrations by Voll M and Wesker K. 3rd ed. New York: Thieme Publishers; 2020.)

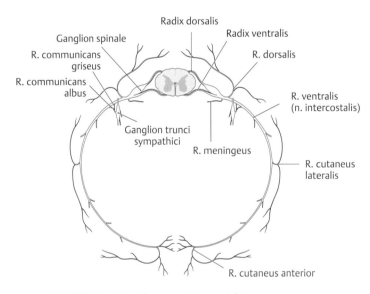

Fig. 6.17 Branches of a nervus intercostalis
(From Gilroy AM et al. Atlas of Anatomy. 4th ed. 2020. Based on: Schuenke M, Schulte E, Schumacher U. THIEME Atlas of Anatomy. General Anatomy and Musculoskeletal System. Illustrations by Voll M and Wesker K. 3rd ed. New York: Thieme Medical Publishers; 2020.)

— Nn. intercostales 7 through 11 continue anteriorly from the intercostal space (spatium intercostale) to innervate the anterior abdominal wall.

— Landmark dermatomes on the thoracic wall include T4 at the nipple and T6 over the proc. xiphoideus.

— Intercostal nerves and vessels are protected within the **sulcus costae** on the deep inferior edge of the ribs (see **Box 6.2**). Within this bundle of neurovascular structures, the nerve runs inferior to its accompanying vessels.

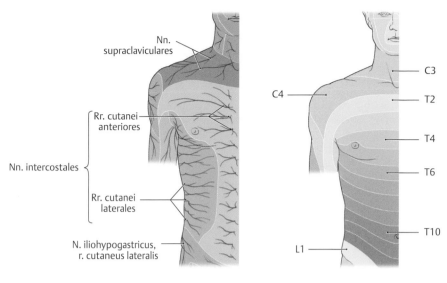

A Sensory nerves of the anterior thoracic wall.

B Dermatomes of the anterior thoracic wall. *Landmarks:* T4 generally includes the nipple; T6 innervates the skin over the proc. xiphoideus.

Fig. 6.18 Cutaneous innervation of the thoracic wall
Anterior view. (From Schuenke M, Schulte E, Schumacher U. THIEME Atlas of Anatomy, Vol 1. Illustrations by Voll M and Wesker K. 3rd ed. New York: Thieme Publishers; 2020.)

BOX 6.2: CLINICAL CORRELATION

INSERTION OF A CHEST TUBE

Abnormal fluid collection in the pleural space (e.g., pleural effusion due to bronchial carcinoma) may necessitate the insertion of a chest tube. Generally, the optimal puncture site in a sitting patient is at the level of the fourth and fifth intercostal space in the mid to anterior axillary line, immediately behind the lateral edge of the m. pectoralis major. The drain should always be introduced at the upper margin of a rib to avoid injuring the a. intercostalis, v. intercostalis, and n. intercostalis.

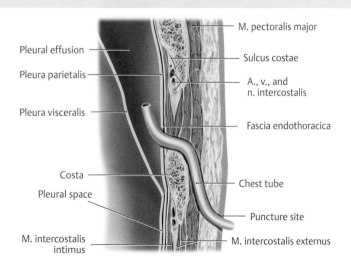

Coronal section, anterior view
(From Gilroy AM et al. Atlas of Anatomy. 4th ed. 2020. Based on: Schuenke M, Schulte E, Schumacher U. THIEME Atlas of Anatomy. General Anatomy and Musculoskeletal System. Illustrations by Voll M and Wesker K. 3rd ed. New York: Thieme Medical Publishers; 2020.)

7 Mediastinum

The **mediastinum** is the region within the thorax between the right and left pulmonary cavities (**Fig 7.1**; see **Table 5.1**). The sternum and the costal cartilages of ribs 1 through 7 form its anterior boundary, and the thoracic vertebrae (vertebrae thoracicae) form its posterior boundary. The mediastinum contains the heart (cor), great vessels, and pericardium, as well as the oesophagus, trachea, thymus, and associated neurovasculature (**Fig. 7.2**).

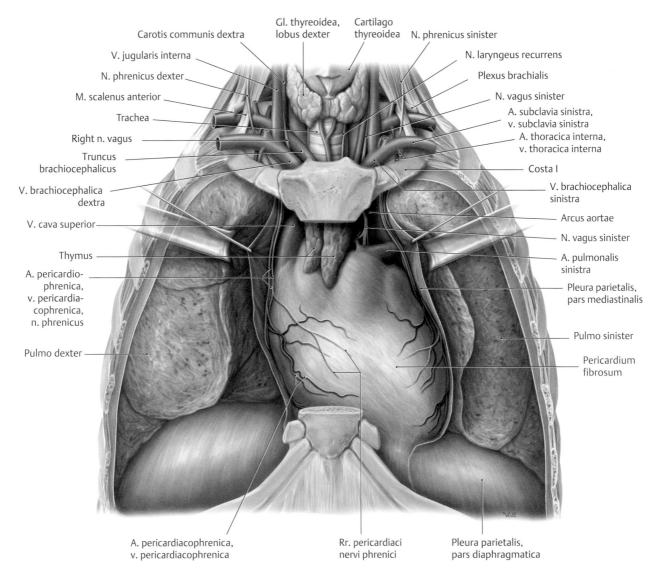

Fig. 7.1 Cavitas thoracica
Opened cavitas thoracica. *Removed:* Thoracic wall; connective tissue of anterior mediastinum. (From Schuenke M, Schulte E, Schumacher U. THIEME Atlas of Anatomy, Vol 2. Illustrations by Voll M and Wesker K. 3rd ed. New York: Thieme Publishers; 2020.)

7.1   Regions of the Mediastinum (Table 7.1)

— A horizontal plane passing through the sternal angle (at the T4–T5 intervertebral disk) divides the region into a **superior mediastinum (mediastinum superius),** bounded above by the superior thoracic aperture, and an **inferior mediastinum (mediastinum inferius)** limited inferiorly by the thoracic diaphragm.

— The inferior mediastinum is further divided into
  • the **anterior mediastinum (mediastinum anterius),** a narrow space posterior to the sternum and anterior to the pericardium;
  • the **middle mediastinum (mediastinum medium),** the largest section of the inferior mediastinum, which contains the pericardium, heart, and major vessels; and
  • the **posterior mediastinum (mediastinum posterius),** a small area posterior to the pericardium and anterior to the 5th through 12th thoracic vertebrae.

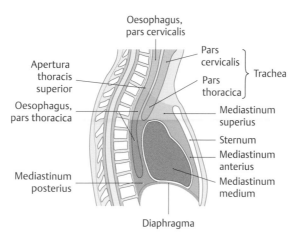

Table 7.1 Contents of the Mediastinum
(From Schuenke M, Schulte E, Schumacher U. THIEME Atlas of Anatomy, Vol 2. Illustrations by Voll M and Wesker K. 3rd ed. New York: Thieme Publishers; 2020.)

| | Mediastinum superius ○ | Mediastinum inferius | | |
		Mediastinum anterius ○	Mediastinum medium ◉	Mediastinum posterius ◉
Organs	• Thymus • Trachea • Oesophagus	• Thymus, inferior aspects (especially in children)	• Cor • Pericardium	• Oesophagus
Arteries	• Arcus aortae • Truncus brachiocephalicus • A. carotis communis sinister • A. subclavia sinister	• Smaller vessels	• Aortae ascendens • Truncus pulmonalis and its branches • Aa. pericardiacophrenicae	• Aorta thoracica and branches
Veins and vasa lymphatica	• V. cava superior • Vv. brachiocephalicae • Ductus thoracicus and ductus lymphaticus dexter	• Smaller veins and vasa lymphatica • Smaller nodi lymphoidei	• V. cava inferior • V. azygos • Vv. pulmonales • Vv. pericardiacophrenicae	• V. azygos • V. hemiazygos • Ductus thoracicus
Nerves	• Nn. vagi • N. laryngeus recurrens sinister • Nn. cardiaci • Nn. phrenici	• None	• Nn. phrenici	• Nn. vagi

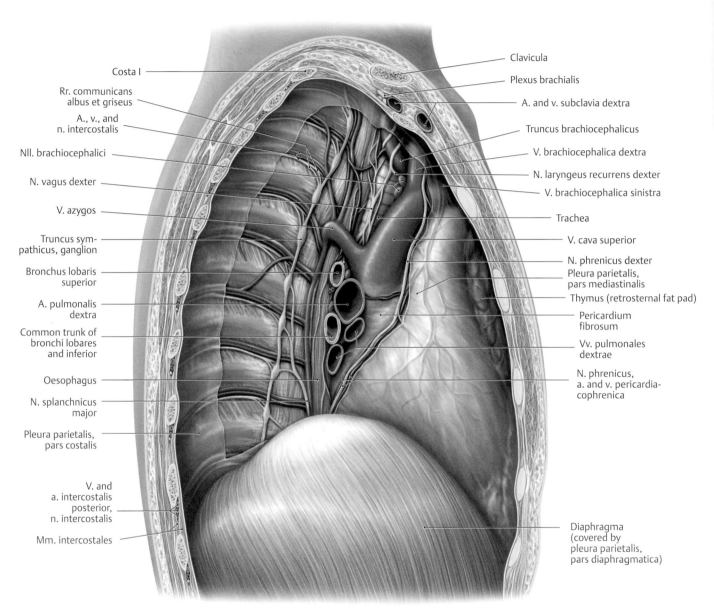

Costa I

Rr. communicans
albus et griseus

A., v., and
n. intercostalis

Nll. brachiocephalici

N. vagus dexter

V. azygos

Truncus sym-
pathicus, ganglion

Bronchus lobaris
superior

A. pulmonalis
dextra

Common trunk of
bronchi lobares
and inferior

Oesophagus

N. splanchnicus
major

Pleura parietalis,
pars costalis

V. and
a. intercostalis
posterior,
n. intercostalis

Mm. intercostales

Clavicula

Plexus brachialis

A. and v. subclavia dextra

Truncus brachiocephalicus

V. brachiocephalica dextra

N. laryngeus recurrens dexter

V. brachiocephalica sinistra

Trachea

V. cava superior

N. phrenicus dexter

Pleura parietalis,
pars mediastinalis

Thymus (retrosternal fat pad)

Pericardium
fibrosum

Vv. pulmonales
dextrae

N. phrenicus,
a. and v. pericardia-
cophrenica

Diaphragma
(covered by
pleura parietalis,
pars diaphragmatica)

A Parasagittal section, right lateral view. Note the many structures passing between the mediastinum superius and mediastinum inferius.

Fig. 7.2 Mediastinum
Divisions of the mediastinum. (From Schuenke M, Schulte E, Schumacher U. THIEME Atlas of Anatomy, Vol 2. Illustrations by Voll M and Wesker K. 3rd ed. New York: Thieme Publishers; 2020.)

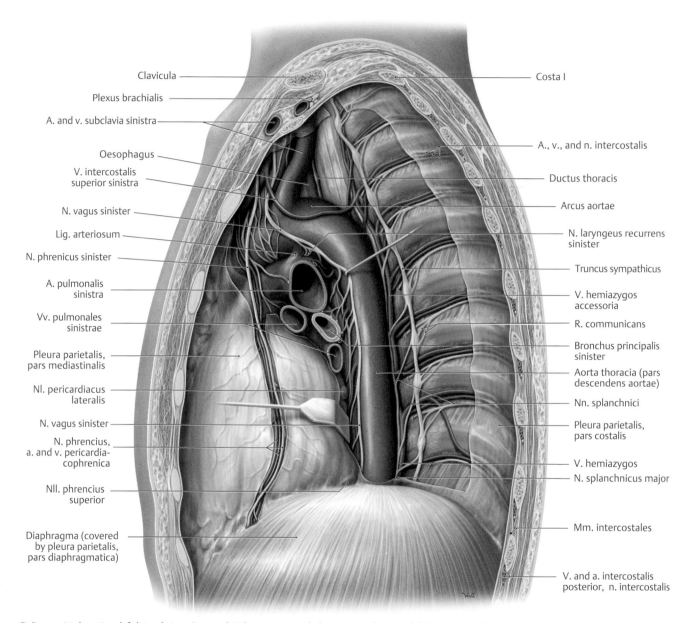

Clavicula — Costa I

Plexus brachialis —

A. and v. subclavia sinistra —

— A., v., and n. intercostalis

Oesophagus —

V. intercostalis — Ductus thoracis
superior sinistra

— Arcus aortae

N. vagus sinister —

— N. laryngeus recurrens
sinister

Lig. arteriosum —

N. phrenicus sinister — — Truncus sympathicus

A. pulmonalis — V. hemiazygos
sinistra accessoria

Vv. pulmonales — — R. communicans
sinistrae

Pleura parietalis, — — Bronchus principalis
pars mediastinalis sinister

Nl. pericardiacus — — Aorta thoracica (pars
lateralis descendens aortae)

N. vagus sinister — — Nn. splanchnici

N. phrencius, — Pleura parietalis,
a. and v. pericardia- pars costalis
cophrenica

Nll. phrencius — — V. hemiazygos
superior — N. splanchnicus major

Diaphragma (covered — — Mm. intercostales
by pleura parietalis,
pars diaphragmatica)

— V. and a. intercostalis
posterior, n. intercostalis

B Parasagittal section, left lateral view. *Removed:* Pulmo sinister and pleura parietalis. *Revealed:* Posterior mediastinal structures.

Fig. 7.2 (*continued*) **Mediastinum**

(From Gilroy AM et al. Atlas of Anatomy. 4th ed. 2020. Based on: Schuenke M, Schulte E, Schumacher U. THIEME Atlas of Anatomy. Internal Organs. Illustrations by Voll M and Wesker K. 3rd ed. New York: Thieme Medical Publishers; 2020.)

7.2   Mediastinum Anterior

Thymus

The thymus is a gland of the immune system, responsible for maturation of T-lymphocytes (**Fig. 7.3**).

— In childhood, the thymus presents as a large bilobed organ that overlies the heart and great vessels in the superior and anterior mediastinum.
— At puberty, high levels of circulating sex hormones cause the gland to atrophy.

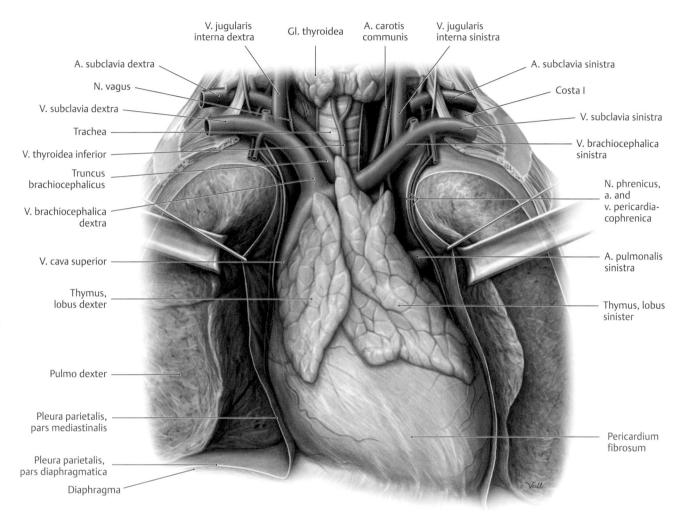

A Anterior view of the mediastinum of a 2-year-old child.

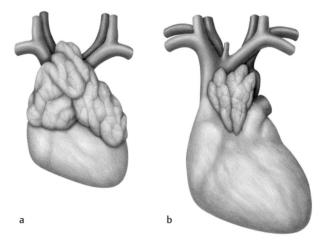

B Size of the thymus in newborns (a) and in adults (b).

Fig. 7.3 The thymus in newborns and adults
The thymus of newborns is much larger than those of adults and extends inferiorly into the anterior part of the mediastinum inferius. Because it atrophies during puberty, the thymus in adults is small and extends only into the mediastinum superius. (From Schuenke M, Schulte E, Schumacher U. THIEME Atlas of Anatomy, Vol 2. Illustrations by Voll M and Wesker K. 3rd ed. New York: Thieme Publishers; 2020.)

7.3 Mediastinum Medius: Pericardium and Cavitas Pericardiaca

Pericardium

The **pericardium**, a double-layered fibroserous membrane, forms the **pericardial sac** that surrounds the heart and the origins of the great vessels (**Figs. 7.4** and **7.5**).

— The pericardium is composed of two layers: an outer fibrous layer and an inner serous layer.

1. The outer **pericardium fibrosum** is composed of tough inelastic connective tissue. It is attached inferiorly to the diaphragma and is continuous superiorly with the tunica adventitia (outer layer) of the great vessels.

2. The thin **pericardium serosum** consists of parietal and visceral layers.

   ○ The **lamina parietalis** of the **pericardium serosum** lines the inner surface of the pericardium fibrosum.

   ○ The **lamina visceralis** of the **pericardium serosum** firmly adheres to the outer surface of the heart as the **epicardium**. This layer is continuous with the lamina parietalis of the pericardium serosum at the root of the great vessels.

— **Aa. pericardiacophrenicae**, branches of the aa. thoracicae internae, provide the main blood supply to the pericardium. Veins that accompany the arteries drain into the v. cava superior.

— The n. vagus (CN X) and n. phrenicus (C3–C5) and branches from the trunci sympathici innervate the pericardium.

— Pericardial pain is often referred via the n. phrenicus to the skin of the ipsilateral supraclavicular region (dermatomes C3–C5).

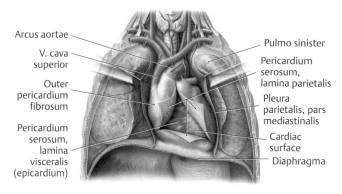

Fig. 7.4 Pericardium
Anterior view of opened thorax. *Removed:* Thymus. *Reflected:* Flaps of the pericardium fibrosum. (From Gilroy AM et al. Atlas of Anatomy. 4th ed. 2020. Based on: Schuenke M, Schulte E, Schumacher U. THIEME Atlas of Anatomy. Internal Organs. Illustrations by Voll M and Wesker K. 3rd ed. New York: Thieme Medical Publishers; 2020.)

BOX 7.1: CLINICAL CORRELATION

PERICARDITIS

Pericarditis is an inflammation of the pericardium, which causes sharp, retrosternal or epigastric pain and a characteristic pericardial friction rub (a sound like the rustle of silk) that is heard on auscultation. This is caused by friction from the roughened layers of the inflamed pericardium rubbing together. Pericarditis can lead to pericardial effusion (fluid in the cavitas pericardiaca) or cardiac tamponade (abnormal accumulation of fluid in the cavitas pericardiaca that prevents venous return to the heart) and may be accompanied by dyspnea (shortness of breath) and peripheral edema (swelling).

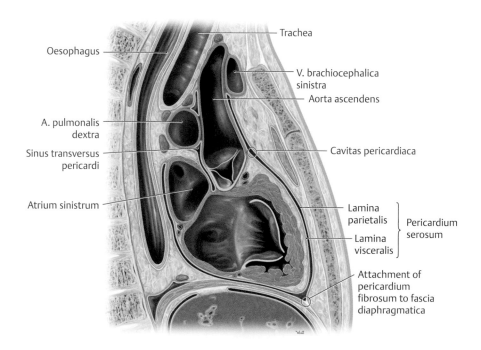

Fig. 7.5 Reflection of pericardium serosum
Sagittal section through the mediastinum. Note the continuity of the pericardium serosum lamina parietalis and pericardium serosum lamina visceralis.
(From Schuenke M, Schulte E, Schumacher U. THIEME Atlas of Anatomy, Vol 2. Illustrations by Voll M and Wesker K. 3rd ed. New York: Thieme Publishers; 2020.)

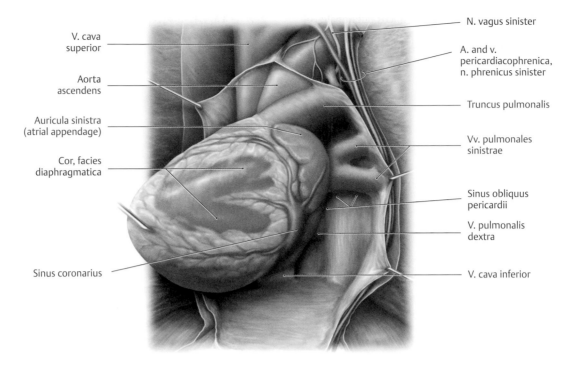

Fig. 7.6 Cavitas pericardiaca posterior
Anterior view. The cor has been elevated to partially visualize the cavitas pericardiaca posterior and the sinus obliquus pericardii. (From Gilroy AM et al. Atlas of Anatomy. 4th ed. 2020. Based on: Schuenke M, Schulte E, Schumacher U. THIEME Atlas of Anatomy. Internal Organs. Illustrations by Voll M and Wesker K. 3rd ed. New York: Thieme Medical Publishers; 2020.)

The Cavitas Pericardiaca

The **cavitas pericardiaca** is the space within the pericardial sac between the lamina parietalis and lamina visceralis of the pericardium serosum (**Figs. 7.6** and **7.7**).

— The cavitas pericardiaca is filled with a thin layer of serous fluid that allows for frictionless movement of the heart.
— Two pericardial recesses form where the pericardium serosum reflects around the roots of the great vessels:
   1. The **sinus transversus pericardii** is a passage between the inflow channels (v. cava superior and vv. pulmonales) and

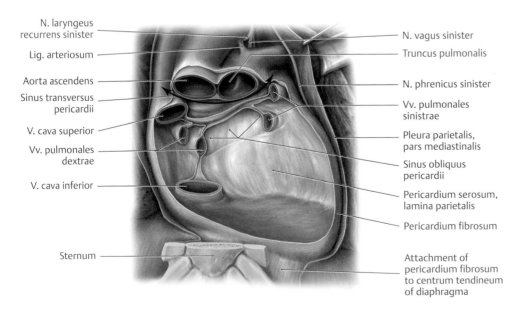

Fig. 7.7 Pericardial recesses
Posterior pericardium, anterior view. *Removed:* Anterior pericardium and cor. *Revealed:* The posterior pericardium and the sinus obliquus pericardii. The *double-headed arrow* indicates the course of the sinus transversus pericardii, the passage between the reflections of the pericardium serosum around the arterial and venous great vessels of the cor. (From Schuenke M, Schulte E, Schumacher U. THIEME Atlas of Anatomy, Vol 2. Illustrations by Voll M and Wesker K. 3rd ed. New York: Thieme Publishers; 2020.)

the outflow channels (aorta and truncus pulmonalis) of the heart.

2. The **sinus obliquus pericardii** is a recess of the cavitas pericardiaca posterior to the heart between the v. pulmonalis dextra and v. pulmonalis sinistra.

BOX 7.3: CLINICAL CORRELATION

SURGICAL SIGNIFICANCE OF THE SINUS TRANSVERSUS PERICARDII
During cardiac surgery, the surgeon is able to isolate (and clamp) the cardiac outflow tracts, the aorta and truncus pulmonalis, from the cardiac inflow tracts, the v. cava superior and vv. pulmonales, by passing the clamps through the sinus transversus pericardii.

7.4 Mediastinum Medius: The Heart

General Features

— The heart is a hollow muscular organ located in the mediastinum medius within the pericardial sac. It rests on the centrum tendineum of the diaphragm and is flanked on either side by the right and left cavitas pleuralis (**Fig. 7.8**).

— The heart has a conical shape. The **base (basis cordis)**, anchored by the great vessels, is on its superior and posterior surfaces. The **apex (apex cordis)**, located approximately at the 5th spatium intercostale, projects anteriorly, inferiorly, and to the left and moves freely within the pericardial sac.

— Internally, the heart is divided into four chambers: the atrium dextrum, atrium sinistrum, ventriculus dexter, and ventriculus sinister.

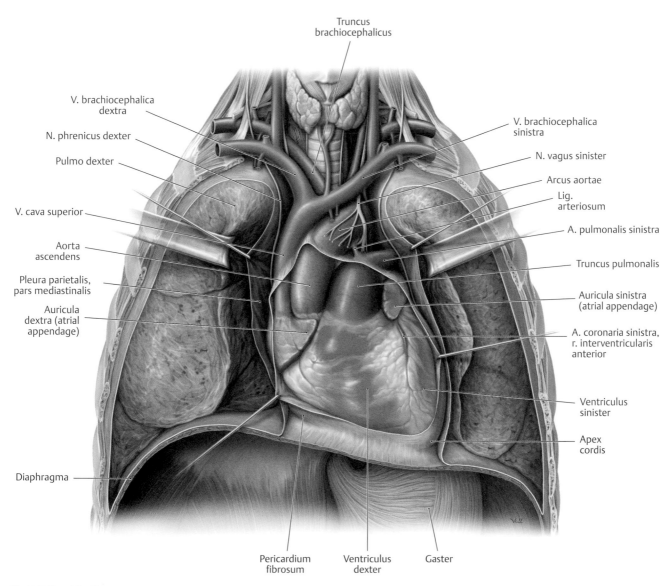

Fig. 7.8 Heart in situ
Anterior view of the opened thorax. *Removed:* Thymus and anterior pericardium. *Revealed:* Heart. (From Schuenke M, Schulte E, Schumacher U. THIEME Atlas of Anatomy, Vol 2. Illustrations by Voll M and Wesker K. 3rd ed. New York: Thieme Publishers; 2020.)

- The atrium dextrum and atrium sinistrum, separated by a **septum interatriale**, are the inflow chambers of the heart, receiving blood from the systemic circulation on the right and pulmonary circulation on the left.
- The ventriculus dexter and ventriculus sinister, separated by a **septum interventriculare**, are the outflow chambers of the heart. Blood flows from the ventriculus dexter into the pulmonary circulation and from the ventriculus sinister into the systemic circulation.
— Two small appendages, the **auricula dextra** and **auricula sinistra,** are extensions of the atria and are visible externally.
— The surfaces of the heart **(Fig. 7.9)** are
  - the **facies sternocostalis** on the anterior side of the heart, formed mostly by the ventriculus dexter with portions of the atrium dextrum and ventriculus sinister;
  - the **basis cordis** on the posterior and superior sides of the heart, formed by the atrium sinistrum and a portion of the atrium dextrum; and
  - the **facies diaphragmatica** on the inferior side of the heart, formed by the ventriculus dexter and ventriculus sinister.
— The borders of the heart define the cardiac shadow that is seen on radiographic images **(Table 7.2)**.
— Three grooves on the external surface of the heart can be used to determine the position of the chambers:

1. The **sulcus coronarius** encircles the heart between the atria and ventricles. Because the heart has an oblique orientation, the sulcus is nearly vertical.
2. The **sulcus interventricularis anterior** is a longitudinal groove on the anterior surface of the heart that marks the position of the septum interventriculare.
3. The **posterior interventricular sulcus** (sulcus interventricularis posterior) is a longitudinal groove on the diaphragmatic surface of the heart that marks the position of the septum interventriculare.
— The **crux cordis** is a point on the posterior surface of the heart where the sulcus coronarius and sulcus interventricularis posterior meet. It marks the junction of the four chambers of the heart.
— The wall of the heart consists of three layers:
1. The **epicardium,** the thin outermost layer, formed by the lamina visceralis of the pericardium serosum
2. The **myocardium,** the thick layer of cardiac muscle, thickest in the walls of the ventricles
3. The **endocardium,** the thin internal layer, which lines the chambers and valves of the heart
— A **cardiac skeleton** of dense fibrous connective tissue forms four **fibrous anuli** (rings) and intervening **trigona** that separate the chambers of the heart, provide anchoring points for cardiac muscle fibers and cardiac valves, and insulate electrical impulses of the heart's conduction system **(Fig. 7.10)**.

Table 7.2 Borders of the Heart

Border	Defining Structures
Right cardiac border	• Atrium dextrum
	• V. cava superior
Apex	• Ventriculus sinister
Left cardiac border	• Arcus aortae ("aortic knob")
	• Truncus pulmonalis
	• Atrium sinistrum
	• Ventriculus sinister
Inferior cardiac border	• Ventriculus sinister
	• Ventriculus dexter

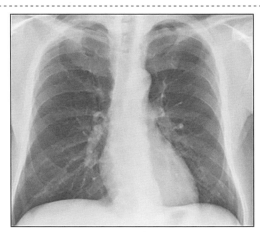

Radiographic appearance of the heart
(From Gunderman R. Essential Radiology, 3rd ed. New York: Thieme Publishers; 2014.)

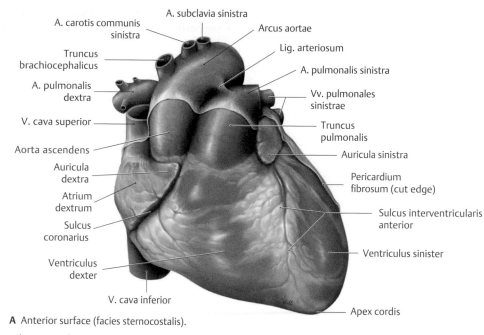

A. carotis communis sinistra

A. subclavia sinistra

Arcus aortae

Truncus brachiocephalicus

Lig. arteriosum

A. pulmonalis dextra

A. pulmonalis sinistra

V. cava superior

Vv. pulmonales sinistrae

Aorta ascendens

Truncus pulmonalis

Auricula dextra

Auricula sinistra

Atrium dextrum

Pericardium fibrosum (cut edge)

Sulcus coronarius

Sulcus interventricularis anterior

Ventriculus dexter

Ventriculus sinister

V. cava inferior

Apex cordis

A Anterior surface (facies sternocostalis).

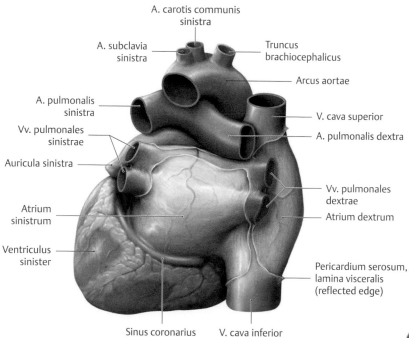

A. carotis communis sinistra

A. subclavia sinistra

Truncus brachiocephalicus

Arcus aortae

A. pulmonalis sinistra

Vv. pulmonales sinistrae

V. cava superior

A. pulmonalis dextra

Auricula sinistra

Atrium sinistrum

Vv. pulmonales dextrae

Ventriculus sinister

Atrium dextrum

Pericardium serosum, lamina visceralis (reflected edge)

Sinus coronarius

V. cava inferior

B Posterior surface (basis cordis).

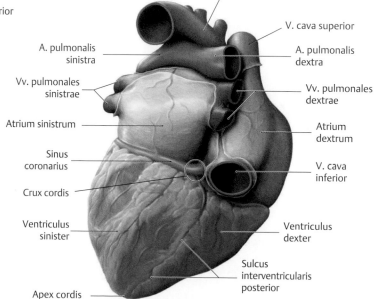

Arcus aortae

V. cava superior

A. pulmonalis sinistra

A. pulmonalis dextra

Vv. pulmonales sinistrae

Vv. pulmonales dextrae

Atrium sinistrum

Atrium dextrum

Sinus coronarius

V. cava inferior

Crux cordis

Ventriculus sinister

Ventriculus dexter

Apex cordis

Sulcus interventricularis posterior

C Inferior surface (facies diaphragmatica).

Fig. 7.9 Surfaces of the heart
The heart has three surfaces: anterior (facies sternocostalis),
posterior (basis cordis), and inferior (facies diaphragmatica).
(From Schuenke M, Schulte E, Schumacher U. THIEME Atlas of
Anatomy, Vol 2. Illustrations by Voll M and Wesker K. 3rd ed.
New York: Thieme Publishers; 2020.)

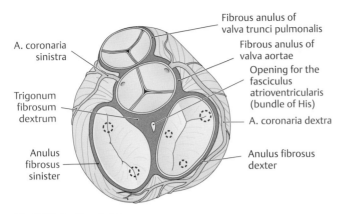

Fig. 7.10 Cardiac skeleton
Superior view. *Red dotted circles* indicate attachment sites of mm. papillares on valves. (From Schuenke M, Schulte E, Schumacher U. THIEME Atlas of Anatomy, Vol 2. Illustrations by Voll M and Wesker K. 3rd ed. New York: Thieme Publishers; 2020.)

The Atria (Figs. 7.11 and 7.12)

The **atria** are the thin-walled inflow chambers of the heart.
— The atrium dextrum receives the v. cava superior and v. cava inferior from the systemic circulation and the vv. cardiacae from the heart. The atrium sinistrum receives the vv. pulmonales from the lungs.
— Each atrium is associated with an auricula, a small pouch that expands the capacity of the atrium and whose roughened walls contain mm. pectinati.
— A depression on the right ride of the septum interatriale, the **oval fossa** (fossa ovalis), is a remnant of the **oval foramen** (foramen ovale), an opening through which blood was shunted from the atrium dextrum to atrium sinistrum in the prenatal circulation.
— The atrium dextrum is divided into two parts by a muscular ridge, the **terminal crest** (crista terminalis). The ridge is evident on the outside of the heart as the **terminal sulcus** (sulcus terminalis)**.** The two parts of the atrium dextrum are

1. the **venous sinus** (sinus venarum), a smooth-walled region on the posterior wall that contains the openings of the v. cava superior, v. cava inferior, sinus coronarius, and vv. cardiacae anteriores; and
2. the **atrium proper,** the anterior muscular portion that, like the auricula dextra, contains mm. pectinati.
— The atrium sinistrum is smaller but thicker walled than the atrium dextrum and receives the four to five vv. pulmonales from the lungs. The atrial walls are smooth, with the mm. pectinati confined to the auricula sinistra.

The Ventricles (Ventriculi) (Figs. 7.11 and 7.12)

The ventricles (ventriculi) are thick-walled chambers that connect to the outflow channels of the heart: the ventriculus dexter to the a. pulmonalis and the ventriculus sinister to the aorta.
— The walls of the ventricles are marked with a meshwork of thick muscular ridges known as **trabeculae carneae.**
— Most of the septum interventriculare is muscular, but there is a small membranous part at the superior end that is a common site of septal defects.
— The ventriculus dexter is the smaller and thinner walled of the two ventricles. A muscular ridge, the **supraventricular crest** (crista supraventricularis), separates it into two parts:
1. The **ventriculus dexter proper**, the inflow portion of the ventricle that receives blood from the atrium dextrum
   ○ An **m. papillaris anterior** and **m. papillaris posterior** arise from its floor, and a **m. papillaris septalis** arises from the septum interventriculare.
   ○ A muscular **septomarginal trabecula** (trabecula septomarginalis) or **moderator band** extends from the septum to the base of the m. papillaris anterior and carries a part of the electrical conduction system (the right branch of the atrioventricular bundle) that facilitates the coordinated contraction of the m. papillaris.
2. The **conus arteriosus** (infundibulum), the smooth-walled outflow channel through which blood flows into the truncus pulmonalis

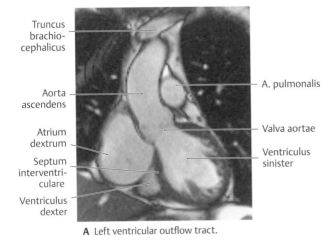

A Left ventricular outflow tract.

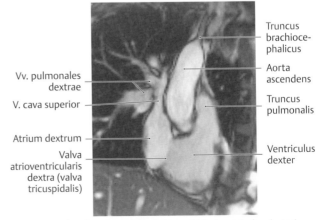

B Two chamber view of the right ventricle (ventriculus dexter).

Fig. 7.11 MRI of the heart
(From Moeller TB, Reif E. Pocket Atlas of Sectional Anatomy, Vol 2, 3rd ed. New York: Thieme; 2007.)

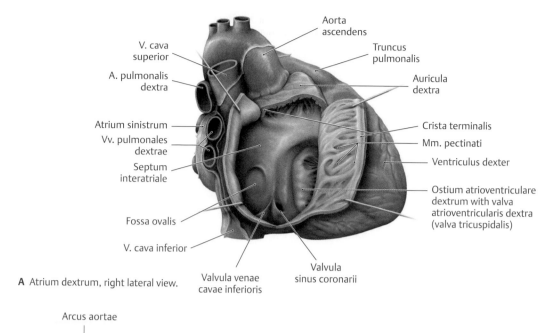

Aorta
ascendens

V. cava
superior

A. pulmonalis
dextra

Truncus
pulmonalis

Auricula
dextra

Atrium sinistrum

Vv. pulmonales
dextrae

Septum
interatriale

Crista terminalis

Mm. pectinati

Ventriculus dexter

Ostium atrioventriculare
dextrum with valva
atrioventricularis dextra
(valva tricuspidalis)

Fossa ovalis

V. cava inferior

Valvula venae
cavae inferioris

Valvula
sinus coronarii

A Atrium dextrum, right lateral view.

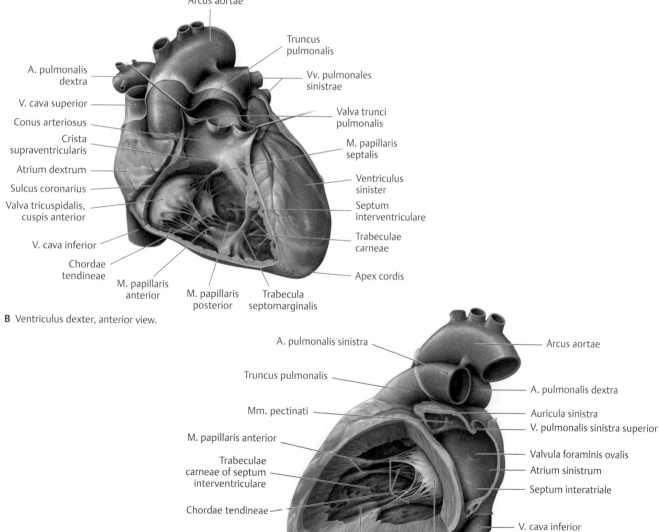

Arcus aortae

Truncus
pulmonalis

A. pulmonalis
dextra

Vv. pulmonales
sinistrae

V. cava superior

Conus arteriosus

Crista
supraventricularis

Atrium dextrum

Sulcus coronarius

Valva tricuspidalis,
cuspis anterior

V. cava inferior

Chordae
tendineae

M. papillaris
anterior

M. papillaris
posterior

Trabecula
septomarginalis

Valva trunci
pulmonalis

M. papillaris
septalis

Ventriculus
sinister

Septum
interventriculare

Trabeculae
carneae

Apex cordis

B Ventriculus dexter, anterior view.

A. pulmonalis sinistra

Truncus pulmonalis

Mm. pectinati

M. papillaris anterior

Trabeculae
carneae of septum
interventriculare

Chordae tendineae

Apex cordis

M. papillaris
posterior

Valva mitralis
(valva atrioventricularis sinistra)

Arcus aortae

A. pulmonalis dextra

Auricula sinistra

V. pulmonalis sinistra superior

Valvula foraminis ovalis

Atrium sinistrum

Septum interatriale

V. cava inferior

Fig. 7.12 Chambers of the heart
(From Schuenke M, Schulte E,
Schumacher U. THIEME Atlas of
Anatomy, Vol 2. Illustrations by Voll M
and Wesker K. 3rd ed. New York:
Thieme Publishers; 2020.)

C Atrium sinistrum and ventriculus sinister, left lateral view. Note the irregular trabeculae carneae characteristic of the ventricular wall.

— The ventriculus sinister, which includes the apex of the heart, is the thickest-walled chamber of the heart. Similar to the ventriculus dexter, the ventriculus sinister is divided into inflow and outflow portions:
1. The **ventriculus sinister proper,** which receives blood from the atrium sinistrum. A large m. papillaris anterior and small m. papillaris posterior arise from its floor
2. The **vestibulum aortae,** the smooth-walled outflow channel through which blood flows into the aorta

---

BOX 7.4: DEVELOPMENTAL CORRELATION

TETRALOGY OF FALLOT
Tetralogy of Fallot is a rare combination of four congenital cardiac defects: pulmonary stenosis, overriding aorta, ventricular septal defect (VSD), and right ventricular hypertrophy. Symptoms include cyanosis, dyspnea (shortness of breath), fainting, finger clubbing, fatigue, and prolonged crying in infants.

Valves of the Heart

There are two types of cardiac valves: atrioventricular and semilunar (**Fig. 7.13**).
1. **Atrioventricular valves** separate the atria from the ventricles and prevent regurgitation of blood into the atria during contraction of the ventricles.
   • The atrioventricular valves are made up of cusps, thin leaflets with free inner margins and outer margins that are attached to the fibrous rings of the cardiac skeleton.
   • Slender threads called **tendinous cords** (chordae tendineae) attach the free edges of the valve leaflets to the mm. papillares in the ventricles. These cords maintain closure of the valves and prevent regurgitation of blood during ventricular contraction. Each cusp attaches to tendinous cords from more than one mm. papillares.

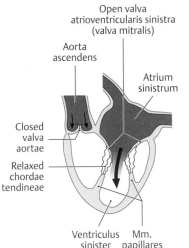

A Blood flow through the left side of the heart during ventricular diastole (relaxation of the ventriculi), anterior view. *Closed:* Valva aortae and valva trunci pulmonalis. *Open:* Valvae atrioventriculares.

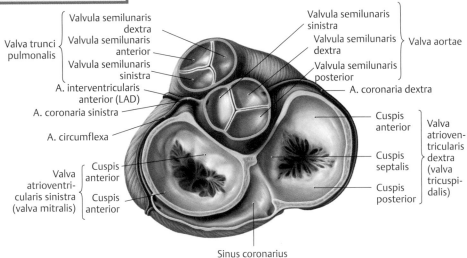

B Superior view of cardiac valves during ventricular diastole. *Closed:* Valva aortae and valva trunci pulmonalis. *Open:* Valvae atrioventriculares. *Removed:* Atria and great arteries.

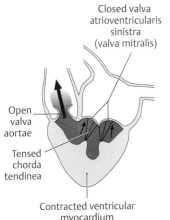

C Blood flow through the left side of the heart during ventricular systole (contraction of the ventriculi). *Closed:* Valvae atrioventriculares. *Open:* Valva aortae and valva trunci pulmonalis.

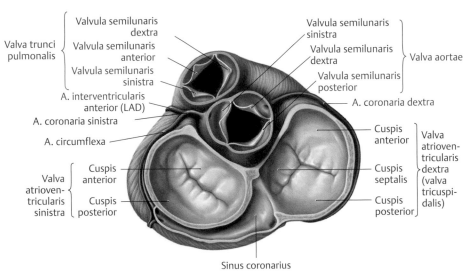

D Superior view of cardiac valves during ventricular systole. *Closed:* Valvae atrioventriculares. *Open:* Valva aortae and valva trunci pulmonalis. *Removed:* Atria and great arteries.

Fig. 7.13 Cardiac valves
(From Gilroy AM et al. Atlas of Anatomy. 4th ed. 2020. Based on: Schuenke M, Schulte E, Schumacher U. THIEME Atlas of Anatomy. Internal Organs. Illustrations by Voll M and Wesker K. 3rd ed. New York: Thieme Medical Publishers; 2020.)

- The atrioventricular valves include
  - the **valva tricuspidalis**, which separates the atrium dextrum from the ventriculus dexter and is composed of a cuspis anterior, cuspis posterior, and cuspis septalis; and
  - the **valva mitralis**, which separates the atrium sinistrum from the ventriculus sinister and is composed of cuspis anterior and cuspis posterior. The cuspis anterior is immediately adjacent to, and continuous with, the wall of the aorta.

BOX 7.5: CLINICAL CORRELATION

MITRAL VALVE PROLAPSE
Mitral valve prolapse is a condition in which one or both leaflets of the valva mitralis prolapse (evert) into the atrium sinistrum, allowing regurgitation of blood through the valva mitralis during systole. This condition is usually asymptomatic but is noted by a midsystolic click (valve prolapsing) and murmur (regurgitation).

---

2. **Semilunar valves** prevent outflow from the ventricles as the chambers fill and backflow of blood into the ventricles after it has been expelled.
   - Each valve is composed of three valvulae semilunares with free inner margins and attached outer margins. A **sinus,** or pocket, is created between each valvula and the vessel wall. The thickened free margin of the valvula, the **lunula**, is the point of contact of the valvulae. A **nodulus** marks the center of the lunula.
   - The semilunar valves include the following:
     - The **pulmonary semilunar valve (valva trunci pulmonalis),** is located in the truncus pulmonalis at the top of the conus arteriosus, where it moderates blood flow through the right ventricular outflow channel. Its valvulae are in the anterior, right, and left positions.
     - The **aortic semilunar valve (valva aortae)** is located within the aorta immediately adjacent to the valva mitralis, where it moderates blood flow through the left ventricular outflow channel. Its valvulae are in the posterior, right, and left positions. The aa. coronariae arise from the sinuses above the valvulae.

BOX 7.6: CLINICAL CORRELATION

AORTIC VALVE STENOSIS
Stenosis of the valva aortae is the most common valve abnormality. Calcifications of the valve leaflets narrow the outflow tract and lead to overload of the ventriculus sinister, resulting in left ventricular hypertrophy.

Heart Sounds and Auscultation Sites

When the heart valves close, they produce characteristic sounds described as "lub dub."
- Closure of the valva tricuspidalis and valva mitralis during contraction of the ventricles produces the first sound ("lub").
- Closure of the valva trunci pulmonalis and valva aortae as the ventricles relax produces the second sound ("dub").
- The sounds, carried by the blood as it flows into the next vessel or chamber, are best distinguished at **auscultation sites** downstream from the valves (**Table 7.3**).

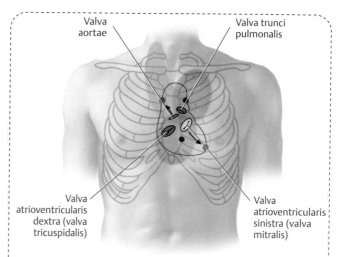

Table 7.3 Position and Auscultation Sites of Cardiac Valves
(From Schuenke M, Schulte E, Schumacher U. THIEME Atlas of Anatomy, Vol 2. Illustrations by Voll M and Wesker K. 3rd ed. New York: Thieme Publishers; 2020.)

Valve	Anatomical Projection	Auscultation Site
Valva aortae	Left sternal border (at level of costa III)	Right 2nd spatium intercostale (at sternal margin)
Valva trunci pulmonalis	Left sternal border (at level of 3rd cartilago costalis)	Left 2nd spatium intercostale (at sternal margin)
Valva atrioventricularis sinistra (valva mitralis)	Left 4th/5th cartilago costalis	Left 5th spatium intercostale (at linea medioclavicularis) or apex cordis
Valva atrioventricularis dextra (valva tricuspidalis)	Sternum (at level of 5th cartilago costalis)	Left 5th spatium intercostale (at sternal margin)

Note: Auscultation sites of the cardiac valves, indicated by *colored dots.* Valvular heart disease causes turbulent blood flow through a valve; this produces a murmur that may be detected in the *colored region* around the valve.

Conduction System of the Heart (Fig. 7.14)

The conduction system of the heart generates and transmits impulses that modulate the contraction of the cardiac muscle. It consists of nodes, which initiate the impulses, and conducting fibers, which distribute the impulses to cardiac muscle to effect a coordinated contraction of the heart chambers.
- The **sinoatrial (SA) node (nodus sinuatrialis),** the pacemaker of the heart, initiates and coordinates the timing of the contraction of the heart chambers.
  - At a frequency of 60 to 70 beats per minute, the SA node transmits impulses to both atria and to the nodus atrioventricularis.
  - It is subepicardial, located on the external surface of the heart, just within the myocardium of the atrium dextrum at the junction with the v. cava superior.
  - A branch of the a. coronaria dextra usually supplies the SA node.

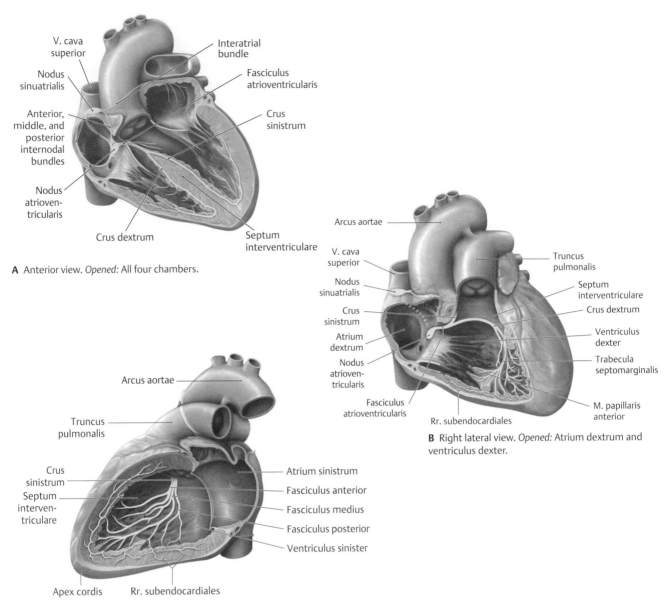

A Anterior view. *Opened:* All four chambers.

B Right lateral view. *Opened:* Atrium dextrum and ventriculus dexter.

C Left lateral view. *Opened:* Atrium sinistrum and ventriculus sinister.

Fig. 7.14 Cardiac conduction system
(From Schuenke M, Schulte E, Schumacher U. THIEME Atlas of Anatomy, Vol 2. Illustrations by Voll M and Wesker K. 3rd ed. New York: Thieme Publishers; 2020.)

— The **atrioventricular (AV) node (nodus atrioventricularis)** is stimulated by the SA node and transmits impulses to the AV bundle (fasciculus atrioventricularis).
  • It is subendocardial, located at the base of the septum interatriale above the cuspis septalis of the valva tricuspidalis.
  • The AV nodal artery, a branch of the a. coronaria dextra, arises near the origin of the r. interventricularis posterior at the crux of the heart.
— The **atrioventricular (AV) bundle (fasciculus atrioventricularis**, or **bundle of His)** arises from cells of the nodus atrioventricularis and transmits impulses to the walls of the ventricles.
  • It runs first along the membranous part of the septum interventriculare and then divides into a **crus dextrum** and **crus sinistrum** that descend to the apex on either side of the muscular part of the septum.

BOX 7.7: CLINICAL CORRELATION

ATRIOVENTRICULAR HEART BLOCK
AV heart block is a partial or complete blockage of the conduction of electrical impulses between the atria and ventricles. This causes bradycardia (slow heartbeat) and arrhythmias (irregular heartbeat) and ultimately prevents the heart from effectively contracting and delivering blood to the body. Although heart block may be congenital, it is frequently the result of damage to the heart muscle after myocardial infarction (MI).

  • The bundle branches end as **Purkinje fibers,** modified cardiac fibers, which ascend within the muscular walls of the ventricles.

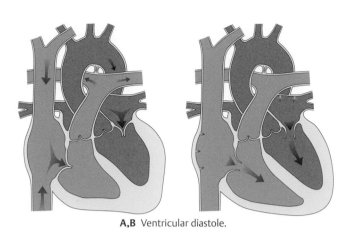

A,B Ventricular diastole.

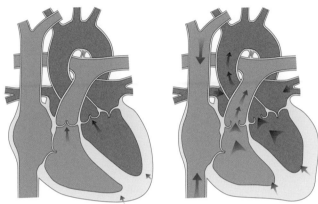

C,D Ventricular systole.

Fig. 7.15 The cardiac cycle
(From Schuenke M, Schulte E, Schumacher U. THIEME Atlas of Anatomy, Vol 2. Illustrations by Voll M and Wesker K. 3rd ed. New York: Thieme Publishers; 2020.)

The Cardiac Cycle

The heart's conduction system moderates the cardiac cycle, the coordinated **systole** (contraction) and **diastole** (relaxation) of the atria and ventricles. **Fig. 7.15** summarizes the sequence of events of the cycle.

1. In the initial phase of diastole, the atria and ventricles are relaxed, and the AV and semilunar valves are closed.
2. In late diastole, the atria fill, the AV valves open, and blood flows passively into the ventricles.
3. Stimulation from the SA node initiates the contraction of the atria, forcing the remaining atrial blood volume into the ventricles.
4. As pressure in the ventricles rises above that in the atria, the AV valves close.
5. Stimulation from the AV node and the AV bundles initiates contraction of the ventricles (ventricular systole).
6. Rising intraventricular pressure forces the semilunar valves to open. Blood is ejected from the ventriculus dexter into the truncus pulmonalis and from the ventriculus sinister into the aorta.
7. Relaxation of the ventricles (ventricular diastole) causes backward flow in the truncus pulmonalis and aorta and closure of the valva trunci pulmonalis and valva aortae.

7.5 Mediastinum Medius: Neurovasculature of the Heart

Aa. Coronariae (Figs. 7.16 and 7.17; Table 7.4)

The **a. coronaria dextra** and **a. coronaria sinistra** arise from the aorta ascendens just superior to the valvulae semilunaris dextra and valvulae semilunaris sinistra of the valva aortae. In the initial phase of ventricular diastole, the local surge in aortic pressure

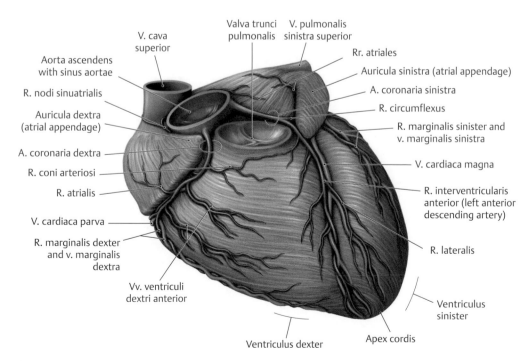

A Anterior view.

Fig. 7.16 Arteriae coronariae and venae cardiacae (*continued on page 110*)
(From Gilroy AM et al. Atlas of Anatomy. 4th ed. 2020. Based on: Schuenke M, Schulte E, Schumacher U. THIEME Atlas of Anatomy. Internal Organs. Illustrations by Voll M and Wesker K. 3rd ed. New York: Thieme Medical Publishers; 2020.)

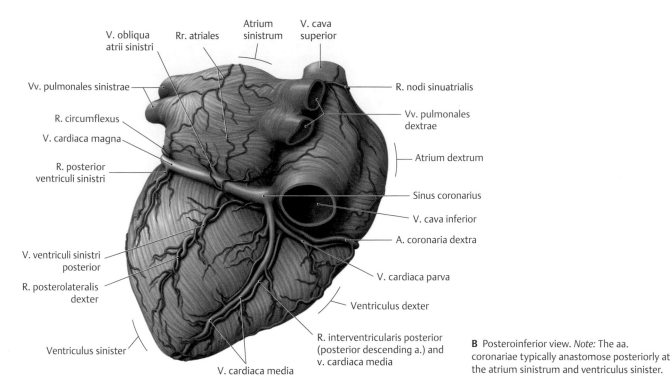

Fig. 7.16 (*continued*) **Arteriae coronariae and venae cardiacae**

B Posteroinferior view. *Note:* The aa. coronariae typically anastomose posteriorly at the atrium sinistrum and ventriculus sinister.

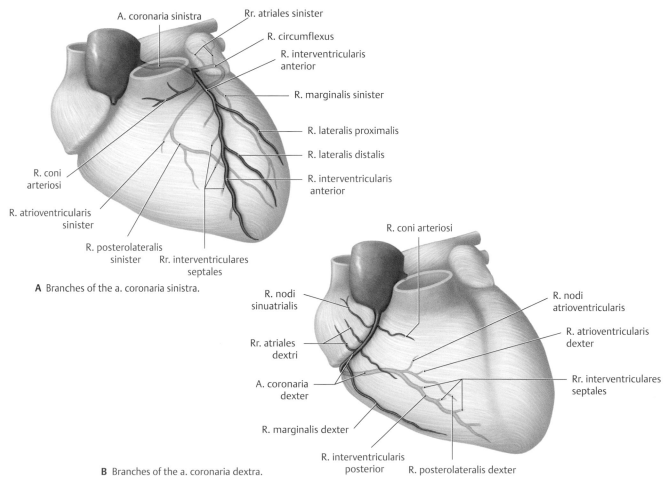

A Branches of the a. coronaria sinistra.

B Branches of the a. coronaria dextra.

Fig. 7.17 Classification of the arteriae coronariae
Anterior view, facies sternocostalis. (From Schuenke M, Schulte E, Schumacher U. THIEME Atlas of Anatomy, Vol 2. Illustrations by Voll M and Wesker K. 3rd ed. New York: Thieme Publishers; 2020.)

Table 7.4 Branches of the Arteriae Coronariae

A. coronaria dexter
— R. nodi sinuatrialis
— Rr. atriales dextri
— R. coni arteriosi dexter
— Rr. ventriculares anteriores
— R. marginalis dexter
— R. nodi atrioventricularis
— R. interventricularis posterior (a. descendens posterior)
— Rr. interventriculares septales

A. coronaria sinistra
— R. interventricularis anterior
  • R. coni arteriosi sinister
  • R. lateralis proximalis (r. diagonalis)
  • R. lateralis distalis (r. diagonalis)
  • Rr. interventriculares septales
— R. circumflexus
  • R. nodi sinuatrialis (in 40%)
  • Left rr. atriales
  • R. marginalis sinister
  • R. posterolateralis sinister
  • R. posterior interventriculi (in about one third of cases)

caused by the backflow closes the valva aortae and drives blood into the aa. coronariae. Blood flow in the arteries is greatest during diastole because of the compression of arteries within the myocardium during systole.

— The a. coronaria dextra and a. coronaria sinistra supply the myocardium and epicardium of the heart.
  • The **a. coronaria dextra** descends within the sulcus coronarius around the right side of the heart. Its major branches and their distribution are
    ○ the **r. nodi sinuatrialis**, which supplies the atrium dextrum and the SA node;
    ○ the **r. marginalis dexter,** which supplies the apex cordis and part of the ventriculus dexter;
    ○ the **r. interventricularis posterior,** which supplies the ventriculus dexter and ventriculus sinister and posterior third of the septum interventriculare and anastomoses with the r. interventricularis of the a. coronaria sinistra near the apex cordis on the facies diaphragmatica; and
    ○ the **AV nodal artery (r. nodi atrioventricularis),** which supplies the AV node.
  • The **a. coronaria sinistra,** typically larger than the a. coronaria dextra, arises from the aorta posterior to the truncus pulmonalis. After a short but variable course, it divides into two large branches, the **left anterior descending (LAD) artery (r. interventricularis anterior),** which descends sulcus interventricularis anterior, and the **r. circumflexus**, which runs around the left side of the heart in the sulcus coronarius. Their branches and distributions include
    ○ the r. interventricularis anterior, which supplies the anterior aspects of the ventriculus dexter and ventriculus sinister and the anterior two thirds of the septum interventriculare, including the AV bundle of the conducting system; and
    ○ the r. circumflexus, which supplies the atrium sinistrum and, via its **r. marginalis sinister**, the

ventriculus sinister. In ~ 40% of the population, an **SA nodal branch** arises to supply the SA node.

— Variation in the coronary circulation is common but the descriptive language is misleading. The word *dominant* refers not to the artery that supplies the greater volume of cardiac tissue (that is almost always the a. coronaria sinistra), but to the artery that gives rise to the r. interventricularis posterior.
  • A right dominant circulation occurs in about two thirds of the population. The r. interventricularis posterior arises from the a. coronaria dextra and supplies the posterior third of the septum interventriculare.
  • A small percentage of people exhibit left dominance in which the r. interventricularis posterior is a branch of the r. circumflexus. In these cases, the entire septum interventriculare and the AV node are supplied by the a. coronaria sinistra.
  • In the shared or "balanced" dominance, seen in a small group of people, branches from both aa. coronariae run in the sulcus interventricularis posterior and jointly supply the septum interventriculare.

BOX 7.8: CLINICAL CORRELATION

ANGINA

Angina (angina pectoris), a sudden, crushing substernal pain, is a result of myocardial ischemia (insufficient blood supply) caused by a narrowing of the aa. coronariae. Exercise following a heavy meal, stress, or even cold weather can trigger an episode. Although angina pain may be severe, it is relieved by a short rest and does not result in infarction of cardiac muscle.

BOX 7.9: CLINICAL CORRELATION

CORONARY ARTERY DISEASE

Coronary artery disease results in ischemia of the myocardium and is a leading cause of death in the United States. In atherosclerosis of the aa. coronariae, lipid deposits build up on the inner wall of the vessel and gradually narrow the lumen. In acute disease a fragment of plaque breaks off and completely obstructs the vessel. This creates a necrotic (dead) area of myocardium known as a myocardial infarction. Chronic disease is characterized by a gradual narrowing (stenosis) of the vessels. Overtime a collateral circulation develops that circumvents the narrowed segment and may prevent, or limit, damage from other ischemic events.

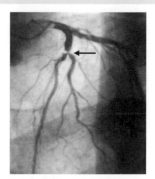

Severe stenosis *(arrow)* of the r. circumflexus
(From Claussen CD, et al. Pareto Reihe Radiologie. Herz/Pareto Series Radiology. Heart. Stuttgart: Thieme; 2007.)

BOX 7.10: CLINICAL CORRELATION

CORONARY ARTERY BYPASS GRAFT
Coronary artery bypass graft (CABG) is a surgical procedure performed to bypass atherosclerotic narrowings of the aa. coronariae that are the cause of anginal pain. If left untreated, these narrow-ings can eventually occlude the vessel and lead to myocardial infarction (MI). The a. thoracica interna and the v. saphena magna are most commonly used as the bypass vessel.

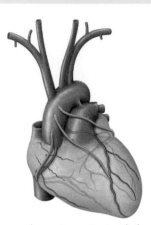

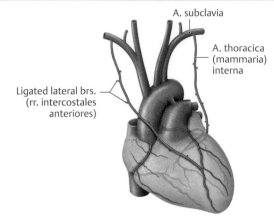

A Aortocoronary venous bypass in a patient with three-vessel disease. Venous grafts are anastomosed to the a. coronaria dextra, and to the rr. interventricularis anterior and circumflexus of the a. coronaria sinistra to bypass stenotic segments of the proximal parts of those vessels.

B Arterial IMA (internal mammary [thoracic] artery) bypass. The distal end of the aa. thoracicae internae are disconnected from their vascular bed and anastomosed to the poststenotic a. coronaria. This bypass method has a significantly lower incidence of long-term postsurgical occlusion and cardiac incidents than venous bypass surgery.

(From Schuenke M, Schulte E, Schumacher U. THIEME Atlas of Anatomy, Vol 2. Illustrations by Voll M and Wesker K. 3rd ed. New York: Thieme Publishers; 2020.)

Vv. Cardiacae (see Fig. 7.18)

— The **sinus coronarius,** which receives most of the venous return from the heart, runs in the sulcus coronarious posterior between the atrium sinistrum and ventriculus sinister. The **thebesian valve (valvula sinus coronarii)** guards the orifice of the sinus coronarius where it drains into the atrium dextrum near the opening of the v. cava inferior (**Figs. 7.9** and **7.12**).

— The large veins of the heart are tributaries of the sinus coronarius.
  • The **v. cardiaca magna** receives the v. interventricularis anterior, v. marginalis sinistra, and v. ventriculi sinistri posterior, which drain the atrium sinistrum and both ventricles.

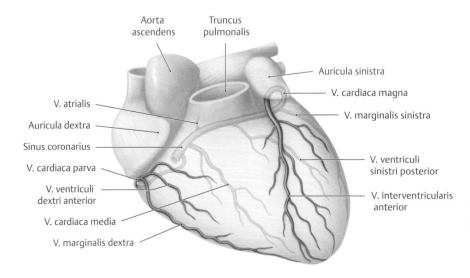

Fig. 7.18 Classification of venae cordis Anterior view, facies sternocostalis. (From Schuenke M, Schulte E, Schumacher U. THIEME Atlas of Anatomy, Vol 2. Illustrations by Voll M and Wesker K. 3rd ed. New York: Thieme Publishers; 2020.)

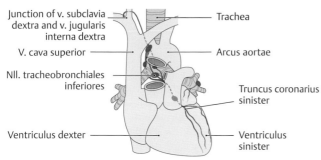

Junction of v. subclavia dextra and v. jugularis interna dextra

V. cava superior

Nll. tracheobronchiales inferiores

Ventriculus dexter

Trachea

Arcus aortae

Truncus coronarius sinister

Ventriculus sinister

A Lymphatic drainage of the left chambers, anterior view.

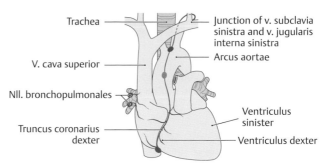

Trachea

V. cava superior

Nll. bronchopulmonales

Truncus coronarius dexter

Junction of v. subclavia sinistra and v. jugularis interna sinistra

Arcus aortae

Ventriculus sinister

Ventriculus dexter

B Lymphatic drainage of the right chambers, anterior view.

Fig. 7.19 Lymphatic drainage of the heart
A unique "crossed" drainage pattern exists in the heart: lymph from the atrium sinistrum and ventriculus sinister drains to the right venous junction, whereas lymph from the atrium dextrum and ventriculus dexter drains to the left venous junction. (From Schuenke M, Schulte E, Schumacher U. THIEME Atlas of Anatomy, Vol 2. Illustrations by Voll M and Wesker K. 3rd ed. New York: Thieme Publishers; 2020.)

- • The **v. cardiaca media (v. interventricularis posterior)** runs in the sulcus interventricularis posterior with the r. interventricularis posterior and drains the posterior part of the septum interventriculare.
- • The **v. cardiaca parva**, which drains the atrium dextrum posterior and the ventriculus dexter, accompanies the a. coronaria dextra in the sulcus coronarius.
- — Vv. cordis anterior drain the anterior surface of the ventriculus dexter and open directly into the atrium dextrum.

Lymphatic Drainage of the Heart

- — Lymphatic vessels of the heart have a crossed drainage pattern. Lymph from the atrium sinistrum and ventriculus sinister drains via a left coronary trunk to nll. trachiobronchiales inferiores. Efferents from these nodes usually drain to the right venous junction via the truncus bronchiomediastinalis. Lymph from the ventriculus dexter and atrium dextrum drains via a right coronary trunk that runs along the aorta ascendens to nll. brachiocephalici near the left venous junction **(Fig. 7.19)**.
- — The pericardium usually drains to the right and left venous junctions via nll. phrenici superiores and trunci bronchomediastinales, but it may also drain superiorly to the nll. brachiocephalici.

Innervation of the Heart

The autonomic nerves of the plexus cardiacus innervate the conduction system of the heart (**Fig. 7.20**, also see Section 5.2); they therefore regulate the heart rate but do not initiate the heartbeat.
- — Sympathetic innervation increases the rate and force of contractions by increasing the response of the SA and AV nodes. It also allows dilation of the aa. coronariae.
- — Parasympathetic innervation decreases the rate of contractions and causes vasoconstriction of the aa. coronariae.

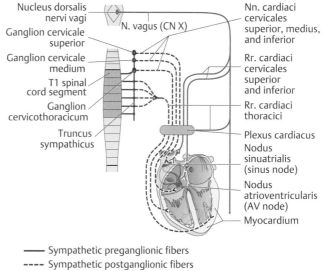

Nucleus dorsalis nervi vagi

Ganglion cervicale superior

Ganglion cervicale medium

T1 spinal cord segment

Ganglion cervicothoracicum

Truncus sympathicus

N. vagus (CN X)

Nn. cardiaci cervicales superior, medius, and inferior

Rr. cardiaci cervicales superior and inferior

Rr. cardiaci thoracici

Plexus cardiacus

Nodus sinuatrialis (sinus node)

Nodus atrioventricularis (AV node)

Myocardium

——— Sympathetic preganglionic fibers
---- Sympathetic postganglionic fibers
——— Parasympathetic preganglionic fibers
---- Parasympathetic postganglionic fibers

Fig. 7.20 Autonomic innervation of the heart
Schematic. (From Gilroy AM et al. Atlas of Anatomy. 4th ed. 2020. Based on: Schuenke M, Schulte E, Schumacher U. THIEME Atlas of Anatomy. Internal Organs. Illustrations by Voll M and Wesker K. 3rd ed. New York: Thieme Medical Publishers; 2020.)

- — Visceral sensory fibers innervating the baroreceptors (receptors that measure blood pressure) and chemoreceptors (receptors that measure blood CO_2) in the heart and arcus aortae travel with the parasympathetic fibers of the n. vagus.
- — Visceral sensory fibers carrying pain sensation travel with sympathetic fibers to the T1–T5 medulla spinalis.

7.6　Prenatal and Neonatal Circulation

Prenatal Circulation

Fetal shunts that direct the flow of blood through the liver, heart, and lungs create a prenatal circulation that differs from that of the adult. The numbered steps in **Fig. 7.21** illustrate the blood flow in the fetal circulation:

1. Fetal blood supplied with oxygen and nutrients in the placenta courses through the v. umbilicalis toward the liver of the fetus.
2. Although a portion of the blood is distributed to the liver, over half bypasses the liver and is redirected through a shunt, the **ductus venosus,** which empties directly into the v. cava inferior. This blood mixes with smaller amounts from the liver and lower parts of the body before entering the atrium dextrum of the heart.
3. The **valvula venae cavae inferioris** (see **Fig. 7.12A**) at the orifice of the v. cava inferior directs this well-oxygenated

mixture across the atrium dextrum into the atrium sinistrum through the foramen ovale on the septum interatriale. The higher systolic pressure in the atrium dextrum relative to that in the atrium sinistrum creates this right-to-left shunt. From the atrium sinistrum, the flow continues into the ventriculus sinister, the aorta, and the systemic circulation of the head and neck. Thus the most highly oxygenated and nutrient-rich blood from the placenta is directed into the aa. coronariae, aa. carotis, and aa. subclaviae to supply the upper body, especially the heart and developing brain.

4. Oxygen-depleted blood entering the atrium dextrum from the v. cava superior is directed downward through the valva tricuspidalis into the ventriculus dexter and out through the truncus pulmonalis.

Because the high vascular resistance in the lungs prevents much blood from entering the aa. pulmonales, most is diverted to the aorta descendens through the **ductus arteriosus,** a connection between the a. pulmonalis sinistra and the arcus aortae.

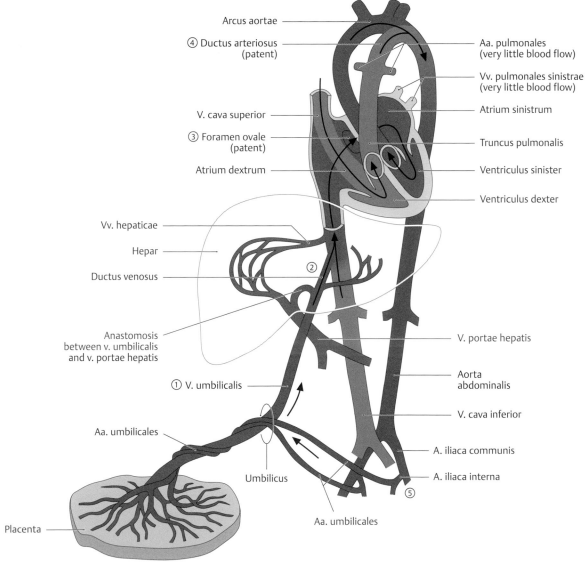

Arcus aortae

④ Ductus arteriosus (patent)

Aa. pulmonales (very little blood flow)

Vv. pulmonales sinistrae (very little blood flow)

V. cava superior

Atrium sinistrum

③ Foramen ovale (patent)

Truncus pulmonalis

Atrium dextrum

Ventriculus sinister

Ventriculus dexter

Vv. hepaticae

Hepar

Ductus venosus

②

V. portae hepatis

Anastomosis between v. umbilicalis and v. portae hepatis

Aorta abdominalis

① V. umbilicalis

V. cava inferior

Aa. umbilicales

A. iliaca communis

Umbilicus

A. iliaca interna

⑤

Aa. umbilicales

Placenta

Fig. 7.21　Prenatal circulation
(After Fritsch H, Kuhnel W. Taschenatlas der Anatomie. Bd.2.7. Aufl. Stuttgart: Thieme Publishers; 2001.)

5. The blood entering the aorta from the ductus arteriosus mixes with some blood from the arcus aortae. This partially oxygenated blood flows into the aorta descendens and is distributed to the lower body, or back to the placenta by way of the paired aa. umbilicales.

Cardiovascular Changes at Birth

At birth, a series of changes occurs in the cardiovascular system (**Fig. 7.22; Table 7.5**).

1. Pressure in the atrium dextrum decreases as a result of
   a. ligation of the v. umbilicalis, which cuts off blood flow from the placenta; and
   b. the onset of pulmonary respiration, which dramatically decreases the pulmonary blood pressure and increases blood flow to the lungs.

Table 7.5 Derivatives of Fetal Circulatory Structures

Fetal Structure	Adult Remnant
Ductus arteriosus	Lig. arteriosum
Foramen ovale	Fossa ovalis
Ductus venosus	Lig. venosum
V. umbilicalis	Lig. teres hepatis
A. umbilicalis	Chorda a. umbilicalis

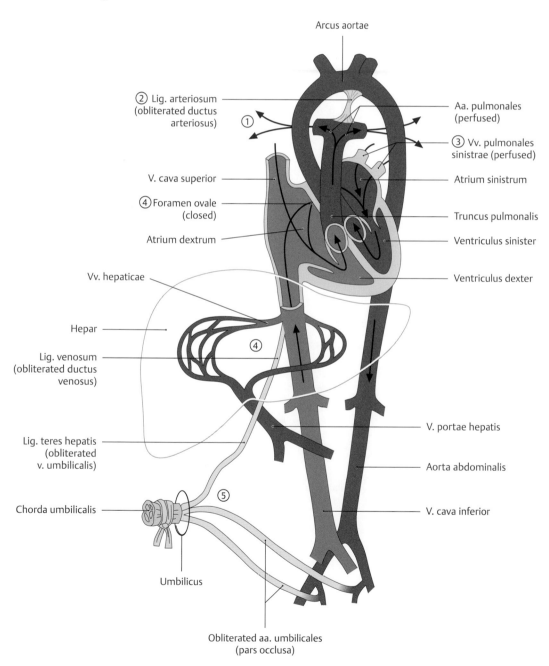

Fig. 7.22 Postnatal circulation
(After Fritsch H, Kuhnel W. Taschenatlas der Anatomie. Bd.2.7. Aufl. Stuttgart: Thieme Publishers; 2001.)

2. As a result of increased flow through the lungs, there is a decreased blood flow through the ductus arteriosus, which constricts within 10 to 15 hours of birth. In the adult, the remnant of this structure is the **lig. arteriosum.**
3. Blood returning to the heart through the vv. pulmonales increases pressure in the atrium sinistrum.
4. Increased pressure in the atrium sinistrum, coupled with a corresponding decrease in pressure in the atrium dextrum, causes a functional closure of the foramen ovale within hours of birth. Complete closure of the foramen ovale usually occurs after several months, forming the **oval fossa** (fossa ovalis) in the adult heart.
5. Functional closure of the aa. umbilicales, vv. umbilicales, and ductus venosus occurs within minutes of birth, although the obliteration of the lumen in each vessel may take several months. The remnants of these vessels in the adult are ligamentous structures.

BOX 7.11: DEVELOPMENTAL CORRELATION

VENTRICULAR SEPTAL DEFECT

Ventricular septal defects (VSDs), the most common of congenital heart defects, usually involve the membranous part of the interventricular septum and are associated with Down syndrome, tetralogy of Fallot, and Turner syndrome. VSDs may also occur traumatically from rupture of the membranous septum following a myocardial infarction. When the VSD is large, the resulting left-to-right shunt increases blood flow through the pulmonary circulation, causing pulmonary hypertension and cardiac failure **(Fig. 7.23B).**

BOX 7.12: DEVELOPMENTAL CORRELATION

PATENT DUCTUS ARTERIOSUS

The opening of the pulmonary circulation at birth causes the ductus arteriosus to constrict, probably in response to an increase in local oxygen tension. If the ductus remains open, as a patent ductus arteriosus (PDA), deoxygenated blood continues to enter the aorta descendens **(Fig. 7.23C)**. There may be no symptoms if the defect is small, but larger defects may cause failure to thrive, dyspnea (shortness of breath), fatigue, tachycardia (increased heart rate), and cyanosis. Because prostaglandins maintain patency of the ductus during fetal life, premature infants whose ductus does not constrict spontaneously at birth may be treated with prostaglandin inhibitors.

BOX 7.13: DEVELOPMENTAL CORRELATION

ATRIAL SEPTAL DEFECT

Atrial septal defects (ASDs) **(Fig. 7.23D)** are among the most common congenital cardiac anomalies and are particularly associated with Down syndrome. Most ASDs result from a failure of the foramen ovale to close at birth, but they may also result from incomplete development of the septal components. ASDs result in left-to-right shunting and an increase in blood volume through the pulmonary circulation. Small ASDs are often asymptomatic, but larger ASDs will cause hypertrophy of the atrium dextrun, ventriculus dexter, and aa. pulmonales due to the fluid overload.

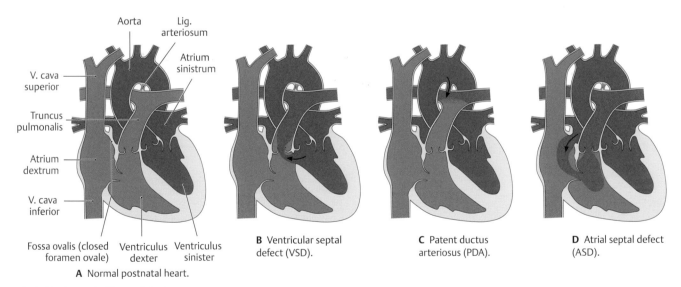

Fig. 7.23 Congenital heart defects
(From Schuenke M, Schulte E, Schumacher U. THIEME Atlas of Anatomy, Vol 2. Illustrations by Voll M and Wesker K. 3rd ed. New York: Thieme Publishers; 2020.)

COARCTATION OF THE AORTA

Coarctation, or stenosis, of the aorta usually occurs in proximity to the lig. arteriosum, where it limits (or obstructs) the normal blood flow from the arcus aortae through the aorta descendens. When the narrowing is distal to the ligamentum (postductal stenosis), an effective collateral circulation links the proximal and distal aortic segments via the aa. thoracicae internae and their intercostal branches. The aa. intercostales may become large and tortuous enough to form notches along the lower margins of the ribs.

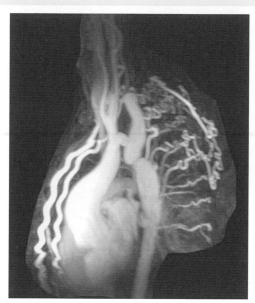

MRI of coarctation in a young child
Note the large aa. thoracicae internae and tortuous aa. intercostales that provide collateral pathways between the thoracic and abdominal parts of the aorta. (From Gunderman R. Essential Radiology, 3rd ed. New York: Thieme; 2014)

7.7 Superior and Posterior Mediastina

Many of the large arteries and veins of the thorax—v. cava superior, v. cava inferior, aorta, a. carotis communis, and a. subclavia—pass through the mediastinum superius and mediastinum posterius en route to the neck or the abdomen or both. They are accompanied by the n. vagus, n. phrenicus, and n. cardiacus. These structures are listed in **Table 7.1** and described in detail in Section 5.2. Only viscera of the superior and posterior mediastina will be discussed in this section.

Oesophagus

The oesophagus, the thoracic segment of the gastrointestinal tract, is a narrow, but highly distensible, muscular tube. It connects the pharynx in the neck to the stomach in the abdomen **(Fig. 7.24)**.

— The oesophagus descends anterior to the corpora vertebrae thoracicae in the mediastinum posterius. Superiorly, it lies posterior to the trachea; inferiorly, it lies posterior to the atrium sinistrum.

— In the upper thorax, the oesophagus descends on the right side of the aorta. Before passing through the hiatus oesophageus of the diaphragma, the oesophagus passes first anterior to, and then to the left of, the aorta.

— The upper oesophagus is composed mostly of striated muscle arranged in inner circular and outer longitudinal layers. Striated muscle is gradually replaced by smooth muscle fibers inferiorly.

— Three constrictions narrow the lumen of the oesophagus **(Fig. 7.25)**:
  1. The **constrictio pharyngo-oesophagealis,** created by the m. cricopharyngeus (part of the m. constrictor pharyngis inferior), which surrounds the upper esophageal opening in the neck
  2. The **constrictio bronchoaortica**, created by the arcus aortae and bronchus principalis sinister
  3. The **constrictio diaphragmatica,** or **cardiac sphincter,** created by circular muscles of the distal oesophagus, folds in the mucosa formed by a submucosal venous plexus, and the muscular hiatus oesophageus of the diaphragma

— The blood supply to the upper, middle, and lower oesophagus arises from vessels in the neck (a. thyroidea inferior), thorax (rr. oesophageales of the aorta descendens), and abdomen (a. gastrica sinistra and a. phrenica inferior sinistra), respectively.

— The veins of upper and middle esophageal segments drain into the azygos system. Veins of the lower esophageal segment drain inferiorly along vv. phrenicae inferiores into the hepatic portal system (the venous drainage for organs of the abdominal gastrointestinal tract). When portal venous flow is obstructed in the liver (such as from cirrhosis), blood can be diverted through the esophageal veins to the azygos system and v. cava superior **(Fig. 7.26)**.

— The **plexus oesophageus,** formed by the nn. vagi dexter and sinister with contributions from the nn. splanchnici major, innervates the oesophagus.

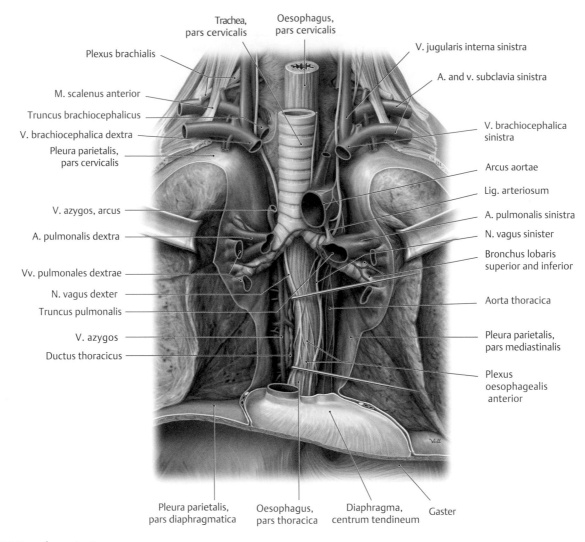

Trachea, pars cervicalis

Oesophagus, pars cervicalis

Plexus brachialis

V. jugularis interna sinistra

M. scalenus anterior

A. and v. subclavia sinistra

Truncus brachiocephalicus

V. brachiocephalica dextra

V. brachiocephalica sinistra

Pleura parietalis, pars cervicalis

Arcus aortae

Lig. arteriosum

V. azygos, arcus

A. pulmonalis sinistra

A. pulmonalis dextra

N. vagus sinister

Vv. pulmonales dextrae

Bronchus lobaris superior and inferior

N. vagus dexter

Aorta thoracica

Truncus pulmonalis

V. azygos

Pleura parietalis, pars mediastinalis

Ductus thoracicus

Plexus oesophagealis anterior

Pleura parietalis, pars diaphragmatica

Oesophagus, pars thoracica

Diaphragma, centrum tendineum

Gaster

Fig. 7.24 Oesophagus in situ
Anterior view. (From Gilroy AM et al. Atlas of Anatomy. 4th ed. 2020. Based on: Schuenke M, Schulte E, Schumacher U. THIEME Atlas of Anatomy. Internal Organs. Illustrations by Voll M and Wesker K. 3rd ed. New York: Thieme Medical Publishers; 2020.)

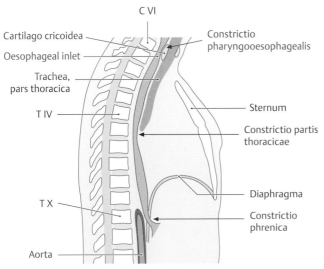

C VI

Cartilago cricoidea

Constrictio pharyngooesophagealis

Oesophageal inlet

Trachea, pars thoracica

Sternum

T IV

Constrictio partis thoracicae

Diaphragma

T X

Constrictio phrenica

Aorta

A Oesophageal constrictions, right lateral view. (From Schuenke M, Schulte E, Schumacher U. THIEME Atlas of Anatomy, Vol 2. Illustrations by Voll M and Wesker K. 3rd ed. New York: Thieme Publishers; 2020.)

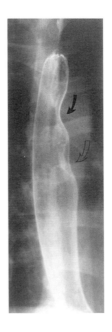

B A double-contrast esophagogram demonstrates normal impressions on the oesophagus by the arcus aortae *(solid arrow)* and the bronchus principalis sinister *(open arrow)*. (From Gunderman R. Essential Radiology, 3rd ed. New York: Thieme Publishers; 2014.)

Fig. 7.25 Oesophagus: location and constrictions

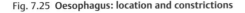

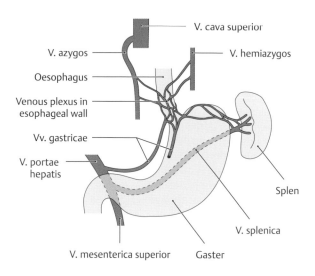

Fig. 7.26 **Oesophageal venous collaterals**
(From Schuenke M, Schulte E, Schumacher U. THIEME Atlas of Anatomy, Vol 2. Illustrations by Voll M and Wesker K. 3rd ed. New York: Thieme Publishers; 2020.)

> **BOX 7.15: CLINICAL CORRELATION**
>
> **ACHALASIA**
> Achalasia is a deficiency of inhibitory neurons in the lower part of the oesophagus. These neurons are responsible for overriding the normal resting tonic contraction of the smooth muscle cells in the lower esophageal sphincter. Their deficiency results in failure of the sphincter to relax during swallowing. As food accumulates above the sphincter, there is an increased risk of aspiration pneumonia.

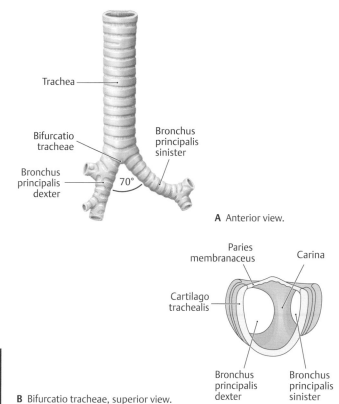

A Anterior view.

B Bifurcatio tracheae, superior view.

Fig. 7.27 **Trachea**
(From Schuenke M, Schulte E, Schumacher U. THIEME Atlas of Anatomy, Vol 2. Illustrations by Voll M and Wesker K. 3rd ed. New York: Thieme Publishers; 2020.)

Trachea and Bronchi

The trachea, located in the mediastinum superius, is the proximal part of the **tracheobronchial tree (arbor tracheobronchialis)**, a passageway for air between the lungs and the external environment. The distal part of this passageway, the **arbor bronchialis,** extends into the lungs and is discussed with the pulmonary cavities in Chapter 8.

— As the trachea descends through the mediastinum superius, slightly to the right of the midline, it lies anterior to the oesophagus and posterior to the great vessels.
— C-shaped cartilaginous rings form the skeleton of the trachea and prevent collapse of the lumen. A muscular membrane connects the ends of the rings posteriorly **(Fig. 7.27)**.

— The **carina,** a wedge-shaped cartilage, marks the bifurcation of the trachea (bifurcatio tracheae) into a **bronchus principalis dexter** and **bronchus principalis sinister** at the T IV–T V vertebral level.
— Of the two bronchi principales, the right is shorter, wider, and more vertical than the left, and therefore is more prone to obstruction by foreign objects.
— Descending branches of the a. thyroidea inferior (a branch of the truncus thyrocervicalis) in the neck as well as aa. bronchiales that arise from the aorta thoracica, supply the trachea. Venous blood drains to the vv. thyroideae inferior.
— Nn. splanchnici thoracici and parasympathetic fibers from the n. vagus (CN X) innervate the trachea via the plexus pulmonalis.

8 Pulmonary Cavities

The right and left pulmonary cavities, which flank the mediastinum laterally and anteriorly, extend superiorly above the costal cartilages of the first rib and inferiorly to the thoracic diaphragm. Each pulmonary cavity contains a lung, bronchial tree with associated neurovasculature, and a pleural sac.

8.1 The Pleura and Cavitas Pleuralis

The Pleura

The **pleura** is a fibroserous membrane that surrounds each lung and lines the pulmonary cavities (**Fig. 8.1**).
- The pleura is composed of two layers:
  - The **pleura parietalis,** which is a continuous layer that lines the inner wall of the cavitas thoracis, the superior surface of the diaphragma, and the mediastinum. Its parts are named according to location: pars costalis, pars diaphragmatica, pars mediastinalis, and cupula pleurae (**Fig. 8.2**).
  - The **pleura visceralis,** which covers the surface of the lung and extends into its fissures.

- The pleura visceralis and pleura parietalis are continuous with one another at the hilum of the lung. Together they form the inner and outer walls of a closed pleural sac that contains a **cavitas pleuralis** (**Fig. 8.3**).
- The **lig. pulmonale** is a double-layered fold of pleura visceralis and pleura parietalis that extends vertically from the hilum to the diaphragma along the mediastinal border of each lung (see **Fig. 8.5B,D**).
- The blood supply and innervation of the pleura are derived from nerves and vessels that supply adjacent structures.
  - Pleura visceralis shares the neurovasculature of the lungs and bronchi.
  - Pleura parietalis shares the neurovasculature of the thoracic wall, pericardium, and diaphragma.

BOX 8.1: CLINICAL CORRELATION

PLEURITIS

Inflammation of the pleura, or pleuritis, creates friction between the pleura visceralis and pleura parietalis that produces a sharp, stabbing pain as the layers glide over one another during respiration. The inflammation may also produce adhesions between the two layers.

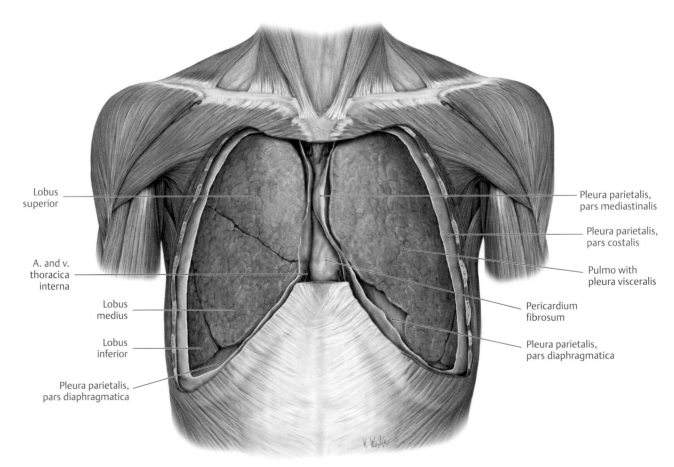

Fig. 8.1 Pulmones in situ
Anterior view. *Removed*: Anterior thoracic wall and pars costalis of the pleura parietalis. (From Gilroy AM et al. Atlas of Anatomy. 4th ed. 2020. Based on: Schuenke M, Schulte E, Schumacher U. THIEME Atlas of Anatomy. Internal Organs. Illustrations by Voll M and Wesker K. 3rd ed. New York: Thieme Medical Publishers; 2020.)

The Cavitas Pleuralis

The **pleural cavity (cavitas pleuralis)**, the cavity within the pleural sac, is the potential space between the pleura visceralis and pleura parietalis (**Fig. 8.3**).

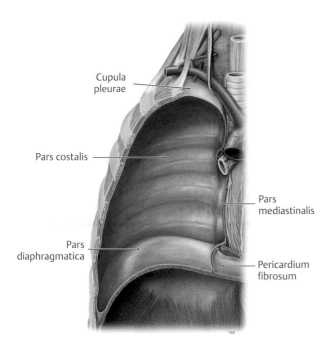

Fig. 8.2 **Parts of the pleura parietalis**
Anterior view. *Opened:* Cavitas pleuralis dexter. (From Gilroy AM et al. Atlas of Anatomy. 4th ed. 2020. Based on: Schuenke M, Schulte E, Schumacher U. THIEME Atlas of Anatomy. Internal Organs. Illustrations by Voll M and Wesker K. 3rd ed. New York: Thieme Medical Publishers; 2020.)

— The cavitas pleuralis contains a thin layer of serous fluid, which lubricates the adjacent pleural surfaces, facilitates the movement of the lung, and maintains surface tension that is crucial to respiration.
— On most surfaces, the two pleural layers approximate one another, but the lung and its pleura visceralis are somewhat smaller than the outer wall of the cavitas pleuralis and its lining of pleura parietalis. Two recesses that form as a result of this discrepancy accommodate the expansion of the lungs during inspiration (**Fig. 8.4**):
   • The **recessus costodiaphragmaticus** forms where the pars diaphragmatica reflects from the perimeter of the diaphragma to meet the pars costalis on the thoracic wall.
   • The **recessus costomediastinalis** forms between the pericardial sac and the sternum, where the pars mediastinalis reflects to meet the pars costalis.

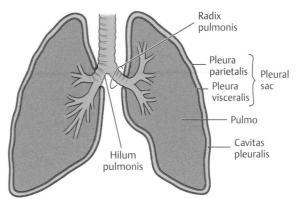

Fig. 8.3 **Pleura and cavitas pleuralis**
Schematic. (From Gilroy AM et al. Atlas of Anatomy. 4th ed. 2020. Based on: Schuenke M, Schulte E, Schumacher U. THIEME Atlas of Anatomy. Internal Organs. Illustrations by Voll M and Wesker K. 3rd ed. New York: Thieme Medical Publishers; 2020.)

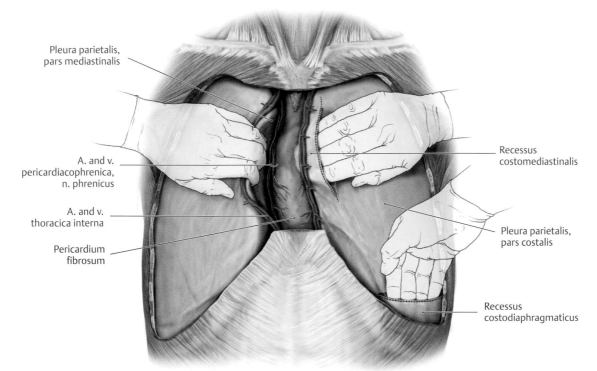

Fig. 8.4 **Recessus costomediastinalis and recessus costodiaphragmaticus**
On the left side of the thorax, the examiner's fingertips are placed in the recessus costomediastinalis and recessus costodiaphragmaticus. These recesses are formed by the acute reflection of the pars costalis of the pleura parietalis onto the pericardium fibrosum (recessus costomediastinalis) or diaphragma (recessus costodiaphragmatica). (From Gilroy AM et al. Atlas of Anatomy. 4th ed. 2020. Based on: Schuenke M, Schulte E, Schumacher U. THIEME Atlas of Anatomy. Internal Organs. Illustrations by Voll M and Wesker K. 3rd ed. New York: Thieme Medical Publishers; 2020.)

BOX 8.2: CLINICAL CORRELATION

PNEUMOTHORAX

Pneumothorax is a condition in which air enters the pleural space. It may result from a tear in the chest wall and pleura parietalis (such as from a stab wound) or a tear of the pleura visceralis (such as from a rupture of a pulmonary lesion). Air in the pleural space decreases the negative pressure that normally keeps the lungs inflated and leads to a partial or complete lung collapse.

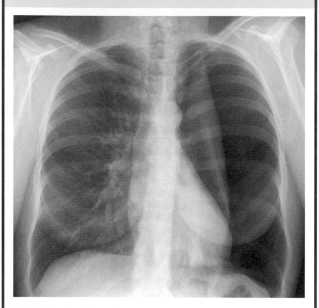

Frontal chest radiograph
Radiograph of a 44-year-old woman demonstrates an absence of pulmonary markings in the lateral half of the left hemithorax and a visceral pleural line that clearly delineates the collapsed left lung from a large left pneumothorax. (From Gunderman R. Essential Radiology, 3rd ed. New York: Thieme Publishers; 2014.)

BOX 8.3: CLINICAL CORRELATION

TENSION PNEUMOTHORAX

Tension pneumothorax is a life-threatening condition in which air accumulates in the pleural space and becomes trapped because the injured tissue acts as a one-way valve. This causes complete collapse of the lung on the affected side and a shifting of the heart to the opposite side, thus compromising venous return and cardiac output. This mediastinal shift also compresses the opposite lung and impairs its ventilatory capacity.

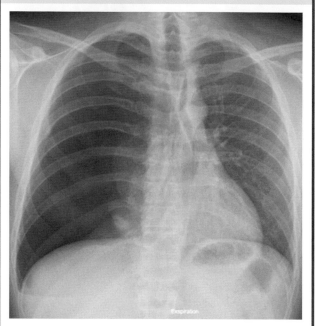

Tension pneumothorax on the right side
The chest radiograph shows almost complete atelectasis of the right lung. The mediastinum is shifted to the left. The intercostal spaces are widened on the right side. (From Krombach GA, Mahnken AH. Body Imaging: Thorax and Abdomen. New York: Thieme Publishers; 2015.)

BOX 8.4: CLINICAL CORRELATION

PLEURAL EFFUSION

Pleural effusion is a condition in which there is excess fluid in the pleural space. Effusions are designated by their protein concentration into transudates (low protein) and exudates (high protein). Transudates are usually caused by congestive heart failure or fluid overload (causing increased venous pressure). Less commonly they are caused by liver failure or renal disease. Exudates may leak from the pleural capillaries in inflammatory states, pneumonia, tuberculosis (TB), and lung cancer. Symptoms include dyspnea (shortness of breath), cough, and dull chest pain. Pleural effusions are treated by draining the fluid through a procedure known as thoracentesis (see Box 6.2 Insertion of a Chest Tube).

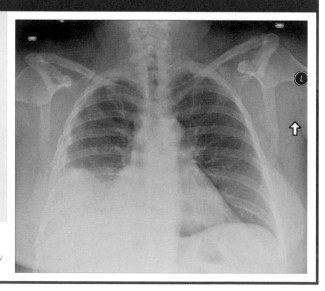

Pleural effusion
This 58-year-old woman's frontal chest radiograph demonstrates a large right pleural effusion. (From Gunderman R. Essential Radiology, 3rd ed. New York: Thieme Publishers; 2014.)

8.2 The Lungs

General Features (Fig. 8.5; Table 8.1)

— Each lung (pulmo) has a facies costalis, facies mediastinalis, and facies diaphragmatica.
— The **apex** of each lung (**apex pulmonis**) projects into the neck above the first cartilago costalis; the **base** of each lung (**basis pulmonis**) rests on the diaphragma.

— The **root** of the lung (**radix pulmonis**), which connects the lung to the mediastinum, contains the pulmonary vessels, nerves, and bronchi. The root enters the lung at the **hilum,** an indentation on the facies mediastinalis (**Fig. 8.6**; see **Fig. 8.3**).
— Fissures, lined by pleura visceralis, divide each lung into lobes: three lobes on the right and two lobes on the left.
— Thin connective tissue septa (intersegmental septa) that are continuous with the pleura visceralis subdivide lobes of the

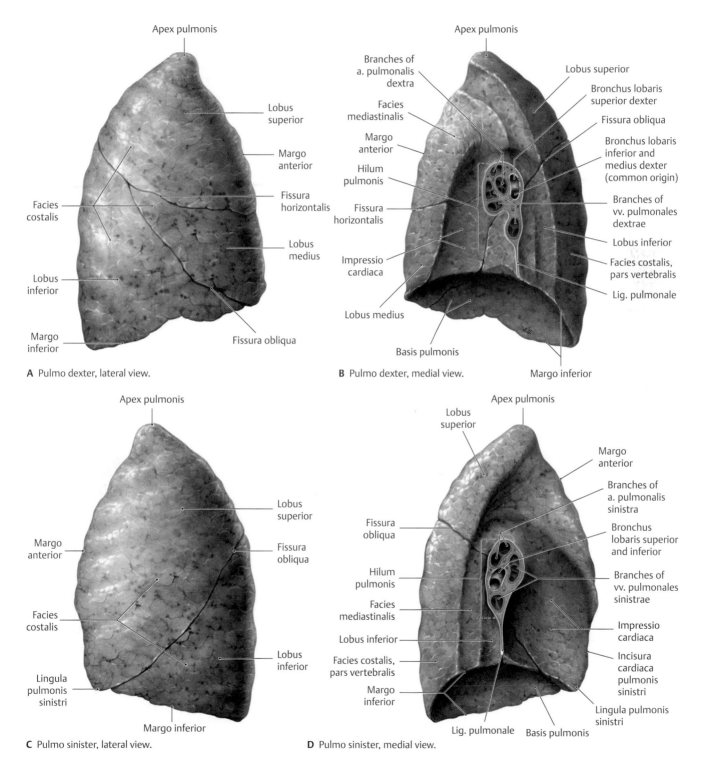

A Pulmo dexter, lateral view.

B Pulmo dexter, medial view.

C Pulmo sinister, lateral view.

D Pulmo sinister, medial view.

Fig. 8.5 Gross anatomy of the pulmones
(From Schuenke M, Schulte E, Schumacher U. THIEME Atlas of Anatomy, Vol 2. Illustrations by Voll M and Wesker K. 3rd ed. New York: Thieme Publishers; 2020.)

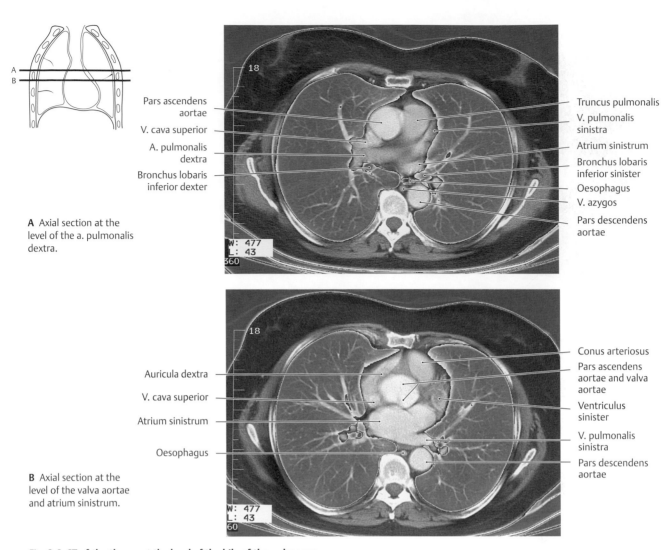

A Axial section at the level of the a. pulmonalis dextra.

Pars ascendens aortae
V. cava superior
A. pulmonalis dextra
Bronchus lobaris inferior dexter

Truncus pulmonalis
V. pulmonalis sinistra
Atrium sinistrum
Bronchus lobaris inferior sinister
Oesophagus
V. azygos
Pars descendens aortae

B Axial section at the level of the valva aortae and atrium sinistrum.

Auricula dextra
V. cava superior
Atrium sinistrum
Oesophagus

Conus arteriosus
Pars ascendens aortae and valva aortae
Ventriculus sinister
V. pulmonalis sinistra
Pars descendens aortae

Fig. 8.6 CT of the thorax at the level of the hila of the pulmones
(From Moeller TB, Reif E. Pocket Atlas of Sectional Anatomy, Vol 2, 3rd ed. New York: Thieme Publishers; 2007.)

Table 8.1 Structure of the Pulmones

	Pulmo dexter	**Pulmo sinister**
Lobi	Superior, medius, inferior	Superior, inferior
Fissurae	Obliqua, horizontalis	Obliqua
Segmenta bronchopulmonalia	10	8–10
Unique Features	Larger and heavier than the left, but shorter and wider due to higher right hemidiaphragm	Lobus superior characterized by the lingula and a deep incisura cardiaca

lungs into discrete pyramidal-shaped units called **segmenta bronchopulmonalia (Fig. 8.7)**.

- Each bronchopulmonary segment (segmentum bronchopulmonalis) is an anatomically and functionally independent respiratory unit. This independence allows the surgical resection of individual segments.
- There are 10 bronchopulmonary segments in the right lung and 8 to 10 segments in the left lung.

Right Lung

- Because the dome of the diaphragma is higher on the right side, the right lung (pulmo dexter) is shorter and wider than the left lung (pulmo sinister).
- Fissura horizontalis and fissura obliqua divide the right lung into lobus superior, lobus medius, and lobus inferior.
- The root of the lung passes under the arcus aortae, posterior to the atrium dextrum, and under the arch of the v. azygos (see **Fig. 7.2A**).
- The bronchus principalis dexter and its branches are the most posterior structures within the root of the lung. The a. pulmonalis passes anterior to the bronchus, and the vv. pulmonales lie anterior and inferior to the artery.

Left Lung

- A fissura obliqua divides the left lung into lobus superior and lobus inferior.
- A deep indentation along the anterior border of the lobus superior, called the **incisura cardiaca,** accommodates the leftward projection of the apex cordis.
- The **lingula pulmonis,** a thin tongue of lung tissue from the lobus superior, forms the inferior border of the incisura

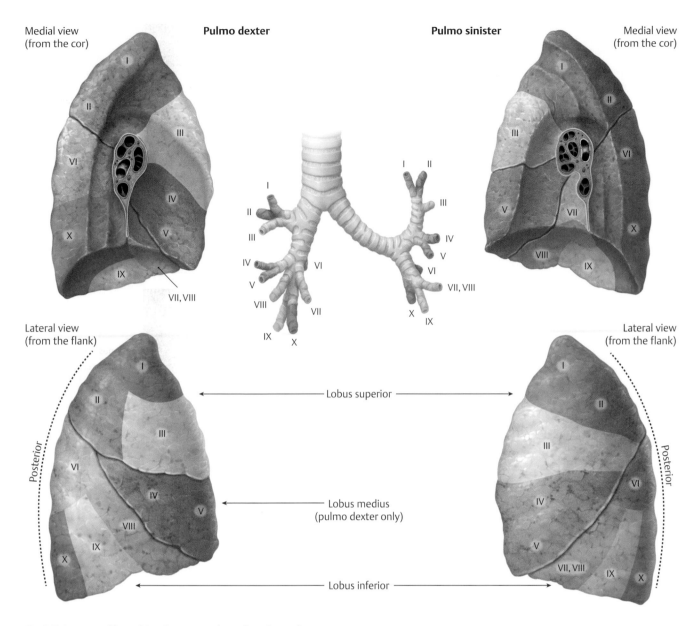

Medial view
(from the cor)

Pulmo dexter

Pulmo sinister

Medial view
(from the cor)

Lateral view
(from the flank)

Posterior

Lobus superior

Lobus medius
(pulmo dexter only)

Lobus inferior

Lateral view
(from the flank)

Posterior

Fig. 8.7 Segmental bronchi and segmenta bronchopulmonalia
(From Krombach GA, Mahnken AH. Body Imaging: Thorax and Abdomen. New York: Thieme Publishers; 2015.)

cardiaca and moves into and out of the recessus costomediastinalis during respiration.

— The arcus aortae crosses over the bronchus principalis sinister, and the aorta descendens passes behind the root of the lung (see **Fig. 7.2B**).

— The a. pulmonalis sinistra arches over the bronchus principalis sinister to become the most superior structure in the root of the lung. Vv. pulmonales pass anterior and inferior to the bronchus.

8.3 The Tracheobronchial Tree

The tracheobronchial tree consists of the trachea and the bronchi in the mediastinum, and the arbor bronchialis (generations of branches formed by successive bifurcations) within the lungs.

(The trachea is discussed in Section 7.7.) The tracheobronchial tree has conducting and respiratory components.

— The trachea and its larger proximal branches form the conducting component, a passageway for air exchange between the lung and the external environment (**Figs. 8.8** and **8.9A**). All except the most distal of these branches have cartilaginous rings or plates in their walls. The branches include

• the **right** and **left main bronchi (bronchus principalis dexter** and **bronchus principalis sinister),** formed by the bifurcatio tracheae in the mediastinum superius. One bronchus principalis enters the hilum of each lung.

• the **bronchi lobares,** which branch from the bronchi principales. One bronchus lobaris enters each lobe of the respective lung (three on the right and two on the left).

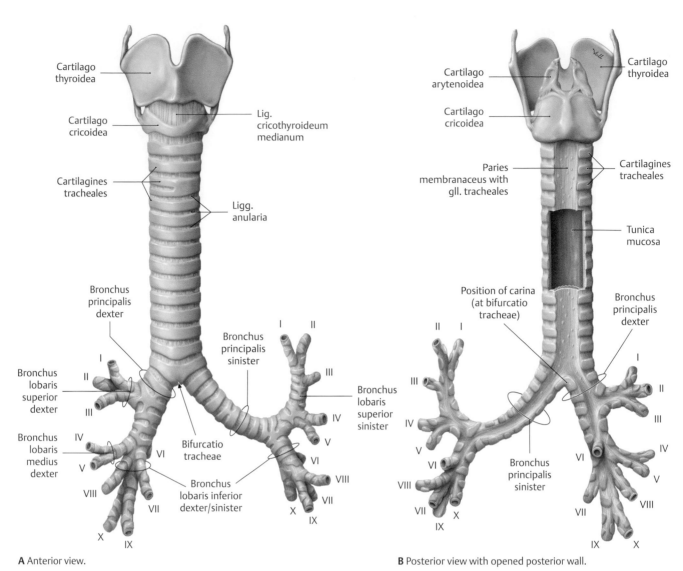

A Anterior view.

B Posterior view with opened posterior wall.

Fig. 8.8 Trachea
The numbers I to IX of the segmental bronchi correspond with segmenta bronchopulmonalia shown in **Fig. 8.7.**
(From Gilroy AM et al. Atlas of Anatomy. 4th ed. 2020. Based on: Schuenke M, Schulte E, Schumacher U. THIEME Atlas of Anatomy. Internal Organs. Illustrations by Voll M and Wesker K. 3rd ed. New York: Thieme Medical Publishers; 2020.)

- the **segmental** (tertiary) **bronchi (bronchi segmentales),** which branch from the lobar bronchi. One segmental bronchus enters each bronchopulmonary segment and divides further into large, and then small, subsegmental bronchi.
- the **conducting bronchioli,** a network of airways without cartilage that are formed as the segmental bronchi subdivide and decrease in size.
- the **terminal bronchioles (bronchioli terminales),** the last branches of the conducting bronchioles and the final part of the conducting airway.
— The respiratory component (seen only histologically), made up of passages distal to the terminal bronchioles, is involved in air conduction as well as in gas exchange (**Fig. 8.9B**).
  - The structures in this part of the arbor bronchialis include the **bronchioli respiratorii, sacculi alveolares,** and **alveoli.**
  - The single-celled walls of the alveoli are designed for efficient gas exchange.

BOX 8.5: CLINICAL CORRELATION

FOREIGN BODY ASPIRATION
Toddlers are at particularly high risk of potentially fatal aspiration of foreign bodies. In general, foreign bodies are more likely to become lodged in the bronchus principalis dexter than the bronchus principalis sinister: the bronchus principalis sinister diverges more sharply at the bifurcatio tracheae to pass more horizontally over the heart, whereas the bronchus principalis dexter is relatively straight and more in line with the trachea.

BOX 8.6: CLINICAL CORRELATION

ATELECTASIS
Atelectasis is the partial or complete collapse of alveoli within the lung and can result from mucus in the airways following surgery (most common), cystic fibrosis, asthma, or obstruction of the airways by a foreign object (e.g., a tumor or blood clot). When severe, it can lead to respiratory failure.

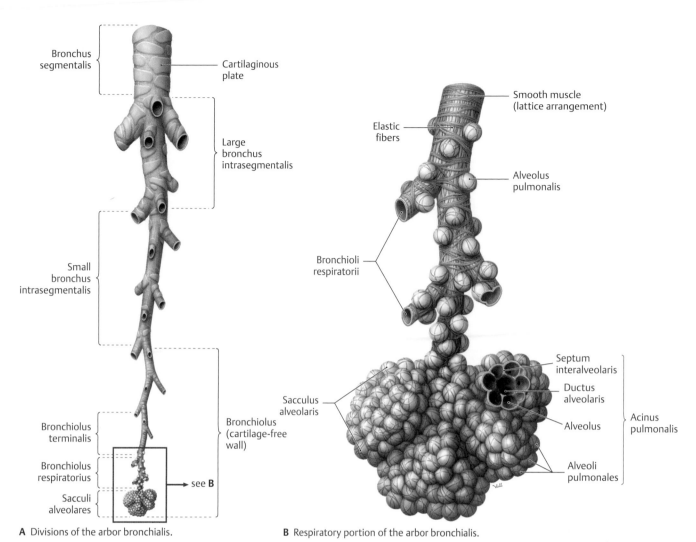

A Divisions of the arbor bronchialis.

B Respiratory portion of the arbor bronchialis.

Fig. 8.9 Arbor bronchialis
(From Schuenke M, Schulte E, Schumacher U. THIEME Atlas of Anatomy, Vol 2. Illustrations by Voll M and Wesker K. 3rd ed. New York: Thieme Publishers; 2020.)

BOX 8.7: DEVELOPMENTAL CORRELATION

NEONATAL RESPIRATORY DISTRESS SYNDROME

Neonatal respiratory distress syndrome (neonatal RDS; also known as hyaline membrane disease), is present in 60% of infants born before 29 weeks due to a deficiency of surfactant. The lung's production of surfactant begins in week 24 but isn't completed until week 36. In premature infants, this deficiency leads to collapse of the alveoli (atelectasis). The use of synthetic surfactant and administration of continuous positive airway pressure (CPAP) can help maintain airway alveolar patency in these infants.

BOX 8.8: CLINICAL CORRELATION

CHRONIC OBSTRUCTIVE PULMONARY DISEASE

Chronic obstructive bronchitis and emphysema, both caused by cigarette smoking, contribute in varying degrees to chronic obstructive pulmonary disease (COPD). Inflammation from chronic bronchitis leads to thickened bronchial tubes, excess mucus production, and a narrowed airway. Emphysema destroys alveolar walls, thereby reducing the capacity for gas exchange, and, as small airways collapse during expiration, air is trapped in the lungs. This chronic hyperinflation of the lungs and the increased work of expiration create a typical barrel chest appearance (increased anteroposterior diameter).

8.4   Mechanics of Respiration

Respiration, the exchange of oxygen and carbon dioxide, requires a continuous flow of air between the lungs and the external environment. It is accomplished through the rhythmic change in thoracic volume and corresponding expansion (during **inspiration**) and contraction (during **expiration**) of the lungs (**Figs. 8.10, 8.11, 8.12**).

— Inspiration requires an expansion of the pulmonary cavities and decrease in intrapleural pressure.
  • During quiet respiration, the diaphragma, the chief respiratory muscle, contracts and flattens, increasing the vertical dimension of the cavity.
  • Forced inspiration engages other respiratory muscles (primarily the mm. intercostales, mm. scaleni, and m. serratus posterior) that elevate the ribs and sternum and expand the cavities horizontally.

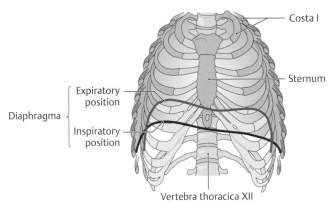

Fig. 8.10 Respiratory changes in thoracic volume
Inspiratory position *(red)*; expiratory position *(blue)*. (From Schuenke M, Schulte E, Schumacher U. THIEME Atlas of Anatomy, Vol 2. Illustrations by Voll M and Wesker K. 3rd ed. New York: Thieme Publishers; 2020.)

Margo inferior pulmonis (full expiration)

Margo inferior pulmonis (full inspiration)

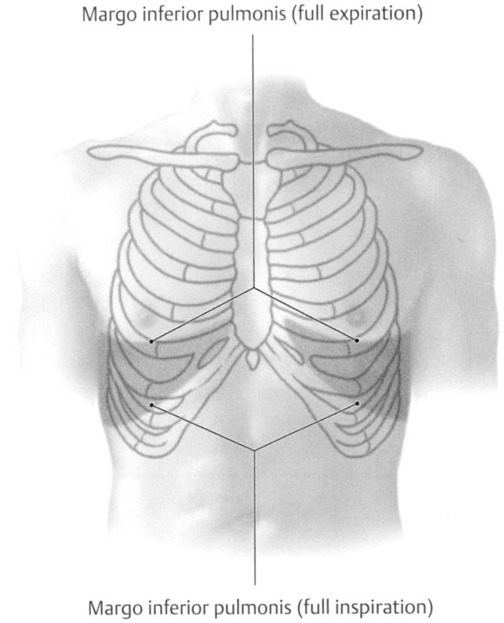

Fig. 8.11 Respiratory changes in lung volume
(From Schuenke M, Schulte E, Schumacher U. THIEME Atlas of Anatomy, Vol 2. Illustrations by Voll M and Wesker K. 3rd ed. New York: Thieme Publishers; 2020.)

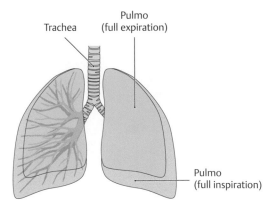

Fig. 8.12 Movements of the pulmo and arbor bronchialis
As the volume of the pulmo changes with the volume of the cavitas thoracica, the entire arbor bronchialis moves within the pulmo. These structural movements are more pronounced in portions of the arbor bronchialis distant from the hilum pulmonis. (From Schuenke M, Schulte E, Schumacher U. THIEME Atlas of Anatomy, Vol 2. Illustrations by Voll M and Wesker K. 3rd ed. New York: Thieme Publishers; 2020.)

  • As the cavities expand, the pleural sac is pulled outward, causing an increase in lung volume and a decrease in intrapleural pressure. When the pressure drops below atmospheric pressure (negative pressure), air is pulled into the respiratory passageways.
— Expiration requires a contraction of the pulmonary cavities and increase in intrapleural pressure.
  • Quiet expiration is a passive process. With relaxation of the diaphragma, there is a decrease in thoracic volume and a corresponding contraction of the lungs. As the intrapleural pressure increases, air is expelled.
  • Forced expiration requires the contraction of mm. abdominis anterior and mm. intercostales to decrease thoracic volume.

8.5   Neurovasculature of the Lungs and Arbor Bronchialis

Arteries of the Lungs and Arbor Bronchialis

— The **aa. pulmonales,** branches of the truncus pulmonalis, transport deoxygenated blood to the capillary network surrounding the respiratory alveoli (**Fig. 8.13**). Within the lungs, branches of the arteries follow the branches of the arbor bronchialis as they ramify within the lobes and bronchopulmonary segments.
— **Aa. bronchiales,** branches of the aorta thoracica, supply the arbor bronchialis, the connective tissue of the lungs, and the pleura visceralis. Typically one branch to the right lung and two to the left lung, these aa. bronchiales travel along the posterior aspect of the bronchi principales and eventually anastomose with distal branches of the aa. pulmonales.

Veins of the Lungs and Arbor Bronchialis

— **Vv. pulmonales** arise from the capillary beds surrounding the alveoli (**Fig. 8.13**). Arising first as small veins that travel within the intersegmental septa carrying oxygenated blood, they receive veins from adjacent bronchopulmonary segments as well as from the pleura visceralis. These veins join to form two vv. pulmonales within each lung, which traverse the hilum and enter the atrium sinistrum of the heart.

BOX 8.9: CLINICAL CORRELATION

PULMONARY EMBOLISM

Pulmonary embolism (PE) is the obstruction of an a. pulmonalis or its branches by fat emboli, air bubbles, or, most commonly, thromboses (blood clots) that have traveled up from the deep veins of the legs. Large obstructions can impede blood flow into the lung and conse- quently cause cor pulmonale, right-sided heart failure. Large obstructions are often fatal, but smaller obstructions may affect only a single bronchopulmonary segment and result in a pulmonary infarction.

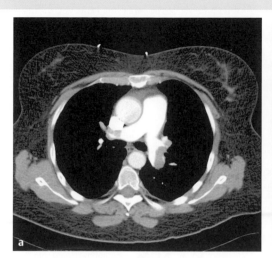
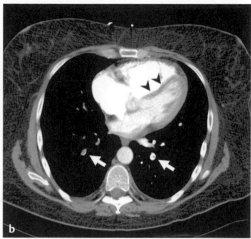

Central pulmonary embolism with subsegmental vascular occlusions. (a) Acute pulmonary embolism with a central embolus. (b) Subsegmental vascular occlusions are also present (*arrows*). The scan additionally shows an enlarged right ventricle with paradoxical bowing of the septum to the left (*arrowheads*) as a sign of a right heart overload. (From Krombach GA, Mahnken AH. Body Imaging: Thorax and Abdomen. New York: Thieme Publishers; 2015.)

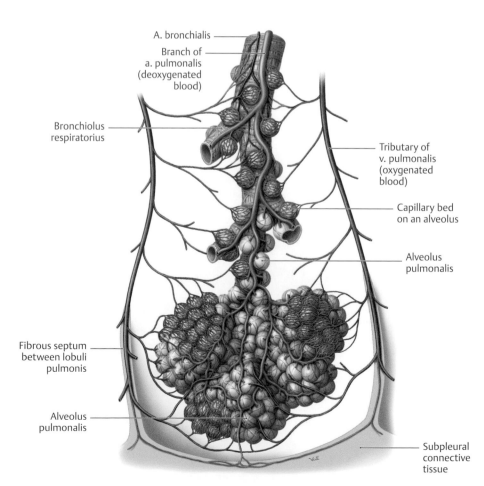

Fig. 8.13 Pulmonary vasculature

Aa. pulmonales *(blue)* carry *deoxygenated* blood and follow the arbor bronchialis. Vv. pulmonales *(red)* are the only veins in the body carrying *oxygenated* blood, which they receive from the alveolar capillaries at the periphery of the lobule. (From Schuenke M, Schulte E, Schumacher U. THIEME Atlas of Anatomy, Vol 2. Illustrations by Voll M and Wesker K. 3rd ed. New York: Thieme Publishers; 2020.)

A. bronchialis

Branch of a. pulmonalis (deoxygenated blood)

Bronchiolus respiratorius

Tributary of v. pulmonalis (oxygenated blood)

Capillary bed on an alveolus

Alveolus pulmonalis

Fibrous septum between lobuli pulmonis

Alveolus pulmonalis

Subpleural connective tissue

— **Vv. bronchiales,** one from each lung, drain only the proximal portion of the root and terminate in the v. azygos and v. hemiazygos accessoria (or vv. intercostales superior).

Lymphatics of the Lungs and Arbor Bronchialis

— The **superficial lymphatic plexus** of the lungs, deep to the pleura visceralis, drains the pleura and the lung tissue.
— The **deep lymphatic plexus,** within the walls of the bronchi, drains structures associated with the lung root.
— Whereas the superficial and deep plexuses eventually drain to the superior and inferior (carinal) **nodi tracheobronchiales**, the deep plexus drains initially to the **nodi bronchopulmonales** along the bronchi lobares (**Fig. 8.14**).

— Lymph from nodi tracheobronchiales drains to **nll. paratracheales** and then to the **trunci lymphatici bronchomediastinales** on either side, which terminate in the junction of the v. subclavia and v. jugularis (jugulosubclavian venous junctions).
— The superior, middle, and inferior lobes of the right lung and the lobus superior of the left lung normally drain along ipsilateral channels. A significant amount of lymph from the lobus inferior of the left lung, however, drains to the right nodi tracheobronchiales, and from there it continues to follow right-sided channels.

A Peribronchial network, coronal section. (From Schuenke M, Schulte E, Schumacher U. THIEME Atlas of Anatomy, Vol 2. Illustrations by Voll M and Wesker K. 3rd ed. New York: Thieme Publishers; 2020.)

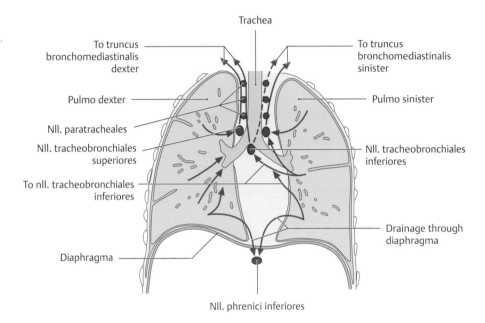

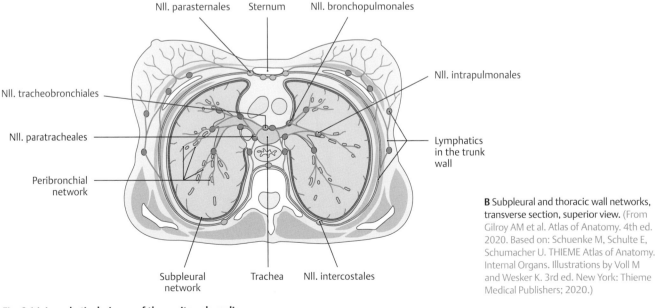

B Subpleural and thoracic wall networks, transverse section, superior view. (From Gilroy AM et al. Atlas of Anatomy. 4th ed. 2020. Based on: Schuenke M, Schulte E, Schumacher U. THIEME Atlas of Anatomy. Internal Organs. Illustrations by Voll M and Wesker K. 3rd ed. New York: Thieme Medical Publishers; 2020.)

Fig. 8.14 **Lymphatic drainage of the cavitas pleuralis**

BOX 8.10: CLINICAL CORRELATION

CARCINOMA OF THE LUNG

Carcinoma of the lung accounts for ~ 20% of all cancers and is mainly caused by cigarette smoking. It arises first in the lining of the bronchi and metastasizes quickly to nll. bronchopulmonales and subsequently to other node groups, including nll. supraclaviculares. It is noteworthy that lymph from most lobes of the lungs drain along ipsilateral channels but that from the left inferior lobe also drains to contralateral nodes, thus facilitating bilateral spread. It can also spread via the blood to the lungs, brain, bone, and glandulae suprarenale. Lung cancer can invade adjacent structures such as the n. phrenicus, resulting in paralysis of a hemidiaphragm, or the n. laryngeus recurrens, resulting in hoarseness due to paralysis of the vocal cord.

Table 8.2 Autonomic Innervation of the Pulmones and Arbor Bronchialis

Target Structures	Sympathetic	Parasympathetic
Bronchial muscles	Inhibitory (bronchodilation)	Motor (bronchoconstriction)
Vasa pulmonales	Motor (vasoconstriction)	Inhibitory (bronchodilation)
Secretory cells of alveoli	Secretomotor	Inhibitory

Nerves of the Lungs and Arbor Bronchialis

— The **plexus pulmonali,** an autonomic nerve plexus that lies anterior and posterior to the root of the lung, innervates the lung, bronchial tree, and visceral pleura (**Fig. 8.15**; **Table 8.2**).
— Visceral afferent fibers carrying pain from the bronchi and pleura visceralis travel with sympathetic nn. splanchnici.

— Visceral sensory fibers from receptors related to cough and stretch reflexes, and receptors for blood pressure and blood gas levels travel with the n. vagus (parasympathetic nerve).
— The pleura parietalis is innervated by somatic nerves of the thoracic wall, and it is extremely sensitive to pain. Nn. intercostales innervate the pars costalis, and nn. phrenici (C3–C5) innervate the pars mediastinalis and pars diaphragmatica.
— Irritation of the pleura parietalis in the areas supplied by the n. phrenicus is referred to the dermatomes C3–C5 on the neck and shoulder.

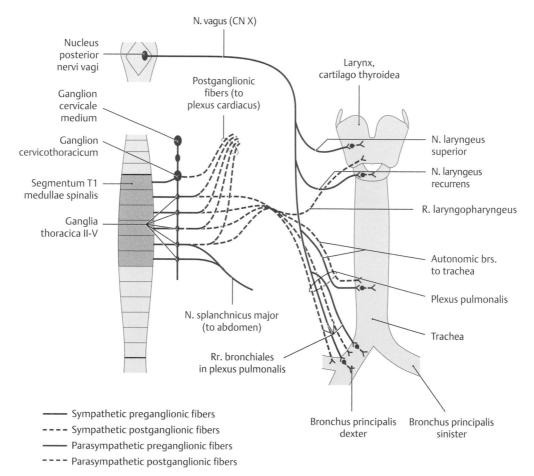

Fig. 8.15 Autonomic innervation of the tracheobronchial tree
Sympathetic innervation (*red*); parasympathetic innervation (*blue*). (From Gilroy AM et al. Atlas of Anatomy. 4th ed. 2020. Based on: Schuenke M, Schulte E, Schumacher U. THIEME Atlas of Anatomy. Internal Organs. Illustrations by Voll M and Wesker K. 3rd ed. New York: Thieme Medical Publishers; 2020.)

9 Clinical Imaging Basics of the Thorax

Radiographs are always the initial choice for imaging of the thorax. The air-filled lungs are perfectly suited for x-rays, making it easy to identify air space abnormalities such as pneumonia, and provide high contrast to the soft tissues of the heart and mediastinum. When more detail of the heart, mediastinum, or lung parenchyma is required (e.g., evaluation of interstitial lung disease), computed tomography (CT) is used. The value of magnetic resonance imaging (MRI) in cardiac imaging is its ability to acquire dynamic images (heart in motion) without radiation. Ultrasound (echocardiography) also has the utility of dynamic imaging without radiation and without the long scan times and issues of claustrophobia associated with MRI. However, the anatomic detail of ultrasound and the ability to assess the coronary vessels is limited when compared with CT and MRI (**Table 9.1**).

The chest x-ray is the starting point of the vast majority of thoracic imaging. When evaluating a chest x-ray (**Fig. 9.1**), the

Table 9.1 Suitability of Imaging Modalities for the Thorax

Modality	Clinical Uses
Radiographs (x-rays)	The mainstay of thoracic imaging and the most common radiologic study performed; excellent for evaluation of the lungs, heart, pulmonary vessels, and pleura
CT (computed tomography)	Exquisite anatomic detail of the lung parenchyma and interstitium
MRI (magnetic resonance imaging)	Best suited for imaging the heart and great vessels; very limited value in evaluating the lungs
Ultrasound	Used primarily for cardiac imaging (echocardiography); provides real-time anatomic and physiologic evaluation of the heart

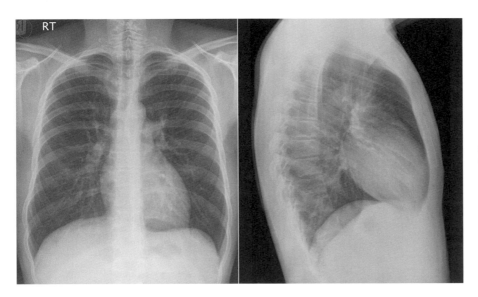

A Frontal and lateral radiographs of the chest (normal).

B Schematic representation of normal anatomic borders seen on frontal and lateral chest radiographs.

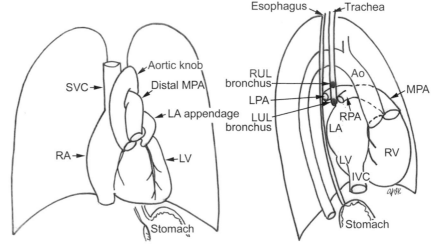

Fig. 9.1 Chest radiograph anatomy

Rendered drawing of chest radiographic anatomy. Ao, ascending aorta (aorta ascendens); IVC, inferior vena cava (v. cava inferior); LA, left atrium (atrium sinistrum); LPA, left pulmonary artery (a. pulmonalis sinistra); LUL, left upper lobar bronchus (bronchus lobaris superior sinister); LV, left ventricle (ventriculus sinister); MPA, main pulmonary artery (truncus pulmonalis); RA, right atrium; RPA, right pulmonary artery (a. pulmonalis dextra); RUL, right upper lobar bronchus (bronchus lobaris superior dexter); RV, right ventricle (ventriculus dexter); SVC, superior vena cava (v. cava superior). (From Yoo S, MacDonald C, Babyn P. Chest Radiographic Interpretation in Pediatric Cardiac Patients. 1st ed. New York: 2010.)

examiner typically follows the airway from the upper trachea down into both lungs and then views each lung in its entirety, sweeping from side to side. The heart borders are evaluated for size and shape, and the smooth surfaces of each hemidiaphragm and mediastinal border are confirmed. Each rib and vertebra is examined (**Fig. 9.2**), and then attention is given to the chest wall and soft tissues. A similar procedure is used to examine the lateral view. The chest x-ray in **Fig. 9.3** is from a patient with cough and fever. Compare the images to the normal radiographs in **Fig. 9.1**. Note the large area of white (opacity) on the right. The lateral view, in conjunction with the frontal view, confirms that this opacity is in the right lung and, more specifically, within the right middle lobe.

Computed tomography scans are excellent for showing details of the soft tissues of the thorax and can be examined in different windows to highlight specific organs (**Fig. 9.4**). CT can also reveal subtle abnormalities of the lungs that would be too small to be seen on a chest x-ray, such as inflammatory or neoplastic small lung nodules or interstitial lung diseases (**Fig. 9.5**). MRI, although not well suited for imaging the lungs, provides very good detail of the heart and allows imaging in specific planes (**Fig. 9.6**). An ultrasound of the heart, or echocardiogram, provides a dynamic view of the heart and is best viewed in "real time." However, standard static "snapshots" can provide important information, such as the four-chamber view (**Fig. 9.7**).

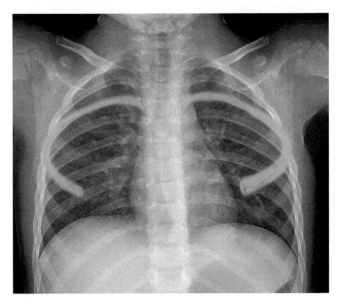

Fig 9.2 Radiograph of the thorax with the 4th ribs highlighted Frontal view.
The ribs extend horizontally from their articulation with the vertebrae and then curve laterally, anteriorly, and inferiorly. When examining a chest radiograph, each rib should be traced over its entire course. Note that the costochondral cartilage is not visible on an x-ray. (Courtesy of Joseph Makris, MD, Baystate Medical Center.)

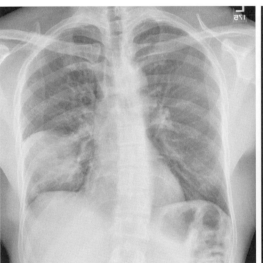
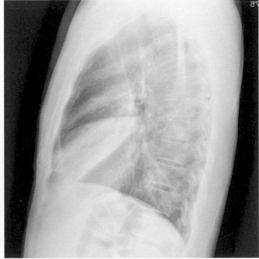

Fig. 9.3 Chest radiographs – right middle lobe pneumonia
Increased opacity (increased white) in the right middle lobe consistent with pneumonia in this patient with cough and fever. Notice the sharp outlines of the abnormal opacity on the lateral view, which represent the fissura obliqua and fissura horizontalis. These are well seen here because the pneumonia fills the right middle lobe. (From Baxter A. Emergency Imaging. A Practical Guide. 1st ed. New York: Thieme; 2015.)

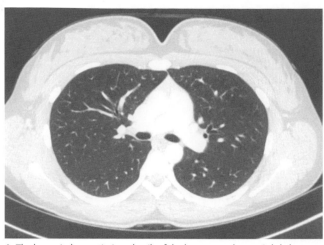 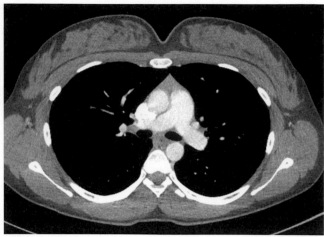

A The lung window optimizes details of the lung parenchyma. Subtle lung disease that may be invisible on a chest x-ray can be detected with chest CT.

B The soft tissue widow optimizes the soft tissue structures, but renders the lung parenchyma black (invisible). The soft tissues of the thoracic wall are well delineated. Also note the detail of the aorta and truncus pulmonalis as they branch.

Fig. 9.4 CT of the thorax, axial images – normal
These images represent the same axial slice from a normal CT scan of the thorax at the level of the truncus pulmonalis. This patient received intravenous contrast causing the blood vessels to appear white. (Courtesy of Joseph Makris, MD, Baystate Medical Center.)

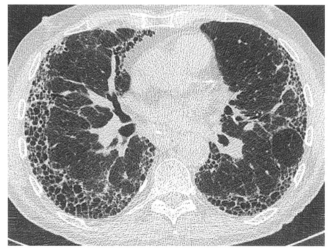

Fig. 9.5 CT of the thorax, axial view – lung disease
A single slice of a chest CT presented in lung windows in a patient with chronic cough and interstitial lung disease. Note the linear/reticular opacities throughout the lungs indicating thickening of the septa, and numerous small cysts in the periphery of the lungs with a "honeycomb" appearance. (From Wormanns D. Diagnostic Imaging of the Chest. 1st ed. New York: Thieme; 2020.)

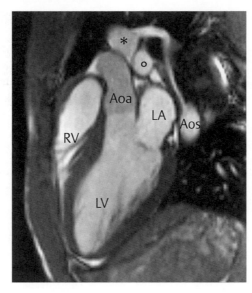

Fig. 9.6 MRI of the heart showing the left ventricular outflow tract
Cardiac MRI scans can be obtained in any plane, with several standard planes selected to optimize specific anatomy. In this example, blood in the vessels and chambers is white and the heart muscle is dark gray. This left ventricular outflow tract view positions the ventriculus sinister and the aorta ascendens in the same plane so the entire outflow tract is visible on a single image. A complete cardiac MRI would contain slices through the entire heart in this plane as well as several other planes. Additionally, MRI allows for dynamic imaging and can produce "cine" (movie) clips of several cardiac cycles showing chamber, wall, and valve motion. Note that dynamic MRIs cannot be seen in "real time" as with ultrasound. *, Superior vena cava (v. cava superior, with termination of v. azygos); •, a. pulmonalis dextra; Aoa, aorta ascendens; Aos, aorta descendens; LA, left atrium (atrium sinistrum); RV, right ventricle (ventriculus dexter); LV, left ventricle (ventriculus sinister). (From Claussen C, Miller S, Riessen R et al. Direct Diagnosis in Radiology. Cardiac Imaging. 1st ed. New York: Thieme; 2007.)

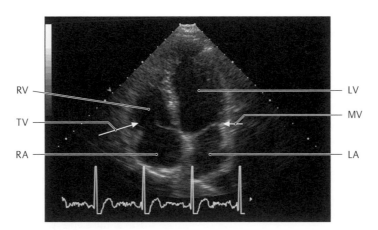

Fig. 9.7 Echocardiogram (heart ultrasound)
Apical four-chamber view taken with the probe positioned at the apex cordis.
Both ventricles (RV, LV), both atria (RA, LA), and the mitral and tricuspid valves (MV, TV) are well seen. Although this is a single static image, the true power of echocardiography is the ability to see heart motion with real-time dynamic images. Ventricular wall motion, valve operation, and blood flow can all be seen and analyzed. The displayed electrocardiogram (ECG) allows the imager to synchronize the heart's motion with its electrical activity. (From Flachskampf F. Kursbuch Echokardiografie, 4th ed. Stuttgart: Thieme Publishers; 2008.)

Unit III   Review Questions: Thorax

1. Which of the following nerves contribute to the n. phrenicus?
   A. Rr. anteriores of nn. spinales C3–C5
   B. Rr. anteriores of nn. spinales C5–T1
   C. Sympathetic fibers from C3–C5 spinal cord segments
   D. Sympathetic fibers from T1–T4 spinal cord segments
   E. Rr. cardiaci from the cervical truncus sympathicus

2. Which of the following is true of bronchopulmonary segments?
   A. Each is served by one terminal bronchiole.
   B. There are three in the right lung and two in the left lung.
   C. Each is supplied by one a. bronchialis.
   D. Each is an anatomically and functionally distinct respiratory unit of the lung.
   E. They have single-celled walls designed for efficient gas exchange.

3. Which of the following structures is/are found in the atrium dextrum?
   A. Chordae tendineae
   B. Fossa ovalis
   C. Valva mitralis
   D. Mm. papillares
   E. Trabeculae carneae

4. The angulus sterni (of Louis) marks the location of the
   A. second costal cartilage
   B. discus intervertebralis T IV–T V
   C. origin of the arcus aortae
   D. bifurcatio tracheae
   E. All of the above

5. You are studying the CT images of your patient who is being treated for lung cancer. You focus on the scan that shows the carina where you note several enlarged lymph nodes. What other structure is most likely visible in this CT image?
   A. Atrium dextrum
   B. Truncus brachiocephalicus
   C. Angulus sterni
   D. Valva tricuspidalis
   E. V. pulmonalis dextra

6. Within hours of arriving home after a 10-hour bus ride, a 77-year-old woman was rushed to the emergency room with shortness of breath, sweating, and nausea. Although she died shortly after being admitted, her workup in the emergency room revealed a pulmonary embolus in her a. pulmonalis sinistra. What other findings would you expect in this patient?
   A. Collapse of the left lung
   B. Acute dilation of the ventriculus dexter
   C. A shift of mediastinal structures to the right side
   D. Hypertrophy of the ventriculus sinister
   E. Dilation of the atrium sinistrum

7. A malignancy involving the lateral breast would *most* likely metastasize first to which of the following groups of nodes?
   A. Parasternal nodes
   B. Abdominal nodes
   C. Deep pectoral nodes
   D. Axillary nodes
   E. Nodes of the contralateral breast

8. What is the surface landmark on the chest that approximates the position of the apex cordis?
   A. Angulus sterni
   B. Left spatium intercostale III
   C. Left spatium intercostale V
   D. Right spatium intercostale V
   E. Proc. xiphoideus of the sternum

9. Dr. P. was performing a cardiac bypass on a 53-year-old man whose a. interventricularis anterior (also known as the left anterior descending artery, LAD) was narrowed near its origin. Although Dr. P. frequently used a saphenous vein graft for this procedure, he chose to use the left a. thoracica interna instead. Leaving its origin intact, he cut its distal connections and anastomosed it to the LAD beyond the narrowed segment. This successfully restored flow to the anterior part of the heart. What path does the blood take through this diverted route?
   A. Arcus aortae to a. subclavia sinistra to a. thoracica interna
   B. Arcus aortae to truncus brachiocephalicus to a. thoracica interna
   C. Arcus aortae to a. thoracica interna
   D. Arcus aortae to a. subclavia sinistra to a. pericardiacophrenica to a. thoracica interna
   E. Arcus aortae to a. axillaris to a. thoracica interna

10. An elderly man who admits to some dizziness and minor chest palpitations during the past week is finally admitted to the emergency department for chest pain and shortness of breath. Imaging reveals a major blockage of his a. coronaria dextra near the crux of the heart just proximal to the origin of the a. interventricularis inferior. Which part of the heart would be affected by the ischemia that results from this blockage?
    A. Sinoatrial (SA) node
    B. Atrioventricular (AV) node
    C. Anterior two thirds of the septum interventriculare
    D. Atrium sinistrum
    E. Ventriculus sinister

11. A woman who had a recent history of a myocardial infarction (MI) complained to her cardiologist of a sharp, stabbing pain behind her sternum that radiated to her shoulder and was accompanied by shortness of breath, particularly when she was lying down. Her physician noted a pericardial friction rub and treated her for pericarditis, an inflammation of her pericardium caused by the recent MI. Pain from her pericardium was transmitted by the
   A. nn. phrenici
   B. plexus cardiacus
   C. plexus pulmonalis
   D. nn. intercostales
   E. None of the above

12. The ductus lymphaticus dexter drains the lymph from
   A. the entire right side of the body
   B. the right side of the thorax, right upper limb, and right side of the head and neck
   C. only the right side of the thorax
   D. only the right side of the head and neck and right upper limb
   E. the right side of the thorax, the abdomen, and the right lower and the right upper limbs

13. Which of the following features are paired with the correct lung?
   A. Lingula—right lung
   B. Fissura horizontalis—left lung
   C. Incisura cardiaca—left lung
   D. Two bronchi lobares—right lung
   E. Shorter and wider than the contralateral lung—left lung

14. Several weeks after suffering a severe myocardial infarction, a man was rushed to the emergency department but died shortly afterward. It was discovered at autopsy that the muscle anchoring one leaflet of his mitral valve had ruptured, probably as a consequence of his earlier heart attack. Which was the affected muscle?
   A. M. papillaris
   B. Trabeculae carneae
   C. M. pectinatus
   D. Crista terminalis
   E. Septomarginal trabecula (trabecula septomarginalis; moderator band)

15. What is the origin of the 3rd through 11th aa. intercostales posteriores?
   A. Aorta descendens
   B. A. thoracica interna
   C. A. thoracica lateralis
   D. A. subclavia
   E. A. epigastrica superior

16. A woman with a history of asthma presents to the emergency department with shortness of breath and wheezing. Drugs and oxygen are administered, but her condition worsens. She is transferred to the intensive care unit and put on a ventilator. Twenty-four hours after admission, she dies from complications of asthma. On autopsy it is found that she has severe inflammation, an increase in smooth muscle, and other pathologic changes around a part of the respiratory tree that does not contain

cartilage. Which part of the airway was most likely affected in this patient?
   A. Trachea
   B. Main (primary) bronchi
   C. Lobar (secondary) bronchi
   D. Segmental (tertiary) bronchi
   E. Bronchioles

17. During the physical examination of a 28-year-old construction worker, you mention that his heart sounds strong and healthy. He asks you to explain what creates the heart sounds. You tell him that the first heart sound (the "lub") is produced by the
   A. closure of the valva tricuspidalis and valva pulmonalis
   B. closure of the valvae atrioventriculares
   C. opening of the semilunar valves
   D. contraction of the ventricles
   E. turbulent flow through the valves

18. All of the following structures are in contact with thoracic corpora vertebrarum except
   A. V. azygos
   B. Trachea
   C. Truncus sympathicus
   D. Ductus thoracicus
   E. Right a. intercostalis posterior

19. What is/are the primary muscle(s) used in quiet respiration?
   A. Mm. intercostales
   B. Mm. scaleni
   C. Diaphragma
   D. M. pectoralis major
   E. Anterior abdominal muscles

20. Which of the following valves is most audible at the right 2nd intercostal space just lateral to the sternum?
   A. Valva aortae
   B. Valva atrioventricularis sinistra
   C. Valva trunci pulmonalis
   D. Valva atrioventricularis dextra
   E. Valvula sinus coronarii

21. During auscultation of the heart, which of the following relationships is *most* likely to be correct in a normal adult?
   A. The left 4th intercostal space at the midaxillary line is the site of auscultation of the valva mitralis.
   B. The left 2nd intercostal space at the sternal border is the site of auscultation of the valva aortae.
   C. The right 3rd intercostal space at the sternal border is the site of auscultation of the valva trunci pulmonalis.
   D. The right 2nd intercostal space at the sternal border is the site of auscultation of the valva aortae.
   E. The right 4th intercostal space at the midclavicular line is the site of auscultation of the valva tricuspidalis.

22. Which of the following events occurs during either quiet or forced expiration?
   A. Collapse of sacculi alveolares
   B. Increase in lung volume
   C. Elevation of the ribs
   D. Increase in intrapleural pressure
   E. Temporary collapse of the segmental bronchi

23. During a routine physical exam of a young woman who is training to compete in the Olympic trials, you scrutinize her cardiac rhythm for abnormalities. Which of the following events normally occur during ventricular diastole?
   A. Contraction of the ventricles
   B. Ejection of blood into the truncus pulmonalis
   C. Opening of the semilunar valves
   D. Filling of the aa. coronariae
   E. Closure of the atrioventricular valves

24. You have been treating a 67-year-old woman for a mediastinal tumor for three months. Following her latest CT scan, it's clear that the tumor has increased in size, despite the chemotherapy, and is now large enough to compress her v. cava superior (superior vena cava syndrome). In spite of this obstruction, veins of her neck and upper limb appear only slightly distended. You know from the CT that the obstruction is located below the junction of the SVC and v. azygos and you are confident that venous blood from the head and upper limb is flowing back to her heart via collateral channels. The backflow of blood through these collateral channels would cause some dilation in collateral vessels. Which of the following would not be affected by this backflow?
   A. Vv. jugulares externae
   B. Vv. pulmonales dextrae
   C. Vv. intercostales posteriores
   D. V. hemiazygos
   E. Vv. thoracicae internae

25. Your 64-year-old neighbor, a retired high school biology teacher, is seemingly recovered from a serious heart attack from several months ago. However, during a recent checkup she was found to have an abnormally slow and irregular heartbeat, a diagnosis of atrioventricular heart block. In an effort to calm her distress and explain her condition, you try to explain how the heart is innervated. Which of the following statements is true of the plexus cardiacus?
   A. It contains postganglionic sympathetic fibers from the cervical and thoracic truncus sympathicus.
   B. Visceral sensory fibers that innervate the baroreceptors (which measure blood pressure) travel with sympathetic fibers.
   C. It contains cardiac branches of the n. vagus, which contain postganglionic sympathetic fibers.
   D. It initiates the heartbeat but does not regulate the heart rate.
   E. Sensations of pain carried on visceral sensory fibers travel with parasympathetic branches of the n. vagi.

26. Your first patient as an Ob/Gyn intern is a 23-year-old woman who gave birth to a premature 5-pound baby girl with Down syndrome. Within the first few days the child is diagnosed with an atrial septal defect (ASD), a common anomaly associated with her congenital defect. Atrial septal defects
   A. cause a right-to-left shunting of blood in the atria
   B. result in a decrease in blood volume in the pulmonary circulation
   C. result from a failure of the ductus arteriosus to constrict
   D. can result from a failure of the foramen ovale to close at birth

   E. can be compensated for by an effective collateral circulation that circumvents the defect

27. The oesophagus is an unusual structure in that it traverses three anatomic regions: the cervical region, the thorax, and the abdomen. Although an important conduit of the gastrointestinal tract, it has no role in digestion. However, it is an organ vulnerable to disease and trauma, and as such, its anatomic relations are significant. Which of the following descriptions of the oesophagus is accurate?
   A. It is innervated by the plexus oesophageus, a parasympathetic nerve plexus.
   B. The upper, middle, and lower oesophageal veins drain solely into the azygos system via posterior intercostal veins.
   C. The arcus aortae and bronchus principalis sinister create the upper oesophageal sphincter, a normal esophageal constriction.
   D. It passes through the hiatus oesophageus in the centrum tendineum of the diaphragma anterior to corpus vertebrae T VIII.
   E. In the thorax, it descends posterior to the trachea and the atrium sinistrum of the heart.

28. A patient with known multisystem disease is admitted to the emergency department with shortness of breath and cough. He is found to have a pleural effusion of the right lung and is treated with the insertion of a chest tube, which drains the fluid. Which of the following is true?
   A. The excess fluid is located in his cavitas pleuralis, which is lined by a thin layer of pleura visceralis surrounded by a tough layer of pleura parietalis.
   B. The fluid is likely to leak into the cavitas pleuralis of his left lung.
   C. The fluid is likely to accumulate in the recessus costodiaphragmaticus.
   D. The chest tube is inserted at the anterior axillary line, in the 5th intercostal space below the rib to avoid damage to the liver.
   E. A pleural effusion is often accompanied by a shift of mediastinal structures, such as the heart, to the opposite side.

29. A patient with cough and fever has a chest x-ray and is diagnosed with complete lobar pneumonia involving the right lower lobe. What usual anatomic outline may become invisible because of the pneumonia?
   A. Right heart border
   B. Right hemidiaphragm
   C. Left hemidiaphragm
   D. Right upper mediastinum
   E. Right breast shadow

30. What would be the best way to detect a cardiac wall motion abnormality in an unstable patient with a recent myocardial infarction (MI)?
   A. Chest x-ray
   B. Chest CT
   C. Ultrasound (echocardiogram)
   D. ECG
   E. MRI

Answers and Explanations

1. **A.** The n. phrenicus is a somatic nerve containing C3–C5 rr. anteriores (Section 5.2).
    B. The rr. anteriores of C5–T1 form the plexus brachialis.
    C. There are no autonomic nerves that arise from the C3–C5 spinal cord.
    D. Sympathetic nn. splanchnici that arise from T1–T4 contribute to the plexus cardiacus and plexus pulmonalis.
    E. Rr. cardiaci from the cervical truncus sympathicus contribute to the plexus cardiacus and are not related to the n. phrenicus.

2. **D.** Bronchopulmonary segments function independently from other segments and are separated from them by thin septa (Section 8.2).
    A. One bronchus segmentalis enters each bronchopulmonary segment and ramifies into many conducting bronchioles, which in turn divide into many terminal bronchioles.
    B. The right lung has 10 bronchopulmonary segments, and the left lung has 8 to 10 segments.
    C. Aa. bronchiales supply the bronchi and connective tissue of the lungs, including the pleura visceralis. Branches of the aa. pulmonales supply the bronchopulmonary segments.
    E. Alveoli, the smallest unit of the respiratory tree, have single-celled walls that facilitate gas exchange.

3. **B.** The fossa ovalis on the septum interatriale is the remnant of the opening between the atria that allows right-to-left shunting in the fetal circulation (Section 7.4).
    A. Chordae tendineae are found in the ventricles.
    C. The valva mitralis (valva atrioventricularis sinistra) separates the atrium sinistrum and ventriculus sinister.
    D. Mm. papillares are found only in the ventricles.
    E. Trabeculae carneae are muscular ridges in the walls of the ventricles.

4. **E.** The sternal angle (angulus sterni) is a palpable bony prominence created at the junction of the body and manubrium of the sternum. It marks the transverse plane that passes through the cartilago costalis II, discus intervertebralis T IV–T V, origin of the arcus aortae, and bifurcation of the trachea (bifurcatio tracheae; Section 6.2).

5. **C.** The carina, at the bifurcatio tracheae, lies approximately at the T IV–T V vertebral level, which is also the level of the angulus sterni (Section 6.2).
    A. The atrium dextrum lies approximately at the level of T VI–T VII, below the carina at the bifurcatio tracheae.
    B. The truncus brachiocephalicus, the first branch of the arcus aortae, lies approximately at the level of T III. The carina lies at the level of the angulus sterni at T IV–T V.
    D. The valva atrioventricularis dextra lies at the level of the cartilago costalis V. The carina lies at the level of the cartilago costalis II and the angulus sterni.
    E. Vv. pulmonales on both sides enter the atrium sinistrum, approximately at the level of T VI–T VII, well below the carina at T IV–T V.

6. **B.** Obstruction of the a. pulmonalis impedes blood flow into the lung and causes pooling of blood in the right side of the heart. This causes acute dilation of the atrium dextrum and ventriculus dexter (Section 8.5).
    A. Collapse of the lung is a symptom of a pneumothorax in which air enters the cavitas pleuralis.

    C. The pressure of a tension pneumothorax can cause the heart to shift to the opposite side.
    D. Hypertrophy of the ventriculus sinister is the result of a chronic condition that causes the myocardium to work harder in response to a fluid overload or an obstruction in the aortic outflow tract. A pulmonary embolism is usually an acute event that causes a fluid overload in the ventriculus dexter but decreases venous return to the ventriculus sinister.
    E. A pulmonary embolism reduces the volume of blood entering the lung from the right side of the heart and therefore results in a diminished venous return to the left side of the heart. The atrium dextrum and ventriculus dexter may be acutely dilated, but the atrium sinistrum and ventriculus sinister are not.

7. **D.** A malignancy involving the lateral breast would most likely metastasize via the axillary nodes (nll. axillares) and then on to nodes around the clavicle and the ipsilateral lymphatic duct (Section 6.1).
    A. Medial portions of the breast may drain to the nll. parasternales. These nodes also receive lymph from the anterior abdominal wall above the umbilicus, the deeper parts of the anterior portion of the thoracic wall, and the superior surface of the liver.
    B. Nodes of the anterior abdominal wall receive lymph from the medial and inferior parts of the breast.
    C. Although some lymph from the breast may drain to deep pectoral nodes posterior to the m. pectoralis, most lymph from the breast drains to nll. axillares.
    E. Lymphatic drainage from the medial breast may drain to the contralateral breast, but lymphatic drainage from the lateral breast most abundantly passes to the nll. axillares.

8. **C.** The apex cordis lies at the level of the 5th intercostal space (spatium intercostale V; Section 7.4).
    A. The angulus sterni is at the level of the cartilago costalis II.
    B. The 3rd intercostal space (spatium intercostale III) is above the level of the heart.
    D. The apex cordis is found at the most inferior and left border of the heart, which lies to the left of the sternum.
    E. The proc. xiphoideus lies in the midline, whereas the apex lies to the left side of the sternum.

9. **A.** The a. thoracica interna is a branch of the a. subclavia sinistra, the third branch of the arcus aortae (Section 5.2).
    B. The a. thoracica interna arises from the a. subclavia.
    C. The a. thoracica interna does not arise directly from the arcus aortae. It is a branch of the a. subclavia.
    D. The aa. pericardiacophrenicae arise from the aa. thoracicae internae to supply the pericardium and diaphragma. They do not contribute to the blood supply of the heart.
    E. The a. thoracica interna arises from the a. subclavia, not the a. axillaris.

10. **B.** The r. nodi atrioventricularis, which branches from the a. coronaria dextra near the origin of the a. interventricularis inferior, usually supplies the AV node (nodus atrioventricularis; Section 7.7).
    A. The SA node (nodus sinuatrialis) is supplied by the SA nodal artery, a branch of the proximal part of the a. coronaria dextra, or by the circumflex branch of the a. coronaria sinistra.

C. The left anterior interventricular artery (LAD; a. interventricularis anterior) supplies the anterior two thirds of the septum interventriculare.

D. The circumflex branch of the a. coronaria sinistra supplies the atrium sinistrum.

E. The marginal branch of the a. coronaria dextra supplies most of the ventriculus dexter. Its origin is well proximal to the crux of the heart and would not be affected by this blockage.

11. **A.** The nn. phrenici (C3–C5) are the primary sensory nerves of the pericardium. Referred pain is often felt in the supraclavicular region, the C3–C5 dermatome (Section 7.3).

B. The plexus cardiacus is a plexus of autonomic fibers that innervate the heart.

C. The plexus pulmonalis, an extension of the plexus cardiacus, regulates the constriction and dilation of the pulmonary vessels and bronchial passages.

D. Nn. intercostales innervate structures of the thoracic and abdominal walls.

E. Not applicable

12. **B.** The ductus lymphaticus dexter drains the lymph from the right side of the thorax, right upper limb, and right side of the head and neck (Section 5.2).

A. Lymph from all structures below the diaphragma drains to the left lymphatic duct (ductus thoracicus).

C. The right side of the head and neck and right upper limb also drain to the ductus lymphaticus dexter.

D. The right side of the thorax also drains to the ductus lymphaticus dexter.

E. Lymph from the abdomen and both lower limbs drains to the ductus thoracicus (left lymphatic duct).

13. **C.** The incisura cardiaca is a deep indentation along the anterior border of the superior lobe of the left lung (Section 8.2).

A. The lingula is a thin tongue of tissue that forms the lower border of the incisura cardiaca of the superior lobe of the left lung.

B. The left lung has only a fissura obliqua that separates the superior and inferior lobes.

D. The right lung has three lobes supplied by three bronchi lobares.

E. The right lung is shorter and wider than the left lung due to the presence of the liver below the right side of the diaphragma.

14. **A.** The mm. papillares of the ventriculus sinister attach to the chordae tendineae of the mitral valve leaflets and prevent them from prolapsing during ventricular systole (Section 7.4).

B. Trabeculae carneae are the thick muscular ridges of the ventricular walls.

C. Mm. pectinati are found in the auricula dextra and auricula sinistra.

D. The terminal crest (crista terminalis) is a muscular ridge within the atrium dextrum that separates its two parts, the sinus venarum cavarum and the atrium proper.

E. The interventricular trabecula septomarginalis is a muscular band that connects the septum interventriculare to the m. papillaris anterior of the ventriculus dexter and carries the right branch of the fasciculus atrioventricularis of the conducting system.

15. **A.** The aorta supplies the 3rd through 11th aa. intercostales posteriores (Section 6.4).

B. The a. thoracica interna supplies the rr. intercostales anteriores.

C. The a. thoracica lateralis originates from the a. axillaris and supplies the m. pectoralis major and m. pectoralis minor, and the mm. serrati anteriores and the rr. mammarii laterales.

D. The a. subclavia supplies only the 1st and 2nd of the aa. intercostales posteriores. It also supplies the a. thoracica interna, a. vertebralis, and a. axillaris, as well as branches to the neck and shoulder.

E. The a. epigastrica superior is a branch of the a. thoracica interna. It supplies the lower anterior intercostal arteries and the anterior abdominal wall.

16. **E.** The bronchioles have no cartilage but do contain a layer of smooth muscle that often hypertrophies (cells increase in size) in severe asthma (Section 8.3).

A. The trachea contains C-shaped cartilage rings.

B. The main bronchi (bronchi principales) contain C-shaped cartilage rings, similar to those in the trachea.

C. Lobar bronchi (bronchi lobares) contain plates of cartilage.

D. Segmental bronchi (bronchi segmentales) contain plates of cartilage.

17. **B.** Closure of tricuspid and mitral (atrioventricular) valves (valvae atrioventriculares) produces the first ("lub") sound (Section 7.4).

A. Closure of the tricuspid valve (valva tricuspidalis) contributes to the first heart sound ("lub"); closure of the pulmonary valve (valva pulmonalis) contributes to the second heart sound ("dub").

C. Opening of the semilunar valves does not produce discernible heart sounds.

D. Contraction of the ventricles does not produce any sound, although it coincides with the closure of the valvae atrioventriculares, which produces the first heart sound.

E. Turbulent flow through the valves, often associated with valvular stenosis and regurgitation, produces a murmur heard on auscultation.

18. **B.** The trachea lies anterior to the oesophagus along its entire length and is not in contact with the corpora vertebrarum (Sections 6.4 and 7.7).

A. The v. azygos ascends along the anterior surface of the vertebrae thoracicae.

C. The trunci sympathici lie along the lateral aspects of the vertebrae thoracicae.

D. The ductus thoracicus ascends along the corpora vertebrarum between the v. azygos and v. hemiazygos.

E. The aa. intercostales posteriores arise from the aorta and cross the corpora vertebrarum to run within the spatia intercostalia on the right side.

19. **C.** During quiet respiration the contraction and relaxation of the diaphragma change the volume of the pulmonary cavities and consequently the expansion and contraction of the lungs (Section 8.4).

A. The mm. intercostales are used to elevate and lower the ribs during forced inspiration and forced expiration.

B. Mm. scaleni are extrinsic muscles of respiration that move the ribs during forced inspiration.

D. The m. pectoralis major moves and stabilizes the upper limb but also assists movements of the ribs during deep inspiration.

E. Anterior abdominal muscles contract during forced expiration.

20. **A.** The valva aortae is most audible at the right 2nd intercostal space just lateral to the sternum (Section 7.4).

B. Sound from the left atrioventricular (AV) valve (valva atrioventricularis sinister) is most audible over the left 5th intercostal space on the midclavicular line.

C. Sound from the pulmonary valve (valva trunci pulmonalis) is most audible over the left 2nd intercostal space just lateral to the sternum.

D. Sound from the right AV valve (valva atrioventricularis dexter) is most audible from the left 5th intercostal space at the sternal margin.

E. There is usually no audible sound from the valve of the coronary sinus (sinus coronarius).

21. **D.** The right 2nd intercostal space at the sternal border is the site of auscultation of the valva aortae (Section 7.4).

A. The left 5th intercostal space at the midclavicular line is the site of auscultation of the mitral valve (valva mitralis).

B. The left 2nd intercostal space at the sternal border is the site of auscultation of the valva aortae.

C. The left 2nd intercostal space at the sternal border is the site of auscultation of the valva trunci pulmonalis.

E. The left 5th intercostal space at the sternal border is the site of auscultation of the tricuspid valve (valva tricuspidis).

22. **D.** During expiration, the contraction of the pulmonary cavity causes an increase in intrapleural pressure, which forces air to be expelled from the lung (Section 8.4).

A. Surfactant lining the walls of the alveoli prevents them from collapsing during expiration.

B. During inspiration the thoracic cavity expands, pulling the pleural sac outward and causing an increase in lung volume.

C. The elevation of the ribs increases the size of the thoracic cavity during inspiration.

E. Incomplete cartilaginous rings in the walls of the bronchi prevent them from collapsing during expiration.

23. **D.** At the beginning of ventricular diastole (relaxation of the ventricles), the semilunar valves close, and backflow in the aorta fills the aa. coronariae (Section 7.4).

A. The ventricles contract during ventricular systole.

B. Blood from the ventriculus dexter is ejected into the truncus pulmonalis during ventricular systole.

C. The semilunar valves open during ventricular systole to allow blood to flow into the aorta and truncus pulmonalis.

E. During the initial phase of ventricular systole, as ventricular pressure increases, the atrioventricular valves close.

24. **B.** Backflow through collateral channels would affect veins that are part of the azygos and caval systems. Blood would eventually drain from the v. cava inferior to the right side of the heart, so the pulmonary and cardiac circulations would remain unaffected (Section 5.1).

A. Vv. jugulares externae drain into the azygos system via the vv. jugulares internae and vv. brachiocephalicae.

C. Reverse flow through the v. azygos into the vv. intercostales posteriores would cause dilation of these vessels.

D. As in all parts of the azygos system, the v. hemiazygos would dilate with increased flow.

E. The reverse flow in the vv. subclaviae into their tributaries, including the vv. thoracicae internae, would result in dilation of these vessels.

25. **A.** Postganglionic sympathetic nerves arise from the cervical and thoracic truncus sympathicus as the superior, middle, and inferior cervical cardiac nerves (Sections 7.4 and 7.5).

B. Visceral sensory fibers that innervate both the baroreceptors and chemoreceptors of the heart travel with the parasympathetic fibers of the n. vagus.

C. The cardiac branches of the n. vagus contain only parasympathetic fibers.

D. The plexus cardiacus regulates the heart rate, but the SA node (nodus sinuatrialis) initiates and coordinates the timing of the contraction of the heart's chambers.

E. Pain sensation from the heart is carried by visceral sensory fibers that travel with sympathetic fibers to the T1–T5 spinal cord.

26. **D.** At birth, the foramen ovale, a normal opening between the right and left atria during fetal growth, closes, thus forcing blood into the pulmonary circulation. Failure to do so results in an opening known as an atrial septal defect (Section 7.6).

A. Because of the reduced pressure in the atrium dextrum compared to that in the atrium sinistrum, an ASD results in a left-to right-shunt.

B. The increased flow into the atrium dextrum results in an increased flow through the truncus pulmonalis and pulmonary circulation.

C. Failure of the ductus arteriosus to constrict is known as a patent ductus arteriosus, a condition unrelated to an ASD.

E. There is no collateral circulation that compensates for the defect in the septum interatriale.

27. **E.** Superiorly, the esophagus lies posterior to the trachea, inferiorly it passes posterior to the atrium sinistrum (Section 7.7).

A. The plexus oesophageus receives parasympathetic fibers from the nn. vagi as well as sympathetic innervation from nn. splanchnici thoracici.

B. The lower esophageal veins anastomose inferiorly with vv. phrenicae inferiores, which are tributaries of the portal system that drains the gastrointestinal system. This is an important anastomosis between the caval and the portal venous systems.

C. The upper esophageal sphincter is created by the m. cricopharyngeus in the neck.

D. The hiatus oesophageus is formed by the crura of the diaphragma at the T X vertebral level.

28. **C.** The recessus costodiaphragmaticus is a lower recess of the cavitas pleuralis, where the fluid is likely to accumulate (Section 8.1).

A. The cavitas pleuralis is surrounded by a continuous single layer of pleura. Pleura parietalis lines the outer wall of the cavity, where it is adjacent to the ribs, the diaphragma, and the mediastinum. It is continuous with the Pleura visceralis that covers the surface of the lung.

B. Each cavitas pleuralis is a separate space. There is no communication between the right and the left cavities.

D. A chest tube is always inserted above the rib to avoid damage to the intercostal neurovascular bundle that runs in the groove along the lower edge of the rib.

E. A "mediastinal shift" is a symptom of a tension pneumothorax but not of a pleural effusion.

29. **B.** Lobar consolidations, such as from pneumonia, often cause the "silhouette sign," which results in a normal anatomic border being rendered invisible because the normally air-filled adjacent lung is filled with fluid. The right lower lobe abuts the right hemidiaphragm, thus obscuring it (Chapter 9).

A. The majority of the right heart border abuts the right middle lobe.

C. The left hemidiaphragm would still be outlined by air in the left lower lobe.

D. The right upper mediastinum is not contiguous with the right lower lobe.

E. The right breast shadow would not be affected by an intrapulmonary process.

30. **C.** Ultrasound (echocardiogram) provides real-time evaluation of cardiac anatomy and is excellent for assessment of function including wall motion, contractility, and cardiac output. Ultrasound can be done at the bedside, is relatively fast and inexpensive, and uses no ionizing radiation (Chapter 9).

A. Chest x-ray may show evidence of congestive heart failure but would not identify cardiac abnormalities directly.

B. Cardiac anatomy is well delineated on CT, but function is not.

D. ECG does not show motion abnormalities.

E. Dynamic cardiac MRI is an excellent tool for cardiac anatomic and functional assessment but would not be suitable for an unstable patient. Long scan times with the patient placed in the MRI machine are prohibitive in this setting.

Unit IV Abdomen

10   The Abdominal Wall and Inguinal Region

The abdomen, the region of the trunk between the thorax and the pelvis, contains the largest portion of the **abdominopelvic cavity (cavitas abdominopelvica),** a peritoneal-lined space that it shares with the pelvis **(Fig. 10.1)**. The abdomen houses the primary organs of the gastrointestinal and urinary systems, although some abdominal viscera (e.g., intestinum tenue) typically overflow the boundaries of the abdomen to occupy pelvic spaces, and pelvic viscera, when distended (i.e., vesica urinaria and uterus), can extend superiorly into the abdomen.

The abdominal wall, composed of skin, subcutaneous tissue, and muscles, is supported by its attachments to the ribs, vertebrae lumbales, and bony pelvis. It moves and stabilizes the trunk, supports the abdominal viscera, and creates intra-abdominal pressure that is crucial in digestion and respiration. The muscular abdominal wall provides little protection for underlying viscera, but much of the upper abdominal viscera lies under the dome of the diaphragma, where the viscera are protected by the thoracic skeleton. The bony pelvis protects most viscera in the lower abdomen.

10.1   Regions and Planes of the Abdominal Wall

— In order to describe the location of abdominal viscera, we divide the abdomen into four quadrants or nine regions, using vertical reference lines and standard transverse planes **(Fig. 10.2)**.
— The **planum transpyloricum,** a transverse plane at the level of T XII–L I, measured halfway between the jugular notch (incisura jugularis) and pubic crest (crista pubica), is a useful horizontal plane that provides orientation to the internal anatomy of the abdomen **(Fig. 10.3)**. The T XII–L I plane passes through (or very close to)
  • the pylorus of the stomach,
  • the ampulla of the duodenum,
  • the origin of the truncus coeliacus,
  • the origin of the a. mesenterica superior,
  • the origin of the v. portae hepatis,
  • the neck of the pancreas (collum pancreatis), and
  • the flexura coli sinistra of the intestinum crassum.

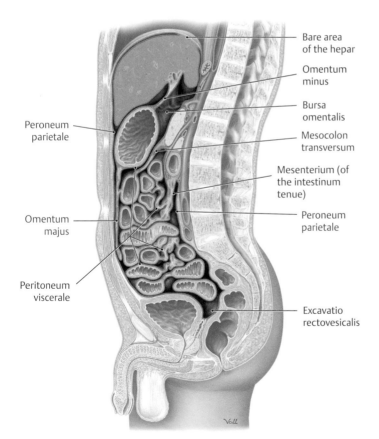

Fig. 10.1 Peritoneal relationships
Midsagittal section through cavitas abdominopelvica in the male, viewed from the left side. The peritoneum is shown *(red)*. (From Gilroy AM et al. Atlas of Anatomy. 4th ed. 2020. Based on: Schuenke M, Schulte E, Schumacher U. THIEME Atlas of Anatomy. Internal Organs. Illustrations by Voll M and Wesker K. 3rd ed. New York: Thieme Medical Publishers; 2020.)

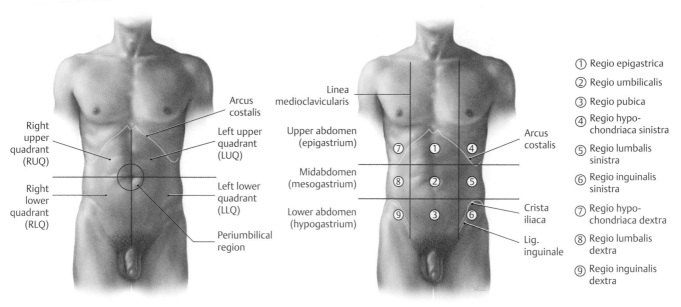

A The abdomen is divided into four quadrants by two perpendicular lines that intersect at the umbilicus.

Fig. 10.2 Criteria for dividing the abdomen into regions
(From Schuenke M, Schulte E, Schumacher U. THIEME Atlas of Anatomy, Vol 1. Illustrations by Voll M and Wesker K. 3rd ed. New York: Thieme Publishers; 2020.)

B Coordinate system composed of two vertical and two horizontal lines divide the abdomen into nine regions, each located in either the upper, middle, or lower abdomen. The two vertical lines are the left and right linea medioclavicularis. One of the two horizontal lines passes through the lowest point of the 10th ribs and the other through the summit of the two cristae iliacae.

- The **superficial fatty layer (panniculus adiposus, Camper's fascia)**, a subcutaneous layer of fat whose thickness varies among individuals and that is continuous with the tela subcutanea of the thorax, back, and lower limb
- The **deep membranous layer (stratum membranosum, Scarpa's fascia)**, a tough fibrous sheet that lies deep to the superficial fatty layer, covers the lower anterior abdominal wall, and extends inferiorly into the perineum, where it is continuous with the **fascia perinei superficialis (Colles' fascia)**.

Muscular Layer: Anterior and Posterior Walls

— Three flat muscles make up most of the muscular layer of the lateral and anterior walls of the abdomen: the **m. obliquus externus abdominis, m. obliquus internus abdominis,** and **m. transversus abdominis**. Their large aponeuroses constitute the most anterior part of the abdominal wall **(Fig. 10.4; Table 10.1)**.
- The thickened inferior edge of the aponeurosis of the m. obliqui externi abdominis forms the **lig. inguinale**, which attaches laterally to the **spina iliaca anterior superior** and medially to the **tuberculum pubicum** of the os pubis. Some fibers of the medial end of the ligament reflect downward as the **lig. lacunare** to attach to the superior edge of the os pubis (see **Fig. 10.14**).
- Inferiorly, the aponeurosis of the m. obliqui interni abdominis and the m. transversus abdominis join to form the **conjoined tendon (tendo conjunctivus),** where they attach to the os pubis.
- In the anterior midline, the aponeuroses of the three muscles overlap those of the contralateral muscles, forming the **linea alba,** a tendinous raphe (junction) that extends from the proc. xiphoideus to the os pubis. The **anulus umbilicalis,** a remnant of the opening for the umbilical cord, interrupts the raphe at its midpoint.

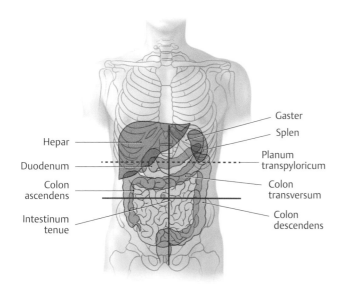

Fig. 10.3 Planum transpyloricum *(dashed red line)* and its relationship to abdominal viscera
Anterior view. (From Schuenke M, Schulte E, Schumacher U. THIEME Atlas of Anatomy, Vol 2. Illustrations by Voll M and Wesker K. 3rd ed. New York: Thieme Publishers; 2020.)

10.2 Structure of the Abdominal Wall

Subcutaneous Layer

— The **subcutaneous layer (tela subcutanea abdominis)**, sometimes referred to as the "superficial fascia," of the abdominal wall, lies deep to the skin and superficial to the muscular layer. It has two components (see **Fig. 10.5**):

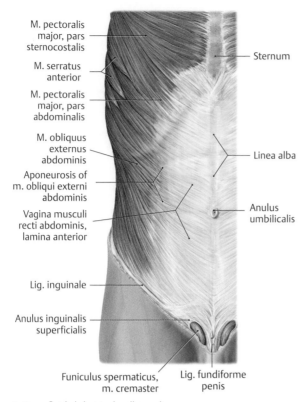

A Superficial abdominal wall muscles.

M. pectoralis major, pars sternocostalis

M. serratus anterior

M. pectoralis major, pars abdominalis

M. obliquus externus abdominis

Aponeurosis of m. obliqui externi abdominis

Vagina musculi recti abdominis, lamina anterior

Lig. inguinale

Anulus inguinalis superficialis

Funiculus spermaticus, m. cremaster

Lig. fundiforme penis

Sternum

Linea alba

Anulus umbilicalis

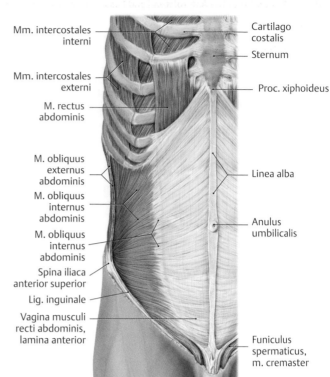

B *Removed:* M. obliquus externus abdominis, m. pectorialis major, and m. serratus anterior.

Mm. intercostales interni

Mm. intercostales externi

M. rectus abdominis

M. obliquus externus abdominis

M. obliquus internus abdominis

M. obliquus internus abdominis

Spina iliaca anterior superior

Lig. inguinale

Vagina musculi recti abdominis, lamina anterior

Cartilago costalis

Sternum

Proc. xiphoideus

Linea alba

Anulus umbilicalis

Funiculus spermaticus, m. cremaster

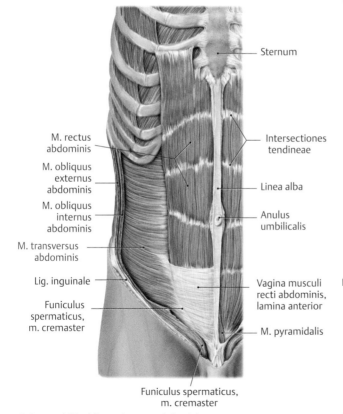

C *Removed:* M. obliquus internus abdominis.

M. rectus abdominis

M. obliquus externus abdominis

M. obliquus internus abdominis

M. transversus abdominis

Lig. inguinale

Funiculus spermaticus, m. cremaster

Funiculus spermaticus, m. cremaster

Sternum

Intersectiones tendineae

Linea alba

Anulus umbilicalis

Vagina musculi recti abdominis, lamina anterior

M. pyramidalis

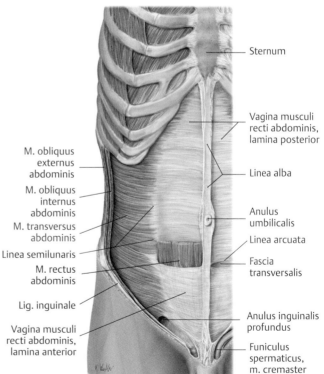

D *Removed:* M. rectus abdominis.

M. obliquus externus abdominis

M. obliquus internus abdominis

M. transversus abdominis

Linea semilunaris

M. rectus abdominis

Lig. inguinale

Vagina musculi recti abdominis, lamina anterior

Sternum

Vagina musculi recti abdominis, lamina posterior

Linea alba

Anulus umbilicalis

Linea arcuata

Fascia transversalis

Anulus inguinalis profundus

Funiculus spermaticus, m. cremaster

Fig. 10.4 Muscles of the anterolateral abdominal wall
Right side, anterior view. (From Schuenke M, Schulte E, Schumacher U. THIEME Atlas of Anatomy, Vol 1. Illustrations by Voll M and Wesker K. 3rd ed. New York: Thieme Publishers; 2020.)

Table 10.1 Muscles of the Anterolateral and Posterior Abdominal Walls

Muscles	Origin	Insertion	Innervation	Action
Anterolateral abdominal wall				
M. obliquus externus abdominis	Costae V–XII (outer surface)	Linea alba, tuberculum pubicum, anterior crista iliaca	Nn. intercostales (T7–T11), n. subcostalis (T12)	*Unilateral*: bends trunk to same side, rotates trunk to opposite side
M. obliquus internus abdominis	Fascia thoracolumbalis (lamina anterior), crista iliaca (linea intermedia), spina iliaca anterior superior, fascia iliopsoas	Costa X–XII (lower borders), linea alba (anterior and posterior layers)	Nn. intercostales (T7–T11), n. subcostalis (T12), n. iliohypogastricus, n. ilioinguinalis	*Bilateral*: flexes trunk, compresses abdomen, stabilizes pelvis
M. transversus abdominis	Cartilagines costales VII–XII (inner surfaces), fascia thoracolumbalis (lamina anterior), crista iliaca, spina iliaca anterior superior (inner lip), fascia iliopsoas	Linea alba, crista pubica		*Unilateral*: rotates trunk to same side *Bilateral*: compresses abdomen
M. rectus abdominis	*Caput laterale:* Crista pubica to tuberculum pubicum *Caput mediale:* Anterior region of symphysis pubica	Cartilagines costales V–VII, proc. xiphoideus sterni	Nn. intercostales (T5–T11), n. subcostalis (T12)	Flexes trunk, compresses abdomen, stabilizes pelvis
M. pyramidalis	Pubis (anterior to m. rectus abdominis)	Linea alba (runs within the vagina musculi recti abdominis)	N. subcostalis (T12)	Tenses linea alba
Posterior abdominal wall				
M. psoas minor	Vertebrae T XII, L I and discus intervertebralis (lateral surfaces)	Linea pectinea, eminentia iliopubica, fascia iliopsoas; lowermost fibers may reach lig. inguinale	Nn. spinales L1–L2 (L3)	Weak flexor of trunk
M. psoas major Superficial layer	Corpora vertebrae T XII–L IV and associated disci intervertebrales (lateral surfaces)	Femur (trochanter minor), joint insertion as m. iliopsoas		Hip joint: flexion and external rotation Lumbar spine (with femur fixed): *Unilateral*: contraction bends trunk laterally *Bilateral*: contraction raises trunk from supine position
Deep layer	L I–L V (procc. costales)			
M. iliacus	Fossa iliaca		N. femoralis (L2–L4)	
M. quadratus lumborum	Crista iliaca and lig. iliolumbale	Costa XII, vertebrae L I–L IV (procc. costales)	N. subcostalis (T12), nn. spinales L1–L4	*Unilateral*: bends trunk to same side *Bilateral*: bearing down and expiration, stabilizes costa XII

— On either side of the anterior midline, an **m. rectus abdominis** and an **m. pyramidalis** is enclosed in a rectus sheath, whose lateral edges are visible externally as the **semilunar lines (lineae semilunares)**. The sheath has anterior and posterior layers, formed by the aponeuroses of the anterolateral muscles as they pass around the mm. recti abdominis to decussate at the linea alba in the midline (**Fig. 10.5** and **10.6**).
  • The anterior layer extends the length of the m. rectus abdominis, but the posterior layer lines only its upper two thirds. The inferior end of the posterior layer is marked by a curved horizontal **linea arcuata**, located at a point one third of the distance between the umbilicus and pubis.
  • Above the linea arcuata, the anterior layer of the sheath is formed by the aponeurosis of the m. obliquus externus abdominis and an anterior leaf of the aponeurosis of the m. obliquus internus abdominis. The posterior layer of the sheath is formed by the aponeurosis of the m. transversus abdominis and posterior leaf of the aponeurosis of the m. obliquus internus abdominis.

  • Below the linea arcuata, the aponeuroses of all three muscles pass anterior to the m. rectus abdominis to form the anterior rectus sheath. In this area, the posterior surface of the m. rectus abdominis is lined only by fascia transversalis (a component of the fascia endoabdominalis) and peritoneum.
— The posterior abdominal wall is the posterior boundary of the cavitas abdominis. Although continuous with the region designated as the "back," which contains the columna vertebralis and paravertebral muscles, the posterior abdominal wall is conceptually considered a separate region.
— Five muscles form most of the posterior abdominal wall: the **m. psoas major**, **m. psoas minor** (sometimes absent), **m. quadratus lumborum**, **m. iliacus**, and **diaphragma** (**Fig. 10.7**).
  • The m. psoas major and m. iliacus unite to form the **m. iliopsoas**, which passes into the thigh and acts on the articulatio coxae.

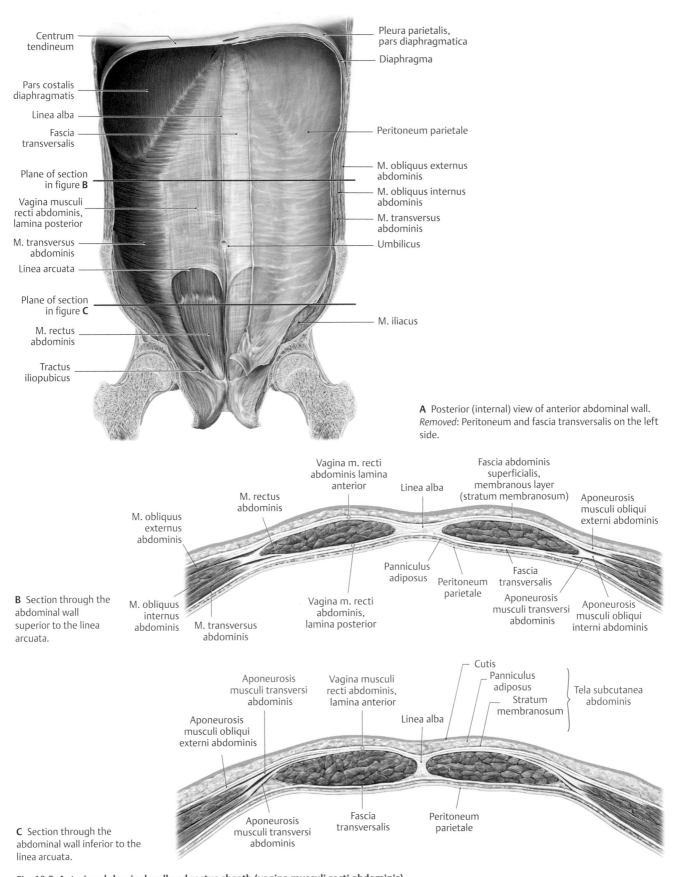

Centrum tendineum

Pars costalis diaphragmatis

Linea alba

Fascia transversalis

Plane of section in figure **B**

Vagina musculi recti abdominis, lamina posterior

M. transversus abdominis

Linea arcuata

Plane of section in figure **C**

M. rectus abdominis

Tractus iliopubicus

Pleura parietalis, pars diaphragmatica

Diaphragma

Peritoneum parietale

M. obliquus externus abdominis

M. obliquus internus abdominis

M. transversus abdominis

Umbilicus

M. iliacus

A Posterior (internal) view of anterior abdominal wall. *Removed*: Peritoneum and fascia transversalis on the left side.

Vagina m. recti abdominis lamina anterior

M. rectus abdominis

M. obliquus externus abdominis

Linea alba

Fascia abdominis superficialis, membranous layer (stratum membranosum)

Aponeurosis musculi obliqui externi abdominis

Panniculus adiposus

Fascia transversalis

Aponeurosis musculi transversi abdominis

Aponeurosis musculi obliqui interni abdominis

Peritoneum parietale

M. obliquus internus abdominis

M. transversus abdominis

Vagina m. recti abdominis, lamina posterior

B Section through the abdominal wall superior to the linea arcuata.

Aponeurosis musculi transversi abdominis

Vagina musculi recti abdominis, lamina anterior

Cutis

Panniculus adiposus

Stratum membranosum

Tela subcutanea abdominis

Aponeurosis musculi obliqui externi abdominis

Linea alba

Aponeurosis musculi transversi abdominis

Fascia transversalis

Peritoneum parietale

C Section through the abdominal wall inferior to the linea arcuata.

Fig. 10.5 Anterior abdominal wall and rectus sheath (vagina musculi recti abdominis)
(From Gilroy AM et al. Atlas of Anatomy. 4th ed. 2020. Based on: Schuenke M, Schulte E, Schumacher U. THIEME Atlas of Anatomy. General Anatomy and Musculoskeletal System. Illustrations by Voll M and Wesker K. 3rd ed. New York: Thieme Medical Publishers; 2020.)

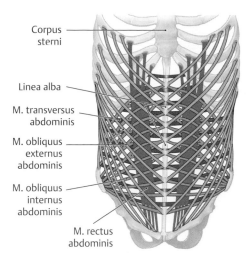

Corpus sterni

Linea alba

M. transversus abdominis

M. obliquus externus abdominis

M. obliquus internus abdominis

M. rectus abdominis

Fig. 10.6 Arrangement of the abdominal wall muscles and rectus sheath
(From Schuenke M, Schulte E, Schumacher U. THIEME Atlas of Anatomy, Vol 1. Illustrations by Voll M and Wesker K. 3rd ed. New York: Thieme Publishers; 2020.)

- The thoracic diaphragm forms part of the superior portion of the posterior abdominal wall.
- The m. transversus abdominis contributes to the lateral part of the posterior abdominal wall.
- Of the posterior wall muscles, only the m. quadratus lumborum is enclosed by the fascia thoracolumbalis (anterior layer), which also encloses the paraspinal muscles of the back. This layer passes posterior to the m. psoas major and laterally fuses with the aponeurosis of the m. transversus abdominis.
— **Fascia endoabdominalis** is a deep fascial layer that lines the internal surface of the abdominal wall muscles. It lies

superficial to (outside of) the peritoneum parietale and in most places is separated from it by a layer of fat called **preperitoneal fat**.

- Each part of the fascia endoabdominalis is named for the muscle it lines: **fascia transversalis (Fig. 10.5)**, **fascia diaphragmatica**, and **fascia iliopsoas, pars psoatica**.
- In the regio inguinalis (groin), a thickened line of the fascia transversalis, the **tractus iliopubicus**, attaches to the inner edge of the lig. inguinale, where it supports the posterior wall of the canalis inguinalis **(Fig. 10.5)**.
- On the posterior wall, the psoas fascia attaches to the lumbar vertebrae medially, and superiorly it blends with the lig. arcuatum mediale of the diaphragm. It extends inferiorly into the thigh with the tendon of the m. iliopsoas. This fascia separates the m. psoas and the plexus lumbalis (see Section 11.2) from viscera in the retroperitoneum of the abdominal cavity.

Internal Surface of the Anterior Abdominal Wall

The internal surface of the anterior abdominal wall is lined with fascia transversalis and peritoneum parietale, with a variable amount of intervening preperitoneal fat **(Figs. 10.8 and 10.9)**.

— **Peritoneal folds** form where structures tent the peritoneum as they course between it and the fascia transversalis. The folds include
- the **plica umbilicalis mediana**, a single midline fold created by the **lig. umbilicale medianum**, a remnant of the **urachus** (a fetal connection between the vesica urinaria and umbilicus);
- the **plicae umbilicales mediales**, paired folds created by the **ligg. umbilicale mediales**, remnants of the aa. umbilicales in the fetus; and
- the **plicae umbilicales laterales**, paired folds created by the **inferior epigastric vessels**.

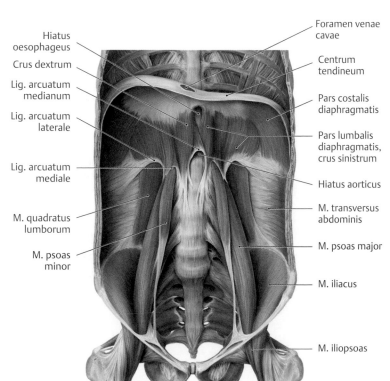

Hiatus oesophageus

Crus dextrum

Lig. arcuatum medianum

Lig. arcuatum laterale

Lig. arcuatum mediale

M. quadratus lumborum

M. psoas minor

Foramen venae cavae

Centrum tendineum

Pars costalis diaphragmatis

Pars lumbalis diaphragmatis, crus sinistrum

Hiatus aorticus

M. transversus abdominis

M. psoas major

M. iliacus

M. iliopsoas

Fig. 10.7 Muscles of the posterior abdominal wall
Coronal section with the diaphragma in the intermediate position, anterior view. (From Gilroy AM et al. Atlas of Anatomy. 4th ed. 2020. Based on: Schuenke M, Schulte E, Schumacher U. THIEME Atlas of Anatomy. General Anatomy and Musculoskeletal System. Illustrations by Voll M and Wesker K. 3rd ed. New York: Thieme Medical Publishers; 2020.)

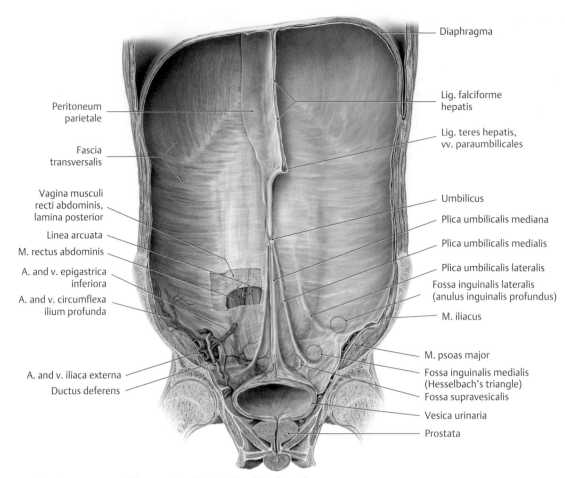

Fig. 10.8 Internal surface anatomy of the anterior abdominal wall in the male
Coronal section through the cavitas abdominopelvica at the level of the hip joints, posterior view. (From Gilroy AM et al. Atlas of Anatomy. 4th ed. 2020. Based on: Schuenke M, Schulte E, Schumacher U. THIEME Atlas of Anatomy. General Anatomy and Musculoskeletal System. Illustrations by Voll M and Wesker K. 3rd ed. New York: Thieme Medical Publishers; 2020.)

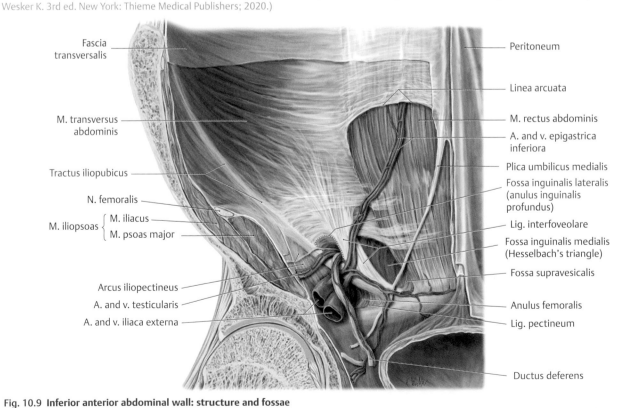

Fig. 10.9 Inferior anterior abdominal wall: structure and fossae
Coronal section, posterior (internal) view of left inferior portion of the anterior abdominal wall. (From Gilroy AM et al. Atlas of Anatomy. 4th ed. 2020. Based on: Schuenke M, Schulte E, Schumacher U. THIEME Atlas of Anatomy. General Anatomy and Musculoskeletal System. Illustrations by Voll M and Wesker K. 3rd ed. New York: Thieme Medical Publishers; 2020.)

— **Peritoneal fossae** are formed between the peritoneal folds and are potential sites of herniation (protrusion of viscera through a wall or tissue). The fossae include
  • the **fossa supravesicalis** between the plica umbilicalis mediana and plica umbilicalis medialis;
  • the **fossa inguinalis medialis,** commonly known as Hesselbach's triangle, between the plica umbilicalis medialis and plica umbilicalis lateralis; and
  • the **fossa inguinalis lateralis,** lateral to the plicae umbilicalis laterales.
— The **lig. falciforme hepatis** is a double-layered peritoneal reflection between the liver and the anterior abdominal wall that extends superiorly from the umbilicus to the roof of the cavitas abdominis. It encloses the lig. teres hepatis (remnant of the v. umbilicalis) and vv. paraumbilicales.

10.3 Neurovasculature of the Abdominal Wall

Arteries of the Abdominal Wall

Arteries of the abdominal wall, which anastomose extensively with one another, arise from the a. thoracica interna, the aorta abdominalis, the a. iliaca externa, and the a. femoralis **(Fig. 10.10)**.
— The branches of each a. thoracica interna are
  • the a. musculophrenica and
  • the a. epigastrica superior, which descends within the vagina musculi recti abdominis posterior to the m. rectus

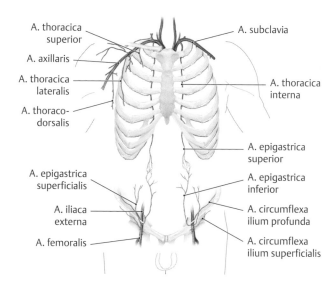

Fig. 10.10 Arteries of the abdominal wall
The a. epigastrica superior and a. epigastrica inferior form a potential anastomosis between the a. subclavia and a. femoralis, which can allow blood to bypass the aorta abdominalis. (From Schuenke M, Schulte E, Schumacher U. THIEME Atlas of Anatomy, Vol 2. Illustrations by Voll M and Wesker K. 2nd ed. New York: Thieme Publishers; 2016.)

abdominis, where it anastomoses with the a. epigastrica inferior.
— The paired segmental branches of the aorta abdominalis are
  • the aa. intercostales, aa. subcostales, and aa. lumbales.
— The branches of the a. iliaca externa are
  • the a. epigastrica inferior and a. circumflexa ilium profunda.
— The branches of the a. femoralis in the thigh that supply the abdominal wall are
  • the **a. epigastrica superficialis** and
  • the **a. circumflexa ilium superficialis**.

Veins of the Abdominal Wall

— The deep veins of the abdominal wall accompany the arteries of similar name and drain to the v. cava superior and v. cava inferior via the v. brachiocephalica, v. azygos, v. hemiazygos, and v. iliaca communis **(Fig 10.11)**.
— An extensive subcutaneous venous network drains superiorly to the v. thoracica interna and **v. thoracica lateralis** of the thorax and inferiorly to the **v. epigastrica inferior** and **v. epigastrica superficialis**.
— Obstruction of the v. cava superior or v. cava inferior may alter the venous flow across the abdominal wall, resulting in the development or enlargement of a superficial anastomosis between the v. axillaris and v. femoralis through the v. thoracoepigastrica (see Section 6.4).

Lymphatic Drainage of the Abdominal Wall

— Lymphatic drainage of the abdominal wall is divided into upper and lower regions by a curved line ("watershed") located between the umbilicus and arcus costalis **(Fig. 10.12)**.
  • From the upper region, lymph drains superiorly to nll. axillares and nll. parasternales before draining superiorly to the right and left jugulosubclavian junctions (venous angles).
  • From the lower region, lymph drains inferiorly to ipsilateral nll. inguinales superficiales. These drain to nll. iliaci externi and nll. iliaci communes and eventually to the ductus thoracicus.

Nerves of the Abdominal Wall

— Nerves of the abdominal wall arise from nn. spinales thoracici and nn. spinales lumbales **(Fig. 10.13)** and include
  • the lower nn. intercostales (T7–T11) and the n. subcostalis (T12) of the thorax, and
  • the n. iliohypogastricus of the plexus lumbalis.
— Dermatomes of the abdominal wall follow the slope of the ribs. Landmark dermatomes that correspond to visible surface features of the abdominal wall include T10 at the umbilicus and L1 at the lig. inguinale and top of the pubis.

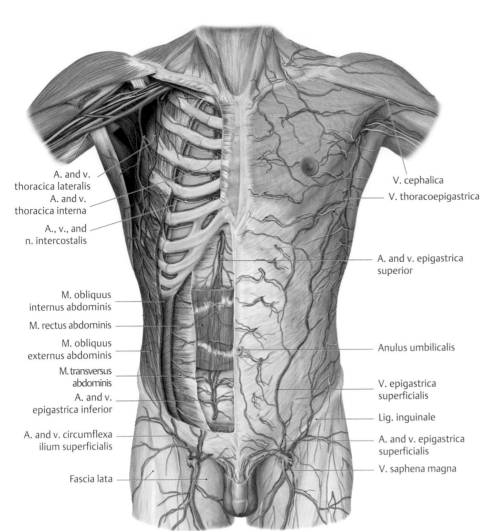

A. and v. thoracica lateralis

A. and v. thoracica interna

A., v., and n. intercostalis

M. obliquus internus abdominis

M. rectus abdominis

M. obliquus externus abdominis

M. transversus abdominis

A. and v. epigastrica inferior

A. and v. circumflexa ilium superficialis

Fascia lata

V. cephalica

V. thoracoepigastrica

A. and v. epigastrica superior

Anulus umbilicalis

V. epigastrica superficialis

Lig. inguinale

A. and v. epigastrica superficialis

V. saphena magna

Fig. 10.11 Neurovascular structures of the anterior trunk wall
Anterior view.
Left side: Superficial dissection. *Right side:* Deep dissection. *Removed:* M. pectoralis major and m. pectoralis minor. *Partially removed:* M. obliquus externus abdominis, m. obliquus internus abdominis, m. transversus abdominis, m. rectus abdominis, and mm. intercostales. (From Schuenke M, Schulte E, Schumacher U. THIEME Atlas of Anatomy, Vol 1. Illustrations by Voll M and Wesker K. 3rd ed. New York: Thieme Publishers; 2020.)

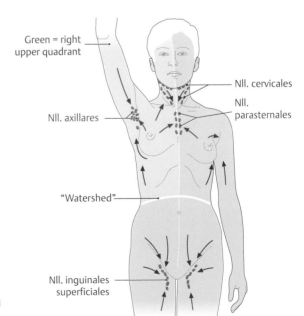

Green = right upper quadrant

Nll. axillares

"Watershed"

Nll. cervicales

Nll. parasternales

Nll. inguinales superficiales

Fig. 10.12 Lymphatic pathways and regional lymph nodes of the anterior trunk wall
Anterior view. *Arrows* indicate the direction of lymph flow. (From Schuenke M, Schulte E, Schumacher U. THIEME Atlas of Anatomy, Vol 1. Illustrations by Voll M and Wesker K. 3rd ed. New York: Thieme Publishers; 2020.)

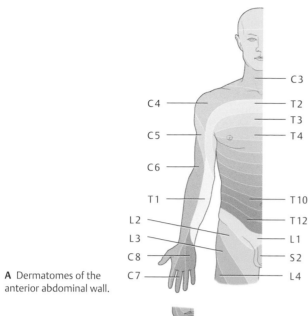

A Dermatomes of the anterior abdominal wall.

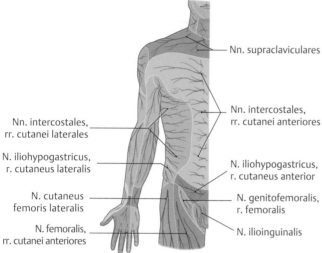

Nn. supraclaviculares

Nn. intercostales, rr. cutanei laterales

N. iliohypogastricus, r. cutaneus lateralis

N. cutaneus femoris lateralis

N. femoralis, rr. cutanei anteriores

Nn. intercostales, rr. cutanei anteriores

N. iliohypogastricus, r. cutaneus anterior

N. genitofemoralis, r. femoralis

N. ilioinguinalis

B Sensory nerves of the anterior abdominal wall.

Fig. 10.13 Cutaneous innervation of the anterior abdominal wall
(From Schuenke M, Schulte E, Schumacher U. THIEME Atlas of Anatomy, Vol 1. Illustrations by Voll M and Wesker K. 3rd ed. New York: Thieme Publishers; 2020.)

10.4 The Inguinal Region

The **inguinal region (regio inguinalis)** describes the inferolateral region of the anterior abdominal wall; the canalis inguinalis; and in males, the funiculus spermaticus.

— The skin and subcutaneous tissue of the abdominal wall continues inferiorly into the thigh below the lig. inguinale and inferomedially into the perineum (see Sections 16.3 and 16.4 for discussions of the perineum).

  • In the female, the skin and both the panniculus adiposus and the stratum membranosum of the subcutaneous tissue form the **labia majora**.

  • In the male, the skin extends into the perineum as the **scrotum**. The fatty layer of the subcutaneous tissue is absent, but the stratum membranosum continues over the penis as the **superficial penile fascia** and lines the scrotum as the **superficial perineal fascia** (Colles' fascia).

— The anterolateral muscles of the abdominal wall and their fasciae form the canalis inguinalis and contribute to the coverings of the funiculus spermaticus.

Canalis Inguinalis

The **inguinal canal (canalis inguinalis)** is an oblique passage through the abdominal wall that allows structures to pass between the abdominal and pelvic cavities and the perineum. Deficiencies in the anterolateral abdominal muscles, their aponeuroses, and their deep fascia create the canalis inguinalis (**Table 10.2**). The canal is present in both males and females, although it is more pronounced in the male.

— The boundaries of the canal are

  • the anterior wall, formed by the aponeurosis of the m. obliquus externus abdominis;

  • the posterior wall, formed by fascia transversalis and tendo conjunctivus;

Table 10.2 Structures and Relations of the Canalis Inguinalis
(From Gilroy AM et al. Atlas of Anatomy. 4th ed. 2020. Based on: Schuenke M, Schulte E, Schumacher U. THIEME Atlas of Anatomy. General Anatomy and Musculoskeletal System. Illustrations by Voll M and Wesker K. 3rd ed. New York: Thieme Medical Publishers; 2020.)

Structures		Formed by
Wall	Anterior wall	① Aponeurosis of m. obliqui externi abdominis
	Roof	② M. obliquus internus abdominis
		③ M. transversus abdominis
	Posterior wall	④ Fascia transversalis
		⑤ Peritoneum parietale
	Floor	⑥ Lig. inguinale (densely interwoven fibers of the lower aponeurosis of m. obliqui externi abdominis and adjacent fascia lata of thigh)
Openings	Anulus inguinalis superficialis	Opening in aponeurosis of m. obliquus obliqui externi abdominis; bounded by crus mediale and crus laterale, fibrae intercrurales, and lig. reflexum
	Anulus inguinalis profundus	Outpouching of the fascia transversalis lateral to the plica umbilicalis lateralis (inferior epigastric vessels)

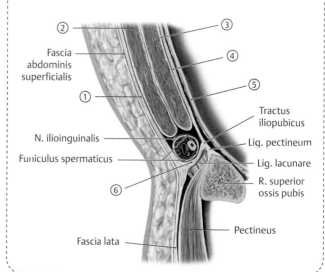

Fascia abdominis superficialis

N. ilioinguinalis

Funiculus spermaticus

Tractus iliopubicus

Lig. pectineum

Lig. lacunare

R. superior ossis pubis

Pectineus

Fascia lata

- the floor, formed by the lig. inguinale; and
- the roof, formed by the arching fibers of the aponeuroses of the m. obliquus internus abdominis and the m. transversus abdominis.
— The canal has two openings:
  - At the medial end of the canal, fibers of the aponeurosis musculi obliqui externi abdominis split to create an opening known as the **anulus inguinalis superficialis**. This ring lies in the anterior wall of the fossa inguinalis medialis.

- At the lateral end of the canalis inguinalis, immediately lateral to the origin of the inferior epigastric vessels, the fascia transversalis evaginates into the canal and creates the **deep inguinal ring (anulus inguinalis profundus)**. This ring lies in the fossa inguinalis lateralis (see **Fig. 10.9**).
— The contents of the canalis inguinalis include the **funiculus spermaticus** in males and the **lig. teres uteri** in females (**Figs. 10.14** and **10.15**; also see Section 15.2).

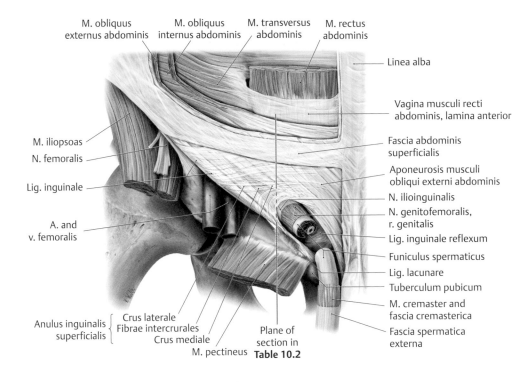

Fig. 10.14 Male regio inguinalis
Right side, anterior view.
(From Schuenke M, Schulte E, Schumacher U. THIEME Atlas of Anatomy, Vol 1. Illustrations by Voll M and Wesker K. 3rd ed. New York: Thieme Publishers; 2020.)

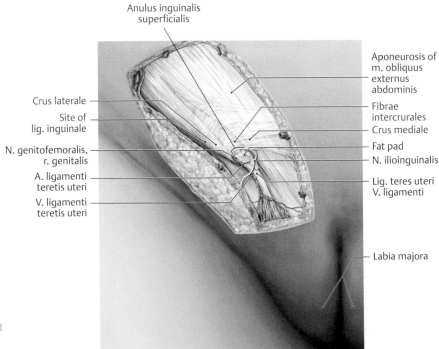

Fig. 10.15 Female regio inguinalis
Right side, anterior view. (From Gilroy AM et al. Atlas of Anatomy. 4th ed. 2020. Based on: Schuenke M, Schulte E, Schumacher U. THIEME Atlas of Anatomy. General Anatomy and Musculoskeletal System. Illustrations by Voll M and Wesker K. 3rd ed. New York: Thieme Medical Publishers; 2020.)

The Funiculus Spermaticus

The funiculus spermaticus forms at the anulus inguinalis profundus, traverses the canalis inguinalis, and exits through the anulus inguinalis superficialis. It enters the scrotum and descends to the posterior surface of the testis (**Fig. 10.16**).

— The structures in the funiculus spermaticus include
  - the ductus deferens;
  - the proc. vaginalis;
  - the a. testicularis and plexus pampiniformis of veins, the a. ductus deferentis, and the a. cremasterica;
  - lymphatic vessels of the testis and funiculus spermaticus; and
  - sympathetic and parasympathetic fibers of the plexus testicularis and the n. genitofemoralis, r. genitalis.

— Derivatives of the muscles and fascia of the abdominal wall surround the contents of the funiculus spermaticus as they pass through the canalis inguinalis. The layers formed by the muscles and fascia are the same as those surrounding the testis (**Table 10.3**):
  - **Fascia spermatica interna** derived from the fascia transversalis
  - **M. cremaster** and **fascia cremasterica** derived from the m. obliquus internus abdominis and fascia
  - **Fascia spermatica externa** derived from the aponeurosis of the m. externus abdominis and fascia.

— The n. ilioinguinalis is not contained within the funiculus spermaticus. However, as it traverses the layers of the abdominal wall, it travels within the canalis inguinalis next to the cord and is enclosed by the external spermatic fascia as it exits the anulus inguinalis superficialis.

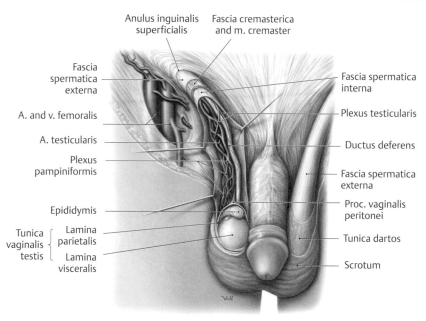

Fascia spermatica externa
Anulus inguinalis superficialis
Fascia cremasterica and m. cremaster
Fascia spermatica interna
A. and v. femoralis
Plexus testicularis
A. testicularis
Ductus deferens
Plexus pampiniformis
Fascia spermatica externa
Epididymis
Proc. vaginalis peritonei
Tunica vaginalis testis { Lamina parietalis / Lamina visceralis
Tunica dartos
Scrotum

Fig. 10.16 Funiculus spermaticus
Male pelvis, anterior view. *Opened:* Canalis inguinalis and coverings of the funiculus spermaticus. (From Gilroy AM et al. Atlas of Anatomy. 4th ed. 2020. Based on: Schuenke M, Schulte E, Schumacher U. THIEME Atlas of Anatomy. General Anatomy and Musculoskeletal System. Illustrations by Voll M and Wesker K. 3rd ed. New York: Thieme Medical Publishers; 2020.)

Table 10.3 Coverings of the Testis
(From Gilroy AM et al. Atlas of Anatomy. 4th ed. 2020. Based on: Schuenke M, Schulte E, Schumacher U. THIEME Atlas of Anatomy. Internal Organs. Illustrations by Voll M and Wesker K. 3rd ed. New York: Thieme Medical Publishers; 2020.)

Covering layer	Derived from
① Scrotal skin	Abdominal skin
② Tunica dartos	Fascia dartos and muscle
③ Fascia spermatica externa	M. obliquus externus abdominis
④ M. cremaster and fascia cremasterica*	M. obliquus internus abdominis
⑤ Fascia spermatica interna	Fascia transversalis
⑥ⓐ Tunica vaginalis, lamina parietalis	Peritoneum
⑥ⓑ Tunica vaginalis, lamina visceralis	

The m. transversus abdominis has no contribution to the funiculus spermaticus or covering of the testis.

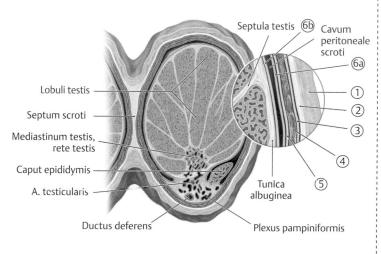

Septula testis ⑥ⓑ
Cavum peritoneale scroti
⑥ⓐ
Lobuli testis
Septum scroti
①
②
Mediastinum testis, rete testis
③
Caput epididymis
④
A. testicularis
Tunica albuginea
⑤
Ductus deferens
Plexus pampiniformis

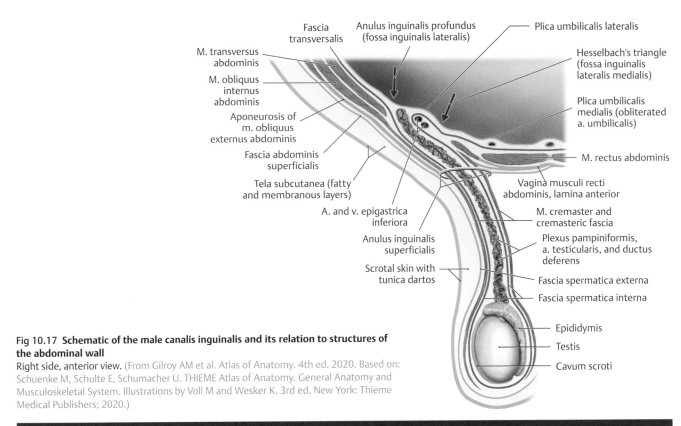

Fig 10.17 Schematic of the male canalis inguinalis and its relation to structures of the abdominal wall

Right side, anterior view. (From Gilroy AM et al. Atlas of Anatomy. 4th ed. 2020. Based on: Schuenke M, Schulte E, Schumacher U. THIEME Atlas of Anatomy. General Anatomy and Musculoskeletal System. Illustrations by Voll M and Wesker K. 3rd ed. New York: Thieme Medical Publishers; 2020.)

BOX 10.1: CLINICAL CORRELATION

INGUINAL HERNIA

Inguinal hernias account for the large majority of abdominal wall hernias, and of those, most occur in males. A hernia is the protrusion of a visceral structure into a space that it does not normally occupy. Inguinal hernias involve the protrusion of peritoneum parietale, peritoneal fat, or the intestinum tenue. Of the two types of inguinal hernias, the indirect hernia can be acquired or congenital and is common in young males, whereas the direct hernia is always acquired and results from a weakening of the abdominal wall and generally occurs in middle-aged males.

During development, a tongue of peritoneum, the proc. vaginalis, evaginates into the newly formed canalis inguinalis and accompanies the testis in its descent into the scrotum. Before birth most of the proc. vaginalis obliterates, closing the communication between it and the cavitas peritonealis. If the proc. vaginalis fails

to obliterate, however, abdominal contents can herniate (indirect hernia) through its opening at the anulus inguinalis profundus in the fossa inguinalis lateralis (lateral to the inferior epigastric vessels) and extend into the scrotum (or labia in females). Herniated viscera travel within the funiculus spermaticus and therefore are covered by the layers of the cord in addition to peritoneum and fascia transversalis.

Direct hernias occur where weakening of the anterior abdominal wall in the fossa inguinalis medialis (medial to the inferior epigastric vessels) allows viscera to protrude through the medial end of the canal, then through an enlarged anulus inguinalis superficialis, and into the scrotum. Since these herniated viscera travel outside the funiculus spermaticus, they are not covered by layers of the funiculus spermaticus but are covered by peritoneum and fascia transversalis of the abdominal wall.

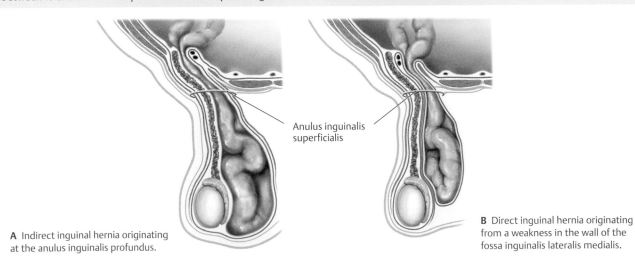

A Indirect inguinal hernia originating at the anulus inguinalis profundus.

B Direct inguinal hernia originating from a weakness in the wall of the fossa inguinalis lateralis medialis.

(From Schuenke M, Schulte E, Schumacher U. THIEME Atlas of Anatomy, Vol 1. Illustrations by Voll M and Wesker K. 3rd ed. New York: Thieme Publishers; 2020.)

The Testes

The testes are paired ovoid reproductive organs, 4 to 5 cm long and 3 cm wide, located in separate compartments within the scrotum. They produce spermatozoa and secrete the male hormone testosterone (**Figs. 10.18** and **10.19**; see also **Table 10.3**).

— An extension of the peritoneum known as the **tunica vaginalis** forms a closed sac that folds around the testis, surrounding it on all sides except on its posterior edge. The tunica vaginalis has an outer lamina parietalis and an inner lamina visceralis that is adherent to the surface of the testis.

— Each testis is enveloped by the **tunica albuginea,** a tough capsule of connective tissue that thickens along the posterior border as the mediastinum of the testis and invaginates to divide the testis into over 200 lobules.

— Sperm develop in the **tubuli seminiferi contorti,** highly coiled tubules within the lobules. They exit the testes through a ductal network, the **rete testis** in the mediastinum, and then pass through **ductuli efferentes testis** to the **epididymis.**

— The a. testicularis, a branch of the aorta abdominalis, supplies the testis. A rich collateral blood supply arises from anastomoses with the a. ductus deferentis, the **a. cremasterica** (a branch of the a. epigastrica inferior), and the **a. pudenda externa** (a branch of the a. femoralis) (**Fig. 10.20**).

— The **plexus pampiniformis** of veins drains the testis and converges to form the v. testicularis. The vv. testiculares drain to the v. cava inferior on the right and to the v. renalis on the left.

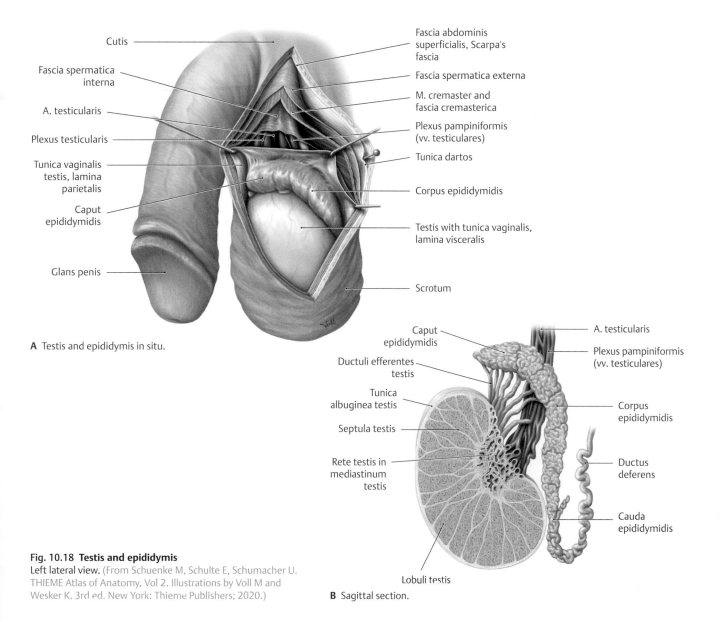

A Testis and epididymis in situ.

B Sagittal section.

Fig. 10.18 Testis and epididymis
Left lateral view. (From Schuenke M, Schulte E, Schumacher U. THIEME Atlas of Anatomy, Vol 2. Illustrations by Voll M and Wesker K, 3rd ed. New York: Thieme Publishers; 2020.)

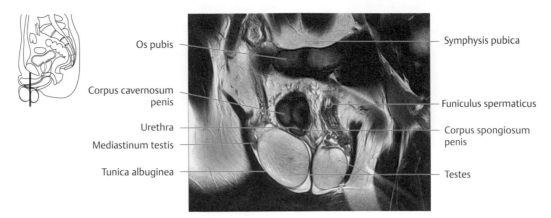

Fig 10.19 MRI of the testes
Coronal section, anterior view. (From Moeller TB, Reif E. Pocket Atlas of Sectional Anatomy, Vol 2, 3rd ed. New York: Thieme Publishers; 2007.)

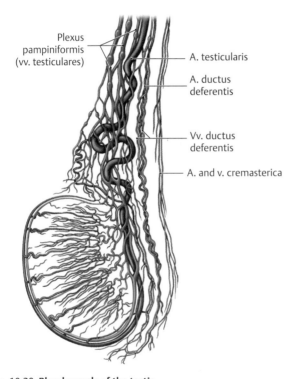

Fig. 10.20 Blood vessels of the testis
Left lateral view. (From Schuenke M, Schulte E, Schumacher U. THIEME Atlas of Anatomy, Vol 1. Illustrations by Voll M and Wesker K. 3rd ed. New York: Thieme Publishers; 2020.)

— The lymph vessels of the testes drain directly to nll. aortici laterales and nll. preaortici.
— The **cremasteric reflex,** initiated by stroking of the inner thigh, contracts the m. cremaster and elevates the testis. The n. ilioinguinalis provides the sensory limb; the r. genitalis of the n. genitofemoralis provides the motor limb.
— The plexus testicularis arises from the plexus aorticus and travels along with the a. testicularis. It contains sympathetic fibers from the T7 nn. spinales, as well as visceral afferent and vagal parasympathetic fibers.

BOX 10.2: CLINICAL CORRELATION

HYDROCELE
The opening into a persistent proc. vaginalis may be small enough to prevent herniation but large enough to form a hydrocele, the accumulation of excess peritoneal fluid. The hydrocele can be confined to the scrotum (hydrocele of the testis) or to the funiculus spermaticus (hydrocele of the cord). Ultrasound or transillumination of the scrotum confirms the presence of excess fluid.

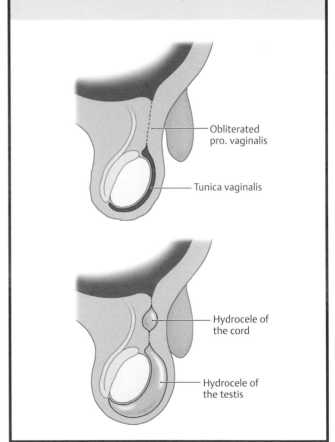

BOX 10.3: CLINICAL CORRELATION

VARICOCELE

The plexus pampiniformis from each testis surrounds the a. testicularis and converges to form a v. testicularis. If the venous valves (valvula venosa) become incompetent, the plexus can become dilated and tortuous, forming a varicocele that is often reported to feel like "a bag of worms." Varicoceles are predominantly on the left side. This is generally attributed to the abrupt termination of the v. testicularis sinistra at the v. renalis sinistra, which may slow venous return.

This 14-year-old boy presented with scrotal discomfort and a palpable mass. This scrotal ultrasound image shows a mass consisting of multiple serpiginous tubules, which indicate a varicocele.
(From Gunderman R. Essential Radiology, 3rd ed. New York: Thieme Publishers; 2014.)

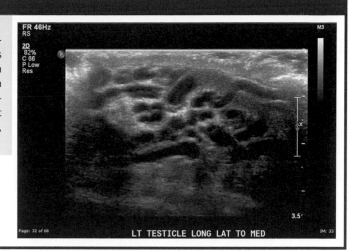

BOX 10.4: CLINICAL CORRELATION

TESTICULAR TORSION

An absent or reduced cremasteric reflex that is accompanied by sudden testicular pain, inflammation and elevation of one testis, nausea, and vomiting may indicate testicular torsion (twisting of a testis). Prompt surgery for testicular torsion (to untwist the affected testis and anchor both testes) may prevent loss of a testis.

BOX 10.5: CLINICAL CORRELATION

TESTICULAR CANCER

Testicular cancer is the most common cancer in males between 15 and 34 years of age. The vast majority of these cancers are seminomas or germ cell tumors that arise in the germ cells that produce immature sperm. Symptoms include a lump in the affected testis (usually only one testis is affected), a feeling of heaviness in the scrotum, pain in the affected testis or scrotum, a sudden collection of fluid in the scrotum, and the development of excess breast tissue (gynecomastia). Testicular cancer commonly metastasizes via lymph nodes to the lungs or via the bloodstream, commonly to the liver, lungs, brain, and spine.

Fig. 10.21 Asymmetric venous drainage of the right and left testes
(From Schuenke M, Schulte E, Schumacher U. THIEME Atlas of Anatomy, Vol 2. Illustrations by Voll M and Wesker K. 3rd ed. New York: Thieme Publishers; 2020.)

The Epididymis and Ductus Deferens

The epididymis and ductus deferens are parts of the male ductal system that transport sperm from the testis to the genital structures in the pelvis (see **Fig. 10.18**).

— The epididymis, a highly coiled tubule where sperm are stored and mature, hugs the posterior surface of the testis. Its expanded head contains the lobules with the efferent ductules, its body is made up of a long convoluted duct, and its tail is continuous with the ductus deferens.

— The **ductus deferens** is a muscular tube that transmits sperm from the scrotum to the pelvis.

• It begins at the cauda epididymidis and continues as part of the funiculus spermaticus through the canalis inguinalis.

• At the anulus inguinalis profundus, the ductus deferens descends into the pelvis posterior to the vesica urinaria, where, near its termination, it enlarges as the **ampulla ductus deferentis** (see **Fig. 15.2**).

• The ampulla joins with the duct of the seminal gland (vesicula seminalis) to form the **ductus ejaculatorius** within the prostata (see Section 15.1).

11   The Cavitas Peritonealis and Neurovasculature of the Abdomen

11.1   The Peritoneum and Cavitas Peritonealis

The **peritoneum**, a thin, transparent serous membrane, lines the cavitas abdominopelvica. The peritoneum parietale and peritoneum viscerale enclose the **cavitas peritonealis**, which contains a thin film of serous fluid that facilitates the movement of the viscera during digestion and respiration (see **Fig. 11.1**).

Peritoneal Relations

— Structures in the abdomen are defined with respect to their relationship to the peritoneum (**Table 11.1**; **Figs. 11.1** and **11.2**).
  • **Intraperitoneal** organs, almost completely enclosed by the visceral layer of the peritoneum, are suspended within the cavitas peritonealis by **mesenteria**, double layers of peritoneum that attach to the body wall.
  • **Extraperitoneal** structures lie posterior or inferior to the cavitas peritonealis.
    ◦ **Primarily retroperitoneal** structures lie posterior to the cavitas peritonealis, are not suspended by a mesenterium, and are covered by peritoneum only on their anterior surface.
    ◦ **Secondarily retroperitoneal** structures were previously intraperitoneal structures that became fixed to the posterior abdominal wall when their mesenterium fused with the peritoneum parietale of the posterior abdominal wall during development.
    ◦ **Subperitoneal structures** include pelvic organs that lie below the peritoneum.
— Organs associated with the gastrointestinal tract are intraperitoneal or secondarily retroperitoneal. Organs of the urinary system are retroperitoneal.

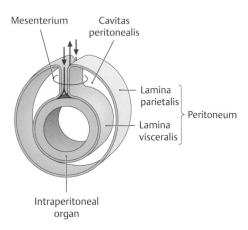

Fig. 11.1 Peritoneum and mesentery
Red and *blue arrows* indicate location of blood vessels. (From Gilroy AM et al. Atlas of Anatomy. 4th ed. 2020. Based on: Schuenke M, Schulte E, Schumacher U. THIEME Atlas of Anatomy. Internal Organs. Illustrations by Voll M and Wesker K. 3rd ed. New York: Thieme Medical Publishers; 2020.)

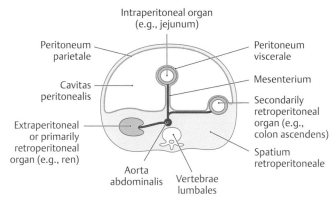

Fig. 11.2 Peritoneal relations of the organs in the abdomen
Transverse section through the abdomen showing the peritoneal relationships of abdominal organs. Viewed from above. (From Gilroy AM et al. Atlas of Anatomy. 4th ed. 2020. Based on: Schuenke M, Schulte E, Schumacher U. THIEME Atlas of Anatomy. Internal Organs. Illustrations by Voll M and Wesker K. 3rd ed. New York: Thieme Medical Publishers; 2020.)

Table 11.1 Organs of the Abdomen

Location		Organs
Intraperitoneal organs: These organs have a mesenterium and are almost completely covered by the peritoneum.		
Abdominal peritoneal cavity		• Gaster
		• Intestinum tenue (jejunum, ileum, some of the pars superior duodeni)
		• Splen
		• Hepar (with the exception of the area nuda)
		• Vesica biliaris
		• Caecum with appendix vermiformis (portions of variable size may be retroperitoneal)
		• Intestinum crassum (colon transversum and colon sigmoideum)
Extraperitoneal organs: These organs either have no mesenterium or lost it during development.		
Retroperitoneum	Primarily retroperitoneal	• Renes
		• Glandulae suprarenales
	Secondarily retroperitoneal	• Duodenum (pars decendens, pars horizontalis, and pars ascendens)
		• Pancreas
		• Colon ascendens and descendens

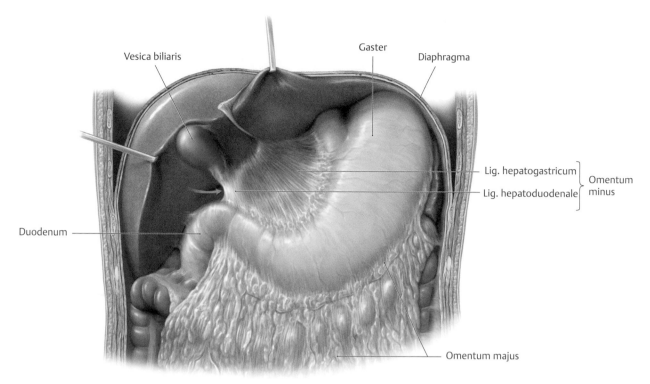

Fig. 11.5 Omentum minus
Anterior view with hepar retracted superiorly. The *arrow* points to the foramen omentale, the opening into the bursa omentalis, posterior to the omentum minus. (From Gilroy AM et al. Atlas of Anatomy. 4th ed. 2020. Based on: Schuenke M, Schulte E, Schumacher U. THIEME Atlas of Anatomy. Internal Organs. Illustrations by Voll M and Wesker K. 3rd ed. New York: Thieme Medical Publishers; 2020.)

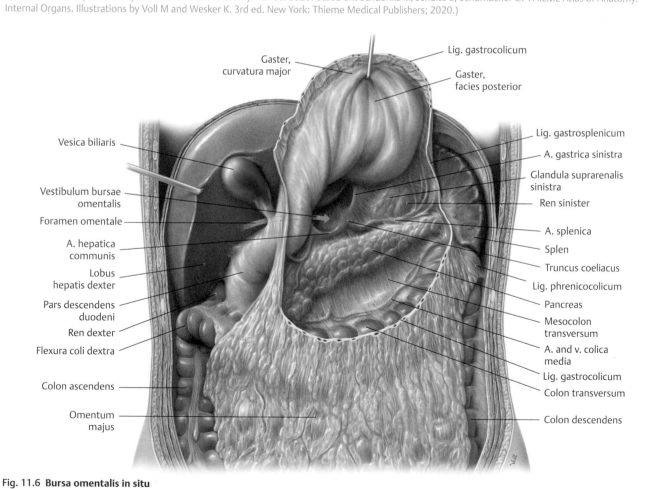

Fig. 11.6 Bursa omentalis in situ
Anterior view. *Divided:* Lig. gastrocolicum. *Retracted:* Hepar. *Reflected:* Gaster. (From Gilroy AM et al. Atlas of Anatomy. 4th ed. 2020. Based on: Schuenke M, Schulte E, Schumacher U. THIEME Atlas of Anatomy. Internal Organs. Illustrations by Voll M and Wesker K. 3rd ed. New York: Thieme Medical Publishers; 2020.)

Subdivisions of the Cavitas Peritonealis

— The cavitas peritonealis is divided into two spaces:
  • The **greater sac**, which includes the entire cavitas peritonealis except that space defined as the lesser sac
  • The **bursa omentalis**, which is a small extension of the cavitas peritonealis that lies behind the stomach and omentum minus (**Table 11.2**; **Figs. 11.6, 11.7, 11.8**). It communicates with the greater sac through a single opening, the **foramen omentale (foramen epiploicum)** (**Table 11.3**).
— Attachments of the peritoneum to the body wall that form during development of the gastrointestinal tract further subdivide the greater sac. These attachments can influence the flow of fluid within the cavity (**Fig. 11.9**).
  • The **recessus subphrenicus** between the diaphragma and liver is limited by the lig. coronarium and separated into right and left spaces by the lig. falciforme hepatis.
  • The **recessus subhepaticus** lies between the liver and the colon transversum. A posterior extension of this space, the **recessus hepatorenalis** (hepatorenal pouch, Morison's pouch), lies between the visceral surface of the liver and the ren dexter and glandula suprarenalis dextra. The recessus hepatorenalis communicates with the recessus subphrenicus dexter.
  • The **supracolic** and **infracolic compartments** are defined by the attachment of the mesocolon transversum on the posterior abdominal wall—with the supracolic compartment above the attachment site and the infracolic compartment below it. The radix mesenterii of the interstinum tenue further divides the infracolic compartment into right and left spaces.
  • The **recessus paracolici**, which lie adjacent to the colon ascendens and colon descendens, allow communication between the supracolic and infracolic compartments.

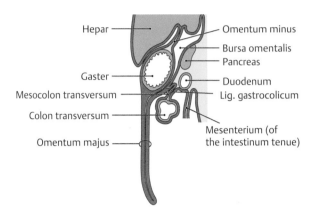

Fig. 11.7 Structure of the omentum majus and omentum minus and their relation to the bursa omentalis
Sagittal section, left lateral view. (From Gilroy AM et al. Atlas of Anatomy. 4th ed. 2020. Based on: Schuenke M, Schulte E, Schumacher U. THIEME Atlas of Anatomy. Internal Organs. Illustrations by Voll M and Wesker K. 3rd ed. New York: Thieme Medical Publishers; 2020.)

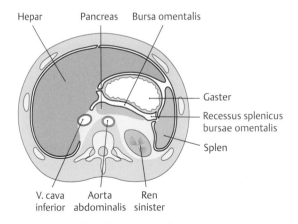

Fig. 11.8 Location of the bursa omentalis
Transverse section, inferior view. (From Gilroy AM et al. Atlas of Anatomy. 4th ed. 2020. Based on: Schuenke M, Schulte E, Schumacher U. THIEME Atlas of Anatomy. Internal Organs. Illustrations by Voll M and Wesker K. 3rd ed. New York: Thieme Medical Publishers; 2020.)

Table 11.2 Boundaries of the Bursa Omentalis (Lesser Sac)

Direction	Boundary	Recess
Anterior	Omentum minus, lig. gastrocolicum	—
Inferior	Mesocolon transversum	Recessus inferior
Superior	Hepar (with lobus caudatus)	Recessus superior
Posterior	Pancreas, aorta (pars abdominalis), truncus coeliacus, a. and v. splenica, gastrosplenic fold, left suprarenal lig. gastrosplenicum, glandula suprarenalis sinistra, ren sinistra (extremitas superior)	—
Right	Hepar, bulbus duodeni	—
Left	Splen, lig. gastrosplenicum	Recessus splenicus

Table 11.3 Boundaries of the Foramen Omentale

The communication between the greater and lesser sacs is the foramen epiploicum (foramen omentale) (see arrow in **Figs. 11.5** and **11.6**).

Direction	Boundary
Anterior	Lig. hepatoduodenale with v. portae hepatis, a. hepatica propria, and ductus choledochus
Inferior	Duodenum (pars superior)
Posterior	V. cava inferior, diaphragm (crus dexter)
Superior	Hepar (lobus caudatus)

BOX 11.1: CLINICAL CORRELATION

PERITONEAL INFECTIONS AND ABSCESSES

The flow of fluid in the cavitas peritonealis can spread intraperitoneal infections and determine the sites of peritoneal abscess formation. Fluid commonly collects in the right and left recessus subphrenicus, although abscesses are more likely to form on the right side due to duodenal or appendiceal ruptures. Fluid in the supracolic compartment, such as recessus subphrenicus and the bursa omentalis, can drain to the recessus hepatorenalis, the lowest part of the cavitas abdominis in the supine patient. Therefore, this is a common site of pus accumulation and abscess formation. In the infracolic compartment, the sulci paracolici direct peritoneal fluid and infections toward the pelvis (see **Figs. 11.9** and **11.10**).

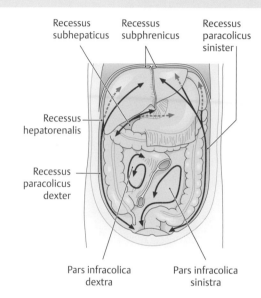

Recessus subhepaticus   Recessus subphrenicus   Recessus paracolicus sinister

Recessus hepatorenalis

Recessus paracolicus dexter

Pars infracolica dextra   Pars infracolica sinistra

Drainage spaces within the cavitas peritonealis
Anterior view. (From Schuenke M, Schulte E, Schumacher U. THIEME Atlas of Anatomy, Vol 2. Illustrations by Voll M and Wesker K. 3rd ed. New York: Thieme Publishers; 2020.)

BOX 11.2: CLINICAL CORRELATION

PERITONITIS AND ASCITES

Bacterial contamination of the peritoneum following surgery or rupture of an inflamed organ (duodenum, vesica biliaris, appendix vermiformis) results in peritonitis, inflammation of the peritoneum. It is accompanied by severe abdominal pain, tenderness, nausea, and fever and can be fatal when generalized throughout the cavitas peritonealis. It often results in ascites, the accumulation of excess peritoneal fluid due to a change in concentration gradients that results in loss of capillary fluid. Ascites can also accompany other pathologic conditions, such as metastatic liver cancer and portal hypertension. In these cases, many liters of ascitic fluid can accumulate in the peritoneal cavity. The fluid is aspirated by paracentesis. The needle is carefully inserted into the abdominal wall so as to avoid the vesica urinaria and inferior epigastric vessels.

Posterior Wall and Retroperitoneum

— The posterior wall of the cavitas abdominis is continuous with the area designated as the "back" but is generally accepted as a separate defined area that is composed of the posterior abdominal wall muscles and their fascia. The retroperitoneum is considered part of the posterior wall.

— The retroperitoneum is a space, or compartment, on the anterior surface of the posterior wall that contains specific retroperitoneal viscera. It is bound anteriorly by the peritoneum parietale and superiorly by the diaphragma. Laterally it's continuous with the extraperitoneal space of the anterior and lateral abdominal wall, and inferiorly it's continuous with the intraperitoneal space of the pelvis.

 • Retroperitoneal organs include the kidneys, ureters, and gll. suprarenales, along with their neurovasculature.

 • Some components of the gastrointestinal tract have become retroperitonealized during development by losing part of their peritoneal covering. These include the second to fourth parts of the duodenum, the pancreas, and colon ascendens and colon descendens.

Hepatic surface of diaphragma   V. cava inferior   Mesocolon transversum (radix)

Lig. hepatoduodenale

Ren dexter

Duodenum

Site of attachment of colon ascendens

Mesenterium (radix)

Recessus ileocaecalis superior

Recessus ileocaecalis inferior

Splen

Ren sinister

Recessus duodenalis superior

Recessus duodenalis inferior

Site of attachment of colon descendens

Sulcus paracolicus sinister

Mesocolon sigmoideum (radix)

Recessus retrocaecalis   Excavatio rectovesicalis   Recessus intersigmoideus

Fig. 11.9 Recesses within the cavitas peritonealis
Posterior wall of the cavitas peritonealis, anterior view. The mesenteric roots and sites of organ attachment create bounded spaces (recesses or sulci) where peritoneal fluid can flow freely. (From Gilroy AM et al. Atlas of Anatomy. 4th ed. 2020. Based on: Schuenke M, Schulte E, Schumacher U. THIEME Atlas of Anatomy. Internal Organs. Illustrations by Voll M and Wesker K. 3rd ed. New York: Thieme Medical Publishers; 2020.)

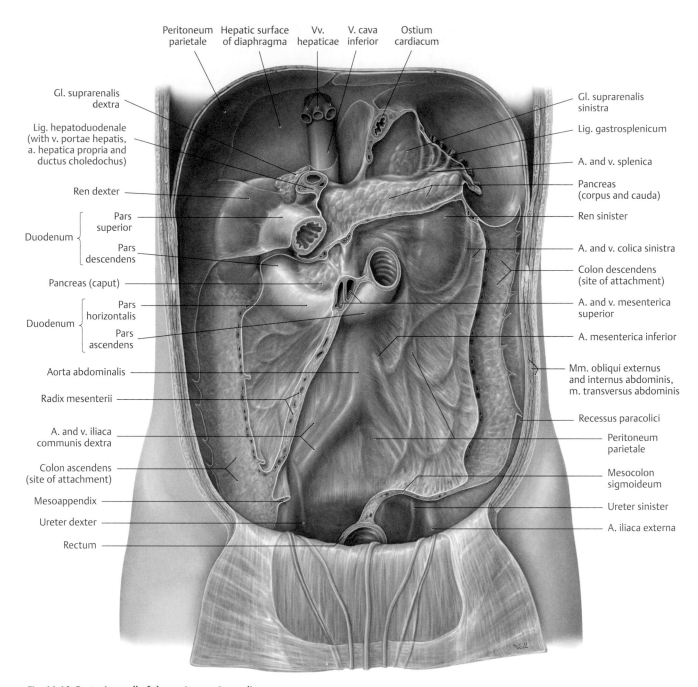

Fig. 11.10 Posterior wall of the cavitas peritonealis
Anterior view. *Removed:* All intraperitoneal organs. (From Schuenke M, Schulte E, Schumacher U. THIEME Atlas of Anatomy, Vol 2. Illustrations by Voll M and Wesker K. 3rd ed. New York: Thieme Publishers; 2020.)

- The retroperitoneum contains the major neurovascular structures of the abdomen, including the aorta and its branches, v. cava inferior and its tributaries, v. azygos and v. hemiazygos, the nll. preaortici and nll. aortici laterales and ductus thoracicus, and the plexus lumbalis and autonomic plexus of the abdomen.
- Mesenteries of the small intestine and large intestine, as well as the peritoneal ligaments associated with the liver and spleen, attach to the retroperitoneum.
- The retroperitoneum is divided into a series of compartments defined by fascia that is variable and often difficult to discern. The perirenal and pararenal spaces

around the kidneys are examples of these. The importance of this organization is appreciated when considering the containment of disease process or hemorrhage.

Neurovasculature of the Peritoneum

The **peritoneum parietale** and **peritoneum viscerale** derive their blood supply, lymphatic drainage, and innervation from different sources.

- Peritoneum parietale derives its neurovasculature from vessels and nerves of the body wall.

- Its sensitivity to pain, pressure, and temperature is well localized (felt acutely) through somatic nerves of the overlying muscles and skin.
— Pertioneum viscerale derives its neurovasculature from the underlying organs.
  - Autonomic nerves mediate sensitivity to stretching and chemical irritation, but the peritoneum viscerale lacks sensitivity to touch and temperature.
  - Sensation is poorly localized and is usually referred to regions that reflect the embryologic origins of the underlying organ.
    ◦ Sensation from foregut structures is referred to the epigastric region.
    ◦ Sensation from midgut structures is referred to the umbilical region.
    ◦ Sensation from hindgut structures is referred to the pubic region.

11.2 Neurovasculature of the Abdomen

Arteries of the Abdomen

— The **aorta abdominalis** supplies abdominal viscera and most of the anterior abdominal wall (**Fig. 11.11**).

- It enters the abdomen at T XII through the hiatus aorticus of the diaphragma and descends along the columna vertebralis to the left of the midline.
- It terminates at the vertebra L IV, where it bifurcates into two **aa. iliacae communes**.
- A single **a. sacralis mediana** arises near the bifurcation.
— **Table 11.4** lists major branches of the aorta abdominalis.
  - Paired parietal (segmental) branches supply the structures of the posterior abdominal wall. These include the **aa. phrenicae inferiores** and **aa. lumbales**.
  - Paired visceral branches supply organs of the retroperitoneum. These are the **aa. suprarenales mediae, aa. testiculares/ovaricae**, and **aa. renales**.
  - Three unpaired visceral branches supply the intestines and accessory organs of the gastrointestinal tract:
    1. The **truncus coeliacus**, a short trunk that arises at T XII/L I and supplies the abdominal foregut. Its branches, the **a. splenica**, **a. gastrica sinistra**, and **a. hepatica communis**, anastomose extensively with each other (**Figs. 11.12, 11.13, 11.14, 11.15**).
    2. The **a. mesenterica superior**, which arises at L I, posterior to the neck of the pancreas. It supplies midgut structures, and its major branches include the

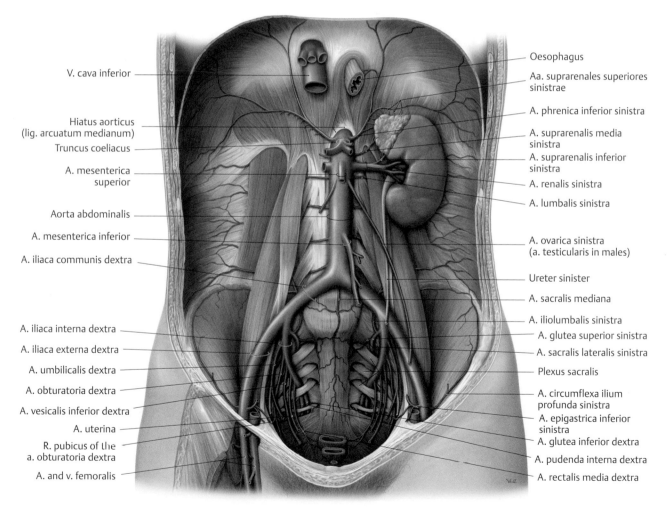

Fig. 11.11 Aorta abdominalis
Female abdomen, anterior view. *Removed:* Abdominal organs and peritoneum. The aorta abdominalis is the distal continuation of the aorta thoracica. It enters the abdomen at the T XII level and bifurcates into the aa. iliacae communes at L 4. (From Schuenke M, Schulte E, Schumacher U. THIEME Atlas of Anatomy, Vol 2. Illustrations by Voll M and Wesker K. 3rd ed. New York: Thieme Publishers; 2020.)

a. pancreaticoduodenalis inferior, a. colica media, a. colica dextra, and a. ileocolica, as well as a series of aa. jejunales and ileales (Figs. **11.16** and **11.17**).

3. The **a. mesenterica inferior**, which arises at L III and has the smallest caliber of the three visceral trunks. It supplies the hindgut through the **a. colica sinistra**, **aa. sigmoideae**, and **a. rectalis superior** (Figs. **11.18** and **11.19**).

- Aa. iliacae communes pass along the brim of the pelvis and terminate by bifurcating into two major branches (see **Fig. 11.11**):
  - The **a. iliaca interna**, which descends into the pelvis.
  - The **a. iliaca externa**, which gives off the **a. epigastrica inferior** and **a. circumflexa ilium profunda** before passing into the lower limb as the **a. femoralis**.

— Important anastomoses connect the three unpaired visceral branches of the aorta and provide a collateral blood supply to the intestinal organs.
- The truncus coeliacus and a. mesenterica superior anastomose in the caput pancreatis through the **aa. pancreaticoduodenales** and in the corpus pancreatis and cauda pancreatis through **a. pancreatica dorsalis** and **a. pancreatica inferior** (Fig. **11.15**).

- The a. mesenterica superior and a. mesenterica inferior anastomose near the junction of the colon transversum and colon descendens through the a. colica media and a. colica sinistra. The **a. marginalis coli** runs along the mesenteric border of the large intestine and connects the a. ileocolica and a. colica dextra, a. colica media, and a. colica sinistra.
- The a. mesenterica inferior anastomoses with arteries of the rectum through the **a. rectalis superior** (see **Fig. 14.19**).

BOX 11.3: CLINICAL CORRELATION

ABDOMINAL AORTIC ANEURYSM

Abdominal aortic aneurysms (AAAs) most commonly occur between the aa. renales and the bifurcatio aortae. When small they can remain asymptomatic, but large aneurysms can be palpated through the abdominal wall to the left of the midline. Ruptured AAAs present with severe abdominal pain that radiates to the abdomen or back. Mortality rates for ruptured aneurysms approach 90% due to overwhelming hemorrhage.

Table 11.4 Branches of the Aorta Abdominalis

The aorta abdominalis gives rise to three major unpaired trunks (bold) and the unpaired a. sacralis mediana, as well as six paired branches.

Branch from Aorta Abdominalis	Branches	
Aa. phrenicae inferiores (paired)	Aa. suprarenales superiores	
Truncus coeliacus	A. gastrica sinistra	
	A. splenica	
	A. hepatica communis	A. hepatica propria
		A. gastrica dextra
		A. gastroduodenalis
Aa. suprarenales mediae (paired)		
A. mesenterica superior	A. pancreaticoduodenalis inferior	
	A. colica media	
	A. colica dextra	
	Aa. jejunales and ileales	
	A. ileocolica	
Aa. renales (paired)	Aa. suprarenales inferiores	
Aa. lumbales (1st–4th, paired)		
Aa. testiculares/ovaricae (paired)		
A. mesenterica inferior	A. colica sinistra	
	Aa. sigmoideae	
	A. rectalis superior	
Aa. iliacae communes (paired)	A. iliaca externa	
	A. iliaca interna	
A. sacralis mediana		

Fig. 11.12 Truncus coeliacus: Gaster, hepar, and vesica biliaris

Anterior view. *Opened:* Omentum minus. *Incised:* Greater omentum. The truncus coeliacus arises from the aorta abdominalis at about the level of L I. (From Schuenke M, Schulte E, Schumacher U. THIEME Atlas of Anatomy, Vol 2. Illustrations by Voll M and Wesker K. 3rd ed. New York: Thieme Publishers; 2020.)

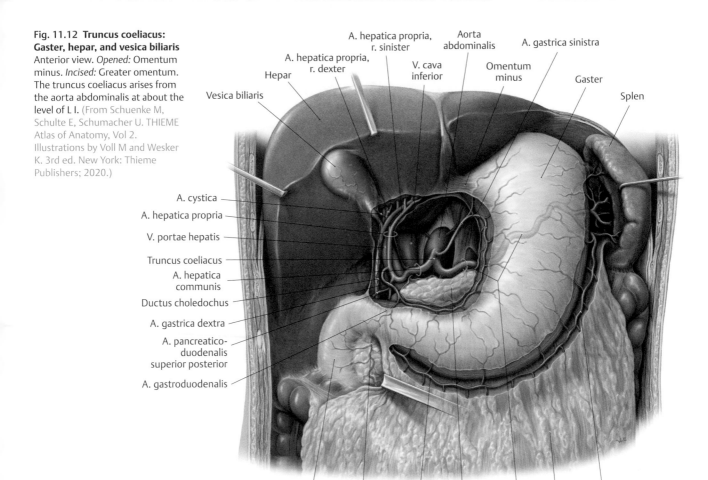

Fig. 11.13 Distribution of the truncus coeliacus and anastomoses between its branches

(From Schuenke M, Schulte E, Schumacher U. THIEME Atlas of Anatomy, Vol 2. Illustrations by Voll M and Wesker K. 3rd ed. New York: Thieme Publishers; 2020.)

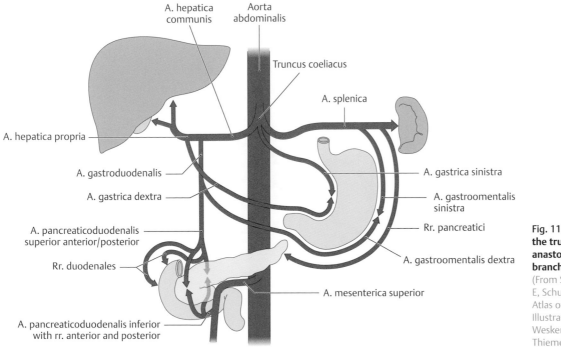

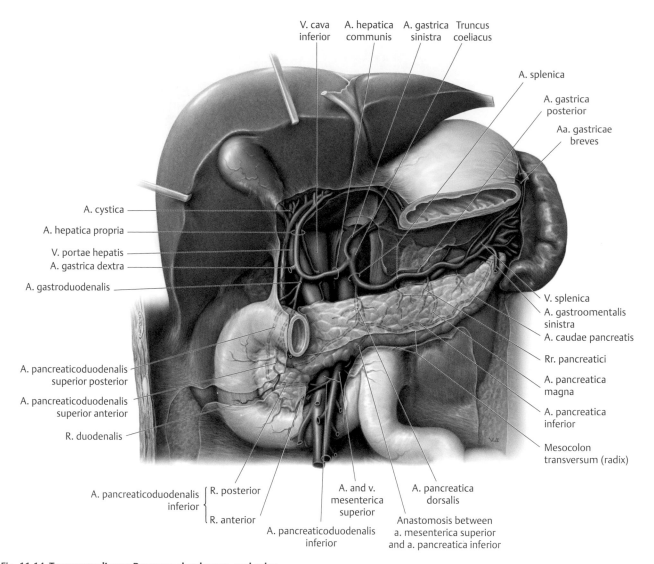

Fig. 11.14 Truncus coeliacus: Pancreas, duodenum, and splen
Anterior view. *Removed:* Gaster (corpus) and omentum minus. (From Schuenke M, Schulte E, Schumacher U. THIEME Atlas of Anatomy, Vol 2. Illustrations by Voll M and Wesker K. 3rd ed. New York: Thieme Publishers; 2020.)

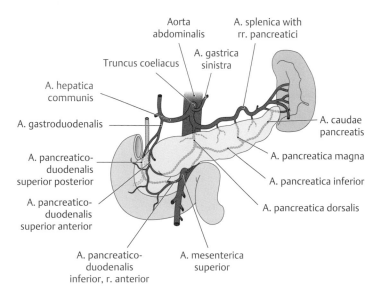

Fig. 11.15 The pancreaticoduodenal arcade, an anastomosis between branches of the truncus coeliacus and arteria mesenterica superior
(From Gilroy AM et al. Atlas of Anatomy. 4th ed. 2020. Based on: Schuenke M, Schulte E, Schumacher U. THIEME Atlas of Anatomy. Internal Organs. Illustrations by Voll M and Wesker K. 3rd ed. New York: Thieme Medical Publishers; 2020.)

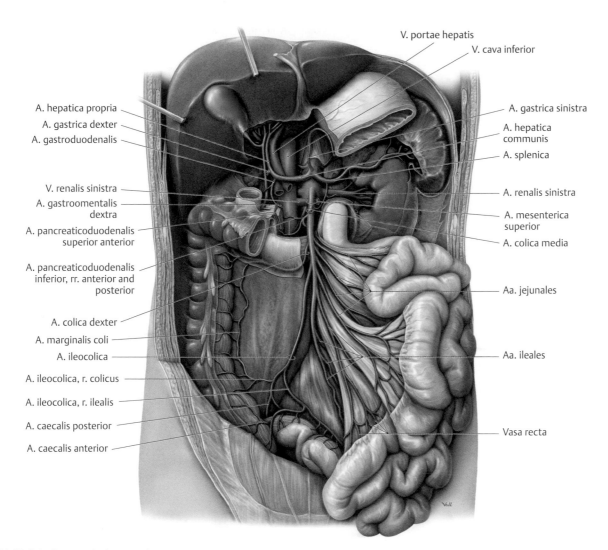

Fig. 11.16 Arteria mesenterica superior
Anterior view. *Partially removed:* Gaster and peritoneum. *Note:* The a. colica media has been truncated. The a. mesenterica superior arises from the aorta opposite L II. (From Schuenke M, Schulte E, Schumacher U. THIEME Atlas of Anatomy, Vol 2. Illustrations by Voll M and Wesker K. 3rd ed. New York: Thieme Publishers; 2020.)

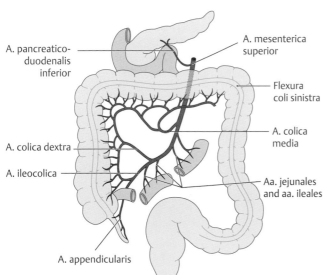

BOX 11.4: CLINICAL CORRELATION

MESENTERIC ISCHEMIA
A decrease in blood flow to the intestine (ischemia) can result from occlusion of the a. mesenterica superior by a thrombus or embolus (acute) or may be secondary to severe atherosclerosis (chronic). In the acute condition, the embolus can obstruct the a. mesenterica superior at its origin or, if small enough, may travel further to obstruct a more peripheral branch. Acute ischemia results in necrosis of the affected part of the intestine. Chronic ischemia is less threatening since obstruction of the vessels occurs gradually, allowing the formation of collateral vessels that will supply the affected intestine. Because of the extensive anastomoses between intestinal arteries, chronic vascular ischemia is rare. Symptoms occur only if two of the three major vessels (truncus coeliacus or a. mesenterica superior or a. mesenterica inferior) are compromised.

Fig. 11.17 Distribution of the arteria mesenterica superior
(From Gilroy AM et al. Atlas of Anatomy. 4th ed. 2020. Based on: Schuenke M, Schulte E, Schumacher U. THIEME Atlas of Anatomy. Internal Organs. Illustrations by Voll M and Wesker K. 3rd ed. New York: Thieme Medical Publishers; 2020.)

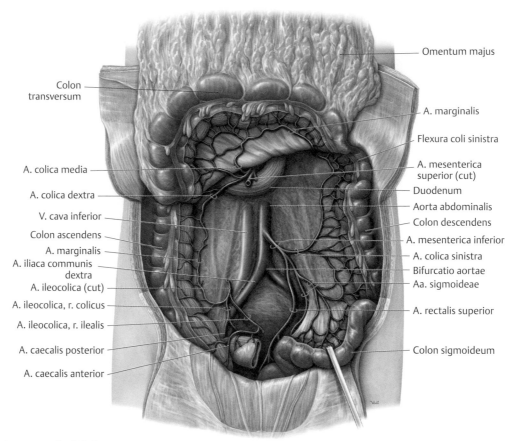

Colon transversum — A. colica media — A. colica dextra — V. cava inferior — Colon ascendens — A. marginalis — A. iliaca communis dextra — A. ileocolica (cut) — A. ileocolica, r. colicus — A. ileocolica, r. ilealis — A. caecalis posterior — A. caecalis anterior

Omentum majus — A. marginalis — Flexura coli sinistra — A. mesenterica superior (cut) — Duodenum — Aorta abdominalis — Colon descendens — A. mesenterica inferior — A. colica sinistra — Bifurcatio aortae — Aa. sigmoideae — A. rectalis superior — Colon sigmoideum

Fig. 11.18 Arteria mesenterica inferior
Anterior view. *Removed:* Jejunum and ileum. *Reflected:* Colon transversum. The a. mesenterica inferior arises from the aorta opposite LIII. (From Schuenke M, Schulte E, Schumacher U. THIEME Atlas of Anatomy, Vol 2. Illustrations by Voll M and Wesker K. 3rd ed. New York: Thieme Publishers; 2020.)

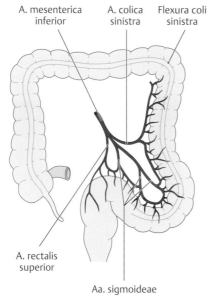

A. mesenterica inferior — A. colica sinistra — Flexura coli sinistra — A. rectalis superior — Aa. sigmoideae

Fig. 11.19 Distribution of the arteria mesenterica inferior
(From Gilroy AM et al. Atlas of Anatomy. 4th ed. 2020. Based on: Schuenke M, Schulte E, Schumacher U. THIEME Atlas of Anatomy. Internal Organs. Illustrations by Voll M and Wesker K. 3rd ed. New York: Thieme Medical Publishers; 2020.)

BOX 11.5: CLINICAL CORRELATION

ANATOMOSES BETWEEN ARTERIES OF THE LARGE INTESTINE

Anastomoses between branches of the a. mesenterica superior and a. mesenterica inferior can compensate for abnormally low blood flow in either of the arteries. Two of these anastomoses, although variable, are of significant value:

Riolan's arcade (arc of Riolan) – connects the a. colica media and a. colica sinistra close to their origins from the a. mesenterica superior and a. mesenterica inferior, respectively.

A. marginalis (of Drummond) – connects all arteries of the colon that run along the periphery of the mesenterium close to the intestinal tube.

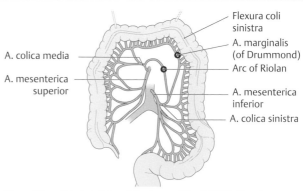

Flexura coli sinistra — A. marginalis (of Drummond) — Arc of Riolan — A. mesenterica inferior — A. colica sinistra — A. colica media — A. mesenterica superior

(From Gilroy AM et al. Atlas of Anatomy. 4th ed. 2020. Based on: Schuenke M, Schulte E, Schumacher U. THIEME Atlas of Anatomy. Internal Organs. Illustrations by Voll M and Wesker K. 3rd ed. New York: Thieme Medical Publishers; 2020.)

Veins of the Abdomen

Venous drainage of the abdomen and pelvis is accomplished through two systems, the **systemic (caval) system** and the **hepatic portal system (Fig. 11.20)**.

1. Organs that drain directly into the **v. cava inferior** or its tributaries make up the systemic (caval) venous system.
   - The v. cava inferior receives blood from retroperitoneal and pelvic organs, walls of the abdomen and pelvis, and the lower limbs **(Fig. 11.21)**.
     - It originates at the L V vertebral level where the vv. iliacae communes merge.
     - It ascends along the right side of the columna vertebralis, passes posterior to the liver, and pierces the centrum tendineum of the diaphragm at the T VIII vertebral level where it enters the atrium dextrum of the heart.
   - **Table 11.5** lists the direct tributaries of the v. cava inferior.
     - Paired vv. iliacae communes drain the **vv. iliacae externae** and **vv. iliacae internae**.
     - Paired **vv. phrenicae inferiores** and **vv. lumbales** drain the posterior abdominal wall and diaphragm and accompany the arteries of similar name.
     - Veins of the retroperitoneal organs include the **v. renalis dextra** and **v. renalis sinistra**, the **v. suprarenalis dextra**, and the **v. testicularis dextra** or **v. ovarica dextra** (right gonadal vein). The v. suprarenalis sinistra and gonadal vein on the left side drain to the v. renalis sinistra.
     - Typically three **vv. hepaticae** enter the IVC from the liver immediately below the diaphragm.
   - Paired **vv. lumbales ascendentes** communicate with the vv. lumbales and are continuous with the v. azygos and v. hemiazygos of the thorax. These communications between the vv. lumbales, vv. lumbales ascendentes, v. azygos, and v. hemiazygos function as a collateral pathway between the v. cava inferior and v. cava superior.
2. Organs that drain into the **v. portae hepatis** or its tributaries and pass through the liver before entering the v. cava inferior make up the hepatic portal system.
   - The v. portae hepatis shunts nutrient-rich venous blood from the capillary beds of the gastrointestinal tract and its associated organs (liver, gallbladder, pancreas, and spleen) to sinusoids of the liver **(Fig. 11.22)**. This blood eventually enters the v. cava inferior through the vv. hepaticae.
   - Tributaries of the v. portae hepatis are listed in **Table 11.6** and include the following:
     - The **v. splenica**, which drains the spleen, and the **v. mesenterica superior**, which drains the small intestine and most of the large intestine. These two veins unite behind the collum pancreatis to form the v. portae hepatis.
     - The **v. mesenterica inferior**, which drains the hindgut portion of the gastrointestinal tract. It usually joins the v. splenica but may empty directly into the v. portae hepatis.
     - Veins from the lower oesophagus, stomach, pancreas, duodenum, and gallbladder
   - Normal connections between the systemic (caval) venous system and portal venous system, called **portosystemic pathways (Fig. 11.23)**, can become abnormally dilated when there is an obstruction of the portal or systemic circulations (e.g., cirrhosis of the liver or pregnancy). These dilations are most prominent in
     1. **venae oesophageales**,
     2. **venae paraumbilicales** through the vv. epigastricae superiores and vv. epigastricae superiores of the abdominal wall,
     3. **venae colici** in the retroperitoneum, and
     4. **venae rectales** of the rectum and canalis analis.

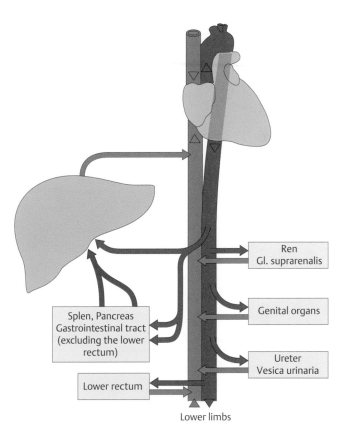

Fig. 11.20 Schematic of systemic and portal venous systems
(From Schuenke M, Schulte E, Schumacher U. THIEME Atlas of Anatomy, Vol 2. Illustrations by Voll M and Wesker K. 3rd ed. New York: Thieme Publishers; 2020.)

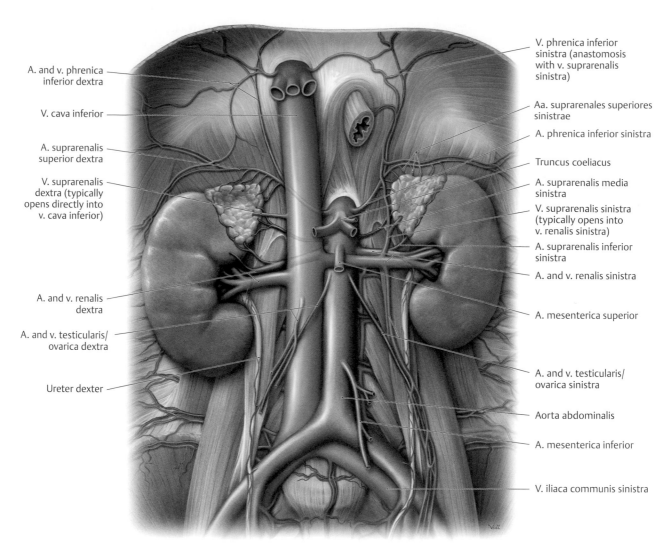

A. and v. phrenica inferior dextra

V. cava inferior

A. suprarenalis superior dextra

V. suprarenalis dextra (typically opens directly into v. cava inferior)

A. and v. renalis dextra

A. and v. testicularis/ ovarica dextra

Ureter dexter

V. phrenica inferior sinistra (anastomosis with v. suprarenalis sinistra)

Aa. suprarenales superiores sinistrae

A. phrenica inferior sinistra

Truncus coeliacus

A. suprarenalis media sinistra

V. suprarenalis sinistra (typically opens into v. renalis sinistra)

A. suprarenalis inferior sinistra

A. and v. renalis sinistra

A. mesenterica superior

A. and v. testicularis/ ovarica sinistra

Aorta abdominalis

A. mesenterica inferior

V. iliaca communis sinistra

Fig. 11.21 Vena cava inferior
Anterior view. *Removed:* All organs except the renes and gll. suprarenalis. (From Schuenke M, Schulte E, Schumacher U. THIEME Atlas of Anatomy, Vol 2. Illustrations by Voll M and Wesker K. 3rd ed. New York: Thieme Publishers; 2020.)

Table 11.5 Tributaries of the Vena Cava Inferior

①R	①L	Vv. phrenicae inferiores (paired)
	②	Vv. hepaticae (3)
③R	③L	Vv. suprarenales (the right vein is a direct tributary)
④R	④L	Vv. renales (paired)
⑤R	⑤L	Vv. testiculares/ovaricae (the right vena is a direct tributary)
⑥R	⑥L	Vv. lumbales ascendens (paired), not direct tributaries
⑦R	⑦L	Vv. lumbales
⑧R	⑧L	Vv. iliacae communes (paired)
	⑨	V. sacralis mediana

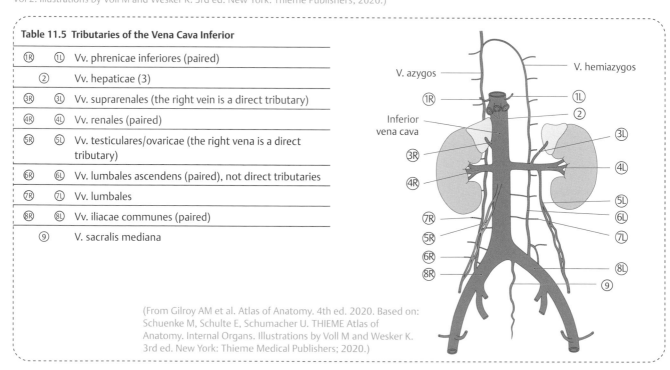

(From Gilroy AM et al. Atlas of Anatomy. 4th ed. 2020. Based on: Schuenke M, Schulte E, Schumacher U. THIEME Atlas of Anatomy. Internal Organs. Illustrations by Voll M and Wesker K. 3rd ed. New York: Thieme Medical Publishers; 2020.)

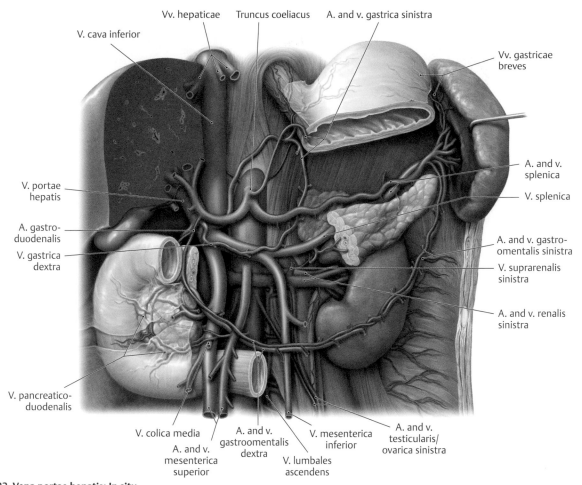

Fig. 11.22 Vena portae hepatis: In situ
Anterior view. *Partially removed:* Gaster, pancreas, and peritoneum. (From Schuenke M, Schulte E, Schumacher U. THIEME Atlas of Anatomy, Vol 2. Illustrations by Voll M and Wesker K. 3rd ed. New York: Thieme Publishers; 2020.)

Table 11.6 Tributaries of the Vena Portae Hepatis

- **Vena mesenterica superior** with its tributaries:
  ① Vv. pancreaticoduodenales
  ② Vv. pancreaticae
  ③ V. gastroomentalis dextra
  ④ Vv. jejunales and vv. ileales
  ⑤ V. ileocolica
  ⑥ V. colica dextra
  ⑦ V. colica media

- **Vena mesenterica inferior** with its tributaries:
  ⑧ V. colica sinistra
  ⑨ Vv. sigmoideae
  ⑩ V. rectalis superior

- **Vena splenica** with its tributaries:
  ⑪ V. gastroomentalis sinistra
  ⑫ Vv. pancreaticae
  ⑬ Vv. gastricae breves

- **Direct tributaries**
  ⑭ V. cystica
  ⑮ V. gastrica sinistra (with vv. oesophageales)
  ⑯ V. gastrica dextra
  ⑰ V. pancreaticoduodenalis superior posterior
  — Vv. paraumbilicales **(see Fig. 11.23)**

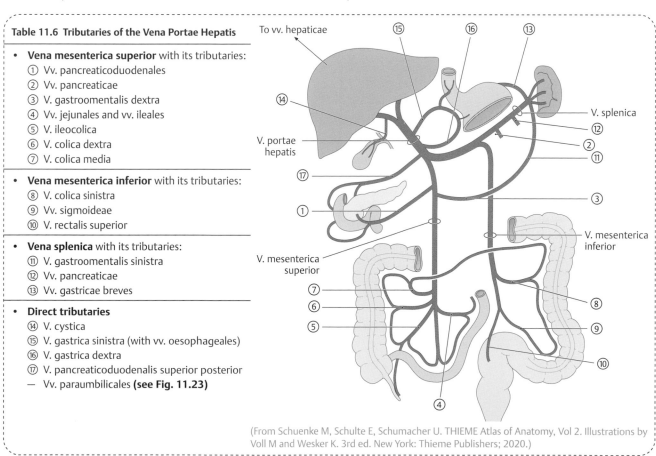

(From Schuenke M, Schulte E, Schumacher U. THIEME Atlas of Anatomy, Vol 2. Illustrations by Voll M and Wesker K. 3rd ed. New York: Thieme Publishers; 2020.)

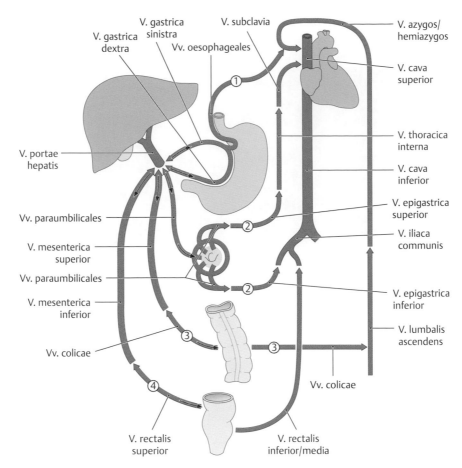

Fig. 11.23 Portosystemic pathways
When the portal system is compromised, the v. portae hepatis can divert blood away from the liver back to its supplying veins, which return this nutrient-rich blood to the heart via the vv. cavae. *Red arrows* indicate flow reversal in the *(1)* vv. oesophageales, *(2)* vv. paraumbilicales, *(3)* vv. colicae, and *(4)* vv. rectales media and inferior. (From Schuenke M, Schulte E, Schumacher U. THIEME Atlas of Anatomy, Vol 2. Illustrations by Voll M and Wesker K. 3rd ed. New York: Thieme Publishers; 2020.)

BOX 11.6: CLINICAL CORRELATION

OESOPHAGEAL VARICES
Submucosal veins of the oesophagus drain superiorly to the systemic system (through the vv. azygos) and inferiorly to the portal system. When flow through the v. portae hepatis is obstructed (as in portal hypertension), these portosystemic anastomoses allow blood in the lower oesophagus to drain to the systemic veins. The oesophageal varices, enlarged veins that result from this increased flow, bulge into the esophageal lumen and can rupture, causing severe hemorrhaging.

BOX 11.7: CLINICAL CORRELATION

PORTAL HYPERTENSION AND SURGICAL PORTOCAVAL SHUNTS
Portal hypertension occurs secondary to liver disease (e.g., cirrhosis) or thrombosis of the v. portae hepatis. Increased resistance to the flow of blood in the portal system forces portal blood through portosystemic (portocaval) anastomoses to the systemic circulation, reversing flow in some venous pathways. Symptoms of portal hypertension include ascites, caput medusa (enlargement of vv. paraumbilicales on the anterior abdominal wall), varices of the vv. rectales (hemorrhoids), and esophageal varices. Symptoms may be relieved by surgically creating a portocaval shunt between the portal and systemic circulations (v. portae hepatis to v. cava inferior or v. splenica to v. renalis sinistra).

Lymphatic Drainage of the Abdomen

Lymph from abdominal and pelvic regions drains through lymphatic vessels that usually accompany the arteries supplying those regions. The lymph passes through one or more lymph node groups that can include primary, or regional, nodes and secondary, or collecting, nodes. These latter groups receive lymph from multiple regions and in the abdomen and pelvis and are known as **nodi lymphoidei lumbales**. They surround the aorta and v. cava inferior and are subdivided by location **(Fig. 11.24)**. Lymph drains from these nodes into either the **trunci lumbales** or **trunci intestinales**, which converge in the upper abdomen to form the **cisterna chyli** and the thoracic duct.

— Groups of nll. lumbales drain all of the abdominal viscera (except a small hepatic segment, which can drain to nodes of the diaphragma) and most of the abdominal wall **(Fig. 11.25; Table 11.7)**. They include:
  • **Nll. preaortici**, which lie anterior to the aorta abdominalis. They receive lymph from the gastrointestinal tract (as far as the midrectum) and associated organs.

Nodes surrounding the base of the major arteries form collecting nodal groups, such as the **nll. mesenterici superiores** and **nll. mesenterici inferiores**. These drain to **nll. coeliaci**, which drain to trunci intestinales.
  • **Nll. aortici laterales** (nll. lumbales dextri and sinistri), which lie along the medial border of the mm. psoae, the crura of the diaphragma, and along the v. cava inferior. They drain the abdominal and pelvic walls and the viscera of the retroperitoneum, including the ovaries and testes. They also receive lymph from the nll. iliaci communes, which drain the pelvic viscera and the lower limb. Drainage from nll. aortici laterales forms a truncus lumbalis on each side.

— **Nll. iliaci communes** drain organs of the pelvis and the lower limbs. Lymph from these nodes drain to the right and left nll. lumbales.

— The cisterna chyli is an elongated, lobulated, thin-walled dilation that, when present, gives rise to the ductus thoracicus. It lies to the right of the corpus vertebrae T XII and receives the trunci lumbales and trunci intestinales.

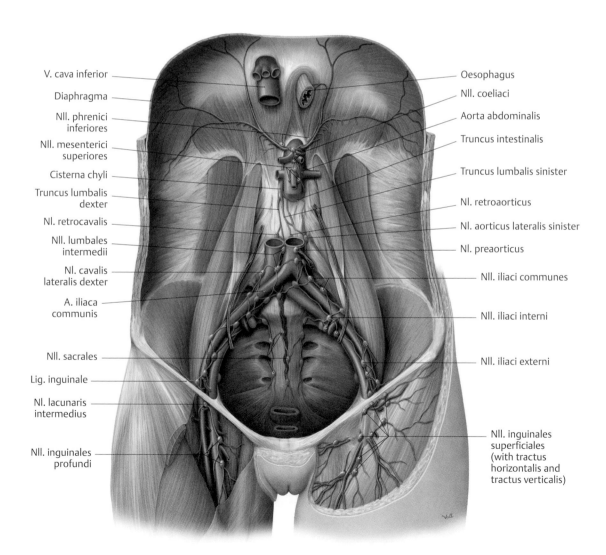

Fig. 11.24 Nll. parietales in the abdomen and pelvis
Anterior view. *Removed*: All visceral structures except vessels. (From Schuenke M, Schulte E, Schumacher U. THIEME Atlas of Anatomy, Vol 2. Illustrations by Voll M and Wesker K. 3rd ed. New York: Thieme Publishers; 2020.)

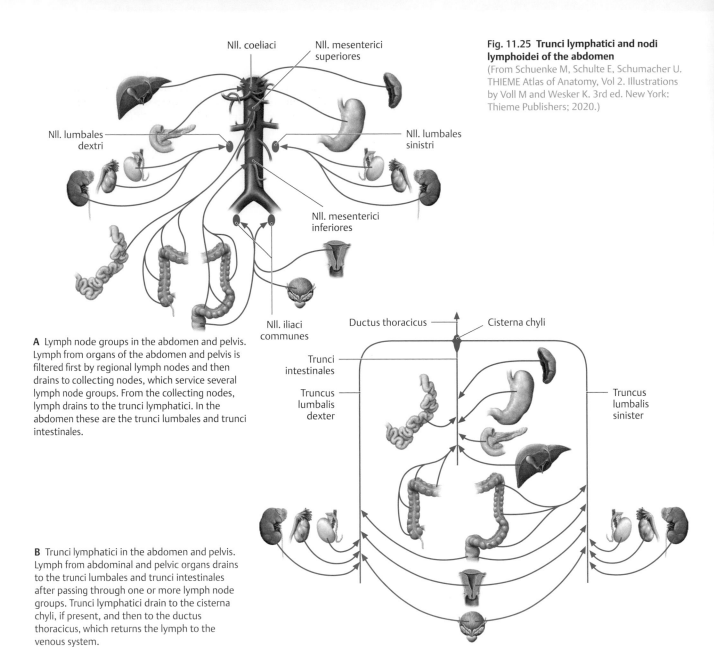

Fig. 11.25 Trunci lymphatici and nodi lymphoidei of the abdomen
(From Schuenke M, Schulte E, Schumacher U. THIEME Atlas of Anatomy, Vol 2. Illustrations by Voll M and Wesker K. 3rd ed. New York: Thieme Publishers; 2020.)

A Lymph node groups in the abdomen and pelvis. Lymph from organs of the abdomen and pelvis is filtered first by regional lymph nodes and then drains to collecting nodes, which service several lymph node groups. From the collecting nodes, lymph drains to the trunci lymphatici. In the abdomen these are the trunci lumbales and trunci intestinales.

B Trunci lymphatici in the abdomen and pelvis. Lymph from abdominal and pelvic organs drains to the trunci lumbales and trunci intestinales after passing through one or more lymph node groups. Trunci lymphatici drain to the cisterna chyli, if present, and then to the ductus thoracicus, which returns the lymph to the venous system.

Table 11.7 Lymph Node Groups and Tributary Regions

Lymph Node Groups and Collecting Lymph Nodes	Location	Organs or Organ Segments that Drain to These Lymph Node Groups (Tributary Regions)
Nll. coeliaci	Around the truncus coeliacus	Distal third of oesophagus, gaster, omentum majus, duodenum (pars superior and pars descendens), pancreas, splen, hepar, and vesica urinaria
Nll. mesenterici superiores	At the origin of the a. mesenterica superior	Second through fourth parts of duodenum, jejunum and ileum, caecum with appendix vermiformis, colon ascendens, colon transversum (proximal two-thirds)
Nll. mesenterici inferiores	At the origin of the a. mesenterica inferior	Colon transversum (distal third), colon descendens, colon sigmoideum, rectum (proximal part)
Nll. lumbales (dextri, intermedi, sinistri)	Around the pars abdominalis aortae and v. cava inferior	Diaphragma (abdominal side), renes, gll. suprarenales, testis and epididymis, ovarium, tuba uterina, fundus uteri, ureteres, spatium retroperitoneale
Nll. iliaci	Around the aa. and vv. iliacae	Rectum (anal end), vesica urinaria and urethra, corpus uteri and cervix uteri, ductus deferens, gl. seminalis, prostata, external genitalia (via nll. inguinales)

Nerves of the Abdomen

— Lower nn. intercostales (T7–T11) and the **n. subcostalis** (T12) continue anteroinferiorly from their position on the thoracic wall to innervate most of the muscles and skin of the anterolateral abdominal wall.
— The **plexus lumbalis** is a somatic nerve plexus formed by the rami anteriores of nn. spinales T12–L4. Its branches pass laterally through the m. psoas major and onto the posterior abdominal wall **(Fig. 11.26)**. Most nerves of this plexus innervate the lower limb (see Section 21.4 and **Table 21.1**). Branches that innervate the abdominal wall and inguinal region include

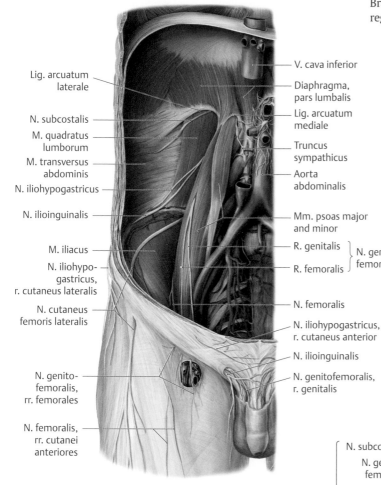

Labels (left to right):
- Lig. arcuatum laterale
- N. subcostalis
- M. quadratus lumborum
- M. transversus abdominis
- N. iliohypogastricus
- N. ilioinguinalis
- M. iliacus
- N. iliohypogastricus, r. cutaneus lateralis
- N. cutaneus femoris lateralis
- N. genitofemoralis, rr. femorales
- N. femoralis, rr. cutanei anteriores

- V. cava inferior
- Diaphragma, pars lumbalis
- Lig. arcuatum mediale
- Truncus sympathicus
- Aorta abdominalis
- Mm. psoas major and minor
- R. genitalis } N. genitofemoralis
- R. femoralis
- N. femoralis
- N. iliohypogastricus, r. cutaneus anterior
- N. ilioinguinalis
- N. genitofemoralis, r. genitalis

A Lumbar plexus in situ.

Fig. 11.26 Nerves of the plexus lumbalis
Anterior view. (From Gilroy AM et al. Atlas of Anatomy. 4th ed. 2020. Based on: Schuenke M, Schulte E, Schumacher U. THIEME Atlas of Anatomy. Internal Organs. Illustrations by Voll M and Wesker K. 3rd ed. New York: Thieme Medical Publishers; 2020.)

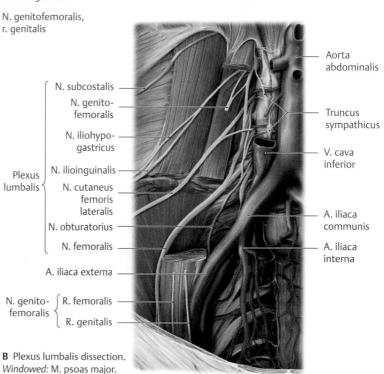

Labels:
- Plexus lumbalis {
  - N. subcostalis
  - N. genitofemoralis
  - N. iliohypogastricus
  - N. ilioinguinalis
  - N. cutaneus femoris lateralis
  - N. obturatorius
  - N. femoralis
- A. iliaca externa
- N. genitofemoralis { R. femoralis, R. genitalis

- Aorta abdominalis
- Truncus sympathicus
- V. cava inferior
- A. iliaca communis
- A. iliaca interna

B Plexus lumbalis dissection.
Windowed: M. psoas major.

- **n. iliohypogastricus** and **n. ilioinguinalis** (L1), which innervate the skin and muscles of the inferior anterior abdominal wall and the skin over the inguinal and pubic regions;
- **n. genitofemoralis** (L1–L2), whose genital branch innervates the m. cremaster surrounding the funiculus spermaticus and the skin over the scrotum and labia; and
- short muscular branches (T12–L4) that innervate the muscles of the posterior abdominal wall.
— **Trunci sympathici lumbales**, the continuations of the trunci sympathici thoracici, descend along the lateral aspect of the

bodies of the lumbar vertebrae and give off three to four **nn. splanchnici lumbales**, which join the autonomic plexuses of the abdomen.
— Plexus autonomici form along the aorta and travel with the major abdominal arteries to innervate the abdominal viscera (**Figs. 11.27, 11.28, 11.29, 11.30, 11.31, 11.32; Tables 11.8 and 11.9**). The plexuses contain combinations of
- preganglionic sympathetic nerves that synapse in the ganglia associated with the plexuses. (Note that the sympathetic nerves innervating the medulla glandulae suprarenalis are an exception and do not synapse in these ganglia.) The preganglionic sympathetic nerves arise from

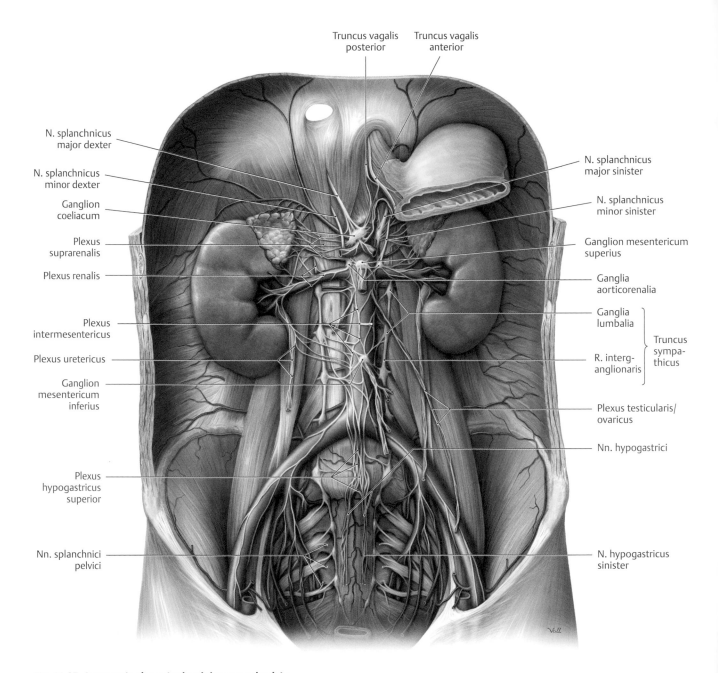

Fig. 11.27 Autonomic plexus in the abdomen and pelvis
Anterior view of the male abdomen. *Removed:* Peritoneum and majority of the gaster. (From Schuenke M, Schulte E, Schumacher U. THIEME Atlas of Anatomy, Vol 2. Illustrations by Voll M and Wesker K. 3rd ed. New York: Thieme Publishers; 2020.)

- nn. splanchnici thoracici (T5–T12), which contribute to the plexus coeliacus, plexus mesentericus superior, and plexus renalis
  - nn. splanchnici lumbales (T11–L2), which contribute to the plexus mesentericus inferior, plexus hypogastricus superior, and plexus hypogastricus inferior
- preganglionic parasympathetic nerves, which pass through the plexuses and synapse in ganglia near their target organ. They arise from either
  - the n. vagus (n. cranialis X), which enter the abdomen as the truncus vagalis anterior and truncus vagalis posterior from the plexus oesophageus. They supply most of the abdominal viscera, including the digestive tract, except for its most distal segment (the colon descendens to the canalis analis). They contribute to all of the abdominal plexuses except the plexus mesentericus inferior, plexus hypogastricus superior, and plexus hypogastricus inferior.
    or
  - the **nn. splanchnici pelvici** (S2–S4), which ascend from the pelvis to innervate the colon descendens and colon

sigmoideum in the abdomen. They also innervate viscera of the pelvis. These fibers contribute to the plexus hypogastricus inferior.

— Although most abdominal plexuses contain both sympathetic and parasympathetic nerves, the plexus mesentericus inferior and plexus hypogastricus superior contain only sympathetic fibers. Viscera supplied by these plexuses receive parasympathetic innervation via nn. splanchnici pelvici and the plexus hypogastricus inferior.

— When pain arising from viscera (visceral pain) and pain arising from somatic structures (somatic pain) are conveyed to the same area of the spinal cord, the convergence of these visceral and somatic fibers confuses the relationship between the visceral pain's actual origin and its perceived origin. This phenomenon is known as **referred pain**. The perceived origin of visceral pain from a specific organ is consistently projected to a well-defined area of the skin. Thus, a knowledge of cutaneous zones of referred pain is instrumental in identifying underlying problems.

Table 11.8 Plexus Autonomici in the Abdomen and Pelvis

Ganglia	Subplexus	Distribution	
Plexus coeliacus			
Ganglion coeliacum	Plexus hepaticus	• Hepar, vesica biliaris	
	Plexus gastricus	• Gaster	
	Plexus splenicus	• Splen	
	Plexus pancreaticus	• Pancreas	
Plexus mesentericus superior			
Ganglion mesentericum superius		• Pancreas (caput) • Duodenum • Jejunum • Ileum	• Caecum • Colon (to flexura coli sinistra) • Ovarium
Plexus suprarenalis and renalis			
Ganglia aorticorenalia	Plexus uretericus	• Glandula suprarenalis • Ren • Ureter proximalis	
Plexus ovaricus/testicularis		• Ovarium/testis	
Plexus mesentericus inferior			
Ganglion mesentericum inferius	Plexus colica sinister	• Flexura coli sinistra	
	Plexus rectalis superior	• Colon descendens and colon sigmoideum • Upper rectum	
Plexus hypogastricus superior	Nn. hypogastrici	• Viscera pelvis	
Plexus hypogastricus inferior			
Ganglion pelvicum	Plexus rectalis medius and inferior	• Middle and lower rectum	
	Plexus prostaticus	• Prostata • Glandula vesiculosa • Gll. bulbourethrales	• Ductus ejaculatorius • Penis • Urethra
	Plexus deferentialis	• Ductus deferens • Epididymis	
	Plexus uterovaginalis	• Uterus • Tuba uterina	• Vagina • Ovarium
	Plexus vesicalis	• Vesica urinaria	
	Plexus uretericus	• Ureteres (ascending from pelvis)	

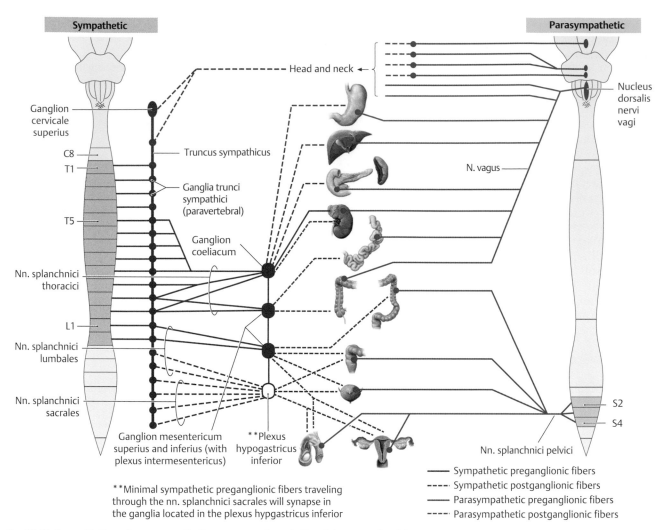

Fig. 11.28 Sympathetic and parasympathetic nervous systems in the abdomen and pelvis
(From Gilroy AM et al. Atlas of Anatomy. 4th ed. 2020. Based on: Schuenke M, Schulte E, Schumacher U. THIEME Atlas of Anatomy. Internal Organs. Illustrations by Voll M and Wesker K. 3rd ed. New York: Thieme Medical Publishers; 2020.)

Table 11.9 Effects of the Autonomic Nervous System in the Abdomen and Pelvis

Organ (Organ System)		Sympathetic Effect	Parasympathetic Effect
Gastrointestinal tract	Longitudinal and circular muscle fibers	↓ Motility	↑ Motility
	Mm. sphincteri	Contraction	Relaxation
	Glands	↓ Secretions	↑ Secretions
Capsula splenica		Contraction	No effect
Hepar		↑ Glycogenolysis/gluconeogenesis	
Pancreas	Pars endocrina	↓ Insulin secretion	
	Pars exocrina	↓ Secretion	↑ Secretion
Vesica urinaria	M. detrusor vesicae	Relaxation	Contraction
	Functional bladder sphincter	Contraction	Inhibits contraction
Gll. seminales and ductus deferentes		Contraction (ejaculation)	No effect
Uterus		Contraction or relaxation, depending on hormonal status	
Arteries		Vasoconstriction	Vasodilation of the arteries of the penis and clitoris (erection)
Glandula suprarenalis (medulla)		Release of adrenalin	No effect
Urinary tract	Renes	Vasoconstriction (↓ urine formation)	Vasodilation

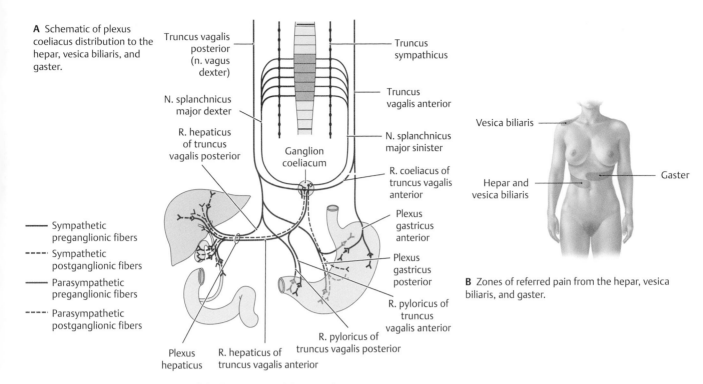

A Schematic of plexus coeliacus distribution to the hepar, vesica biliaris, and gaster.

Truncus vagalis posterior (n. vagus dexter)

N. splanchnicus major dexter

R. hepaticus of truncus vagalis posterior

Ganglion coeliacum

Truncus sympathicus

Truncus vagalis anterior

N. splanchnicus major sinister

R. coeliacus of truncus vagalis anterior

Plexus gastricus anterior

Plexus gastricus posterior

R. pyloricus of truncus vagalis anterior

R. pyloricus of truncus vagalis posterior

Plexus hepaticus

R. hepaticus of truncus vagalis anterior

—— Sympathetic preganglionic fibers

---- Sympathetic postganglionic fibers

—— Parasympathetic preganglionic fibers

---- Parasympathetic postganglionic fibers

Vesica biliaris

Hepar and vesica biliaris

Gaster

B Zones of referred pain from the hepar, vesica biliaris, and gaster.

Fig. 11.29 Autonomic innervation of the hepar, vesica biliaris, and gaster
(From Gilroy AM et al. Atlas of Anatomy. 4th ed. 2020. Based on: Schuenke M, Schulte E, Schumacher U. THIEME Atlas of Anatomy. Internal Organs. Illustrations by Voll M and Wesker K. 3rd ed. New York: Thieme Medical Publishers; 2020.)

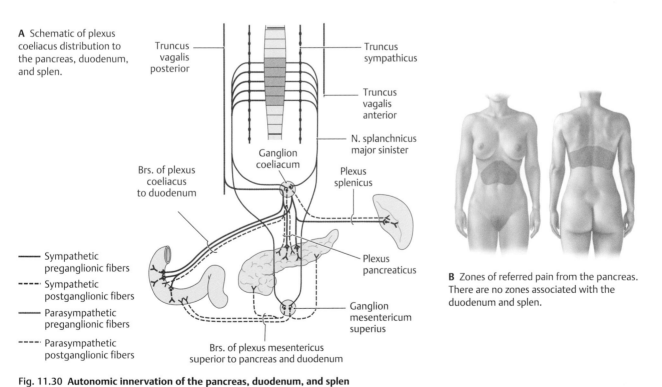

A Schematic of plexus coeliacus distribution to the pancreas, duodenum, and splen.

Truncus vagalis posterior

Brs. of plexus coeliacus to duodenum

Ganglion coeliacum

Truncus sympathicus

Truncus vagalis anterior

N. splanchnicus major sinister

Plexus splenicus

Plexus pancreaticus

Ganglion mesentericum superius

Brs. of plexus mesentericus superior to pancreas and duodenum

—— Sympathetic preganglionic fibers

---- Sympathetic postganglionic fibers

—— Parasympathetic preganglionic fibers

---- Parasympathetic postganglionic fibers

B Zones of referred pain from the pancreas. There are no zones associated with the duodenum and splen.

Fig. 11.30 Autonomic innervation of the pancreas, duodenum, and splen
(From Gilroy AM et al. Atlas of Anatomy. 4th ed. 2020. Based on: Schuenke M, Schulte E, Schumacher U. THIEME Atlas of Anatomy. Internal Organs. Illustrations by Voll M and Wesker K. 3rd ed. New York: Thieme Medical Publishers; 2020.)

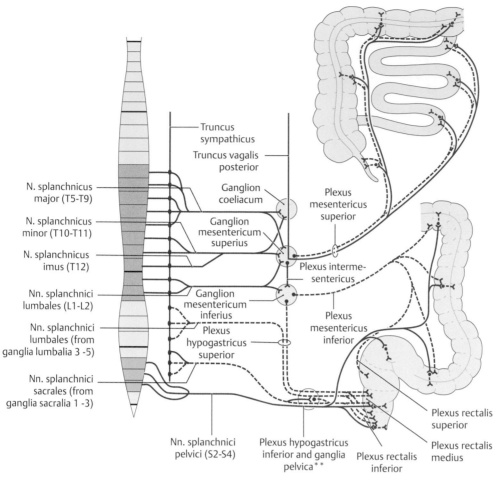

- —— Sympathetic preganglionic fibers
- ----- Sympathetic postganglionic fibers
- —— Parasympathetic preganglionic fibers
- ----- Parasympathetic postganglionic fibers

**Minimal sympathetic preganglionic fibers traveling through the nn. splanchnici sacrales will synapse in the ganglia located in the plexus hypogastricus inferior.

A Schematic of plexus mesentericus superior, plexus mesentericus inferior, and plexus hypogastricus inferior distribution.

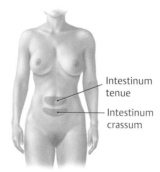

B Zones of referred pain from the small intestine and large intestine.

Fig. 11.31 Autonomic innervation of the intraperitoneal organs
(From Gilroy AM et al. Atlas of Anatomy. 4th ed. 2020. Based on: Schuenke M, Schulte E, Schumacher U. THIEME Atlas of Anatomy. Internal Organs. Illustrations by Voll M and Wesker K. 3rd ed. New York: Thieme Medical Publishers; 2020.)

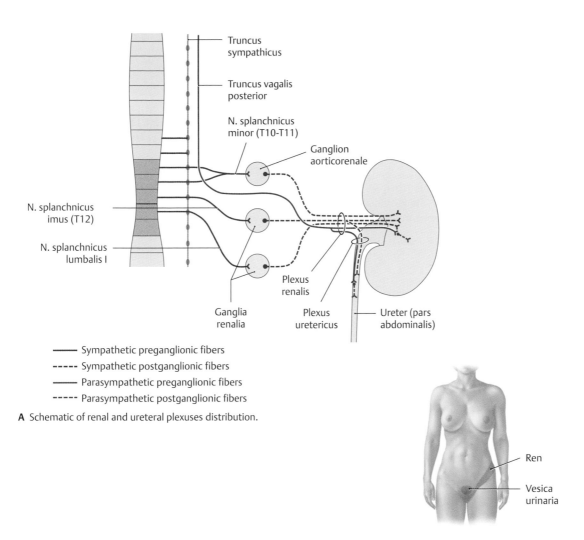

Truncus sympathicus

Truncus vagalis posterior

N. splanchnicus minor (T10-T11)

Ganglion aorticorenale

N. splanchnicus imus (T12)

N. splanchnicus lumbalis I

Plexus renalis

Ganglia renalia

Plexus uretericus

Ureter (pars abdominalis)

—— Sympathetic preganglionic fibers
- - - - Sympathetic postganglionic fibers
—— Parasympathetic preganglionic fibers
- - - - Parasympathetic postganglionic fibers

A Schematic of renal and ureteral plexuses distribution.

Ren

Vesica urinaria

B Zones of referred pain from the ren sinister and vesica urinaria.

Fig. 11.32 Autonomic innervation of the renes and upper ureteres
(From Gilroy AM, MacPherson BR, Wikenheiser JC. Atlas of Anatomy. Illustrations by Voll M and Wesker K. 4th ed. New York: Thieme Publishers; 2020.)

12 Abdominal Viscera

The cavitas peritonealis of the abdomen contains the primary and accessory organs of the gastrointestinal tract. The primary organs are the stomach (gaster), small intestine (intestinum tenue), and large intestine (intestinum crassum). The accessory organs are the liver (hepar), gallbladder (vesica biliaris), pancreas, and spleen (splen). The kidneys (renes), proximal ureters (ureteres), and adrenal glands (glandulae suprarenales) are found outside the cavitas peritonealis within the spatium retroperitoneale on the posterior abdominal wall **(Fig. 12.1)**.

12.1 Organs of the Peritoneal Cavity— Gastrointestinal Tract

Divisions of the Gastrointestinal Tract

The three divisions of the embryonic gastrointestinal tract are retained in the adult system and reflected in its blood supply and innervation. These divisions are

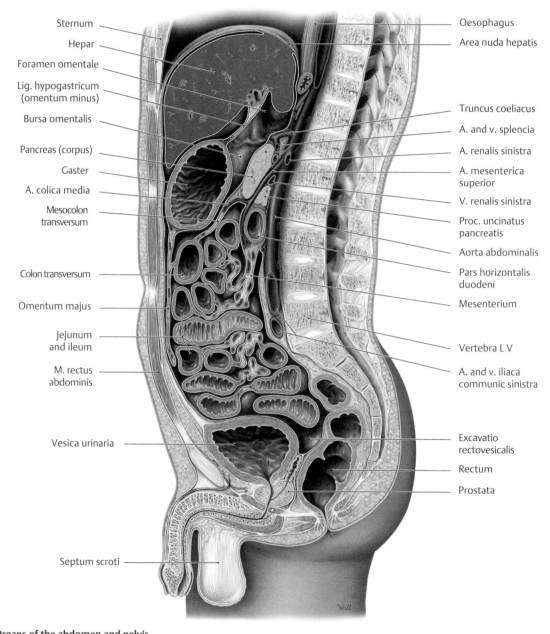

Fig. 12.1 Organs of the abdomen and pelvis
Midsagittal section through male pelvis, viewed from the left side. (From Schuenke M, Schulte E, Schumacher U. THIEME Atlas of Anatomy, Vol 2. Illustrations by Voll M and Wesker K. 3rd ed. New York: Thieme Publishers; 2020.)

- the **foregut (praeenteron)**, which consists of the distal oesophagus, the stomach, the proximal half of the duodenum, the liver, the gallbladder, and the superior part of the pancreas;
- the **midgut (mesenteron)**, which includes the distal half of the duodenum, the jejunum, ileum, caecum, and appendix vermiformis, and the ascending colon and proximal two thirds of the colon transversum; and
- the **hindgut (metenteron)**, which includes the distal third of the colon transversum, the colon descendens and colon sigmoideum the rectum, and the upper part of the canalis analis.

Stomach (Gaster)

The **stomach (gaster)**, a hollow reservoir that stores, churns, and initiates digestion of food, communicates with the oesophagus

---

BOX 12.1: DEVELOPMENTAL CORRELATION

ROTATION OF THE MIDGUT TUBE

Development of the mesenteron is characterized by rapid elongation of the gut and its mesenterium, resulting in the formation of the primary intestinal loop. The loop is attached anteriorly to the yolk sac by the ductus omphaloentericus (yolk stalk) and posteriorly to the posterior abdominal wall by the a. mesenterica superior. As a result of this rapid elongation and expansion of the liver, the cavitas abdominis becomes too small to contain all the intestinal loops, and they physiologically herniate into the proximal part of the funiculus umbilicalis. Coincident with growth in length, the primary intestinal loop rotates 270 degrees counterclockwise (if viewed from the front) around the axis established by the attachment of the a. mesenterica superior. Rotation occurs during herniation (approximately 90 degrees) and during the return of the intestinal loops into the cavitas abdominis (remaining 180 degrees), which is thought to occur when the relative size of the liver and kidney decreases. Malrotation of the midgut can result in congenital abnormalities such as volvulus (twisting) of the intestine.

BOX 12.2: DEVELOPMENTAL CORRELATION

LOCALIZATION OF PAIN FROM FOREGUT, MIDGUT, AND HINDGUT DERIVATIVES

Pain from gastrointestinal organs follows pathways determined by embryologic origin. Pain from foregut structures is localized to the spigastric region (regio epigastrica), pain from structures of the mesenteron localizes in the periumbilical region (regio umbilicalus), and pain arising from structures of the metenteron localizes in the hypogastric region (hypogastrium).

---

proximally and the duodenum of the small intestine distally (**Figs. 12.2, 12.3, 12.4**).

- It is normally J-shaped and lies in the left upper quadrant, although its shape and position vary among individuals and can change depending on its contents.
- The stomach has four parts:
    1. The **cardia**, which surrounds the opening to the oesophagus
    2. The **fundus gastricus**, the superior portion that rises above and to the left of the opening between the oesophagus and stomach (**ostium cardiacum**)
    3. The **corpus gastricum**, the large expanded portion below the fundus
    4. The **pars pylorica**, which is the outflow channel made up of the wide **antrum pyloricum**, a narrow **canalis pyloricus**, and the **pars pylorica** or sphincteric region, which contains an **m. sphincter pylori** that surrounds the ostium pyloricum into the first part of the duodenum.
- The stomach has a curvatura minor and a curvatura major.
    - The **curvatura minor** makes up the superior concave border. An **incisura angularis** (or incisure) along the curvature marks the junction of the corpus gastricum and pars pylorica.
    - The **curvatura major** makes up the inferior convex border.
- Although hollow organs of the gastrointestinal tract generally have walls composed of two muscular layers, the stomach is unique in having three layers: an outer longitudinal layer,

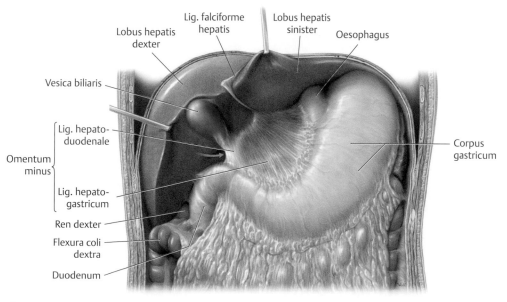

Fig 12.2 Gaster in situ
Anterior view of upper abdomen. The hepar has been reflected superiorly to expose the gaster and omentum minus. (From Gilroy AM et al. Atlas of Anatomy. 4th ed. 2020. Based on: Schuenke M, Schulte E, Schumacher U. THIEME Atlas of Anatomy. Internal Organs. Illustrations by Voll M and Wesker K. 3rd ed. New York: Thieme Medical Publishers; 2020.)

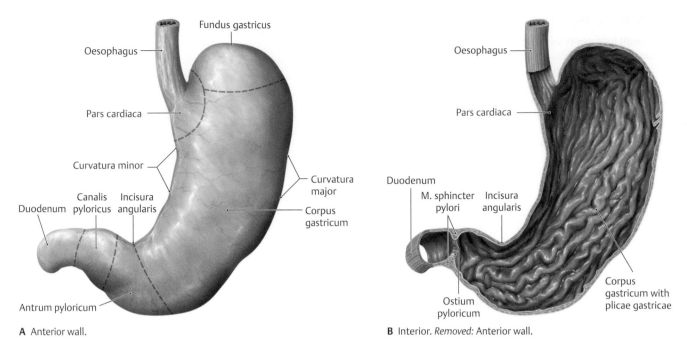

A Anterior wall.

B Interior. *Removed:* Anterior wall.

Fig. 12.3 Gaster
Anterior view. (From Schuenke M, Schulte E, Schumacher U. THIEME Atlas of Anatomy, Vol 2. Illustrations by Voll M and Wesker K. 3rd ed. New York: Thieme Publishers; 2020.)

a middle circular layer, and inner oblique layer. These enable the stomach to create powerful churning movements that break apart large food particles.

— The inner surface of the stomach is highly distensible; in adults, the stomach can accommodate 2 to 3 liters. **Rugae** (longitudinal folds, plicae gastricae) of the tunica mucosa, formed during contraction of the stomach, are most prominent in the pars pylorica and along the curvatura major. Gastric filling causes the mucosal folds to disappear.

— The layers of peritoneum on the stomach's anterior and posterior surfaces unite along the curvatura minor to form the omentum minus; along the curvatura major they unite to form the omentum majus (see **Figs. 12.1** and **12.2**).

— Anteriorly, the stomach is in contact with the abdominal wall, the diaphragma, and the left lobe of the liver. Posteriorly, it forms the anterior wall of the bursa omentalis.

— When the body is supine, the stomach rests on the pancreas, the spleen, the left kidney, the left gl. suprarenalis, and the colon transversum and its mesentery.

— A. gastrica dextra and a. gastrica sinistra, **a. gastroomentalis dextra** and **a. gastroomentalis sinistra**, and **aa. gastricae breves** (all derived from branches of the truncus coeliacus) supply the stomach (see **Figs. 11.12** and **11.14**).

— Veins that accompany the arteries of the stomach drain to the hepatic portal venous system.

— Lymph vessels drain to nll. gastrici and nll. gastroomentales, which drain to the nll. coeliaci.

— The plexus coeliacus innervates the stomach (see **Fig. 11.30**).

  • Sympathetic nerves promote vasoconstriction and inhibit peristalsis.

  • Parasympathetic nerves stimulate gastric secretion.

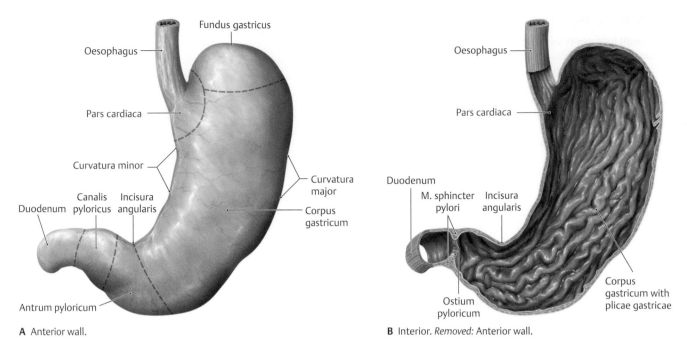

Fig. 12.4 Radiograph of double contrast barium enema of the stomach
Anterior view. (From Gunderman R. Essential Radiology, 3rd ed. New York: Thieme Publishers; 2014)

BOX 12. 3: CLINICAL CORRELATION

GASTRIC ULCERS
Gastric ulcers are open lesions of the tunica mucosa that are believed to be initiated by increased acid secretion and exacerbated by the presence of the bacterium *Helicobacter pylori*. Gastric ulcers can cause hemorrhaging if they erode into gastric arteries. Posteriorly located ulcers can erode into the pancreas and a. splenica, causing severe hemorrhaging. Patients with chronic ulcers may undergo a vagotomy, the surgical sectioning of the n. vagus, which may curtail the production of gastric acid.

Small Intestine (Intestinum Tenue)

The **small intestine (intestinum tenue)** extends from the ostium pyloricum of the stomach to the ostium ileale at the ileocecal junction and is the primary site of digestion and absorption of digested products. It is made up of three sections, the **duodenum**, which is mostly retroperitoneal, and the **jejunum** and **ileum,** which are suspended by the mesentery of the small intestine.

— The duodenum, the first and shortest section, forms a C-shaped curve around the head of the pancreas and has four parts (**Figs. 12.5, 12.6, 12.7**):

1. The **pars superior (first part)** is at the level of the vertebra L I.
   - The proximal 2-cm segment, called the **bulbus duodeni** or ampulla, is suspended from a mesenterium.
2. The **pars descendens (second part)** extends along the right side of the vertebral bodies L I–L III.
   - This is the site of the junction of the praeenteron and mesenteron.
   - The **hepatopancreatic duct**, formed by the ductus choledochus and ductus pancreaticus, enters the duodenum through the **papilla duodeni major** on the posteromedial wall. Superior to that, the **ductus pancreaticus accessorius** enters through the **papilla duodeni minor**.
3. The **pars horizontalis (third part)** crosses to the left, anterior to the v. cava inferior, the aorta, and vertebra L III, along the inferior border of the pancreas.
   - The root of the mesenterium of the small intestine (radix mesenterii) and superior mesenteric vessels cross anteriorly.

4. The **pars ascendens (fourth part)** ascends along the left side of the aorta to the level of the vertebra L II at the inferior border of the pancreas.
   - It joins the jejunum at the flexura duodenojejunalis, which is suspended from the posterior abdominal wall by the **lig. suspensorium duodeni** (ligament of Treitz)

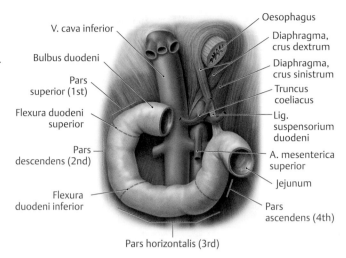

Fig. 12.5 Parts of the duodenum
Anterior view. (From Gilroy AM et al. Atlas of Anatomy. 4th ed. 2020. Based on: Schuenke M, Schulte E, Schumacher U. THIEME Atlas of Anatomy. Internal Organs. Illustrations by Voll M and Wesker K. 3rd ed. New York: Thieme Medical Publishers; 2020.)

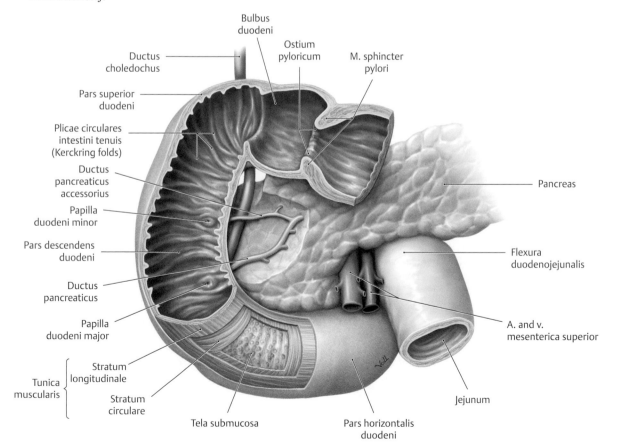

Fig. 12.6 Duodenum
Anterior view with the anterior wall opened. (From Schuenke M, Schulte E, Schumacher U. THIEME Atlas of Anatomy, Vol 2. Illustrations by Voll M and Wesker K. 3rd ed. New York: Thieme Publishers; 2020.)

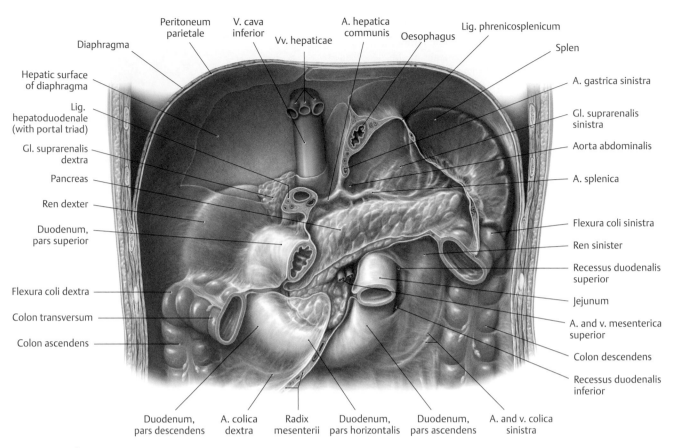

Fig. 12.7 Duodenum in situ
Anterior view. *Removed:* Gaster, hepar, small intestine, and large portion of the colon transversum. (From Schuenke M, Schulte E, Schumacher U. THIEME Atlas of Anatomy, Vol 2. Illustrations by Voll M and Wesker K. 3rd ed. New York: Thieme Publishers; 2020.)

BOX 12.4: CLINICAL CORRELATION

DUODENAL (PEPTIC) ULCERS
Duodenal ulcers usually occur within a few centimeters of the pylorus on its posterior wall. Perforation of the duodenum can lead to peritonitis and ulceration of adjacent organs. Severe hemorrhaging results if the ulcer erodes through the a. gastroduodenalis, which runs along the posterior side of the duodenum.

— The jejunum, the proximal two fifths of the intraperitoneal portion of the small intestine, is suspended by the mesenterium and is located predominantly in the left upper quadrant (**Figs. 12.8, 12.9, 12.10, 12.11**).
  • It is thicker walled and larger in diameter than the ileum.
  • Tall, closely packed **circular folds** (**plicae circulares**) line its inner surface, increasing its surface area for absorption.
  • Widely spaced arterial arcades within its mesenterium give rise to long, straight arteries, the **vasa recta** (see **Fig. 11.16**).
— The ileum, which makes up the distal three fifths of the intraperitoneal portion of the small intestine, is also suspended by the mesenterium of the small intestine. The ileum extends from the end of the jejunum to its junction with the cecum (**ileocecal junction**) and resides in the lower left quadrant and the greater pelvis (**Figs. 12.8, 12.9, 12.10, 12.11**).
  • It is longer in length than the jejunum.
  • Lymphoid nodules (**noduli lymphoidei aggregati, Peyer's patches**) bulge outward from the connective tissue layer underlying the epithelium (lamina propria).

• Circular folds (plicae circulares) are low and sparse.
• The ileum has more fat, denser arterial arcades, and shorter vasa recta in its mesentery than the jejunum.
— The blood supply, lymphatic drainage, and innervation of the parts of the small intestine reflect their development from the embryonic praeenteron and mesenteron (see Section 11.2).
  • The section that extends from the m. sphincter pylori to below the papilla duodeni major (praeenteron) is supplied by the **aa. pancreaticoduodenales superiores** from the **a. gastroduodenalis** (supplied through the truncus coeliacus).
  • The mesenteron (distal part of the pars descendens duodeni, the jejunum, and the ileum) is supplied by the **aa. pancreaticoduodenales inferiores, aa. jejunales**, and **aa. ileales**, branches of the a. mesenterica superior.
  • Veins of similar names accompany the arteries and terminate in the hepatic portal system.
  • Lymph vessels from the small intestine follow the course of the arteries and drain into the nll. coeliaci and nll. mesenterici superiores.
  • The plexus coeliacus (to praeenteron) and plexus mesentericus superior (to mesenteron) innervate the small intestine.
    ○ Sympathetic innervation inhibits intestinal mobility, secretion, and vasodilation.
    ○ Parasympathetic innervation restores normal digestive activity following sympathetic stimulation.
    ○ Visceral sensory fibers transmit feelings of distension (often perceived as cramping), but the intestine is insensitive to most pain stimuli.

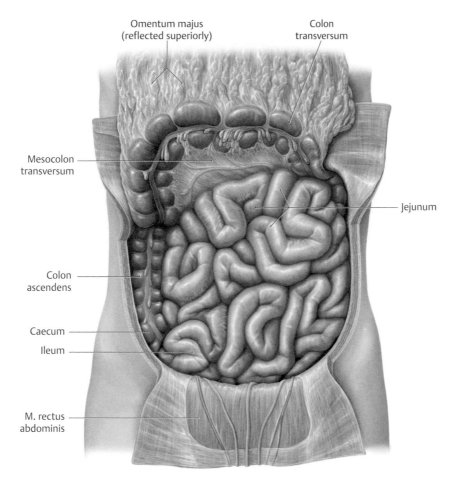

Fig. 12.8 Jejunum and ileum in situ
Anterior view. *Reflected:* Colon transversum and omentum majus. (From Schuenke M, Schulte E, Schumacher U. THIEME Atlas of Anatomy, Vol 2. Illustrations by Voll M and Wesker K. 3rd ed. New York: Thieme Publishers; 2020.)

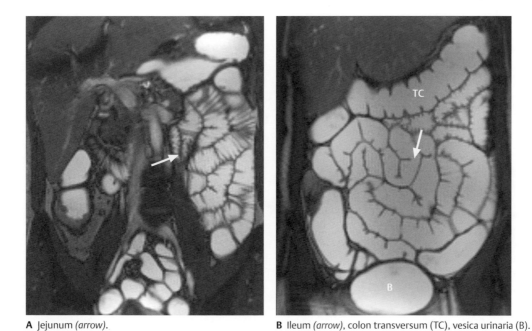

A Jejunum *(arrow)*.

B Ileum *(arrow)*, colon transversum (TC), vesica urinaria (B).

Fig. 12.9 MRI of the small intestine
Coronal view. Sectional imaging modalities like CT and MR have mostly replaced conventional radiographs in the evaluation of gastrointestinal disease.
(From Krombach GA, Mahnken AH. Body Imaging: Thorax and Abdomen. New York: Thieme Publishers; 2015.)

Fig. 12.10 Mesentery of the small intestine
Anterior view. *Removed:* Gaster, jejunum, and ileum. *Reflected:* Hepar. (From Schuenke M, Schulte E, Schumacher U. THIEME Atlas of Anatomy, Vol 2. Illustrations by Voll M and Wesker K. 3rd ed. New York: Thieme Publishers; 2020.)

Duodenum, pars superior

Gaster, pars pylorica

Omentum majus

Colon transversum

Duodenum, pars horizontalis

Mesenterium (cut edge)

Colon ascendens

Pars terminalis ilei

Splen

Pancreas

Mesocolon transversum (radix)

Flexura duodenojejunalis

Colon descendens

Mesocolon sigmoideum (cut edge)

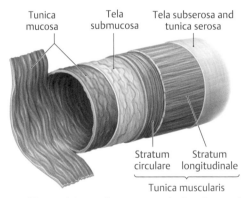

Tunica mucosa

Tela submucosa

Tela subserosa and tunica serosa

Stratum circulare

Stratum longitudinale

Tunica muscularis

A Wall layers of the small intestine are displayed in a "telescoped" cross section and the tunica mucosa has been incised longitudinally and opened.

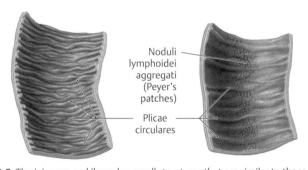

Noduli lymphoidei aggregati (Peyer's patches)

Plicae circulares

B,C The jejunum and ileum have wall structures that are similar to those of other hollow organs of the gastrointestinal tract, but local differences can be seen in the plicae circulares.

Fig. 12.11 Wall structure of the small intestine
(From Schuenke M, Schulte E, Schumacher U. THIEME Atlas of Anatomy, Vol 2. Illustrations by Voll M and Wesker K. 3rd ed. New York: Thieme Publishers; 2020.)

BOX 12.5: DEVELOPMENTAL CORRELATION

ILEAL DIVERTICULUM
Ileal diverticulum (also known as Meckel's diverticulum), the most common congenital abnormality of the bowel, is an outpouching of the ileum that is a remnant of the omphalomesenteric duct (yolk stalk) that fails to resorb. The diverticulum may be unattached distally or connect to the umbilicus via a fibrous cord or fistula. They are present in ~ 2% of the population, are located ~ 2 feet proximal to the ileocecal junction, and often contain two or more types of mucosa. The diverticulum can contain gastric, pancreatic, jejunal, or colonic tissue. An ileal diverticulum is usually asymptomatic but when inflamed may mimic acute appendicitis.

Ventral body wall

Meckel's diverticulum

Umbilicus

Ileum

Obliterated vitelline duct

(From Schuenke M, Schulte E, Schumacher U. THIEME Atlas of Anatomy, Vol 2. Illustrations by Voll M and Wesker K. 3rd ed. New York: Thieme Publishers; 2020.)

Large Intestine (Intestinum Crassum)

The **large intestine (intestinum crassum)** extends from the caecum to the canalis analis **(Figs. 12.12, 12.13, 12.14)**. It converts liquid feces to a semisolid state through the absorption of water, electrolytes, and salts. It also stores and lubricates fecal matter. Although it consists of five parts, only the **caecum, appendix vermiformis**, and **colon** reside in the abdomen. The **rectum** and **canalis analis** are described in Chapter 15, Pelvic Viscera.

— The caecum is a blind pouch located in the right lower quadrant.
- • It is attached proximally in an end-to-side fashion to the pars terminalis ilei and is continuous distally with the colon ascendens.
- • It lacks a mesenterium but is surrounded by peritoneum and therefore is fairly mobile.

— The appendix vermiformis is a blind muscular diverticulum (outpouching) that opens into the posteromedial wall of the caecum below the **ostium ileale**.
- • Its walls contain large masses of lymphoid tissue (nodi lymphoidei aggregati appendicis vermiformis).
- • Its mesoappendix (mesenterium) suspends it from the ileum.
- • Its position is highly variable, but it is often retrocecal (posterior to the caecum).

— The colon has four parts that frame the abdominal viscera:
1. The **colon ascendens** ascends from the caecum in the right lower quadrant to the **right colic flexure** (hepatic flexure, **flexura coli dextra**) under the liver.
2. The **colon transversum** crosses the abdomen from the flexura coli dextra to the left upper quadrant, where it terminates at the **left colic flexure** (splenic flexure, **flexura coli sinistra**).
3. The **colon descendens** descends along the left side of the abdomen to the left lower quadrant.
4. The **colon sigmoideum** crosses the fossa iliaca to join the rectum in the pelvis.

— The appendix vermiformis, colon transversum, and colon sigmoideum are intraperitoneal. Each is suspended by its respective **mesocolon** (mesenterium). The flexura coli sinistra is attached to the diaphragma by the **lig. phrenicocolicum**.

— The colon ascendens and colon descendens are secondarily retroperitoneal and therefore lack mesenteries.

— External features of the colon distinguish it from the small intestine:
- • **Taeniae coli**, three longitudinal bands (taenia mesocolica, taenia omentalis, and taenia libera), formed by the outer muscular layer,
- • **Haustra**, outpouchings of the intestinal wall visible between the taeniae coli,

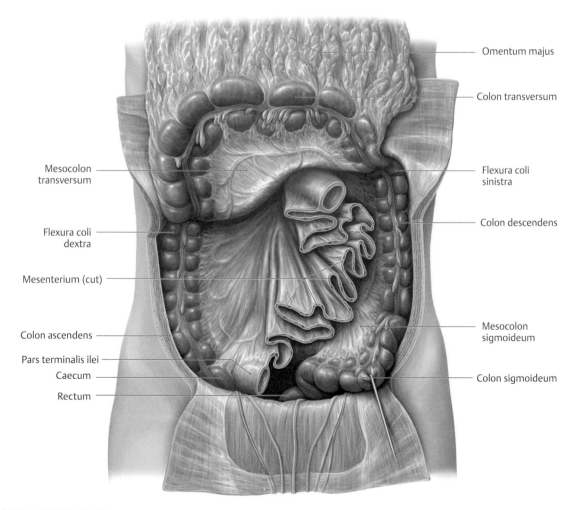

Fig 12.12 Large intestine in situ
Anterior view. *Reflected:* Colon transversum and omentum majus. *Removed:* Intraperitoneal small intestine. (From Schuenke M, Schulte E, Schumacher U. THIEME Atlas of Anatomy, Vol 2. Illustrations by Voll M and Wesker K. 3rd ed. New York: Thieme Publishers; 2020.)

Fig. 12.13 Large intestine
Anterior view. (From Gilroy AM
et al. Atlas of Anatomy. 4th ed.
2020. Based on: Schuenke M,
Schulte E, Schumacher U. THIEME
Atlas of Anatomy. Internal Organs.
Illustrations by Voll M and Wesker
K. 3rd ed. New York: Thieme
Medical Publishers; 2020.)

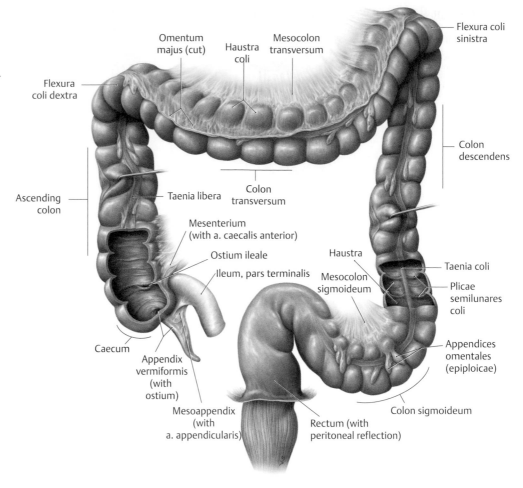

Fig. 12.14 Radiograph of double contrast barium enema of the large intestine
Anterior view. (From Moeller TB, Reif E. Pocket Atlas of Sectional Anatomy, Vol 2, 3rd ed. New
York: Thieme; 2007.)

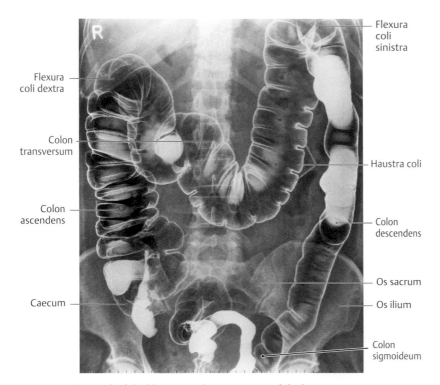

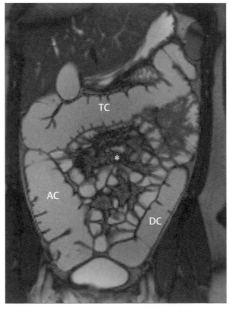

Fig. 12.15 MRI of the large intestine
Colon ascendens (AC), colon descendens (DC),
colon transversum (TC), * small intestine and
mesenteric structures. (From Gilroy AM et al. Atlas
of Anatomy. 4th ed. 2020. Based on: Schuenke M,
Schulte E, Schumacher U. THIEME Atlas of
Anatomy. Internal Organs. Illustrations by Voll M
and Wesker K. 3rd ed. New York: Thieme Medical
Publishers; 2020.)

- **Appendices omentales (epiploicae)**, small sacs of fat aligned along the taeniae.
- The blood supply, lymphatic drainage, and innervation of the parts of the large intestine reflect their development from the embryonic mesenteron and metenteron (see Section 11.2).
  - The a. ileocolica, a. colica dextra, and a. colica media from the a. mesenterica superior supply the caecum, colon ascendens, and proximal two thirds of the colon transversum (mesenteron).
  - The a. colica sinistra and aa. sigmoideae from the a. mesenterica inferior supply the distal third of the colon transversum, and the colon descendens and colon sigmoideum (metenteron). The a. rectalis superior supplies the upper rectum in the pelvis.
  - The a. marginalis coli runs along the mesenteric border of the large intestine, anastomosing branches of the a. mesenterica superior with those of the a. mesenterica inferior. In turn, the a. rectalis superior anastomoses with a. rectalis media and a. rectalis inferior in the pelvis.
  - Veins of the colon follow the arteries and drain into the hepatic portal system.

- Lymph vessels follow arterial pathways to drain into nll. mesenterici superiores or nll. mesenterici inferiores.
- The plexus mesentericus superior (mesenteron) and plexus mesentericus inferior (metenteron) innervate the large intestine.

BOX 12.6: CLINICAL CORRELATION

INFLAMMATORY BOWEL DISEASE

There are two types of inflammatory bowel disease (IBD): Crohn's disease and ulcerative colitis. Crohn's disease is a chronic inflammatory disease that can affect the entire gastrointestinal (GI) tract but most commonly affects the terminal ileum and colon. It causes ulcers, fistulas (abnormal communications), and granulomata, producing symptoms such as fever, diarrhea, weight loss, and abdominal pain. Ulcerative colitis is a recurrent inflammatory disease of the colon and rectum that produces bloody diarrhea, weight loss, fever, and abdominal pain. These diseases are treated with drugs that reduce the inflammatory response.

BOX 12.7: CLINICAL CORRELATION

APPENDICITIS AND VARIABLE POSITION OF THE APPENDIX VERMIFORMIS

Anomalies in the rotation of the embryonic gut can result in several positional variations of the caecum and appendix vermiformis. This can influence the accurate interpretation of symptoms of appendicitis. Inflammation of an appendix in the typical position is felt initially as vague pain in the periumbilical region, transmitted via visceral fibers from the T10 spinal cord segment. As the inflammation irritates the overlying peritoneum parietale, tenderness can be elicited by pressure at two points:

McBurney point: located one third of the distance along a line from the spina iliaca anterior superior to the umbilicus.

Lanz point: located one third of the distance along a line from the spina iliaca anterior superior dextra to the similar landmark on the left side.

If the position of the appendix is atypical, tenderness may be felt at other abdominal sites, thus complicating the diagnosis.

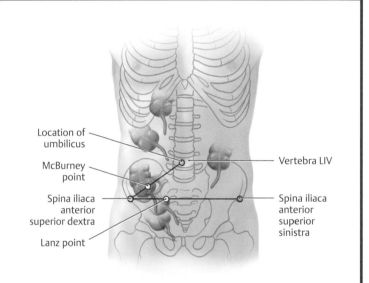

(From Schuenke M, Schulte E, Schumacher U. THIEME Atlas of Anatomy, Vol 2. Illustrations by Voll M and Wesker K. 3rd ed. New York: Thieme Publishers; 2020.)

BOX 12.8: CLINICAL CORRELATION

COLON CARCINOMA

Malignant tumors of the colon and rectum are among the most frequent solid tumors. More than 90% occur in patients over the age of 50. In early stages, the tumor may be asymptomatic; later symptoms include loss of appetite, changes in bowel movements, and weight loss. Blood in the stools is particularly incriminating, necessitating a thorough examination. Hemorrhoids are not a sufficient explanation for blood in stools unless all other tests (including a colonoscopy) are negative.

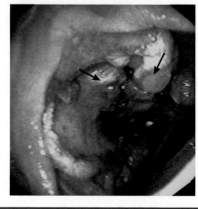

Colonoscopy of colon carcinoma. The tumor *(black arrows)* partially blocks the lumen of the colon. (From Gilroy AM et al. Atlas of Anatomy. 4th ed. 2020. Based on: Schuenke M, Schulte E, Schumacher U. THIEME Atlas of Anatomy. Internal Organs. Illustrations by Voll M and Wesker K. 3rd ed. New York: Thieme Medical Publishers; 2020.)

12.2   Organs of the Peritoneal Cavity— Accessory Organs of the Gastrointestinal Tract

Liver (Hepar)

The **liver (hepar)** is located in the right upper quadrant under the right hemidiaphragm and extends inferiorly to the arcus costalis **(Fig. 12.16)**. It has a primary role in carbohydrate, protein, and fat metabolism. It also produces and secretes bile and bile pigments; detoxifies substances absorbed by the gastrointestinal tract; and stores vitamins and minerals, such as iron. In the fetus, the liver is the site of hematopoiesis (red blood cell production).

— Externally, ligaments and fissures divide the liver into four anatomic (topographic) lobes: the **lobus hepatis dexter, lobus hepatis sinister, lobus caudatus**, and **lobus quadratus (Fig. 12.17)**.

— The liver's diaphragmatic surface conforms to the shape of the diaphragma and is marked by the **area nuda**, which lacks peritoneum and is in direct contact with the diaphragma.

— The liver's visceral (inferior) surface has three prominent fissures:

1. The left sagittal fissure or umbilical fissure (fissura umbilicalis) accommodates
   ◦ the **lig. teres hepatis** anteriorly between the lobus hepatis sinister and lobus quadratus. The lig. teres hepatis is a remnant of the fetal v. umbilicalis.
   ◦ the **ligamentum venosum** posteriorly between the lobus hepatis sinister and lobus caudatus. The lig. venosum is a remnant of the fetal ductus venosus.
2. The right sagittal fissure or main portal fissure (fissura portalis principalis) accommodates
   ◦ the gallbladder anteriorly between the lubus hepatis dexter and lobus quadratus and
   ◦ the v. cava inferior posteriorly between the lobus hepatis dexter and lobus caudatus.

3. The transverse fissure or right portal fissure (fissura portalis dextra) accommodates
   ◦ the **porta hepatis**, or hilum of the liver. Structures of the **portal triad** (a. hepatica propria, v. portae hepatis, and **ductus choledochus**) enter or exit here.

— The liver is intraperitoneal, covered by peritoneum except at the area nuda, fossa vesicae biliaris, and porta hepatis. Peritoneal reflections include
   • **lig. coronarium hepatis** and **ligg. triangulares**, single-layered reflections between the liver and diaphragm that surround the area nuda;
   • the lig. falciforme, a double layer of peritoneum, which attaches the liver to the anterior abdominal wall and contains the lig. teres hepatis in its free edge; and
   • the lig. hepatogastricum and lig. hepatoduodenale (both parts of the omentum minus), which attach the liver to the stomach and proximal duodenum.

— A subperitoneal fibrous capsule, **Glisson's capsule**, covers the surface of the liver.

— Internally, branching of the intrahepatic blood vessels divides the liver into eight functional segments (designated as I through VIII) **(Fig. 12.18, Table 12.1)**. This segmental arrangement of the blood supply facilitates the resection of individual diseased segments.

— The liver has a dual blood supply: the v. portae hepatis and the proper a. hepatica propria (see Section 11.2). Both vessels divide to form primary and secondary branches that supply the liver segments.
   • The v. portae hepatis, carrying nutrient-rich blood from the digestive tract, provides 75 to 80% of the blood volume to the liver.
   • The a. hepatica propria, supplied by the truncus coeliacus via the a. hepatica communis, contributes 20 to 25% of the blood volume to the liver.

— V. hepatica dextra, v. hepatica sinistra, and v. hepatica intermedia run intersegmentally, draining adjacent segments, and open into the v. cava inferior immediately below the diaphragma.

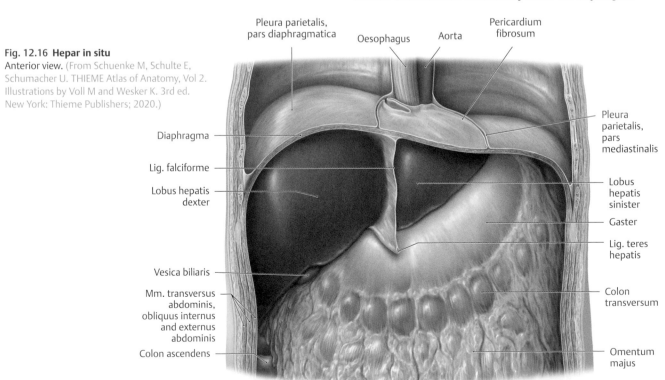

Fig. 12.16 Hepar in situ
Anterior view. (From Schuenke M, Schulte E, Schumacher U. THIEME Atlas of Anatomy, Vol 2. Illustrations by Voll M and Wesker K. 3rd ed. New York: Thieme Publishers; 2020.)

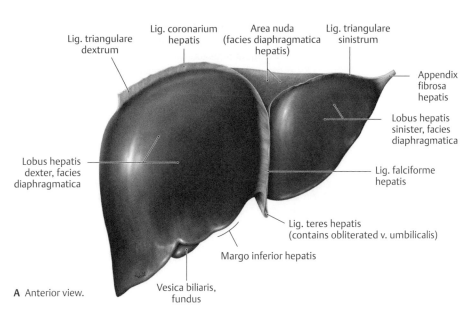

A Anterior view.

Lig. triangulare dextrum

Lig. coronarium hepatis

Area nuda (facies diaphragmatica hepatis)

Lig. triangulare sinistrum

Appendix fibrosa hepatis

Lobus hepatis sinister, facies diaphragmatica

Lig. falciforme hepatis

Lobus hepatis dexter, facies diaphragmatica

Lig. teres hepatis (contains obliterated v. umbilicalis)

Margo inferior hepatis

Vesica biliaris, fundus

Fig. 12.17 Surfaces of the hepar
The hepar is divided by its ligaments into four lobes: right, left, caudate, and quadrate. (From Schuenke M, Schulte E, Schumacher U. THIEME Atlas of Anatomy, Vol 2. Illustrations by Voll M and Wesker K. 3rd ed. New York: Thieme Publishers; 2020.)

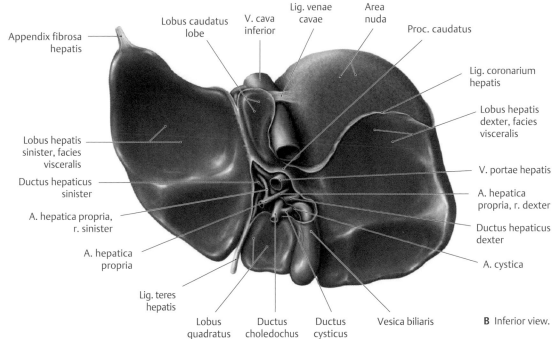

B Inferior view.

Appendix fibrosa hepatis

Lobus caudatus lobe

V. cava inferior

Lig. venae cavae

Area nuda

Proc. caudatus

Lig. coronarium hepatis

Lobus hepatis dexter, facies visceralis

Lobus hepatis sinister, facies visceralis

Ductus hepaticus sinister

A. hepatica propria, r. sinister

A. hepatica propria

V. portae hepatis

A. hepatica propria, r. dexter

Ductus hepaticus dexter

A. cystica

Lig. teres hepatis

Lobus quadratus

Ductus choledochus

Ductus cysticus

Vesica biliaris

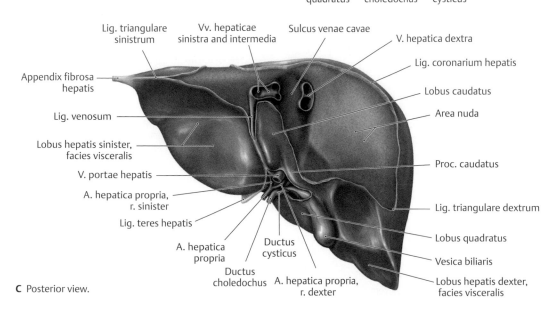

C Posterior view.

Lig. triangulare sinistrum

Vv. hepaticae sinistra and intermedia

Sulcus venae cavae

V. hepatica dextra

Lig. coronarium hepatis

Lobus caudatus

Area nuda

Proc. caudatus

Lig. triangulare dextrum

Lobus quadratus

Vesica biliaris

Lobus hepatis dexter, facies visceralis

Appendix fibrosa hepatis

Lig. venosum

Lobus hepatis sinister, facies visceralis

V. portae hepatis

A. hepatica propria, r. sinister

Lig. teres hepatis

A. hepatica propria

Ductus cysticus

Ductus choledochus

A. hepatica propria, r. dexter

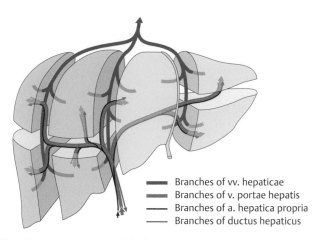

Branches of vv. hepaticae
Branches of v. portae hepatis
Branches of a. hepatica propria
Branches of ductus hepaticus

Fig. 12.18 Segmentation of the hepar
Anterior view. Branches of the a. hepatica, v. portae hepatis, and ductus hepaticus communis divide the hepar into segments. (From Schuenke M, Schulte E, Schumacher U. THIEME Atlas of Anatomy, Vol 2. Illustrations by Voll M and Wesker K. 2nd ed. New York: Thieme Publishers; 2016.)

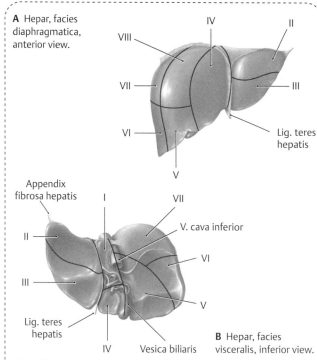

A Hepar, facies diaphragmatica, anterior view.

Lig. teres hepatis

Appendix fibrosa hepatis
V. cava inferior
Lig. teres hepatis
Vesica biliaris
B Hepar, facies visceralis, inferior view.

(From Schuenke M, Schulte E, Schumacher U. THIEME Atlas of Anatomy, Vol 2. Illustrations by Voll M and Wesker K. 3rd ed. New York: Thieme Publishers; 2020.)

Table 12.1 Hepatic Segments

Part	Division	Segment	
Pars hepatis sinistra	Pars posterior	I	Lobus caudatus
	Left lateral division	II	Posterius laterale sinistrum
		III	Anterius laterale sinistrum
	Left medial division	IV	Mediale sinistrum
Pars hepatis dextra	Right medial division	V	Anterius mediale dextrum
		VI	Anterius laterale dextrum
	Right lateral division	VII	Posterius laterale dextrum
		VIII	Posterius mediale dextrum

— The liver has superficial and deep lymphatic drainages.
  • The superficial lymphatic plexus, found within the capsula fibrosa, drains the anterior liver surfaces to nll. hepatici (and eventually into the nll. coeliaci) and drains the posterior surfaces toward the area nuda, which flow into nll. phrenici or nll. mediastinales posteriores.
  • The deep plexus, which accompanies vessels within the liver segments, drains most of the liver, flowing first into nll. hepatici in the porta hepatis and omentum minus, before draining to the nll. coeliaci.

BOX 12.9: CLINICAL CORRELATION

CIRRHOSIS OF THE LIVER
Cirrhosis, most commonly caused by chronic alcoholism, is characterized by a progressive fibrosis of hepatic tissue around the intrahepatic vessels and biliary ducts that impedes blood flow. The liver becomes hard and nodular in appearance. Symptoms include ascites, splenomegaly, peripheral edema, oesophageal varices, and other signs of portal hypertension.

— The plexus hepaticus, a division of the plexus coeliacus, travels along the vessels of the portal triad to innervate the liver.

Gallbladder and Extrahepatic Biliary System

The **gallbladder (vesica biliaris)** is a pear-shaped sac that lies in a fossa on the visceral surface of the liver (**Figs. 12.17** and **12.19**). It stores the bile produced and secreted by the liver and concentrates it by absorbing salts and water. Hormonal or neural stimulation causes the vesica biliaris to release bile into the **extrahepatic bile ducts** (**Fig. 12.20**).
— The vesica biliaris has four parts (**Fig. 12.21**):
  1. The **fundus vesicae biliaris**, the expanded distal end that is in contact with the anterior abdominal wall
  2. The **body (corpus vesicae biliaris)**, the main portion
  3. The **infundibulum vesicae biliaris** between the corpus vesicae biliaris and collum vesicae biliaris
  4. The **neck (collum vesicae biliaris)**, the narrow distal segment that joins with the ductus cysticus
— The extrahepatic biliary system of ducts transports bile from the liver and vesica biliaris to the duodenum. It consists of
  • the **ductus hepaticus communis** formed by the junction of the ductus hepaticus dexter and ductus hepaticus sinister, which drain the liver;
  • the **ductus cysticus**, which drains the vesica biliaris and communicates with the ductus hepaticus communis from the liver (a **spiral valve**, **plica spiralis**, in the collum vesicae biliaris keeps the ductus cysticus open); and
  • the **ductus choledochus**, formed by the junction of the ductus hepaticus communis and ductus cysticus, which drains bile into the second part of the duodenum.
— The ductus choledochus passes posterior to the first part of the duodenum and posterior to, or through, the head of the pancreas. It ends at the **ampulla hepatopancreatica** (of Vater), a dilation of the distal end of the duct, where it joins with the **ductus pancreaticus** of the pancreas.
— A muscular **sphincter** (of Oddi, sphincter ampullae) surrounds the ampulla hepatopancreatica as it traverses the medial wall of the duodenum through the papilla duodeni major and opens into the pars descendens (**Fig. 12.22**).
— The **a. cystica**, usually a branch of the a. hepatica dextra, supplies the vesica biliaris.

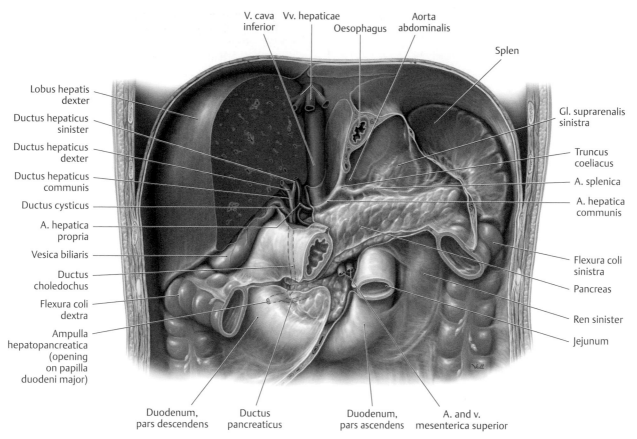

Fig. 12.19 Biliary tract in situ
Anterior view. *Removed:* Gaster, small intestine, colon transversum, and large portions of the hepar. The vesica biliaris is intraperitoneal, covered by peritoneum viscerale where it is not attached to the hepar. (From Gilroy AM et al. Atlas of Anatomy. 4th ed. 2020. Based on: Schuenke M, Schulte E, Schumacher U. THIEME Atlas of Anatomy. Internal Organs. Illustrations by Voll M and Wesker K. 3rd ed. New York: Thieme Medical Publishers; 2020.)

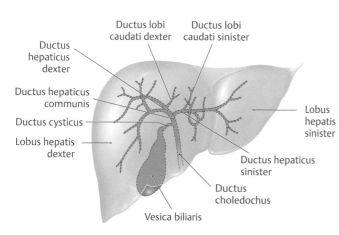

Fig 12.20 Hepatic bile ducts
Projection onto the surface of the hepar, anterior view. (From Schuenke M, Schulte E, Schumacher U. THIEME Atlas of Anatomy, Vol 2. Illustrations by Voll M and Wesker K. 3rd ed. New York: Thieme Publishers; 2020.)

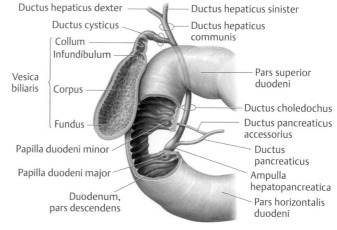

Fig. 9.21 Extrahepatic bile ducts and vesica biliaris
Anterior view. *Opened:* Vesica biliaris and duodenum. (From Schuenke M, Schulte E, Schumacher U. THIEME Atlas of Anatomy, Vol 2. Illustrations by Voll M and Wesker K. 3rd ed. New York: Thieme Publishers; 2020.)

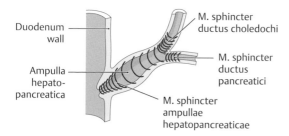

Fig. 12.22 Biliary sphincter system
Sphincters of the ductus pancreaticus and ductus choledochus. (From Schuenke M, Schulte E, Schumacher U. THIEME Atlas of Anatomy, Vol 2. Illustrations by Voll M and Wesker K. 3rd ed. New York: Thieme Publishers; 2020.)

BOX 12.10: CLINICAL CORRELATION

GALLSTONES

Gallstones are concretions of cholesterol crystals that lodge within the biliary tree. They occur most commonly in women over the age of 40. Gallstones can remain asymptomatic, but when they obstruct the ampulla hepatopancreatica, they impede the flow of bile and pancreatic secretions, which may cause bile to enter the pancreas, leading to pancreatitis. Gallstones that obstruct the ductus cysticus lead to biliary colic, characterized by severe waves of pain, cholecystitis, and jaundice. Stones that accumulate in the fundus of a diseased vesica biliaris (also known as Hartmann's pouch) may ulcerate through the wall of the fundus into the colon transversum. These can pass naturally via the rectum, or they may pass into the small intestine where they can obstruct the ostium ileale, producing an intestinal obstruction (gallstone ileus). Pain arising from gallstones originates in the epigastrium or right hypochondrium, but may also be referred to the posterior thoracic wall or right shoulder due to irritation of the diaphragma.

BOX 12.11: CLINICAL CORRELATION

CHOLECYSTECTOMY AND THE CYSTOHEPATIC TRIANGLE (OF CALOT)

Ninety-five percent of injuries to extrahepatic bile ducts are sustained intraoperatively, most commonly during removal of the vesica biliaris (cholecystectomy), which includes transection of the a. cystica and ductus cysticus. The cystohepatic triangle serves as a guide for accurate identification of these structures, whose anatomy can be highly variable. The borders of this space are the ductus cysticus inferiorly, the ductus hepaticus communis medially, and the visceral surface of the liver superiorly.

BOX 12.12: CLINICAL CORRELATION

IMPLICATIONS OF THE SHARED EMPTYING OF THE DUCTUS CHOLEDOCHUS AND DUCTUS PANCREATICUS

The ductus choledochus and ductus pancreaticus both empty into the papilla major duodeni. This has important clinical implications (e.g., a tumor at the caput pancreatis may obstruct the ductus choledochus, causing biliary reflux into the liver and jaundice). Similarly, a gallstone that lodges in the ductus choledochus may obstruct the terminal part of the ductus pancreaticus, causing acute pancreatitis.

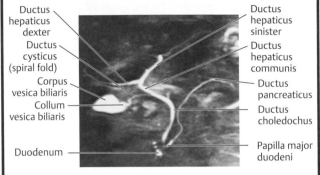

MR cholangiopancreatography
(From Moeller TB, Reif E. Pocket Atlas of Sectional Anatomy, Vol 2, 3rd ed. New York: Thieme Publishers; 2007.)

- Sympathetic stimulation inhibits bile secretion.
- Parasympathetic stimulation causes the vesica biliaris to contract and release bile.

Pancreas

The **pancreas** is a lobulated gland that has dual functions. As an exocrine gland it synthesizes digestive enzymes, and as an endocrine gland it produces and secretes the hormones insulin and glucagon (**Figs. 12.19, 12.23, 12.24, 12.25**).

— Venous blood from the vesica biliaris drains into vv. hepaticae in the liver, which drain into the v. cava inferior.
— The plexus nervosus hepaticus innervates the gallbladder.

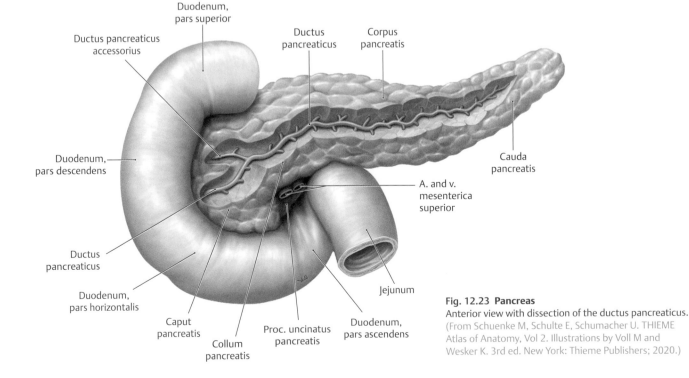

Fig. 12.23 Pancreas
Anterior view with dissection of the ductus pancreaticus.
(From Schuenke M, Schulte E, Schumacher U. THIEME Atlas of Anatomy, Vol 2. Illustrations by Voll M and Wesker K. 3rd ed. New York: Thieme Publishers; 2020.)

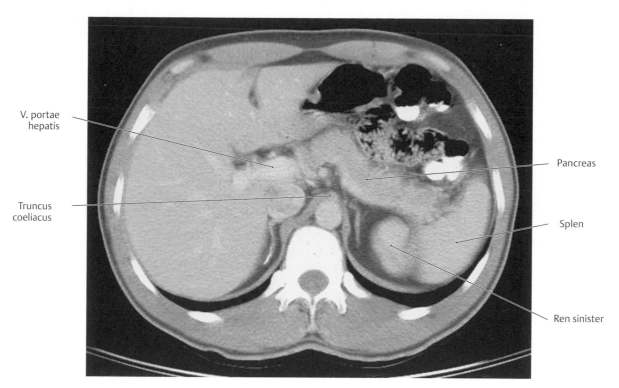

Fig 12.24 CT of the abdomen at the vertebra L I level
(From Moeller TB, Reif E. Pocket Atlas of Sectional Anatomy, Vol 2, 3rd ed. New York: Thieme Publishers; 2007.)

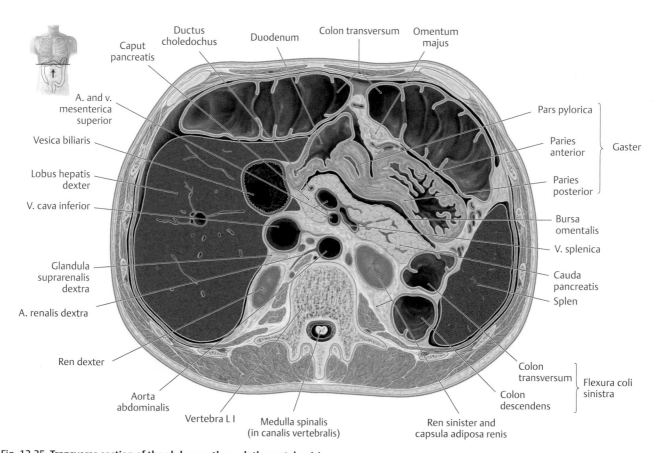

Fig. 12.25 Transverse section of the abdomen through the vertebra L I
Inferior view. (From Schuenke M, Schulte E, Schumacher U. THIEME Atlas of Anatomy, Vol 2. Illustrations by Voll M and Wesker K. 3rd ed. New York: Thieme Publishers; 2020.)

— It is secondarily retroperitoneal and lies on the posterior wall of the bursa omentalis.
— It crosses the midline with its head within the "C" of the duodenum and its tail touching the hilum splenicum.
— The four parts of the pancreas are the **head** (caput pancreatis) and **uncinate process** (proc. uncinatus pancreatis), the **neck** (collum pancreatis), the **body** (corpus pancreatis), and the **tail** (cauda pancreatis).
— The **ductus pancreaticus** (of Wirsung) traverses the length of the gland to join with the ductus choledochus at the ampulla hepatopancreatica. Together they drain into the pars descendens of the duodenum at the **papilla duodeni major** (see **Figs. 12.21** and **12.22**).
— When present, a **ductus pancreaticus accessorius** (of Santorini) may drain to the pars descendens of the duodenum at the **papilla duodeni minor**, 2 cm proximal to the drainage site of the ductus pancreaticus.
— Because of its central location in the upper abdomen, the pancreas is related topographically to many of the major abdominal vascular structures (see **Fig. 11.23**):
  • The caput pancreatis lies anterior to the a. renalis dextra and v. renalis dextra, v. renalis sinistra, and v. cava inferior.
  • The collum pancreatis and corpus pancreatis cross anterior to the aorta abdominalis, a. mesenterica superior and v. mesenterica superior, and v. portae hepatis. The truncus coeliacus arises from the aorta immediately superior to this.
  • The cauda pancreatis crosses anterior to the ren sinister and extends to the hilum splenicum. The a. splenica runs along its superior border, and the v. splenica courses behind it.
— Branches of the truncus coeliacus and a. mesenterica superior supply the pancreas (see Section 11.2).

  • Rr. pancreaticoduodenales of the a. gastroduodenalis (from the truncus coeliacus) and a. mesenterica superior supply the caput pancreatis.
  • Branches of the a. splenica supply the collum pancreatis, corpus pancreatis, and cauda pancreatis.
— Venous blood drains into the v. splenica and v. mesenterica superior, which merge to form the hepatic portal system.
— Lymphatic drainage is as varied as its blood supply but generally follows arterial pathways, ultimately draining into nll. coeliaci and nll. mesenterici superior.
— The plexus coeliacus and plexus mesentericus superior innervate the pancreas.

Spleen (Splen)

The **spleen (splen)** is an intraperitoneal organ located in the hypochondriac region of the left upper quadrant (**Figs. 12.25,**

12.26, 12.27). It functions as a lymphoid gland and as a filter for old or abnormal red blood cells.
— Nestled under the dome of the diaphragma, the spleen does not normally project below the arcus costalis and therefore is not palpable on examination.
— The convex surface admits the splenic vessels and nerves at the **hilum splenicum**.
— The spleen is connected to adjacent organs by peritoneal ligaments.
  • The **lig. splenorenale**, which contains the branches of the splenic vessels and the cauda pancreatis, connects the spleen to the kidney.
  • The **lig. gastrosplenicum**, which contains the short gastric and left gastroomental vessels, connects the spleen to the stomach.
  • The **lig. splenocolicum** connects the spleen to the flexura coli sinistra.
  • The **lig. phrenicosplenicum** connects the spleen to the diaphragma.
— Although it is sheltered by the 9th, 10th, and 11th ribs, the spleen is particularly vulnerable to lacerations from fractured ribs, and because of its dense vascularity, it bleeds profusely.
— Accessory spleens are common (20%) and are most often found within the lig. gastrosplenicum, near the hilum splenicum or cauda pancreatis.
— The a. splenica, a large tortuous branch of the truncus coeliacus, divides within the lig. splenorenale at the hilum splenicum (see Section 11.2).
— The spleen is vulnerable to infarction (interruption of the blood supply causing tissue death) because the a. splenica has no collateral arteries and is the gland's sole blood supply.
— The v. splenica courses behind the pancreas, where it joins with the v. mesenterica superior to form the v. portae hepatis.
— The plexus splenicus, a derivative of the plexus coeliacus, innervates the spleen.

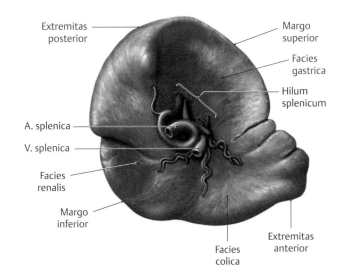

Fig. 12.26 Splen
Visceral surface. (From Schuenke M, Schulte E, Schumacher U. THIEME Atlas of Anatomy, Vol 2. Illustrations by Voll M and Wesker K. 3rd ed. New York: Thieme Publishers; 2020.)

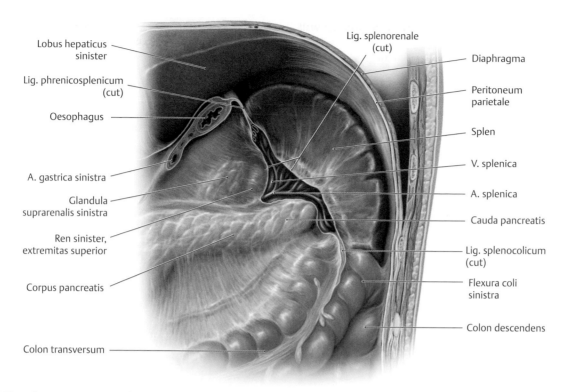

Fig. 12.27 The splen in situ: peritoneal relationships
Anterior view into the left upper quadrant (LUQ) with the gaster removed. (From Schuenke M, Schulte E, Schumacher U. THIEME Atlas of Anatomy, Vol 2. Illustrations by Voll M and Wesker K. 3rd ed. New York: Thieme Publishers; 2020.)

BOX 12.14: CLINICAL CORRELATION

SPLENIC TRAUMA AND SPLENECTOMY

Although the spleen appears to be well protected by the lower ribs on the posterior wall, it is the most frequently injured abdominal organ. It is particularly vulnerable to rupture from left-sided trauma that fractures the lower ribs. An enlarged spleen (splenomegaly) that projects below the costal margin may be vulnerable during blunt abdominal trauma that can rupture the thin splenic capsule. Splenic rupture results in severe hemorrhage and may require a total or partial splenectomy. During a total splenectomy the cauda pancreatis is vulnerable to injury where it passes through the splenorenal ligament with the splenic vessels.

BOX 12.15: DEVELOPMENTAL CORRELATION

ACCESSORY SPLEENS

Accessory spleens are small nodules of splenic tissue, usually ~ 1 cm in diameter, that form separately from the main spleen. They are usually located at the hilum splenicum (commonly) near the cauda pancreatis, in the lig. gastrosplenicum or lig. splenorenale, in the mesenterium, or near the ovarium or testis.

12.3 Organs of the Retroperitoneum

Kidneys (Renes)

The **kidneys (renes)** are generally smooth-sided, reddish brown organs ~ 11 cm in length. They are retroperitoneal and lie anterior to the mm. quadratus lumborum on each side of the columna vertebralis between T XII and L III (**Figs. 12.28** and **12.29**). The kidneys regulate blood pressure and the ionic balance and water con-

tent of the blood; they also eliminate metabolic waste and produce urine.

— The right kidney
  • lies anterior to the costa XII, slightly lower than the left, because of the presence of the large lobus dexter hepatis.
  • lies posterior to the right gl. suprarenalis, liver, pars descendens duodeni, and flexura dextra coli of the large intestine.

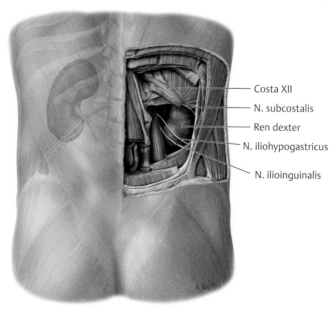

Fig. 12.28 Renes in situ
Posterior view with the trunk wall opened. (From Schuenke M, Schulte E, Schumacher U. THIEME Atlas of Anatomy, Vol 2. Illustrations by Voll M and Wesker K. 3rd ed. New York: Thieme Publishers; 2020.)

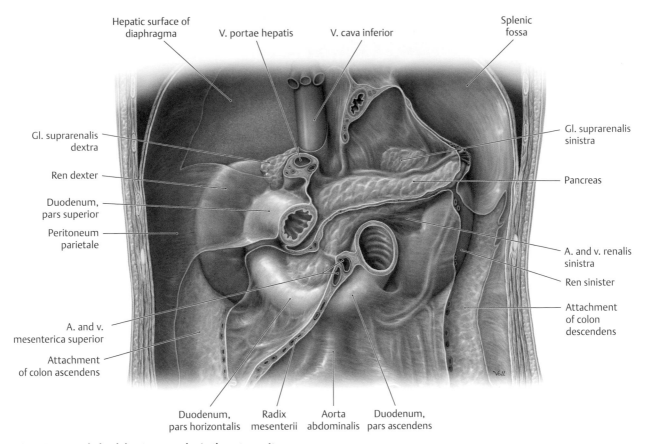

Fig. 12.29 Renes and glandulae suprarenales in the retroperitoneum
Anterior view. Both the renes and glandulae suprarenales are retroperitoneal. *Removed:* Intraperitoneal organs, along with portions of the colon ascendens and colon descendens. (From Schuenke M, Schulte E, Schumacher U. THIEME Atlas of Anatomy, Vol 2. Illustrations by Voll M and Wesker K. 3rd ed. New York: Thieme Publishers; 2020.)

— The left kidney
  • lies anterior to costae XI and XII;
  • lies posterior to the gl. suprarenalis sinistra, spleen, cauda pancreatis, and flexura coli sinistra.
— A **fascia renalis** surrounds each kidney and its associated gl. suprarenalis, renal vessels, ureter, and capsula adiposa renis (**Fig. 12.30**). Pararenal fat (corpus adiposum pararenale) lies outside this space and is thickest posteriorly.

— Deep to the fascia renalis, a thin **capsula fibrosa renis** completely invests each kidney (**Fig. 12.31A**).
— The lateral edge of the kidney (margo lateralis renis) is smooth and concave; the medial border (margo medialis renis) has a vertical hilum that is pierced by the v. renalis, a. renalis, and pelvis renalis. The hilum expands within the kidney as the **sinus renalis**.

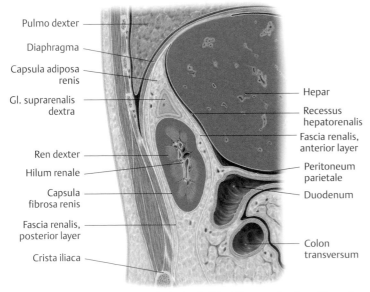

A Sagittal section at approximately the level of the hilum renale, viewed from the right side.

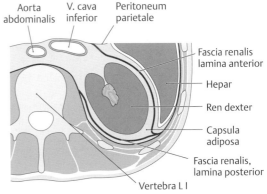

B Transverse section through the abdomen at approximately the L I/L II level, viewed from above.

Fig. 12.30 Ren dexter in the renal bed
(From Gilroy AM et al. Atlas of Anatomy. 4th ed. 2020. Based on: Schuenke M, Schulte E, Schumacher U. THIEME Atlas of Anatomy. Internal Organs. Illustrations by Voll M and Wesker K. 3rd ed. New York: Thieme Medical Publishers; 2020.)

— Internally, the kidney consists of cortical and medullary regions that contain up to 2 million nephrons, the renal functional units **(Fig. 12.30)**.
  • The cortex renalis, the outer region, lies deep to the capsula fibrosa renis and extends into the medullary region as **renal columns (columnae renales)**.
  • The medulla renalis, the inner region, is arranged in **renal pyramids (pyramides renales)** with the broad base facing outward and the apex fitting into a cup-shaped **calix renalis minor**.
  • Up to 11 minor calyces merge to form two or three **calices renales major**, which combine to form the **pelvis renalis**. At the hilum renale the pelvis renalis narrows to form the ureter.
— A single a. renalis, a direct branch of the aorta abdominalis at L II, normally supplies each kidney **(Figs. 12.31** and **12.32)**.
  • The a. renalis dextra is longer than the a. renalis sinistra and passes posterior to the v. cava inferior.
  • The artery divides near the hilum to supply anterior and posterior segments of the kidney, which are separated by an avascular longitudinal plane (Brodel's white line).

— A single v. renalis from each kidney drains to the v. cava inferior (**Figs. 12.31** and **12.32**).
  • Both vv. renales receive a tributary from the ureter, but only the v. renalis sinistra receives the v. suprarenalis sinistra and v. testicularis sinistra or v. ovarica sinistra. On the right these veins drain directly into the v. cava inferior.
  • The v. renalis sinistra is longer than the v. renalis dextra and passes anterior to the aorta immediately inferior to the origin of the a. mesenterica superior.
  • The longer length of the v. renalis sinistra makes the left kidney the preferred choice for organ donation.
— The plexus renalis, an extension of the plexus coeliacus, forms a dense periarterial plexus along the aa. renales (see Section 11.2).
  • Pain from renal disease is referred along the T12–L2 dermatomes to the lumbar and inguinal regions and the upper part of the anterior thigh.

BOX 12.16: CLINICAL CORRELATION

RENAL VEIN ENTRAPMENT
The v. renalis sinistra crosses the midline in the narrow angle between the downwardly directed a. mesenterica superior and the aorta abdominalis. Pathologic conditions (atherosclerosis, aneurysms) of the arteries or downward pressure on the a. mesenterica superior can compress the v. renalis. This is sometimes called the nutcracker syndrome.

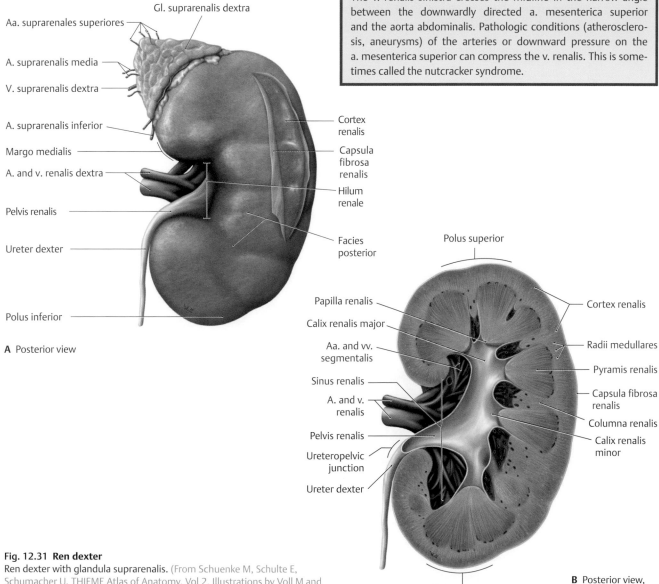

Fig. 12.31 Ren dexter
Ren dexter with glandula suprarenalis. (From Schuenke M, Schulte E, Schumacher U. THIEME Atlas of Anatomy, Vol 2. Illustrations by Voll M and Wesker K. 3rd ed. New York: Thieme Publishers; 2020.)

A Posterior view

B Posterior view, midsagittal section

BOX 12.17: DEVELOPMENTAL CORRELATION

COMMON RENAL ANOMALIES

Variations in renal vessels are common and usually asymptomatic. Kidneys develop in the pelvis and ascend to their location in the lumbar region between the 6th and 9th fetal weeks. As they ascend, more superior renal arteries and veins replace the inferior renal vessels. In ~ 30% of the population, failure of these inferior vessels to degenerate results in multiple renal arteries and veins.

In some cases, one kidney may fail to ascend (a), resulting in a pelvic kidney. In other cases, the inferior poles of the kidneys may fuse to form a single U-shaped structure (b), although they remain functionally separate. These "horseshoe kidneys" (ren unguliformis) get trapped in their ascent under the a. mesenterica inferior and remain at the L III or L IV level.

Gll. suprarenales

Ren pelvicus, dexter

Ren unguliformis

a   b

(From Schuenke M, Schulte E, Schumacher U. THIEME Atlas of Anatomy, Vol 2. Illustrations by Voll M and Wesker K. 3rd ed. New York: Thieme Publishers; 2020.)

Ureters (Ureteres)

The **ureters (ureteres)** are muscular tubes, 25 to 30 cm in length, that convey urine from the kidneys to the vesica urinaria through peristaltic (wavelike) action (**Figs. 12.32** and **12.33**). Both the pars abdominalis and the pars pelvica ureteris are retroperito-

neal along their entire course. The pelvic ureter is discussed further in Chapter 15, Pelvic Viscera.

— Near the hilum renale, the pelvis renalis narrows to join with the origin of the ureter at the **ureteropelvic junction (Fig. 12.31)**.

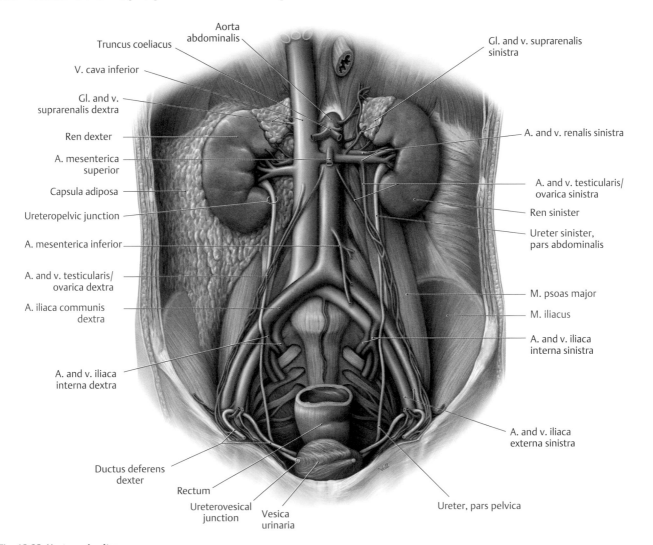

Fig. 12.32 Ureteres in situ
Retroperitoneum of male abdomen, anterior view. *Removed:* Nonurinary organs and rectal stump. (From Schuenke M, Schulte E, Schumacher U. THIEME Atlas of Anatomy, Vol 2. Illustrations by Voll M and Wesker K. 3rd ed. New York: Thieme Publishers; 2020.)

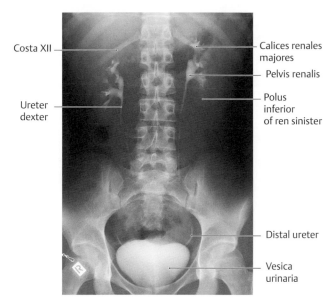

Fig. 12.33 **Radiograph of intravenous pyelogram**
Anterior view. (From Moeller TB, Reif E. Pocket Atlas of Sectional Anatomy, Vol 2, 3rd ed. New York: Thieme Publishers; 2007.)

Labels (img_2): Costa XII — Calices renales majores — Pelvis renalis — Ureter dexter — Polus inferior of ren sinister — Distal ureter — Vesica urinaria

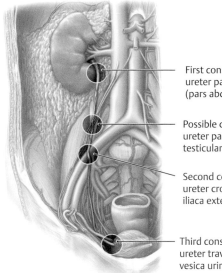

Fig.12.34 **Anatomic constrictions of the ureter**
Right side, anterior view. (From Schuenke M, Schulte E, Schumacher U. THIEME Atlas of Anatomy, Vol 2. Illustrations by Voll M and Wesker K. 3rd ed. New York: Thieme Publishers; 2020.)

Labels (img_1): First constriction: ureter passes over polus inferior (pars abdominalis) — Possible constriction where ureter passes behind a. and v. testicularia/ovarica — Second constriction: ureter crosses over a. and v. iliaca externa (pars pelvica) — Third constriction: ureter traverses the wall of vesica urinaria (pars intramuralis)

— The pars abdominalis of the ureter descends along the anterior surface of the m. psoas where it is crossed by the gonadal vessels.

— The ureter crosses over the pelvic brim to enter the pelvis at the bifurcation of the a. iliaca communis into the a. iliaca interna and a. iliaca externa.

— The pars pelvica of the ureter travels anteriorly along the lateral pelvic wall before it enters the vesica urinaria at the **ureterovesical junction**.

— Constrictions of the ureter, caused by ureteral narrowing or compression by adjacent structures, can occur near its origin and along its length (**Fig. 12.34**).

— Branches from several arteries form a delicate anastomosis along the length of the ureter (see Section 11.2).

   • In the abdomen, this network of vessels usually includes contributions from the aorta abdominalis and the a. renalis, a. testiculars/ovarica, and a. iliaca communis.

   • Branches of the aa. vesicales superiores, a. vesicalis inferior, and a. uterina supply the pelvic ureter.

— The veins of the ureter accompany the arteries.

— Contributions from the plexus renalis, plexus aorticus abdominalis, and plexus hypogastricus superior innervate the pars abdominalis ureteris. The plexus hypogastricus inferior innervates the pars pelvica ureteris (see Section 10.6).

— Pain from the ureter is relayed along sympathetic routes to spinal cord segments T11–L2 and is referred to the corresponding dermatomes of the lower abdominal wall, inguinal region, and medial aspects of the thigh.

BOX 12.18: CLINICAL CORRELATION

CALCULI OF THE KIDNEY AND URETER
Calculi (stones) formed in the urine can become lodged in the calices renales, pelvis renalis, or ureter. Calculi lodged in the ureters distend the ureteric walls and cause intense intermittent pain as peristaltic contractions move the calculi inferiorly. As the calculi move toward the pelvis, pain moves from the lumbar to inguinal regions (T11–L2 dermatomes) and may extend into the scrotum and anterior thigh with branches of the n. genitofemoralis.

Suprarenal Glands (Gll. Suprarenales)

The paired **suprarenal glands** (adrenal glands, gll. suprarenales) are located in the spatium retroperitoneale, where they cap the superior pole of each kidney and lie anterior to the crura diaphragma. The gll. suprarenales are neuroendocrine glands that respond to stress.

— Capsula adiposa renis and fascia renalis surround both glands; a septum of the fascia separates them from the kidney.

— The gl. suprarenalis dextra is pyramidal, and the left is crescent shaped (**Figs. 12.35** and **12.36**).

— The glands are composed of an outer cortex and an inner medulla. Both parts act as endocrine glands (i.e., secrete hormones) but differ from each other developmentally and functionally.

— The **cortex glandulae suprarenalis**
   • is derived from mesoderm;
   • is stimulated by hormones such as adrenocorticotropic hormone (ACTH); and
   • secretes hormones (corticosteroids and androgens), which influence blood pressure and blood volume by regulating sodium and water retention in the kidneys.

— The **medulla glandulae suprarenalis**
   • is primarily composed of nervous tissue that is derived from neural crest cells (embryonic cells that migrate from the developing neural tube and give rise to a variety of structures associated with the peripheral nervous system);
   • is stimulated by preganglionic sympathetic fibers from the plexus coeliacus; and
   • contains **chromaffin cells** that function like sympathetic ganglia and secrete hormones (catecholamines) that increase heart rate, blood pressure, blood flow, and respiration.

— Veins and lymphatic vessels exit at the hilum glandulae suprarenalis on the anterior surface, but arteries and nerves access the glands at multiple points.

— Each gl. suprarenalis has multiple aa. suprarenales superiores, a. suprarenalis media, and a. suprarenalis inferior, which

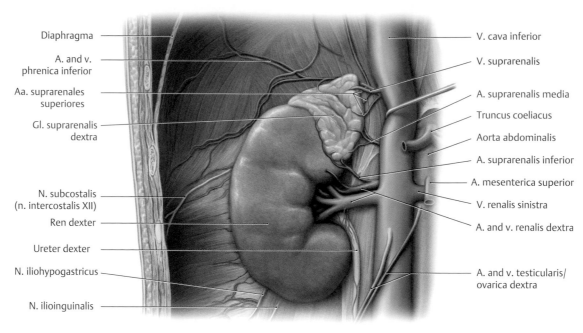

Fig. 12.35 Ren dexter and glandula suprarenalis
Anterior view. *Removed:* Capsula adiposa. *Retracted:* Vena cava inferior. (From Schuenke M, Schulte E, Schumacher U. THIEME Atlas of Anatomy, Vol 2. Illustrations by Voll M and Wesker K. 3rd ed. New York: Thieme Publishers; 2020.)

branch from the a. phrenica inferior, aorta abdominalis, and a. renalis, respectively.

— A single v. suprarenalis drains each gland. The v. suprarenalis dextra drains to the v. cava inferior; the v. suprarenalis sinistra may join with v. phrenica inferior before draining to the v. renalis sinistra.

— Preganglionic sympathetic fibers of the n. splanchnicus major combine with fibers of the plexus coeliacus to form the plexus suprarenalis, but they do not synapse on the ganglia coeliaca. These preganglionic fibers, which may be considered homologous with postganglionic sympathetic neurons, terminate directly on the chromaffin cells of the medulla.

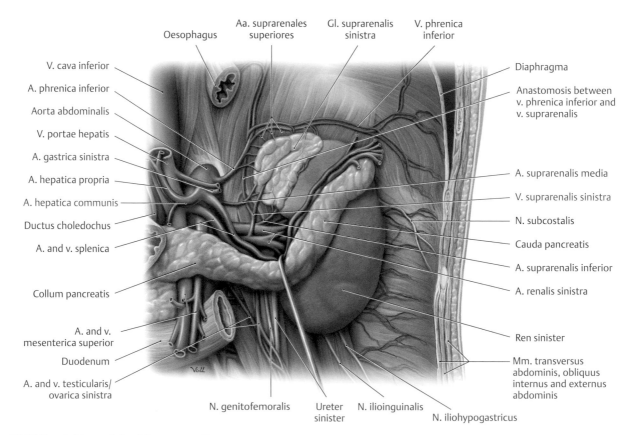

Fig. 12.36 Ren sinister and glandula suprarenalis
Anterior view. *Removed:* Capsula adiposa. *Retracted:* Pancreas. (From Schuenke M, Schulte E, Schumacher U. THIEME Atlas of Anatomy, Vol 2. Illustrations by Voll M and Wesker K. 3rd ed. New York: Thieme Publishers; 2020.)

13 Clinical Imaging Basics of the Abdomen

In patients with acute abdominal pain, radiographs are a quick and inexpensive first imaging step that give an overview of the bowel gas pattern and can identify abdominal emergencies such as a bowel obstruction or a perforated bowel. However, x-rays usually lack the specificity to identify specific pathology.

Computed tomography (CT) on the other hand shows anatomic detail of all of the internal organs and can usually provide a diagnosis of most intra-abdominal pathology. The speed and overall ease of obtaining CT scans make it ideal for emergent conditions. Magnetic resonance imaging (MRI) also shows high detail within the abdomen but is usually reserved for non-emergent situations due to long scanning time. When an abnormality of the biliary system or urinary tract is considered, ultrasound is often the best imaging test. Lack of radiation, easy access and overall low cost of ultrasound make it suitable for both emergent and non-emergent evaluation (**Table 13.1**). In pediatrics, ultrasound offers additional utility as a first-line imaging tool in the evaluation of children with abdominal pain, specifically for evaluation of the appendix (**Fig. 13.1**).

Standard radiographic (x-rays) views of the abdomen include frontal (anteroposterior, AP) views in supine and upright positions (**Fig. 13.2**). Changes in position should redistribute bowel gas in a normal patient. When evaluating abdominal radiographs, a systematic approach is important and should include

- evaluating the pattern of gas distribution in the bowel,
- gross estimation of organ size and location, assessment for abnormal calcifications (only the bones should be calcified, i.e., white), and
- assessment for abnormal air (outside of the bowel).

An abnormal bowel gas pattern can be a sign of a serious underlying condition, and the ability to recognize such patterns is an important skill to develop. All students should become familiar with both normal and abnormal patterns as a speedy diagnosis can be critical (**Figs. 13.2** and **13.3**). Details of abdominal structures can be enhanced by the use of barium (ingested by the patient), used in fluoroscopic studies (**Fig. 13.4**), and by oral or intravenous contrast used for abdominal CT scans (**Fig. 13.5**). In MRI studies, intra-abdominal fat can act as a natural "contrast agent" by outlining the organs (**Fig. 13.6**). Ultrasound often utilizes adjacent structures to better see specific target organs (**Fig. 13.7**).

Table 13.1 Suitability of Imaging Modalities for the Abdomen

Modality	Clinical Uses
Radiographs	
• X-ray	Abdominal x-ray ("KUB": kidneys, ureters, and bladder) is often the first choice in patients with acute abdominal pain to assess for bowel obstruction and/or bowel perforation. Radiography is readily available and a radiograph can be obtained very quickly. Although many patients will require more advanced imaging and/or other testing, the abdominal radiograph can provide crucial information and lead to therapeutic decisions.
• Fluoroscopy	"Real-time" radiography: x-rays viewed dynamically on a computer screen as the image is obtained; most often used to image the gastrointestinal (GI) tract with the aid of intraluminal contrast material (usually barium). The advent of direct visualization with endoscopy has minimized the use of this modality.
CT (computed tomography)	Provides cross-sectional anatomic detail not possible with plain radiographs. Most accurate imaging for evaluation of solid organs, ducts, and blood vessels.
MRI (magnetic resonance imaging)	Very useful for evaluating solid organs and is becoming increasingly more useful for evaluation of the bowel. The drawback of MRI is the long exam time and expense.
Ultrasound	Usually first line of imaging for evaluation of the biliary system and the kidneys.

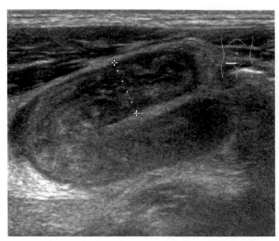 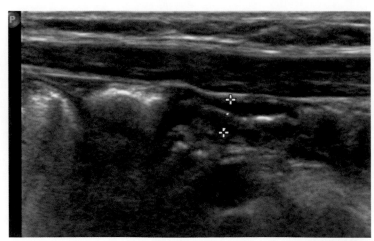

A Normal appendix for comparison. (Courtesy of Joseph Makris, MD, Baystate Medical Center.)

B Acute appendicitis. The tubular blind ending structure is a thickened/inflamed appendix. (Courtesy of Joseph Makris, MD, Baystate Health Care.)

Fig. 13.1 Abdominal ultrasound
Focused ultrasound of the right lower quadrant of the abdomen in children with abdominal pain.

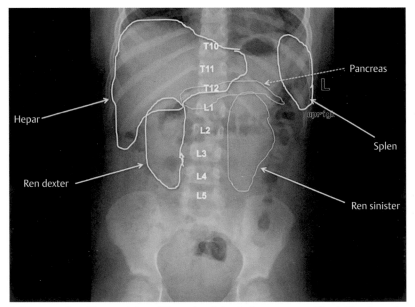 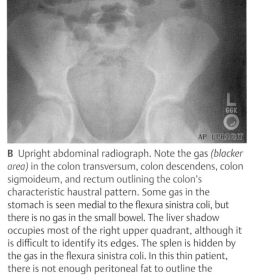

A The normal positions and sizes of the major abdominal organs are outlined. (Courtesy of Joseph Makris, MD, Baystate Medical Center.)

Fig. 13.2 Abdominal radiographs
Anterior view.

B Upright abdominal radiograph. Note the gas *(blacker area)* in the colon transversum, colon descendens, colon sigmoideum, and rectum outlining the colon's characteristic haustral pattern. Some gas in the stomach is seen medial to the flexura sinistra coli, but there is no gas in the small bowel. The liver shadow occupies most of the right upper quadrant, although it is difficult to identify its edges. The splen is hidden by the gas in the flexura sinistra coli. In this thin patient, there is not enough peritoneal fat to outline the kidneys. (Courtesy of Joseph Makris, MD, Baystate Medical Center.)

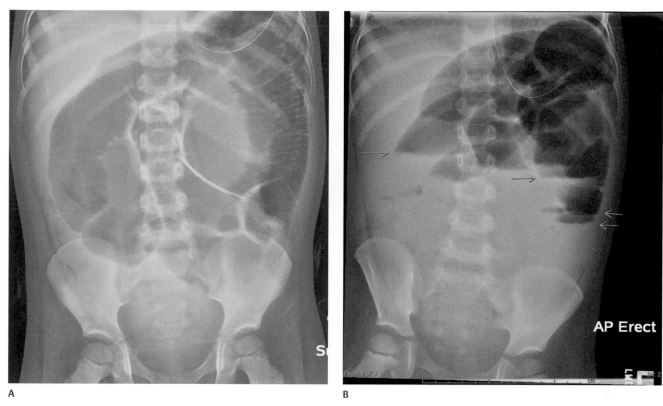

A

B

Fig. 13.3 Bowel obstruction in a young child
Supine (**A**) and upright (**B**) radiographs show several loops of gas-filled and dilated bowel. Notice that the abnormal bowel loops form C shapes and appear to be stacked upon each other. Also, note the straight horizontal lines that form in the upright position at the inferior aspect of the gas-filled bowel (*arrows*). These are air-fluid levels. (Courtesy of Joseph Makris, MD, Baystate Medical Center.)

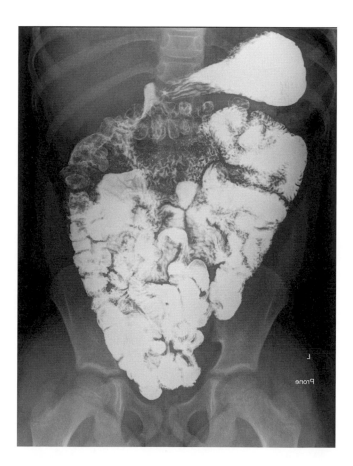

Fig. 13.4 Abdominal radiograph with barium
Anterior view.
The barium has progressed through the bowel, coating its walls, to the level of the colon ascendens. Note that the loops of the small intestine in the left upper quadrant (jejunum) have many more folds per length of bowel than does the bowel in the lower abdomen (ileum). This beautifully illustrates the physiologic and anatomic properties relating to absorption of nutrients in the proximal and distal small intestine (form follows function). (Courtesy of Joseph Makris, MD, Baystate Medical Center.)

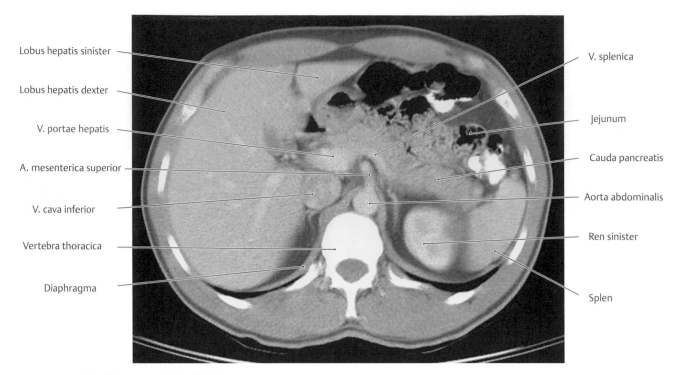

Fig. 13.5 CT of the abdomen at the level of the upper renes
Inferior view.
Oral contrast is used to highlight the bowel *(bright white)*; intravenous contrast is used to enhance the appearance of vessels and organs. This image demonstrates the cortical phase of enhancement; the cortex renis is whiter than the remainder of the kidneys. The full capability of CT is realized when scrolling through a full set of axial images on a computer screen and cross-referencing the axial images with the full data set of sagittal and coronal reformatted images. (From Moeller TB, Reif E. Pocket Atlas of Sectional Anatomy, Vol 2, 3rd ed. New York: Thieme Publishers; 2007.)

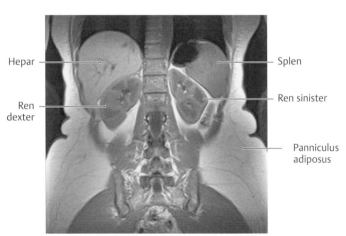

Fig. 13.6 MRI of the abdomen
Coronal section.
In this image fat is *bright,* air is *black,* and the soft tissues are shades of *gray*. Fluid is *darker gray*. Note the architecture of the normal kidney, with darker pyramides (darker because fluid content is greater there than in the cortex). The kidneys are surrounded by retroperitoneal fat. (From Moeller T, et al. Pocket Atlas of Sectional Anatomy, Vol. II: Thorax, Abdomen, Heart, and Pelvis, 3rd ed. Stuttgart: Thieme; 2007.)

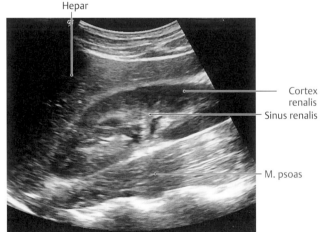

Fig. 13.7 Ultrasound of the right kidney
Sagittal section.
The probe is positioned on the anterior abdominal wall and the liver is used as a "window" to view the kidney. The echogenic *(whiter)* sinus renalis is easily seen within the cortex renalis. (From Block B. Color Atlas of Ultrasound Anatomy, 2nd ed. New York: Thieme; 2012.)

Unit IV   Review Questions: Abdomen

1. An arteriogram performed on one of your patients revealed significant arterial disease (atherosclerosis) of the proximal 3 cm of the a. mesenterica superior, which narrowed the angle between the artery and the aorta. What structure normally crosses the aorta below the artery and is at risk of compression in this patient?
   A. V. renalis sinistra
   B. Second part of the duodenum
   C. Jejunum
   D. Colon transversum
   E. Pancreas

2. A 12-year-old girl is seen in the emergency department for the suspicion of appendicitis. However, her pain is vague, and she does not complain when you gently press on her abdominal wall in the lower right quadrant. You are undeterred in your diagnosis, however, because you know that pain from an inflamed appendix refers first to another area of the abdomen based on its embryonic origins. Which of the following is true regarding referred pain from the appendix?
   A. As part of the embryonic praeenteron, pain is referred to the epigastric region.
   B. As part of the embryonic mesenteron, pain is referred to the epigastric region.
   C. As part of the embryonic mesenteron, pain is referred to the periumbilical region.
   D. As part of the embryonic metenteron, pain is referred to the hypogastric region.
   E. As part of the embryonic metenteron, pain is referred to the periumbilical region.

3. A renal abscess can irritate the nerves of the posterior abdominal wall. This is often referred to the dermatome that runs just above the lig. inguinale from the crista iliaca to the os pubis. Which nerves transmit this irritation?
   A. N. cutaneus femoris lateralis
   B. N. ilioinguinalis and n. iliohypogastricus
   C. N. femoralis
   D. N. phrenicus inferior
   E. N. intercostalis T10

4. Which of the following is true regarding the a. renalis and v. renalis?
   A. The a. renalis dextra passes posterior to the v. cava inferior.
   B. Both vv. renales receive tributaries from the gll. suprarenales.
   C. The v. renalis sinistra is shorter than the v. renalis dextra.
   D. Aa. renales are the most anterior structure in the hilum renalis.
   E. Aa. renales arise from the aorta at the L IV vertebral level.

5. During a colectomy on a patient with colon cancer, you ask a medical student to describe characteristics of the colon descendens. Her correct answer would include that it

A. is supplied primarily by branches of the a. mesenterica superior
B. receives parasympathetic innervation by the n. vagus
C. is marked by three taeniae coli on its outer surface
D. is primarily retroperitoneal
E. is derived from the embryonic mesenteron

6. The m. obliquus externus abdominis and aponeurosis contribute to the formation of all except which of the following structures?
   A. Anulus umbilicalis
   B. Linea alba
   C. Tendo conjunctivus
   D. Lig. inguinale
   E. Anulus inguinalis superficialis

7. Which of the following is true regarding the relations of the pancreas?
   A. The a. splenica runs along its inferior border.
   B. The v. portae hepatis forms anterior to the neck and body.
   C. The neck crosses the midline slightly superior to the planum transpyloricum.
   D. The ductus pancreaticus accessorius drains inferiorly to the horizontal part of the duodenum.
   E. It lies on the posterior wall of the bursa omentalis.

8. The artery that supplies blood directly to the pyloric region of the stomach is the
   A. a. gastrica sinistra
   B. a. gastrica brevis
   C. a. gastrica dextra
   D. a. gastroomentalis sinistra
   E. a. pancreaticoduodenalis superior

9. Inferior to the linea arcuata, the posterior layer of the vagina musculi recti abdominis is composed of the
   A. aponeurosis of the m. obliquus externus abdominis
   B. aponeurosis of the m. obliquus internus abdominis
   C. aponeurosis of the m. transversus abdominis
   D. fascia transversalis
   E. All of the above

10. One of your elderly patients has lost significant weight and complains of abdominal pain following meals. You know that his a. mesenterica inferior was ligated several years ago as part of an aortic aneurysm repair, and imaging reveals that his a. mesenterica superior is now severely narrowed at its origin. As a result, anastomosing vessels between the truncus coeliacus and the a. mesenterica superior are enlarged. What vessels are involved in this anastomosis?
    A. A. marginalis
    B. Aa. pancreaticoduodenales
    C. A. gastroomentalis
    D. A. hepatica propria
    E. A. gastrica sinistra

11. A 46-year-old woman is admitted to the emergency department with acute abdominal pain due to peritonitis from a ruptured duodenal ulcer. Imaging reveals an abscess in one of the peritoneal recesses. Which of the following is the lowest space within the cavitas peritonealis where fluid accumulation and abscess formation are most likely to occur in a bedridden patient?
    A. Bursa omentalis
    B. Infracolic compartment
    C. Sulcus paracolicus sinister
    D. Recessus subphrenicus
    E. Recessus hepatorenalis

12. A young mother is determined to get into shape following the birth of her first child. She was humiliated in aerobics class when she could no longer do the required sit-ups. Strengthening which of the following muscles would help her accomplish this exercise?
    A. M. obliquus externus abdominis
    B. M. obliquus internus abdominis
    C. M. rectus abdominis
    D. M. psoas major
    E. All of the above

13. Your 45-year-old brother was taken to the emergency department for severe pain that radiated along his lower abdominal wall, inguinal region, and scrotum. Ultrasound revealed a large calculus lodged in his right ureter. From your understanding of ureteric anatomy, select the INCORRECT statement.
    A. The calculus is likely to be lodged in one of the ureter's normal anatomic constrictions, which include the ureterovesical and ureteropelvic junctions.
    B. Pain associated with the calculus is relayed to the medulla spinalis via sympathetic routes.
    C. Pain from the ureter is felt along the T11–L2 dermatomes.
    D. Ureters convey urine from the kidneys to the vesica urinaria through peristaltic action of their muscular walls.
    E. Rr. ureterici of the aa. renales are the primary blood supply to the pelvic ureter.

14. In patients who have conditions that affect the cavitas peritonealis, such as an inflammation due to a perforated gastric ulcer, the abdominal wall muscles, in a "defense" reflex, become rigid and can be encountered as such during physical examination. Which of the following nerves contribute sensory and motor branches to this defense mechanism?
    A. N. phrenicus
    B. N. vagus
    C. Nn. intercostales
    D. Nn. splanchnici lumbales
    E. N. splanchnicus major

15. A pediatric surgeon is performing an appendectomy on a 10-year-old child, but upon entering the abdomen he finds a healthy appendix. With further exploration he finds an inflamed finger of bowel originating from the ileum ~ 2 feet from the ostium ileale. It is connected to the umbilicus by a fibrous stalk. What embryonic structure failed to degenerate in this patient?
    A. Ductus venosus
    B. V. umbilicalis
    C. A. umbilicalis
    D. Ductus omphaloentericus
    E. Urachus

16. One of your patients suffers from multisystem disease as a result of his poor diet and long-term alcoholism. He exhibits many symptoms of chronic portal hypertension, but you suspect that some of his other symptoms have a different underlying cause. Which of the following symptoms are probably not associated with his portal hypertension?
    A. Oesophageal varices
    B. Enlarged spleen
    C. Rectal varices
    D. Renal calculi
    E. Ascites (fluid in the cavitas peritonealis)

17. A 6-month-old boy underwent surgery for an indirect inguinal hernia. The surgeon opened the superficial inguinal ring and located the hernia sac, which protruded through the abdominal wall
    A. below the lig. inguinale
    B. medial to the a. epigastrica inferior and v. epigastrica inferior
    C. within the trigonum inguinale
    D. at the anulus inguinalis profundus
    E. above the tendo conjunctivus

18. Which of the following is a characteristic of the gl. suprarenalis?
    A. It's a secondarily intraperitoneal organ.
    B. Its cortex is composed of nervous tissue derived from neural crest cells.
    C. It's supplied by a single a. suprarenalis, which arises from the a. renalis.
    D. Its medulla is innervated by preganglionic sympathetic neurons that synapse directly on the chromaffin cells of the medulla.
    E. It sits on the polus superior of each kidney but remains outside of the capsula adiposa and fascia renalis that encompass the kidney.

19. Your neighbor was recently diagnosed with liver cancer. His doctor explained that, because the primary tumor was in the area nuda, it metastasized quickly to the mediastinum posterius and nll. supraclaviculares. You recall that, although most lymph from the liver drains toward the nll. coeliaci and trunci lymphatici intestinales, the area nuda drains to trunci lymphatici bronchomediastinales in the thorax. What is the area nuda?
    A. An area on the facies diaphragmatica bounded by lig. coronarium hepatis and lig. triangulare
    B. The area of liver that lines the fossa vesicae biliaris
    C. An area on the facies visceralis surrounding the porta hepatis
    D. The space between the leaflets of the lig. falciforme
    E. A subperitoneal capsula fibrosa that covers the surface of the liver

20. A 58-year-old postal worker complained to his physician that he noticed a swelling in his scrotum that felt similar to "a bag of worms," that was present during the day but disappeared in the morning. On examination you are able to diagnose a varicocele of the plexus pampiniformis that drains his left testis. What is the venous drainage of the testes?

   A. The right testis drains to the v. cava inferior; the left testis drains to the v. iliaca communis sinistra.
   B. The right testis drains to the v. cava inferior; the left testis drains to the v. renalis sinistra.
   C. The right testis drains to the v. renalis dextra; the left testis drains to the v. cava inferior.
   D. Both testes drain to ipsilateral vv. renales.
   E. Both testes drain to the v. cava inferior.

21. In portal hypertension portocaval anastomoses allow portal blood to divert into the systemic system. These anastomoses might involve the

   A. v. pancreaticoduodenalis
   B. vv. paraumbilicales
   C. v. renalis
   D. v. testicularis
   E. None of the above

22. The ductus choleoduchus is most often formed by the

   A. ductus hepaticus dexter and ductus hepaticus sinister
   B. ductus cysticus and ductus hepaticus communis
   C. ductus pancreaticus and ductus hepaticus communis
   D. ductus hepatopancreaticus and ductus cysticus
   E. ductus pancreaticus and ductus cysticus

23. Within the testis, sperm develop in the

   A. epididymis
   B. tunica albuginea
   C. ductus deferens
   D. rete testis
   E. tubuli seminiferi

24. A 34-year-old male with a remote history of abdominal surgery presents to the emergency department with severe abdominal pain, vomiting, and lethargy. What should be the first imaging study performed?

   A. CT
   B. Ultrasound
   C. Chest x-rays
   D. Abdominal x-rays
   E. MRI

25. A man presented to his physician's office with the complaint of severe intermittent pain in the upper right quadrant of his abdomen. You recognize his condition as biliary colic due to gallstones lodged at the entrance to the gallbladder. What valve or sphincter maintains the opening of the ductus cysticus?

   A. Spiral valve
   B. Ostium ileale
   C. M. sphincter pylori
   D. M. sphincter ampullae
   E. Papilla duodeni major

26. You routinely perform vasectomies at the free clinic in your area. You make a small incision at the top of the scrotum to access the funiculus spermaticus. Ligation of which of the cord structures would be most effective in preventing the transmission of sperm?

   A. A. testicularis
   B. Plexus pampiniformis
   C. Urachus
   D. Ductus deferens
   E. Epididymis

27. What anatomic feature of the gallbladder makes it highly suitable for ultrasound evaluation?

   A. It lies on the surface of the liver
   B. It stores bile
   C. A and B
   D. It is pear shaped
   E. It is retroperitoneal

28. Which of the following structures forms as an intraperitoneal organ but becomes secondarily retroperitoneal during later development?

   A. Aorta
   B. Pancreas
   C. Spleen
   D. Colon transversum
   E. Ren

29. Which of the following are reflections or remnants of peritoneum?

   A. Gerota's fascia
   B. Tunica albuginea
   C. Capsula fibrosa perivascularis
   D. Omentum minus
   E. Lig. umbilicale medianum

30. Which of the following are tributaries of the inferior vena cava?

   A. V. mesenterica inferior
   B. V. lumbalis
   C. V. gastrica dextra
   D. V. colica sinistra
   E. V. rectalis superior

Answers and Explanations

1. **A.** The v. renalis sinistra passes under the a. mesenterica superior as it crosses the aorta and can be compressed in the narrow angle (Section 12.3).

   B. The second part of the duodenum lies on the right side of the columna vertebralis and does not cross the aorta.

   C. The jejunum is suspended by the mesenterium that contains the a. mesenterica superior.

   D. The colon transversum is suspended from the mesocolon transversum and lies anterior to the a. mesenterica superior.

   E. The pancreas lies anterior to the a. mesenterica superior.

2. **C.** The appendix is derived from the embryonic mesenteron, which refers pain to the periumbilical region (Section 12.1).
      A. The appendix is derived from the embryonic mesenteron, not the praeenteron.
      B. Structures of the mesenteron refer pain to the periumbilical region; structures of the praeenteron refer pain to the epigastric region.
      D. The appendix is derived from the embryonic mesenteron, not the metenteron.
      E. Pain from the appendix is referred to the periumbilical region, but it is not part of the embryonic metenteron.

3. **B.** The pain is felt in the L1 dermatome innervated by the n. ilioinguinalis and n. iliohypogastricus (Section 10.3).
      A. The n. cutaneus femoris lateralis transmits sensation from the lateral thigh.
      C. The n. femoralis transmits sensation from the anterior thigh.
      D. The n. phrenicus inferior transmits sensation from the inferior surface of the diaphragma.
      E. The n. intercostalis T10 transmits sensation from the T10 dermatome at the level of the umbilicus.

4. **A.** The a. renalis dextra is longer than the a. renalis sinistra and passes posterior to the v. cava inferior (Section 12.3).
      B. The gl. suprarenalis sinistra drains into the v. renalis sinistra, but the gl. suprarenalis dextra drains into the v. cava inferior.
      C. The v. renalis sinistra crosses the aorta and is longer than the v. renalis dextra.
      D. At the hilum renalis, the vv. renales are anterior to the aa. renales. The pelvis renalis is the most posterior structure.
      E. Aa. renales arise from the aorta at L I/L II.

5. **C.** The taeniae coli, three longitudinal bands of muscle, are characteristics of the entire large intestine (Section 12.1).
      A. Branches of the a. mesenterica inferior supply the colon descendens.
      B. Nn. splanchnici pelvici provide parasympathetic innervation to the colon descendens.
      D. The colon descendens forms with the gastrointestinal tract as an intraperitoneal organ and loses its mesenterium during later development, becoming secondarily retroperitoneal.
      E. The colon descendens is part of the embryonic metenteron.

6. **C.** The conjoined tendon is formed by the aponeuroses of the m. obliquus internus abdominis and m. transversus abdominis (Section 10.2).
      A. The anulus umbilicalis, a remnant of the opening for the umbilical cord (chorda umbilicalis), interrupts the linea alba at the L IV vertebral level.
      B. The linea alba is a tendinous raphe formed in the midline by the aponeuroses of the three anterior abdominal wall muscles.
      D. The lower edge of the m. obliquus externus abdominis is thickened and curved inward to form the lig. inguinale.
      E. The anulus inguinalis superficialis is a defect in the aponeurosis of the m. obliquus externus abdominis that allows passage of the funiculus spermaticus.

7. **E.** The pancreas lies behind the stomach on the posterior wall of the bursa omentalis (Section 12.2).
      A. The a. splenica runs along the superior border of the pancreas.
      B. The v. portae hepatis forms by the union of the v. splenica and v. mesenterica superior posterior to the collum pancreatis.
      C. The collum pancreatis and cauda pancreatis cross the midline slightly below the planum transpyloricum at approximately the L II vertebral level.
      D. The ductus pancreaticus accessorius drains into the pars descendens duodeni, superior to the drainage of the main ductus pancreaticus.

8. **C.** The a. gastrica dextra, a branch of the a. hepatica propria, supplies the pyloric region (Sections 11.2 and 12.1).
      A. The a. gastrica sinistra supplies blood to the cardiac part of the stomach and the gastroesophageal sphincter.
      B. The aa. gastricae breves supply blood to the fundus of the stomach.
      D. The a. gastroomentalis sinistra supplies blood to the greater curvature of the stomach and the omentum majus.
      E. The a. pancreaticoduodenalis superior supplies blood to the pars descendens duodeni and the caput pancreatis.

9. **D.** Inferior to the linea arcuata, the posterior wall of the vagina musculi recti abdominis is composed of fascia transversalis (Section 10.2).
      A. The m. obliquus externus abdominis only contributes to the anterior layer of the vagina musculi recti abdominis.
      B. The m. obliquus internus abdominis forms part of the posterior layer of the vagina musculi recti abdominis above the linea arcuata and part of the vagina musculi recti abdominis below the linea arcuata.
      C. The m. transversus abdominis forms part of the anterior layer of vagina musculi recti abdominis below the linea arcuata.
      E. Not applicable.

10. **B.** The aa. pancreaticoduodenales superiores arise from the a. gastroduodenalis (a secondary branch of the truncus coeliacus). The aa. pancreaticoduodenales inferiores arises from the a. mesenterica superior. These vessels anastomose within the caput pancreatis and can enlarge significantly to form an effective collateral pathway (Section 11.2).
      A. The a. marginalis establishes a collateral circulation between the a. mesenterica superior and a. mesenterica inferior but does not communicate directly with branches of the truncus coeliacus.
      C. The aa. gastroomentales anastomose with the a. gastroduodenalis and a. splenica but do not communicate with the a. mesenterica superior.
      D. The a. hepatica propria anastomoses with the a. gastrica sinistra through its right gastric branch but it does not communicate directly with the a. mesenterica superior.
      E. The a. gastrica sinistra anastomoses with the aa. hepaticae and a. splenica but does not communicate directly with the a. mesenterica superior.

11. E. The recessus hepatorenalis, which is continuous with the recessus subphrenicus, is the lowest and most gravity-dependent space in the cavitas peritonealis. Therefore, it is a common site for fluid collection and abscess formation (Section 11.1).

A. Fluid from the bursa omentalis flows into the recessus hepatorenalis.

B. The infracolic compartment lies below the mesocolon transversum and is separated into right and left sides by the mesenterium of the small intestine. Fluid in this space can drain to the recessus paracolici and the pelvis.

C. Fluid in the recessus paracolicus sinister would likely drain to the pelvis.

D. Fluid in the recessus subphrenicus drains to the more gravity-dependent recessus hepatorenalis in the supine patient.

12. E. The m. obliquus externus abdominis, m. obliquus internus abdominis, and m. rectus abdominis flex the trunk when acting bilaterally and help stabilize the pelvis. The m. psoas major assists in raising the trunk from the supine position (Section 10.2).

A. The m. obliquus externus abdominis flexes the trunk when acting bilaterally and helps stabilize the pelvis. B through D are also correct (E).

B. The m. obliquus internus abdominis flexes the trunk when acting bilaterally and helps stabilize the pelvis. A, C, and D are also correct (E).

C. The m. rectus abdominis flexes the trunk, compresses the abdomen, and stabilizes the pelvis. A, B, and D are also correct (E).

D. The m. psoas major flexes the hip and assists in raising the trunk from the supine position. A through C are also correct (E).

13. E. The pelvic ureter is supplied by aa. vesicales superiores, a. vesicalis inferior, and a. uterina (Section 12.3).

A. Calculi can be lodged in several natural constrictions of the ureter, including where it passes behind the gonadal vessels or across the a. iliaca communis, as well as at the ureterovesical and ureteropelvic junctions.

B. Distension of the ureteric walls sends pain signals to the T11–L2 medulla spinalis via sympathetic nerves.

C. Pain is felt first in the lower lumbar region and moves downward to the inguinal region and medial thigh, the areas that represent the T11–L2 dermatomes.

D. The muscular walls of the ureter function through peristaltic action.

14. C. The nn. intercostales are instrumental in the ability to sense, and react to, abdominal pain as they innervate the peritoneum parietale (sensory branches) and the abdominal wall muscles (motor branches). Inflammation of the peritoneum parietale can cause severe pain. The peritoneum viscerale is not very sensitive (Section 11.1).

A. The n. phrenicus innervates the diaphragm but does not contribute to the innervation of the abdominal wall muscles.

B. The n. vagus innervates neither the peritoneum nor the abdominal wall muscles.

D. Nn. splanchnici lumbales carry sympathetic fibers that innervate abdominal viscera.

E. The n. splanchnicus thoracicus major carries only sympathetic fibers, which innervate abdominal viscera.

15. D. The ductus omphaloentericus (yolk stalk) has failed to regress and remains as an ileal (Meckel's) diverticulum (Section 12.1).

A. The ductus venosus diverts blood in the v. umbilicalis into the v. cava inferior in the fetus.

B. The remnant of the v. umbilicalis, the ligamentum teres, runs in the inferior edge of the lig. falciforme, which connects the liver to the anterior abdominal wall.

C. The lig. umbilicale medianum on the anterior abdominal wall is the remnant of the a. umbilicalis.

E. The urachus, the remnant of the fetal allantois, extends superiorly on the anterior abdominal wall from the apex of the vesica urinaria to the umbilicus, as the lig. umbilicale medianum.

16. D. Renal calculi form in the kidney from concentrated urine and are associated with inflammatory bowel disease and other pathology but are not a symptom of portal hypertension (Section 12.2).

A. Oesophageal veins that drain superiorly to the azygos (systemic) system and inferiorly to the portal system form an important portocaval anastomosis. Varices of these veins are a typical symptom of portal hypertension.

B. In portal hypertension, flow through the v. splenica slows, causing the spleen to enlarge abnormally (splenomegaly).

C. Vv. rectales drain superiorly to the portal system and inferiorly to the systemic system. In portal hypertension they enlarge (forming varices) to accommodate the greater flow into the systemic system.

E. Ascites is a typical symptom of portal hypertension due to liver disease.

17. D. Indirect inguinal hernias pass through the anulus inguinalis profundus, which is lateral to the a. and v. epigastrica inferior and superior to the lig. inguinale (Section 10.4).

A. Inguinal hernias are located above the lig. inguinale; femoral hernias are located below the ligament.

B. Indirect inguinal hernias are located lateral to the a. epigastrica inferior and v. epigastrica inferior; direct inguinal hernias are located medial to the vessels.

C. Direct inguinal hernias protrude through the trigonum inguinale; indirect inguinal hernias protrude through the anulus inguinalis profundus lateral to the trigonum.

E. The aponeuroses of the m. obliquus internus abdominis and m. transversus abdominis form the conjoined tendon where they attach to the ramus superior ossis pubis. This is not a common site for hernias.

18. D. The medulla contains chromaffin cells that function as sympathetic ganglia where preganglionic sympathetic fibers from the plexus coeliacus synapse (Section 12.3).

A. The gll. suprarenales develop within the retroperitoneum and therefore are primary retroperitoneal organs.

B. The cortex is derived from mesoderm; the medulla is derived from neural crest cells.

C. Each gl. suprarenalis is supplied by multiple arteries arising from the aorta, and a. phrenica inferior and a. renalis.

E. The gll. suprarenales are enclosed by the fascia renalis and capsula adiposa, separated from the kidney only by a thin septum.

19. **A.** The area nuda is an area devoid of peritoneum adjacent to the inferior surface of the diaphragma bounded by the lig. coronarium and lig. triangulare (Section 12.2).
B. The fossa vesicae biliaris on the facies visceralis hepatis is also devoid of peritoneum but is not known as the area nuda.
C. Peritoneum covers the surface of the liver around the porta hepatis, the entry site for the structures of the portal triad.
D. The leaflets of the lig. falciforme do not contain the area nuda, but on the surface of the liver the leaflets separate to form the lig. coronarium, which surrounds the area nuda.
E. The subperitoneal capsula fibrosa of the liver is Glisson's capsule (capsula fibrosa perivascularis), not the area nuda.

20. **B.** The v. testicularis dextra drains into the v. cava inferior, but the v. testicularis sinistra drains into the v. renalis sinistra. The angle at which the v. testicularis sinistra enters the v. renalis sinistra increases its susceptibility to obstruction. This is probably the reason why varicoceles are most commonly found on the left side (Section 10.4).
A. Neither testis drains to the v. iliaca communis.
C. The right testis drains to the v. cava inferior, and the left drains to the v. renalis sinistra.
D. Although the left testis drains to the ipsilateral v. renalis, the right testis drains directly to the v. cava inferior.
E. Although the right testis drains directly to the v. cava inferior, the left testis drains to the ipsilateral v. renalis.

21. **B.** Vv. paraumbilicales anastomose with veins on the anterior abdominal wall and act as a portocaval shunt in severe portal hypertension (Section 11.2).
A. Vv. pancreaticoduodenales drain to the v. portae hepatis but do not anastomose with veins of the systemic system.
C. Vv. renales drain into the v. cava inferior and do not connect to the portal system.
D. Vv. testiculares drain to the systemic system and do not anastomose with the portal system.
E. Not applicable.

22. **B.** The ductus hepaticus communis of the liver joins the ductus cysticus of the gallbladder to form the ductus choledochus (Section 12.2).
A. The ductus hepaticus sinister and ductus hepaticus dexter join to form the ductus hepaticus communis.
C. The ductus pancreaticus joins the ductus hepaticus communis to form the ampulla hepaticopancreatica.
D. The ductus cysticus does not join the ductus hepatopancreaticus. It joins the ductus hepaticus communis to form the ductus choledochus.
E. The ductus pancreaticus does not join the ductus cysticus.

23. **E.** Seminiferous tubules (tubuli seminiferi) are highly coiled structures within the lobes of the testes where sperm develop (Section 10.4).
A. The epididymis is a site of sperm storage and maturation.
B. The tunica albuginea is the tough connective tissue capsule of the testis.
C. The ductus deferens transports sperm along the funiculus spermaticus to the deep pelvis.

D. The rete testis is a network of ducts through which sperm exit the testis.

24. **D.** Abdominal x-rays are the easiest and fastest way to get an overview of the bowel gas pattern and assess for bowel obstruction and/or bowel perforation, both intra-abdominal emergencies that may require immediate surgical intervention (Chapter 13).
A. CT may be a secondary choice in this patient.
B. Ultrasound may be a secondary tool if additional clinical signs point to a liver or biliary abnormality.
C. The patient is not having cardiopulmonary symptoms.
E. MRI is generally too time-consuming in the emergent setting.

25. **A.** The spiral valve in the neck of the gallbladder maintains the opening of the ductus cysticus (Section 12.2).
B. The ostium ileale is located between the ileum and caecum.
C. The m. sphincter pylori is located between the pylorus of the stomach and the first part of the duodenum.
D. The m. sphincter ampullae surrounds the ampulla hepatopancreatica as it enters the descending part of the duodenum at the papilla duodeni major.
E. The papilla duodeni major is an elevation on the medial wall of the pars descendens of the duodenum where the ampulla hepatopancreatica (formed by the union of the ductus choledochus and ductus pancreaticus) enters.

26. **D.** The ductus deferens is the structure within the funiculus spermaticus that transmits sperm (Section 10.4).
A. The a. testicularis does not transmit sperm.
B. The plexus pampiniformis is a venous plexus that drains the testis.
C. The urachus connects the apex of the bladder to the umbilicus and transmits urine in the fetus.
E. The epididymis is a site for sperm maturation and storage located within the scrotal sac on the posterior surface of the testis.

27. **C.** (A and B) The liver is an excellent acoustic "window" and the gallbladder's position within a fossa on the facies visceralis hepatis, as well as physiologically being filled with liquid bile, make ultrasound ideal for its evaluation (Chapter 13).
D. The pear shape is not a factor.
E. The gallbladder is not retroperitoneal.

28. **B.** Most of the pancreas is secondarily retroperitoneal. The cauda pancreatis lies within the lig. splenorenale and is considered intraperitoneal (Sections 11.1 and 12.2).
A. The aorta abdominalis is retroperitoneal and lies on the left side of the vertebral bodies.
C. The spleen is completely intraperitoneal, supported by the lig. gastrosplenicum and lig. splenorenale.
D. The colon transversum is intraperitoneal, supported by its mesocolon transversum.
E. The kidney is a primary retroperitoneal organ, surrounded by perirenal fat (capsula adiposa) and covered by peritoneum only on its anterior surface.

29. **D.** The omentum minus is a two-layer peritoneal membrane that connects the liver to the stomach and duodenum (Section 11.1).

　A. Gerota's fascia (lamina anterior fasciae renalis) is part of the fascia renalis that surrounds the kidney, gl. suprarenalis, a. renalis and v. renalis, and capsula adiposa.

　B. The tunica albuginea is the tough outer fibrous membrane that surrounds the testis and invaginates to form the lobuli testis.

　C. Capsula fibrosa perivascularis is a subperitoneal capsula fibrosa that surrounds the liver.

　E. The lig. umbilicale medianum is the remnant of the a. umbilicalis on the anterior abdominal wall.

30. **B.** The four vv. lumbales on each side drain the posterior abdominal wall and terminate in the v. cava inferior (Section 11.2).

　A. The v. mesenterica inferior terminates either in the v. mesenterica superior or v. splenica, which are tributaries of the v. portae hepatis.

　C. The v. gastrica sinistra drains into the v. portae hepatis.

　D. The v. colica sinistra drains to the v. mesenterica inferior, which is a tributary of the v. portae hepatis.

　E. The v. rectalis superior drains superiorly to the v. mesenterica inferior, which is a tributary of the portal system.

Unit V   Pelvis and Perineum

14 Overview of the Pelvis and Perineum

The pelvic region is the area of the trunk between the abdomen and lower limb. It includes the **cavitas pelvis,** the bowl-shaped space enclosed by the bony pelvis, and the **perineum,** the diamond-shaped area inferior to the pelvic floor (diaphragma pelvis) and between the upper aspects of the thighs.

14.1 General Features

— **Table 14.1** provides an overview of the divisions of the pelvis and perineum.
  • The bony pelvis (pelvis ossea), or pelvic girdle (cingulum pelvicum), encloses the cavitas pelvis. Its superior bony landmark is the crista iliaca (**Fig. 14.1**).
  • The **linea terminalis** at the plane of the **pelvic inlet (apertura pelvis superior)** defines the upper border of the bony **pelvis minor** and separates it from the **pelvis major** above. A **pelvic outlet (apertura pelvis inferior)** defines the lower border of the pelvis minor (**Fig. 14.2**).
  • The muscular floor of the cavitas pelvis, the **diaphragma pelvis**, separates the pelvis minor from the perineum, which lies below it (**Fig. 14.3**).
  • The diamond-shaped perineum is subdivided into an anterior **regio urogenitalis** and a posterior **regio analis** (**Fig. 14.4**).
  • A **membrana perinei** divides the **regio urogenitalis** into two small spaces:
    ◦ an upper **deep pouch (spatium profundum perinei)**, which includes the anterior recesses of the fossae ischioanales and which is bounded by the membrana perinei inferiorly, the inferior fascia of the pelvic diaphragm (fascia diaphragmatis pelvis inferior) superiorly, and the fascia obturatoria laterally and
    ◦ a lower **superficial pouch (spatium superficiale perinei)** bounded superiorly by the membrana perinei,

inferiorly by the superficial fascia perinei, and laterally by the ischiopubic rami (**Fig. 14.3**).

The membrana perinei is not present in the regio analis (see **Fig. 15.24**).

— The apertura pelvis superior and apertura pelvis inferior are apertures of the pelvis ossea (**Fig. 14.5**).
  • The pelvic inlet (linea terminalis), the apertura pelvis superior, is defined by a line that extends from the promontorium of the os sacrum, along the linea arcuata of the os ilium and pecten ossis pubis, to the superior border of the symphysis pubica.
  • The pelvic outlet, apertura pelvis inferior, is defined by a line that connects the os coccygis, ligg. sacrotuberalia, tubera ischiadica, rami ischiopubici, and inferior border of the symphysis pubica.

— The cavities of the pelvis minor and pelvis major are continuous with each other but contain different viscera.
  • The **pelvis minor** lies below the linea terminalis and is bounded inferiorly by the diaphragma pelvis. In the adult, this space houses the bladder, rectum, and pelvic genital structures.

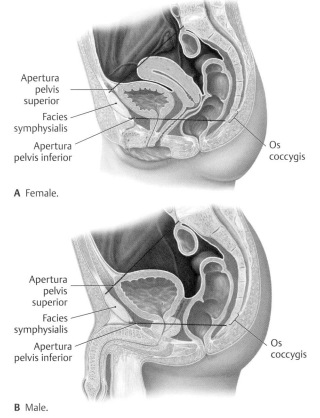

A Female.

B Male.

Fig. 14.2 Pelvis minor and pelvis major
Midsagittal sections, viewed from the left side. (From Gilroy AM et al. Atlas of Anatomy. 4th ed. 2020. Based on: Schuenke M, Schulte E, Schumacher U. THIEME Atlas of Anatomy. General Anatomy and Musculoskeletal System. Illustrations by Voll M and Wesker K. 3rd ed. New York: Thieme Medical Publishers; 2020.)

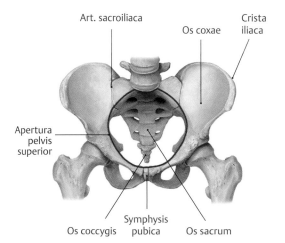

Fig. 14.1 Pelvic girdle
Anterosuperior view. The cingulum pelvicum consists of the two os coxae and the os sacrum. (From Schuenke M, Schulte E, Schumacher U. THIEME Atlas of Anatomy, Vol 1. Illustrations by Voll M and Wesker K. 3rd ed. New York: Thieme Publishers; 2020.)

Table 14.1 Divisions of the Pelvis and Perineum

The levels of the pelvis are determined by bony landmarks (alae ossium ilium and apertura pelvis superior/linea terminalis). The contents of the perineum are separated from the pelvis minor by the diaphragma pelvis and two fascial layers.

Crista iliaca

Pelvis	**Pelvis major**	• Ileum • Caecum and appendix vermiformis • Colon sigmoideum • Aa. and vv. iliacae communes and externae • Rr. plexus lumbalis
	Apertura pelvis superior	
	Pelvis minor	• Distal ureteres • Vesica urinaria • Rectum • ♀: Vagina, uterus, tubae uterinae, and ovaria • ♂: Ductus deferens, gl. vesiculosa, and prostata • A. and v. iliaca interna and branches • Plexus sacralis • Plexus hypogastricus inferior

Diaphragma pelvis (m. levator ani & m. coccygeus)

Perineum	**Spatium profundum perinei**	• Sphincter externus urethrae • Compressor urethrae and sphincter urethrovaginalis (females) • Urethra (pars membranacea in males) • M. transversus profundus perinei (males), smooth muscle (female) • Gl. bulbourethralis (male) • Anterior recess of corpora adiposa fossae ischioanalis • A. and v. pudenda interna, n. pudendus and branches
	Membrana perinei	
	Spatium superficiale perinei	• M. ischiocavernosus, m. bulbospongiosus, and m. transversus perinei • Urethra (pars spongiosum urethrae in males) • Clitoris and radix penis • Bulbi vestibuli • Gll. vestibulares majores • A. and v. pudenda interna, n. pudendus and branches
	Stratum membranosum of the subcutaenous perineal tissue (Colles' fascia)	
	Spatium subcutaneum perinei	• Fat

Cutis

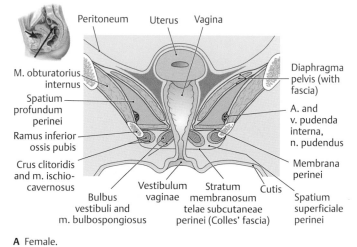

A Female.

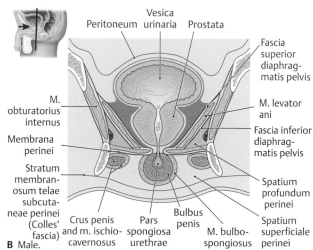

B Male.

Fig. 14.3 Pelvis and regio urogenitalis of the perineum

Coronal section, anterior view. (From Gilroy AM et al. Atlas of Anatomy. 4th ed. 2020. Based on: Schuenke M, Schulte E, Schumacher U. THIEME Atlas of Anatomy. General Anatomy and Musculoskeletal System. Illustrations by Voll M and Wesker K. 3rd ed. New York: Thieme Medical Publishers; 2020.)

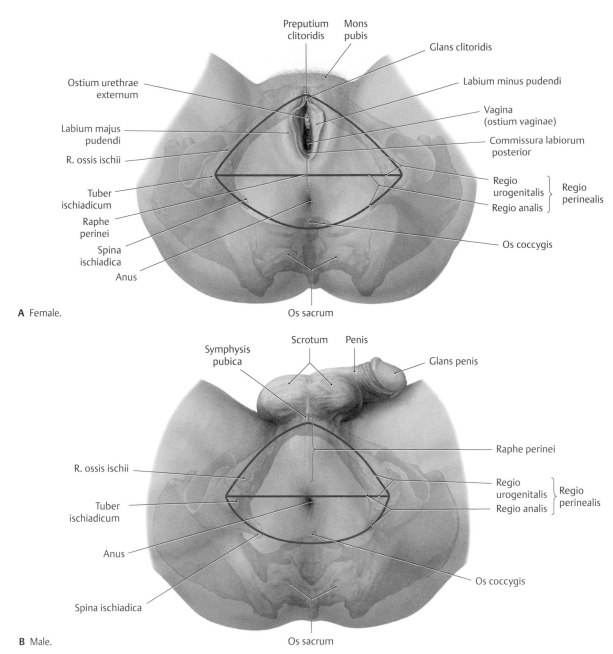

A Female.

B Male.

Fig. 14.4 Regions of the perineum
Lithotomy position, caudal (inferior) view. (From Schuenke M, Schulte E, Schumacher U. THIEME Atlas of Anatomy, Vol 1. Illustrations by Voll M and Wesker K. 3rd ed. New York: Thieme Publishers; 2020.)

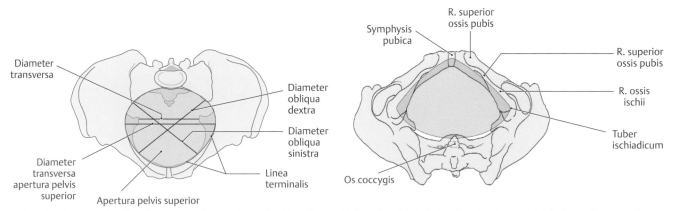

A Female pelvis, superior view. Apertura pelvis superior outlined in *red.*

B Female pelvis, inferior view. Apertura pelvis inferior outlined in *red.*

Fig. 14.5 Apertura pelvis superior and apertura pelvis inferior
(From Schuenke M, Schulte E, Schumacher U. THIEME Atlas of Anatomy, Vol 1. Illustrations by Voll M and Wesker K. 3rd ed. New York: Thieme Publishers; 2020.)

- The **pelvis major** is the lower part of the cavitas abdominis that lies above the linea terminalis and is bounded on each side by the fossa iliaca. It contains the caecum, appendix vermiformis, colon sigmoideum, and loops of the small intestine.
— The peritoneum of the cavitas abdominis continues into the cavitas pelvis.
  - The peritoneum of the anterior abdominal wall drapes over the bladder (vesica urinaria), uterus, rectum, and pelvic walls, but it does not extend as far inferiorly as the diaphragma pelvis.
  - Deep viscera pelvis that lie below the peritoneum occupy a **spatium infraperitoneale** that is continuous with the spatium retroperitoneale of the abdomen (see **Fig. 14.3**).
— The perineum lies inferior to the cavitas pelvis (see **Fig. 14.4**).
  - The apertura pelvis inferior forms the perimeter of the perineum, the diaphragma pelvis forms its roof, and, inferiorly, perineal skin forms its floor.
  - The regio urogenitalis of the perineum contains the external genital structures and openings for the urethra and vagina (in females).

BOX 14.1: CLINICAL CORRELATION

PELVIC DIAMETERS: TRUE CONJUGATE, DIAGONAL CONJUGATE
Pelvic measurements are important obstetric predictors of ease of vaginal delivery. The true (obstetrical) conjugate (conjugata vera obstetrica), the narrowest anteroposterior diameter of the birth canal, is measured from the posterior superior margin of the symphysis pubica to the tip of the promontorium ossis sacri (~ 11 cm). Because this distance is difficult to measure accurately, the diagonal conjugate is used to estimate it. This is measured from the lower border of the symphysis pubica to the tip of the promontorium ossis sacri (~ 12.5 cm).

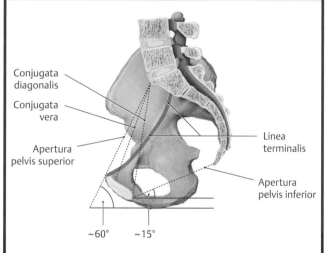

Right hemipelvis
(From Gilroy AM et al. Atlas of Anatomy. 4th ed. 2020. Based on: Schuenke M, Schulte E, Schumacher U. THIEME Atlas of Anatomy. General Anatomy and Musculoskeletal System. Illustrations by Voll M and Wesker K. 3rd ed. New York: Thieme Medical Publishers; 2020.)

- The regio analis of the perineum contains the anal opening and canalis analis, surrounded by the m. sphincter ani externus.
— The **ischioanal fossae (fossae ischioanales)**, wedge-shaped, fat-filled spaces of the regio analis, lie on either side of the canalis analis and extend anteriorly into a small recess of the regio urogenitalis (see **Fig. 15.24**; Section 16.5).

14.2 The Bony Pelvis

The bony pelvis (pelvis ossea), or **pelvic girdle (cingulum pelvicum)**, consists of the os sacrum, the os coccygis, and the two **coxal (hip) bones (ossa coxae)**. It protects the viscera pelvis, stabilizes the back, and provides an attachment site for the lower limbs. Pelvic joints create the circular configuration of the cingulum pelvicum, which is maintained by strong pelvic ligaments (see **Fig. 14.1**).
— The os sacrum and os coccygis, the lowest segments of the columna vertebralis, constitute the posterior wall of the cingulum pelvicum.
— Each os coxae, the lateral parts of the cingulum pelvicum, is formed by the fusion of three bones: the **os ilium, os ischii, and os pubis (Fig. 14.6)**. Features of the ossa coxae **(Fig. 14.7)** include the following:
  - The **r. inferior ossis pubis** and **r. superior ossis pubis**, which join anteriorly but diverge laterally around the large **foramen obturatum**
  - The **spina ischiadica** posteriorly, which separates the **incisura ischiadica major** and **incisura ischiadica minor**
  - The **r. ossis ischii**, which fuses with the **r. inferior ossis pubis** anteriorly and ends as the **tuber ischiadicum** posteriorly
  - The **ala ossis ilii,** which is concave anteriorly, forming the **fossa iliaca.** The superior edge of the ala ossis ilii, the **crista iliaca**, ends anteriorly as the **spina iliaca anterior superior** and posteriorly as the **spina iliaca posterior superior**.
  - A **linea arcuata** on the internal surface, which bisects the os ilium and continues anteriorly to join with the **pecten ossis pubis** of the pubis. Both lines form part of the apertura pelvis superior (also known as the **linea terminalis**).
  - A deep, cup-shaped depression, the **acetabulum,** on the lateral surface, which articulates with the femur of the lower limb

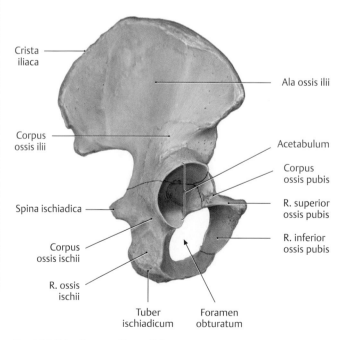

Fig. 14.6 Triradiate cartilage of the os coxae
Right os coxae, lateral view. The os coxae consists of the os ilium, os ischii, and os pubis. (From Schuenke M, Schulte E, Schumacher U. THIEME Atlas of Anatomy, Vol 1. Illustrations by Voll M and Wesker K. 3rd ed. New York: Thieme Publishers; 2020.)

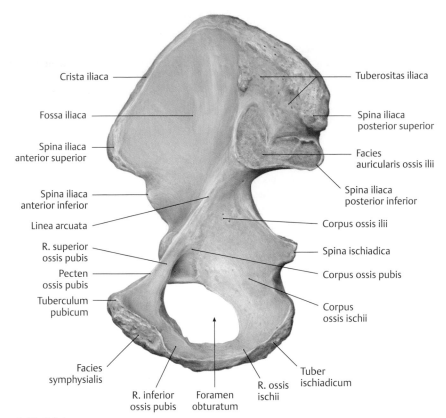

A Medial view.
(From Gilroy AM et al. Atlas of Anatomy. 4th ed. 2020. Based on: Schuenke M, Schulte E, Schumacher U. THIEME Atlas of Anatomy. General Anatomy and Musculoskeletal System. Illustrations by Voll M and Wesker K. 3rd ed. New York: Thieme Medical Publishers; 2020.)

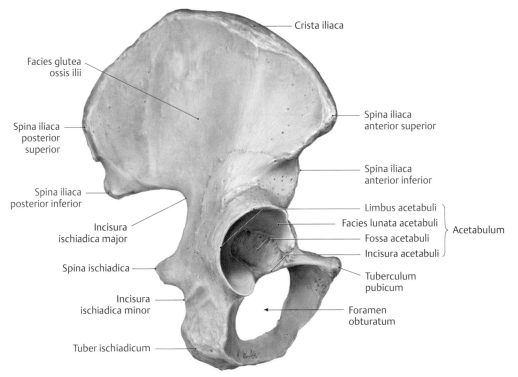

B Lateral view.
(From Schuenke M, Schulte E, Schumacher U. THIEME Atlas of Anatomy, Vol 1. Illustrations by Voll M and Wesker K. 3rd ed. New York: Thieme Publishers; 2020.)

Fig. 14.7 Os coxae
Os coxae dexter (male).

— The joints of the cingulum pelvicum include the following (see **Fig. 14.1**):
  • The paired **artt. sacroiliacae**, which are synovial joints between the auricular surfaces of the os sacrum and the ossa coxae
  • The **symphysis pubica**, an immobile cartilaginous joint in the anterior midline that joins the pubic portions of the ossa coxae with an intervening fibrocartilaginous disk

— Ligaments that support pelvic joints **(Fig. 14.8)** include the following:
  • The strong **ligg. sacroiliaca anteriora**, **ligg. sacroliaca posteriora**, and **ligg. sacroiliaca interossea** that support the artt. sacroiliacae
  • The **ligg. iliolumbales** that stabilize the junction between the vertebrae lumbales and os sacrum

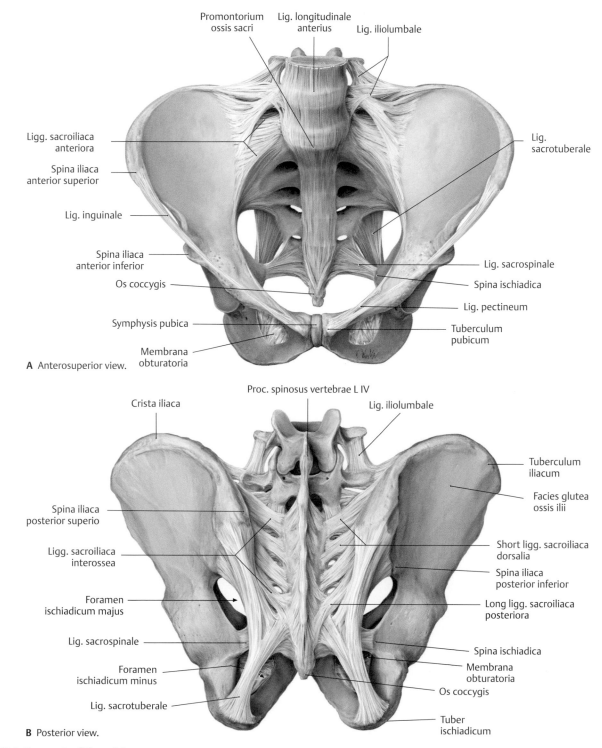

A Anterosuperior view.

B Posterior view.

Fig. 14.8 Ligaments of the pelvis
Male pelvis. (From Gilroy AM et al. Atlas of Anatomy. 4th ed. 2020. Based on: Schuenke M, Schulte E, Schumacher U. THIEME Atlas of Anatomy. General Anatomy and Musculoskeletal System. Illustrations by Voll M and Wesker K. 3rd ed. New York: Thieme Medical Publishers; 2020.)

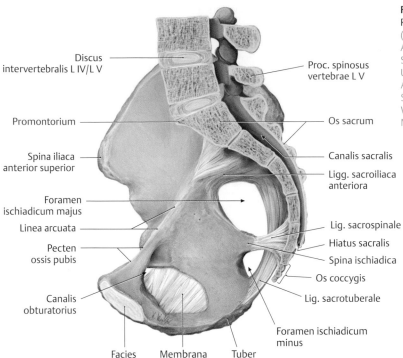

Discus intervertebralis L IV/L V

Promontorium

Spina iliaca anterior superior

Foramen ischiadicum majus

Linea arcuata

Pecten ossis pubis

Canalis obturatorius

Proc. spinosus vertebrae L V

Os sacrum

Canalis sacralis

Ligg. sacroiliaca anteriora

Lig. sacrospinale

Hiatus sacralis

Spina ischiadica

Os coccygis

Lig. sacrotuberale

Foramen ischiadicum minus

Facies symphysialis   Membrana obturatoria   Tuber ischiadicum

Fig. 14.9 Pelvic openings
Right half of male pelvis, medial view.
(From Gilroy AM et al. Atlas of Anatomy. 4th ed. 2020. Based on: Schuenke M, Schulte E, Schumacher U. THIEME Atlas of Anatomy. General Anatomy and Musculoskeletal System. Illustrations by Voll M and Wesker K. 3rd ed. New York: Thieme Medical Publishers; 2020.)

- Two pairs of posterior ligaments that secure the sacrum and hip bone articulations and resist posterior displacement of the os sacrum
    1. The **lig. sacrotuberale** originate on the os sacrum and insert on the tuber ischiadicum.
    2. The **lig. sacrospinale** originate on the os sacrum and insert on the spina ischiadica.

> **BOX 14.2: CLINICAL CORRELATION**
>
> **LAXITY OF LIGAMENTS AND INCEASED MOBILITY DURING PREGNANCY**
> During the final trimester of pregnancy, there is a marked increase in the softness and laxity of the symphysis pubica and ligg. sacroiliaca, which is attributed to increased levels of relaxin and other pregnancy hormones. This often results in some pelvic instability and the characteristic waddling gait of the third trimester. Softening of the pelvic ligaments increases the pelvic diameter, which is of benefit as the neonate negotiates the birth canal. Normal ligament integrity returns within a few months following birth.

- The pelvic bones and ligaments form openings that allow pelvic vessels, nerves, and muscles to connect to adjacent regions **(Fig. 14.9)**.
    - The **foramen ischiadicum majus** is a posterior opening that connects the pelvis to the regio glutealis (the buttocks).
    - The **foramen ischiadicum minus** is a passageway between the lig. sacrotuberale and lig. sacrospinale that connects the regio glutealis and perineum.
    - An **membrana obturatoria** covers most of the bony foramen obturatum, leaving a small **canalis obturatorius** through which the n. obturatorius and obturator vessels pass into the thigh.

14.3 Pelvic Walls and Floor (Table 14.2; Fig. 14.10)

- The muscles that line the pelvic walls pass into the regio glutealis, where they attach to the femur (thigh bone) and act on the hip joint (art. coxae).
    - The **m. piriformis** lines the posterior wall of the pelvis.
        - It passes from the pelvis to the regio glutealis through the foramen ischiadicum majus.
        - It forms the bed for the plexus sacralis and internal iliac vessels on the posterior pelvic wall.
    - The **m. obturatorius internus**, covered by an overlying **fascia obturatoria**, lines the sidewall of the pelvis and perineum.
        - Its tendon passes from the perineum to the regio glutealis through the foramen ischiadicum minus.
        - A thickening of the fascia obturatoria, the **arcus tendineus musculi levatoris ani**, runs from the corpus ossis pubis to the spina ischiadica.
- The funnel-shaped pelvic floor is composed of muscles, collectively known as the **diaphragma pelvis**, that support the viscera pelvis and resist intra-abdominal pressure (i.e., pressure created during coughing, sneezing, forced expiration, defecating, and parturition). The diaphragma pelvis is composed of the **m. levator ani** and the **m. coccygeus**.
    - The m. levator ani forms the largest part of the pelvic floor. The three muscles of the m. levator ani arise from the r. ossis pubis superior and the arcus tendineus. They insert in the midline on the os coccygis and along a tendinous raphe, called the **lig. anococcygeum**.
        - The **m. pubococcygeus** forms the anterior part of the m. levator ani.
        - The **m. iliococcygeus** forms the middle part of the m. levator ani.
        - The **m. puborectalis** forms a muscular sling that loops around the anorectum. Normal tone of the muscle

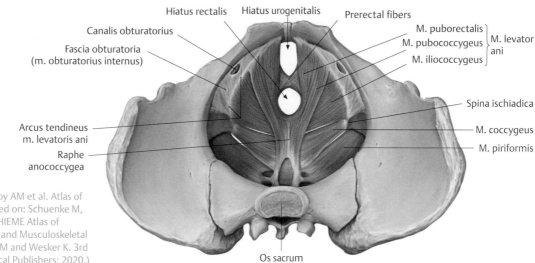

A Superior view. (From Gilroy AM et al. Atlas of Anatomy. 4th ed. 2020. Based on: Schuenke M, Schulte E, Schumacher U. THIEME Atlas of Anatomy. General Anatomy and Musculoskeletal System. Illustrations by Voll M and Wesker K. 3rd ed. New York: Thieme Medical Publishers; 2020.)

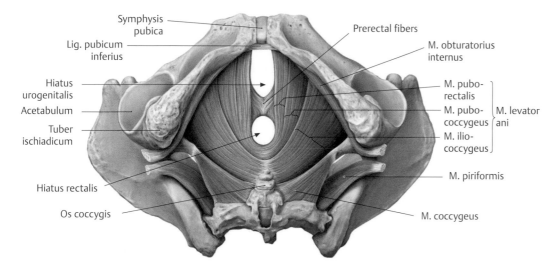

B Inferior view. (From Gilroy AM et al. Atlas of Anatomy. 4th ed. 2020. Based on: Schuenke M, Schulte E, Schumacher U. THIEME Atlas of Anatomy. General Anatomy and Musculoskeletal System. Illustrations by Voll M and Wesker K. 3rd ed. New York: Thieme Medical Publishers; 2020.)

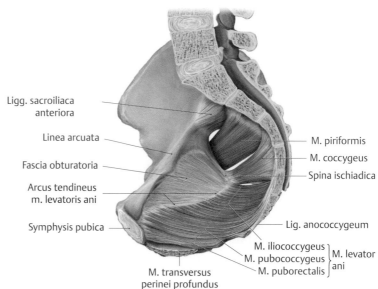

C Medial view of right hemipelvis. (From Schuenke M, Schulte E, Schumacher U. THIEME Atlas of Anatomy, Vol 1. Illustrations by Voll M and Wesker K. 3rd ed. New York: Thieme Publishers; 2020.)

Fig. 14.10 Muscles of the pelvic floor
Female pelvis.

Table 14.2 Muscles of the Pelvic Floor

Muscle		Origin	Insertion	Innervation	Action
Muscles of the diaphragma pelvis					
M. levator ani	M. puborectalis	Ramus superior ossis pubis (both sides of symphysis pubica)	Corpus anococcygeum	Nerve to m. levator ani (S4), n. analis inferior	Diaphragma pelvis: Supports pelvic viscera
	M. pubococcygeus	Os pubis (lateral to origin of m. puborectalis)	Corpus anococcygeum, os coccygis		
	M. iliococcygeus	Internal fascia obturatoria of m. levator ani (arcus tendineus musculi levatoris ani)			
M. ischiococ-cygeus		Lateral surface of os coccygis and S5 segment	Spina ischiadica	Direct brs. from plexus sacralis (S4, S5)	Supports pelvic viscera, flexes os coccygis
Muscles of the pelvic wall (parietal muscles)					
M. piriformis		Os sacrum (facies pelvica)	Femur (apex of trochanter major)	Direct brs. from plexus sacralis (S1, S2)	Hip joint: external rotation, stabilization, and abduction of flexed hip
M. obturatorius internus		Membrana obturatoria and bony boundaries (inner surface)	Femur (trochanter major, medial surface)	Direct brs. from plexus sacralis (L5, S1)	Hip joint: External rotation and abduction of flexed hip

maintains the anterior angle of the anorectum where it passes through the diaphragma pelvis. The muscle relaxes during defecation.

- The m. coccygeus forms the posterior part of the dia-phragma pelvis; it attaches to the os sacrum and spina ischiadica and tightly adheres to the lig. sacrospinale along its entire length.

— The **hiatus urogenitalis**, a gap between the mm. puborectalis either side, allows the passage of the urethra, vagina, and rectum into the perineum.

— The a. glutea inferior, a. glutea superior, and aa. sacrales laterales, branches of the aa. iliacae internae, and the a. sacralis mediana, a branch of the aorta abdominalis, supply most muscles of the pelvic walls and floor (see **Fig. 14.14A**).

— Veins that accompany the arteries and drain the pelvic floor and walls ultimately drain to the vv. iliacae internae, although the vv. sacrales laterales may also drain to the plexus venosus vertebralis internus.

14.4   Pelvic Fascia

Pelvic fascia (fascia pelvis) is a connective tissue layer located between the viscera and the muscular walls and floor of the pel-vis. There are two types, **membranous fascia** and **fascia endopel-vica (Figs. 14.11** and **14.12;** see also **Fig. 14.3**).

— Membranous pelvic fascia, usually a thin layer that adheres to the pelvic walls and viscera, has visceral and parietal layers.

- The **fascia pelvis visceralis** surrounds the individual organs, and when in contact with the peritoneum it lies between the peritoneum viscerale and the organ wall.
- The **fascia pelvis parietalis** lines the inner surface of the muscles of the pelvic walls and floor. It is continuous with the fascia transversalis and fascia psoae of the abdomen and is named regionally for the muscle it covers (i.e., fascia obturatoria).

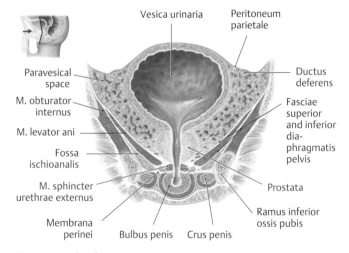

Fig. 14.11   Pelvic fascia
Male pelvis in coronal section, anterior view. (From Gilroy AM et al. Atlas of Anatomy. 4th ed. 2020. Based on: Schuenke M, Schulte E, Schumacher U. THIEME Atlas of Anatomy. General Anatomy and Musculoskeletal System. Illustrations by Voll M and Wesker K. 3rd ed. New York: Thieme Medical Publishers; 2020.)

- Where the viscera pelvis pierce the diaphragma pelvis, the parietal and visceral layers merge to form a **arcus tendineus fasciae pelvis**. This arch runs from the os pubis to the os sacrum on either side of the viscera pelvis. **Ligg. pubovesi-calia** in the female and **ligg. puboprostatica** in the male are extensions of the arcus tendinei that support the bladder and prostate. In females, the **paracolpium**—lateral connections between the visceral fascia and the arcus tendinei—suspends and supports the vagina.

— **Fascia endopelvica** forms a loose connective tissue matrix that fills the spatium subperitoneale between the visceral and parietal layers of the membranous fascia.

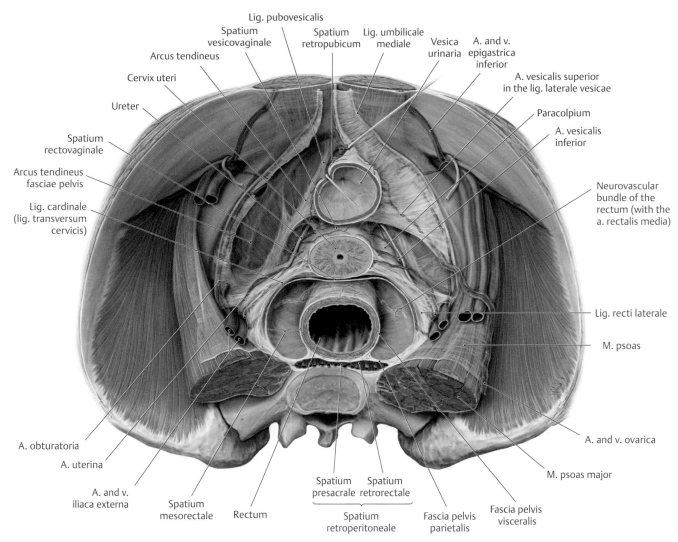

Fig. 14.12 Fascial attachments in the female pelvis
Transverse section through the cervix, superior view. (From Gilroy AM et al. Atlas of Anatomy. 4th ed. 2020. Based on: Schuenke M, Schulte E, Schumacher U. THIEME Atlas of Anatomy. Internal Organs. Illustrations by Voll M and Wesker K. 3rd ed. New York: Thieme Medical Publishers; 2020.)

- Much of this fascia has a cotton candy–like consistency that pads the subperitoneal space but allows for distension of the viscera pelvis (e.g., vagina, rectum).
- Large supporting columns of this connective tissue extend from the pelvic walls to the rectum as the **lig. laterale of the rectum**, and from the pelvic wall to the bladder, the **lig. laterale vesicae**.
- In some areas, the fascia endopelvica forms fibrous condensations [e.g., lig. cardinale (lig. transversum cervicis)] that support the viscera pelvis and their vascular and nerve plexuses.

14.5 Pelvic Spaces

The peritoneum of the abdominal wall covers the superior surface of the bladder, the anterior and posterior surface of the uterus, and the anterolateral surfaces of the rectum. Because the peritoneum does not descend to the pelvic floor, spaces are created above the peritoneum, within the cavitas peritonealis, and below the peritoneum in the spatium infraperitoneale **(Fig. 14.13)**.

— **Peritoneal recesses,** intraperitoneal spaces that are continuous with the cavitas peritonealis of the abdomen and lined by the peritoneum viscerale of the pelvic organs, are normally occupied by loops of small intestine and peritoneal fluid.
  - In males, an **excavatio rectovesicalis** between the bladder and rectum is the lowest point in the male cavitas peritonealis.
  - In females, an **excavatio vesicouterina** forms between the bladder and uterus, and an **excavatio rectouterina** (of Douglas) forms between the uterus and rectum. The excavatio rectouterina is the lowest point of the female cavitas peritonealis.
— **Subperitoneal recesses** are extraperitoneal spaces that are continuous with the spatium retroperitoneale of the abdomen and are filled with fascia endopelvica.
  - The **retropubic space** (prevesical space, space of Retzius, **spatium retropubicum**) lies between the symphysis pubica and the bladder.
  - The **spatium retrorectale** (spatium presacrale) lies between the rectum and os sacrum.

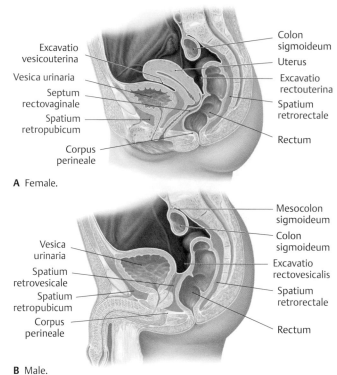

A Female.

B Male.

Fig. 14.13 Peritoneal and subperitoneal spaces in the pelvis
Midsagittal section, viewed from the left side. Subperitoneal spaces shown in *green*. (From Gilroy AM et al. Atlas of Anatomy. 4th ed. 2020. Based on: Schuenke M, Schulte E, Schumacher U. THIEME Atlas of Anatomy. Internal Organs. Illustrations by Voll M and Wesker K. 3rd ed. New York: Thieme Medical Publishers; 2020.)

— A double-layered peritoneal septum descends from the excavatio rectovesicalis (or excavatio rectouterina) to the perineum.
  • In males, this **septum rectovesicale** separates the rectum from the gll. seminales and prostata. Its lower part is often referred to as the **fascia rectoprostatica**.
  • In females, the **septum rectovaginale** separates the rectum from the vagina.

14.6 Neurovasculature of the Pelvis and Perineum

Arteries of the Pelvis and Perineum

Viscera pelvis are well vascularized, primarily by branches of the a. iliaca interna, with abundant ipsilateral and contralateral communications (**Fig. 14.14**).
— The **a. iliaca communis dextra** and **a. iliaca communis sinistra** descend along the linea terminalis before bifurcating into the a. iliaca externa and a. iliaca interna at the level of the discus intervertebralis L V–S I.
— Each **a. iliaca externa** continues along the linea terminalis, lateral to the accompanying vein, and enters the lower limb without contributing branches to viscera pelvis.
— Each **a. iliaca interna** descends into the pelvis minor along the lateral wall before branching into two divisions (**Table 14.3**)
  1. The anterior division supplies most of the pelvic viscera, structures of the perineum, and some muscles in the regio glutealis and thigh.

Table 14.3 Branches of the Arteria Iliaca Interna

Anterior Division		Posterior Division
Visceral branches	**Parietal branches**	**Parietal branches**
• A. umbilicalis—a. vesica superior*	• A. obturatoria • A. glutea inferior	• A. iliolumbalis • Aa. sacrales laterales • A. glutea superior
• A. uterina (female)		
• A. vaginalis (female)		
• A. vesicalis inferior (male)		
• A. rectalis media		
• A. pudenda interna		

*After birth, the distal portion of the a. umbilicalis obliterates, but its remnant remains as the lig. umbilicale medianum on the anterior abdominal wall; the proximal portion remains as the a. vesica superior to the vesica urinaria.

  2. The posterior division contributes only parietal branches that supply muscles of the posterior abdominal wall, lower back, and regio glutealis, as well as spinal branches that supply the meninges of the sacral spinal roots.
— The **a. pudenda interna**, a branch of the a. iliaca interna, supplies most structures in the perineum. It exits the pelvis through the foramen ischiadicum majus and then passes through the foramen ischiadicum minus into the perineum where it runs along the lateral wall of the regio analis to the membrana perinei. Its major branches (**Figs. 14.15** and **14.16**) include the following:
  • The **a. rectalis inferior**, which supplies the m. sphincter ani externus and skin around the anus
  • The **a. perinealis**, which supplies the structures of the spatium superficiale perinei through aa. scrotales posteriores or aa. labiales posteriores
  • The **a. dorsalis penis** or **a. dorsalis clitoridis**, which supplies structures in the spatium profundum perinei and the glans penis or glans clitoridis
— The **a. pudenda externa**, a branch of the a. femoralis in the thigh, supplies superficial tissues of the perineum.
Arteries of the pelvis that arise directly or indirectly from the aorta abdominalis provide an important additional collateral blood supply to pelvic viscera.
— The **aa. ovaricae and aa. testiculares** arise from the aorta abdominalis at L2 and descend along the posterior abdominal wall.
  • The a. ovarica crosses the linea terminalis and enters the pelvis within the **lig. suspensorium ovarii**. In the pelvis it supplies the ovary and tuba uterina and anastomoses with the a. uterina (**Fig. 14.17**).
  • The a. testicularis passes through the canalis inguinalis as part of the funiculus spermaticus to supply the testis. It does not supply any structures within the pelvis (**Fig 14.18**).
— The a. rectalis superior, a branch of the a. mesenterica inferior, supplies the upper rectum and canalis analis and anastomoses with a. rectalis media and a. rectalis inferior in the pelvis and perineum (**Fig. 14.19**).

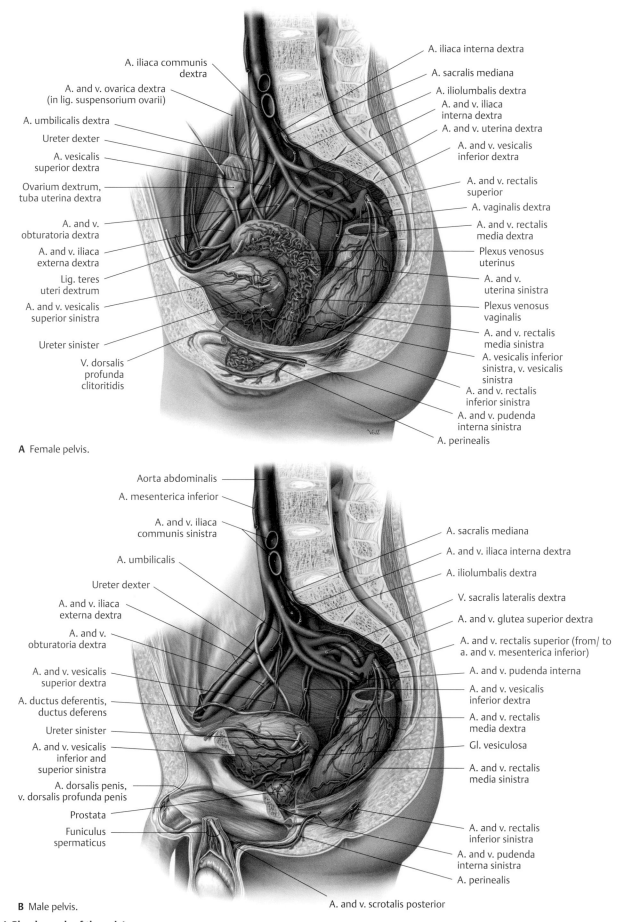

A Female pelvis.

A. iliaca communis dextra
A. and v. ovarica dextra (in lig. suspensorium ovarii)
A. umbilicalis dextra
Ureter dexter
A. vesicalis superior dextra
Ovarium dextrum, tuba uterina dextra
A. and v. obturatoria dextra
A. and v. iliaca externa dextra
Lig. teres uteri dextrum
A. and v. vesicalis superior sinistra
Ureter sinister
V. dorsalis profunda clitoritidis

A. iliaca interna dextra
A. sacralis mediana
A. iliolumbalis dextra
A. and v. iliaca interna dextra
A. and v. uterina dextra
A. and v. vesicalis inferior dextra
A. and v. rectalis superior
A. vaginalis dextra
A. and v. rectalis media dextra
Plexus venosus uterinus
A. and v. uterina sinistra
Plexus venosus vaginalis
A. and v. rectalis media sinistra
A. vesicalis inferior sinistra, v. vesicalis sinistra
A. and v. rectalis inferior sinistra
A. and v. pudenda interna sinistra
A. perinealis

B Male pelvis.

Aorta abdominalis
A. mesenterica inferior
A. and v. iliaca communis sinistra
A. umbilicalis
Ureter dexter
A. and v. iliaca externa dextra
A. and v. obturatoria dextra
A. and v. vesicalis superior dextra
A. ductus deferentis, ductus deferens
Ureter sinister
A. and v. vesicalis inferior and superior sinistra
A. dorsalis penis, v. dorsalis profunda penis
Prostata
Funiculus spermaticus

A. sacralis mediana
A. and v. iliaca interna dextra
A. iliolumbalis dextra
V. sacralis lateralis dextra
A. and v. glutea superior dextra
A. and v. rectalis superior (from/ to a. and v. mesenterica inferior)
A. and v. pudenda interna
A. and v. vesicalis inferior dextra
A. and v. rectalis media dextra
Gl. vesiculosa
A. and v. rectalis media sinistra
A. and v. rectalis inferior sinistra
A. and v. pudenda interna sinistra
A. perinealis
A. and v. scrotalis posterior

Fig. 14.14 Blood vessels of the pelvis
Idealized right hemipelvis, left lateral view. (From Gilroy AM et al. Atlas of Anatomy. 4th ed. 2020. Based on: Schuenke M, Schulte E, Schumacher U. THIEME Atlas of Anatomy. Internal Organs. Illustrations by Voll M and Wesker K. 3rd ed. New York: Thieme Medical Publishers; 2020.)

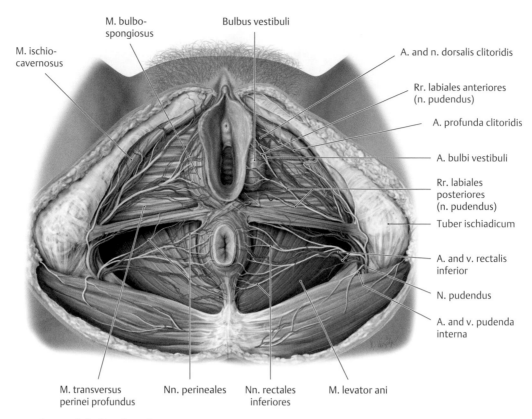

Fig. 14.15 Neurovasculature of the female perineum
Lithotomy position. *Removed:* M. bulbospongiosus sinister and m. ischiocavernosus. (From Schuenke M, Schulte E, Schumacher U. THIEME Atlas of Anatomy, Vol 1. Illustrations by Voll M and Wesker K. 3rd ed. New York: Thieme Publishers; 2020.)

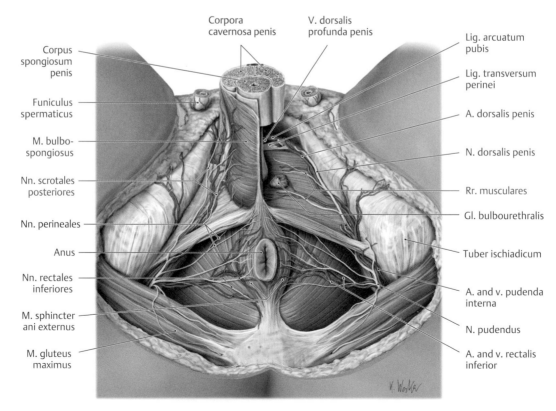

Fig. 14.16 Neurovasculature of the male perineum
Lithotomy position. *Removed from left side:* Membrana perinei, m. bulbospongiosus, and radix penis. (From Schuenke M, Schulte E, Schumacher U. THIEME Atlas of Anatomy, Vol 1. Illustrations by Voll M and Wesker K. 3rd ed. New York: Thieme Publishers; 2020.)

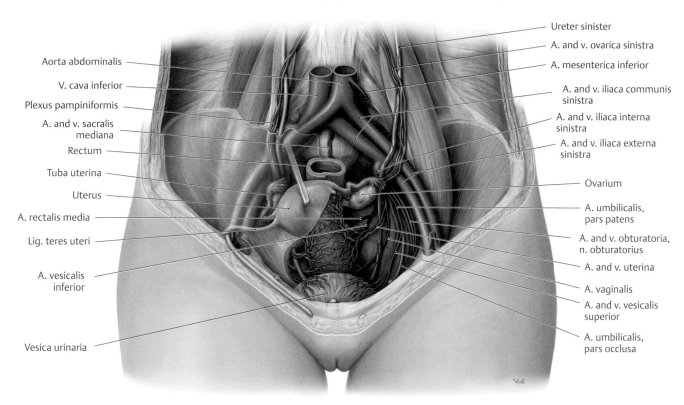

Aorta abdominalis

V. cava inferior

Plexus pampiniformis

A. and v. sacralis mediana

Rectum

Tuba uterina

Uterus

A. rectalis media

Lig. teres uteri

A. vesicalis inferior

Vesica urinaria

Ureter sinister

A. and v. ovarica sinistra

A. mesenterica inferior

A. and v. iliaca communis sinistra

A. and v. iliaca interna sinistra

A. and v. iliaca externa sinistra

Ovarium

A. umbilicalis, pars patens

A. and v. obturatoria, n. obturatorius

A. and v. uterina

A. vaginalis

A. and v. vesicalis superior

A. umbilicalis, pars occlusa

Fig. 14.17 Blood vessels of the female genitalia
Anterior view. *Removed from left side:* Peritoneum. *Displaced:* Uterus. (From Schuenke M, Schulte E, Schumacher U. THIEME Atlas of Anatomy, Vol 2. Illustrations by Voll M and Wesker K. 3rd ed. New York: Thieme Publishers; 2020.)

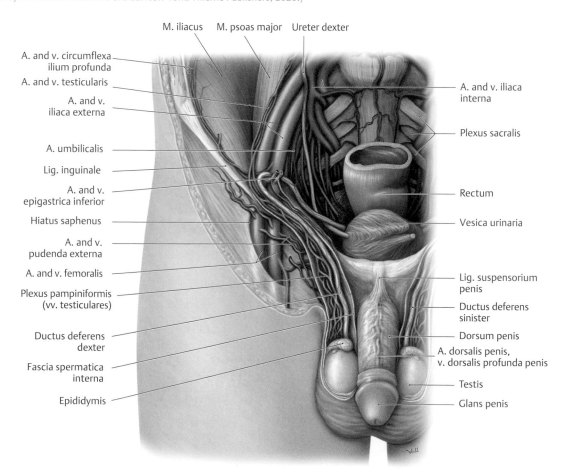

M. iliacus   M. psoas major   Ureter dexter

A. and v. circumflexa ilium profunda

A. and v. testicularis

A. and v. iliaca externa

A. umbilicalis

Lig. inguinale

A. and v. epigastrica inferior

Hiatus saphenus

A. and v. pudenda externa

A. and v. femoralis

Plexus pampiniformis (vv. testiculares)

Ductus deferens dexter

Fascia spermatica interna

Epididymis

A. and v. iliaca interna

Plexus sacralis

Rectum

Vesica urinaria

Lig. suspensorium penis

Ductus deferens sinister

Dorsum penis

A. dorsalis penis, v. dorsalis profunda penis

Testis

Glans penis

Fig. 14.18 Blood vessels of the male genitalia
Anterior view. *Opened:* Canalis inguinalis and coverings of the funiculus spermaticus. (From Schuenke M, Schulte E, Schumacher U. THIEME Atlas of Anatomy, Vol 2. Illustrations by Voll M and Wesker K. 3rd ed. New York: Thieme Publishers; 2020.)

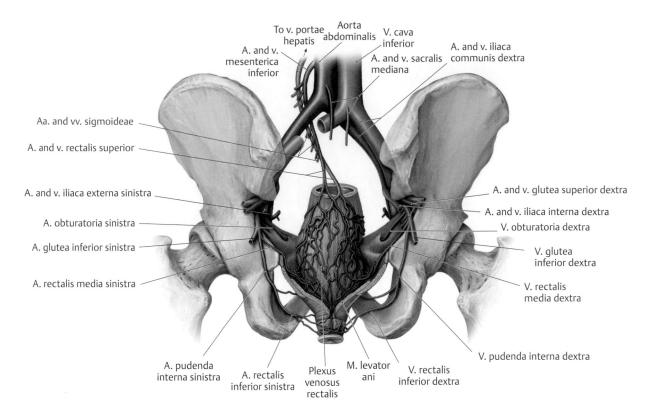

Fig. 14.19 Blood vessels of the rectum
Posterior view. The main blood supply to the rectum is from the a. rectalis superior; the aa. rectales mediae serve as an anastomosis between the a. rectalis superior and a. rectalis inferior. (From Schuenke M, Schulte E, Schumacher U. THIEME Atlas of Anatomy, Vol 2. Illustrations by Voll M and Wesker K. 3rd ed. New York: Thieme Publishers; 2020.)

Veins of the Pelvis and Perineum

Blood from most viscera pelvis drains to a plexus venosus contained either within the fascia visceralis surrounding the organ (bladder, prostate) or within the organ wall (rectum).

— The plexus venosus visceralis in the pelvis communicate freely, and most drain to the inferior vena caval system through tributaries of the vv. iliacae internae that accompany the arteries of similar name and vascular territory (area supplied by a vessel) (see **Fig. 14.14**).

— The **v. pudenda interna** accompanies the a. pudenda interna and drains most structures of the perineum. However, erectile tissues in the regio urogenitalis drain through **vv. dorsales profundi** that pass under the symphysis pubica to join with plexus venosus visceralis in the pelvis.

— The **vv. iliacae internae** ascend from the pelvis to join with the **vv. iliacae externae**. These join to form the **v. iliaca communis dextra** and **v. iliaca communis sinistra**, which converge to form the v. cava inferior at L V.

— There are three alternate venous drainages from viscera pelvis.
  1. Vv. ovaricae drain directly into the v. cava inferior on the right and into the v. renalis on the left, but they also communicate with other pelvic plexus venosus (uterinus, vaginalis), which drain to the vv. iliacae internae (see **Fig. 14.17**).
  2. The v. rectalis superior drains to the hepatic portal system through the v. mesenterica inferior. This drainage establishes an anastomosis between the portal and caval venous systems (a portosystemic anastomosis) with the v. rectalis media and v. rectalis inferior, which are tributaries of the vv. iliacae internae (see **Figs. 14.19**).
  3. The plexus venosus vertebralis, which drains into the azygos system, communicates with pelvic plexus venosus visceralis through tributaries of the vv. iliacae internae (see **Fig. 3.17**).

Lymphatics of the Pelvis and Perineum

Lymph from the pelvis and perineum travels through one or more groups of lymph nodes, all of which ultimately drain into the ductus thoracicus **(Table 14.4)**. The groups of nodes tend to be interconnected but vary in size and number.

There are several general drainage patterns.

— Within the pelvis, lymph drainage usually follows venous pathways, although structures that drain to the nll. iliaci externi do not follow this pattern.

— Nll. iliaci externi receive lymph from the superior parts of the anterior viscera pelvis.

— Nll. iliaci interni receive lymph from deep pelvic and deep perineal structures.

— Nll. sacrales receive lymph from deep posterior viscera pelvis.

— Nll. inguinales superficiales and nll. inguinales superficiales profundi drain most structures of the perineum.

— Nll. inguinales drain to nll. iliaci externi.

— Nll. iliaci externi, nll. iliaci interni, and nll. sacrales drain to nll. iliaci communes, which in turn drain to nll. aortici laterales and trunci lumbales.

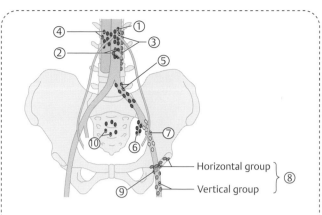

Table 14.4 Lymph Nodes of the Pelvis
(From Gilroy AM et al. Atlas of Anatomy. 4th ed. 2020. Based on: Schuenke M, Schulte E, Schumacher U. THIEME Atlas of Anatomy. Internal Organs. Illustrations by Voll M and Wesker K. 3rd ed. New York: Thieme Medical Publishers; 2020.)

Nll. preaortici	① Nll. mesenterici superiores
	② Nll. mesenterici inferiores
③ Nll. aorticic laterales sinistri	
④ Nll. aorticic (cavales) laterales dextri	
⑤ Nll. iliaci communes	
⑥ Nll. iliaci interni	
⑦ Nll. iliaci externi	
⑧ Nll. inguinales superficiales	Horizontal group
	Vertical group
⑨ Nll. inguinales profundi	
⑩ Nll. sacrales	
Abbreviation: nll., lymph nodes	

Nerves of the Pelvis and Perineum

Nerves of the pelvis and perineum include branches from somatic nerve plexuses as well as autonomic plexuses. Somatic nerves arise from the plexus lumbalis and plexus sacralis.

— The plexus lumbalis (T12–L4) forms on the posterior abdominal wall (see **Fig. 11.26**). Its nerves primarily innervate muscles and skin of the lower abdominal wall and lower limb. However, its n. ilioinguinalis and n. genitofemoralis transmit sensation from the mons pubis and labia and anterior scrotum in the perineum.
   • The n. obturatorius (L2–L4) passes along the sidewall of the pelvis and exits through the canalis obturatorius. Although it does not innervate structures of the pelvis, its location is noteworthy because it can be injured during pelvic surgery.
— The **plexus sacralis** forms on the posterior wall of the pelvis from the rami anteriores of L4–S4. Except for short branches to pelvic floor muscles, branches of the plexus exit the pelvis through the foramen ischiadicum majus, where they innervate structures in the perineum, regio glutealis, and lower limb (see Section 15.4). Its branches in the pelvis include
   • The **n. pudendus** (S2–S4), a branch of the plexus sacralis, is the primary nerve of the perineum. It passes through the foramen ischiadicum majus close to the spina ischiadica and

then into the perineum through the foramen ischiadicum minus, where it courses anteriorly with the a. and v. pudenda interna. The n. pudendus is a mixed somatic nerve (motor and sensory) but also carries postganglionic sympathetic fibers to perineal structures. Its major branches include the following (**Figs. 14.20** and **14.21**):
   ◦ The **n. rectalis inferior**, which innervates the m. sphincter ani externus
   ◦ The **n. perinealis**, which supplies cutaneous branches to the scrotum and labia and motor branches to the muscles of the spatium profundum perinei and spatium superficialis perinei
   ◦ The **n. dorsalis penis (n. dorsalis clitoridis)**, which is the primary sensory nerve to the penis and clitoris, especially to the glans.

Autonomic innervation of the pelvis includes both sympathetic and parasympathetic contributions (**Figs. 14.22, 14.23, 14.24, 14.25**; see also **Table 11.8**).

— **Trunci sympathici sacrales**, the continuations of the trunci sympathici lumbales, descend along the anterior surface of the os sacrum to the os coccygis, where they merge to form a small ganglion, the **ganglion impar**. The primary function of this part of the trunci sympathici is to provide postganglionic sympathetic fibers via nn. splanchnici sacrales to lower limb branches of the plexus sacralis. It contributes a few fibers to the visceral plexuses of the pelvis.
— The **plexus hypogastricus superior**, a continuation of the plexus intermesentericus in the abdomen, receives additional contributions from the two lower nn. splanchnici lumbales (sympathetic). It drapes over the bifurcatio aortae and branches into **n. hypogastricus dexter** and **n. hypogastricus sinister**, which pass into the pelvis.
— The **nn. splanchnici pelvici**, are the pelvic component of the parasympathetic nervous system. They originate from the medulla spinalis sacralis and enter the pelvis with the rami anteriores S2–S4.
— The nn. hypogastrici, joined by nn. splanchnici sacrales (sympathetic) and nn. splanchnici pelvici (parasympathetic), form **plexus hypogastricus inferior dexter** and **plexus hypogastricus inferior sinister**.
— **Plexus rectalis**, **plexus uterovaginalis** (in females), **plexus prostaticus** (in males), and **plexus vesicalis** are derived from the plexus hypogastricus inferior and surround individual pelvic organs.
   • **Nn. cavernosi** arising from the plexus hypogastricus inferior pass through the hiatus urogenitalis carrying parasympathetic nerves to perineal structures. They are responsible for engorgement of the erectile tissue and erection of the penis and clitoris. They are particularly at risk during surgical removal of the prostate.
— Visceral afferent fibers from most structures in the pelvis travel with sympathetic or parasympathetic nerves, depending on the relationship of the viscera to the peritoneum, a division known as the "pelvic pain line."
   • From pelvic viscera in contact with the peritoneum, sensory fibers travel with sympathetic nerves to the plexus hypogastricus superior and medulla spinalis thoracica.
   • From viscera pelvis below the peritoneum, afferent fibers travel with nn. splanchnici pelvici to the medulla spinalis sacralis.
   • Although the rectum is in contact with the peritoneum on most of its surfaces, its visceral afferent fibers also travel with nn. splanchnici pelvici.

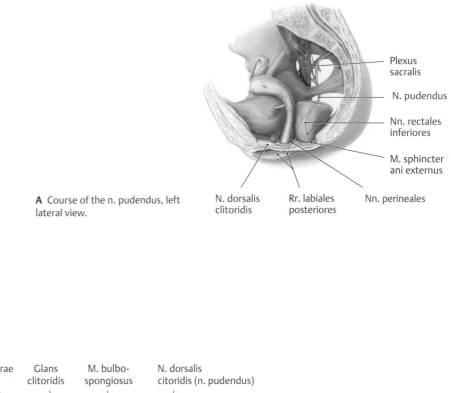

A Course of the n. pudendus, left lateral view.

Plexus sacralis

N. pudendus

Nn. rectales inferiores

M. sphincter ani externus

N. dorsalis clitoridis

Rr. labiales posteriores

Nn. perineales

N. ilioinguinalis and n. genitofemoralis, r. genitalis and r. labialis

N. pudendus

N. cutaneus femoris posterior

Nn. clunium medii

Nn. clunium superiores

Nn. clunium inferiores

Nn. anococcygei

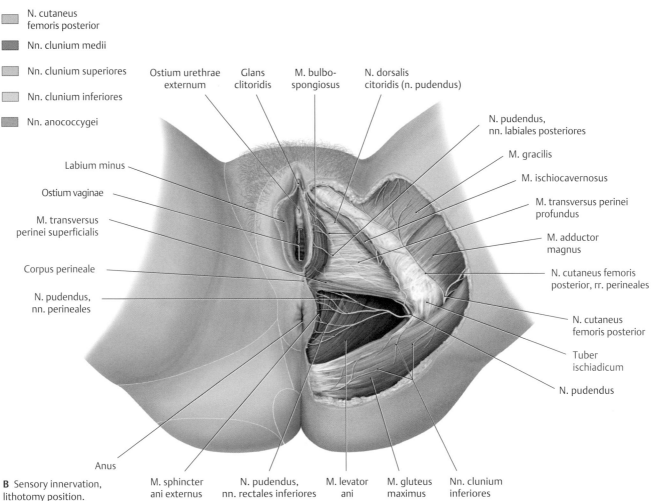

Ostium urethrae externum

Glans clitoridis

M. bulbo-spongiosus

N. dorsalis citoridis (n. pudendus)

Labium minus

Ostium vaginae

M. transversus perinei superficialis

Corpus perineale

N. pudendus, nn. perineales

Anus

N. pudendus, nn. labiales posteriores

M. gracilis

M. ischiocavernosus

M. transversus perinei profundus

M. adductor magnus

N. cutaneus femoris posterior, rr. perineales

N. cutaneus femoris posterior

Tuber ischiadicum

N. pudendus

M. sphincter ani externus

N. pudendus, nn. rectales inferiores

M. levator ani

M. gluteus maximus

Nn. clunium inferiores

B Sensory innervation, lithotomy position.

Fig. 14.20 Nerves of the female perineum and genitalia
(From Schuenke M, Schulte E, Schumacher U. THIEME Atlas of Anatomy, Vol 1. Illustrations by Voll M and Wesker K. 3rd ed. New York: Thieme Publishers; 2020.)

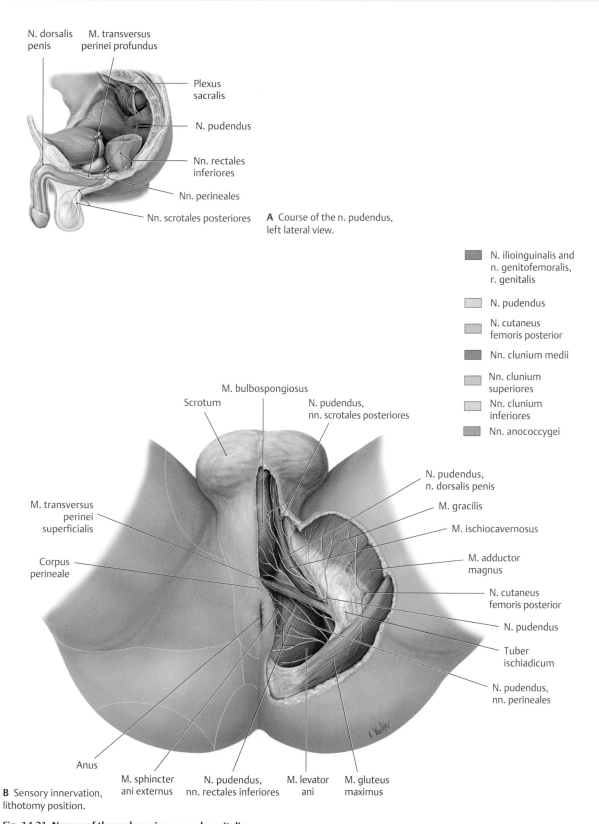

N. dorsalis penis

M. transversus perinei profundus

Plexus sacralis

N. pudendus

Nn. rectales inferiores

Nn. perineales

Nn. scrotales posteriores

A Course of the n. pudendus, left lateral view.

N. ilioinguinalis and n. genitofemoralis, r. genitalis

N. pudendus

N. cutaneus femoris posterior

Nn. clunium medii

Nn. clunium superiores

Nn. clunium inferiores

Nn. anococcygei

M. bulbospongiosus

Scrotum

N. pudendus, nn. scrotales posteriores

N. pudendus, n. dorsalis penis

M. gracilis

M. ischiocavernosus

M. adductor magnus

N. cutaneus femoris posterior

N. pudendus

Tuber ischiadicum

N. pudendus, nn. perineales

M. transversus perinei superficialis

Corpus perineale

Anus

M. sphincter ani externus

N. pudendus, nn. rectales inferiores

M. levator ani

M. gluteus maximus

B Sensory innervation, lithotomy position.

Fig. 14.21 Nerves of the male perineum and genitalia
(From Schuenke M, Schulte E, Schumacher U. THIEME Atlas of Anatomy, Vol 1. Illustrations by Voll M and Wesker K. 3rd ed. New York: Thieme Publishers; 2020.)

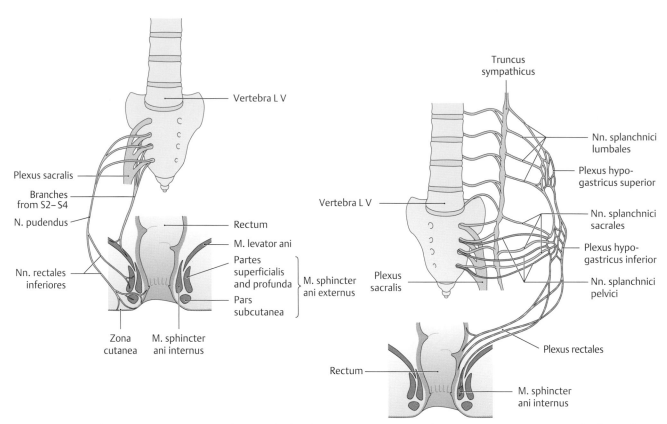

A Somatomotor and somatosensory innervation. The nn. pudendi and nn. rectales inferiores provide active, partly voluntary innervation of the m. sphincter ani externus and m. levator ani, and sensation for the anus and perianal skin.

B Visceromotor and viscerosensory innervation. Nn. splanchnici pelvici (S2–S4) innervate the m. sphincter ani internus, which helps maintain closure of the canalis analis. They also supply sensation to the wall of the rectum, particularly the stretch receptors in the ampulla recti, which when stretched trigger an awareness of the need to defecate.

Fig. 14.22 Innervation of the anal sphincter mechanism
(From Gilroy AM et al. Atlas of Anatomy. 4th ed. 2020. Based on: Schuenke M, Schulte E, Schumacher U. THIEME Atlas of Anatomy. Internal Organs. Illustrations by Voll M and Wesker K. 3rd ed. New York: Thieme Medical Publishers; 2020.)

BOX 14.3: CLINICAL CORRELATION

PUDENDAL NERVE BLOCK
During labor, anesthesia of the n. pudendus can ease perineal pain of delivery. A pudendal block can be administered through the posterior wall of the vagina, with the surgeon aiming the needle toward the spina ischiadica. The block can also be administered externally, inserting the needle through the skin medial to the tuber ischiadicum. Since the n. pudendus innervates only the perineum, the superior vagina and cervix are not affected by the block, and the mother continues to feel the uterine contractions.

BOX 14.4: CLINICAL CORRELATION

PAIN TRANSMISSION DURING LABOR AND DELIVERY
The sensation of pain travels along both visceral sensory and somatic sensory routes during labor and delivery. The dividing line between these routes is the pelvic pain line, which refers to the relation of viscera pelvis to the peritoneum. Pain from the body and fundus of the uterus (intraperitoneal) travel along sympathetic nerves to the Plexus hypogastricus superior, and pain from the cervix and upper two-thirds of the vagina (subperitoneal) along parasympathetic nerves to the medulla spinalis sacralis. Pain from superficial structures, the lower vagina and perineum, travels via branches of the n. pudendus to the plexus sacralis.

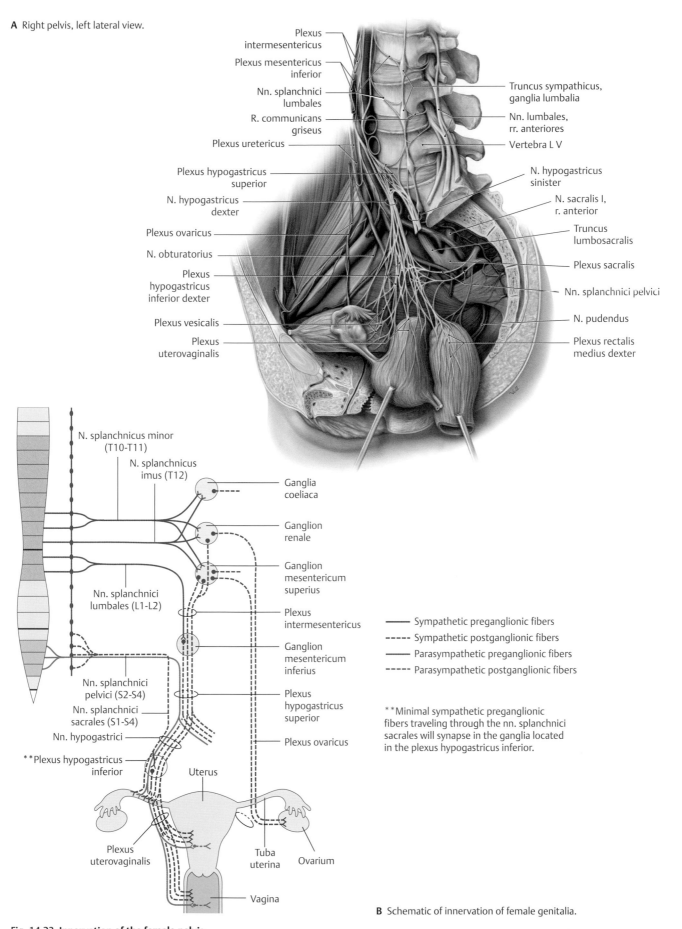

A Right pelvis, left lateral view.

Plexus intermesentericus
Plexus mesentericus inferior
Nn. splanchnici lumbales
R. communicans griseus
Plexus uretericus
Plexus hypogastricus superior
N. hypogastricus dexter
Plexus ovaricus
N. obturatorius
Plexus hypogastricus inferior dexter
Plexus vesicalis
Plexus uterovaginalis

Truncus sympathicus, ganglia lumbalia
Nn. lumbales, rr. anteriores
Vertebra L V
N. hypogastricus sinister
N. sacralis I, r. anterior
Truncus lumbosacralis
Plexus sacralis
Nn. splanchnici pelvici
N. pudendus
Plexus rectalis medius dexter

N. splanchnicus minor (T10-T11)
N. splanchnicus imus (T12)
Nn. splanchnici lumbales (L1-L2)
Nn. splanchnici pelvici (S2-S4)
Nn. splanchnici sacrales (S1-S4)
Nn. hypogastrici
**Plexus hypogastricus inferior
Uterus
Plexus uterovaginalis
Tuba uterina
Ovarium
Vagina

Ganglia coeliaca
Ganglion renale
Ganglion mesentericum superius
Plexus intermesentericus
Ganglion mesentericum inferius
Plexus hypogastricus superior
Plexus ovaricus

—— Sympathetic preganglionic fibers
----- Sympathetic postganglionic fibers
—— Parasympathetic preganglionic fibers
----- Parasympathetic postganglionic fibers

**Minimal sympathetic preganglionic fibers traveling through the nn. splanchnici sacrales will synapse in the ganglia located in the plexus hypogastricus inferior.

B Schematic of innervation of female genitalia.

Fig. 14.23 Innervation of the female pelvis
(From Gilroy AM et al. Atlas of Anatomy. 4th ed. 2020. Based on: Schuenke M, Schulte E, Schumacher U. THIEME Atlas of Anatomy. Internal Organs. Illustrations by Voll M and Wesker K. 3rd ed. New York: Thieme Medical Publishers; 2020.)

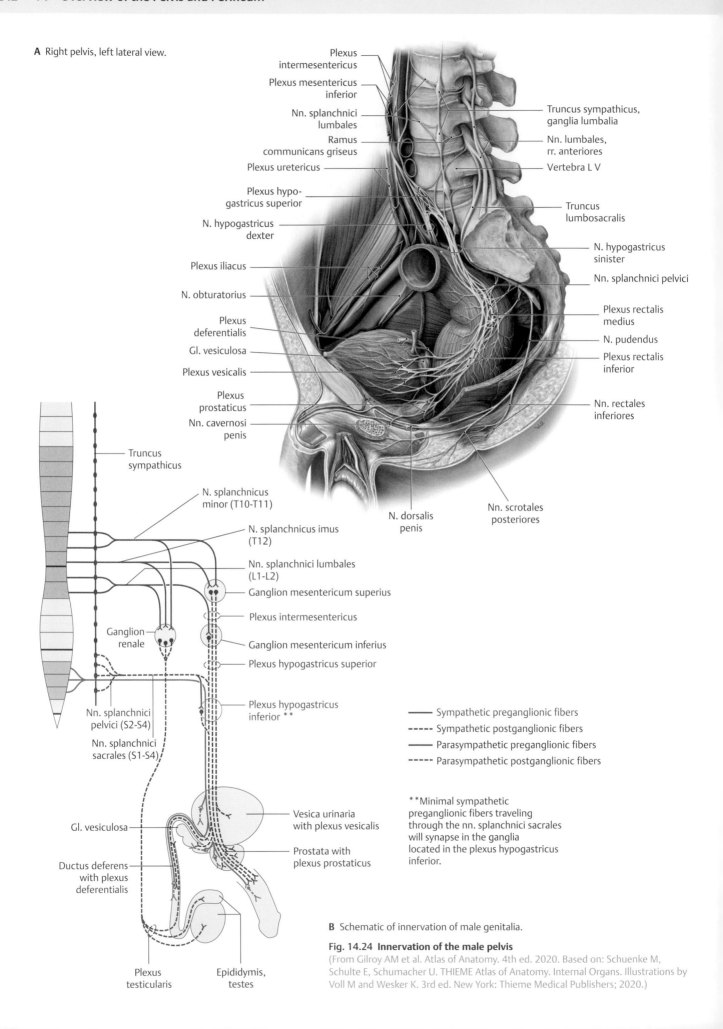

A Right pelvis, left lateral view.

Plexus intermesentericus

Plexus mesentericus inferior

Nn. splanchnici lumbales

Ramus communicans griseus

Plexus uretericus

Plexus hypo- gastricus superior

N. hypogastricus dexter

Plexus iliacus

N. obturatorius

Plexus deferentialis

Gl. vesiculosa

Plexus vesicalis

Plexus prostaticus

Nn. cavernosi penis

Truncus sympathicus, ganglia lumbalia

Nn. lumbales, rr. anteriores

Vertebra L V

Truncus lumbosacralis

N. hypogastricus sinister

Nn. splanchnici pelvici

Plexus rectalis medius

N. pudendus

Plexus rectalis inferior

Nn. rectales inferiores

Nn. scrotales posteriores

N. dorsalis penis

Truncus sympathicus

N. splanchnicus minor (T10-T11)

N. splanchnicus imus (T12)

Nn. splanchnici lumbales (L1-L2)

Ganglion mesentericum superius

Plexus intermesentericus

Ganglion renale

Ganglion mesentericum inferius

Plexus hypogastricus superior

Plexus hypogastricus inferior **

Nn. splanchnici pelvici (S2-S4)

Nn. splanchnici sacrales (S1-S4)

Gl. vesiculosa

Ductus deferens with plexus deferentialis

Vesica urinaria with plexus vesicalis

Prostata with plexus prostaticus

Plexus testicularis

Epididymis, testes

——— Sympathetic preganglionic fibers

- - - - Sympathetic postganglionic fibers

——— Parasympathetic preganglionic fibers

- - - - Parasympathetic postganglionic fibers

**Minimal sympathetic preganglionic fibers traveling through the nn. splanchnici sacrales will synapse in the ganglia located in the plexus hypogastricus inferior.

B Schematic of innervation of male genitalia.

Fig. 14.24 Innervation of the male pelvis
(From Gilroy AM et al. Atlas of Anatomy. 4th ed. 2020. Based on: Schuenke M, Schulte E, Schumacher U. THIEME Atlas of Anatomy. Internal Organs. Illustrations by Voll M and Wesker K. 3rd ed. New York: Thieme Medical Publishers; 2020.)

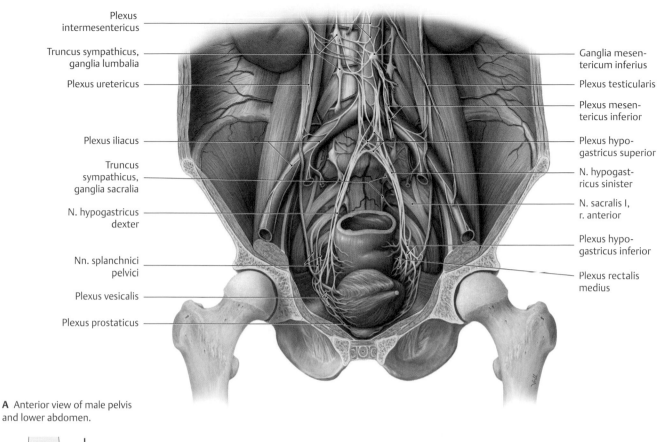

Plexus intermesentericus

Truncus sympathicus, ganglia lumbalia

Plexus uretericus

Plexus iliacus

Truncus sympathicus, ganglia sacralia

N. hypogastricus dexter

Nn. splanchnici pelvici

Plexus vesicalis

Plexus prostaticus

Ganglia mesentericum inferius

Plexus testicularis

Plexus mesentericus inferior

Plexus hypogastricus superior

N. hypogastricus sinister

N. sacralis I, r. anterior

Plexus hypogastricus inferior

Plexus rectalis medius

A Anterior view of male pelvis and lower abdomen.

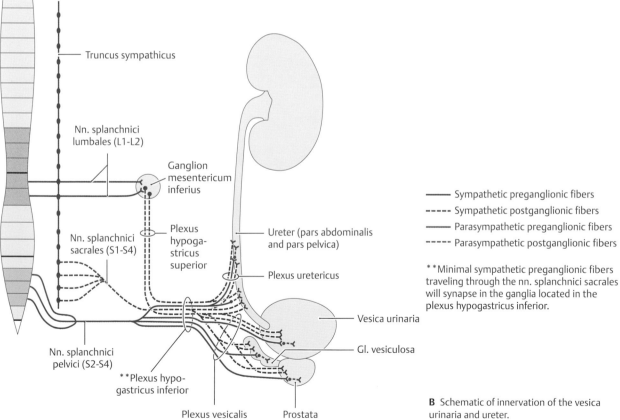

Truncus sympathicus

Nn. splanchnici lumbales (L1-L2)

Ganglion mesentericum inferius

Nn. splanchnici sacrales (S1-S4)

Plexus hypogastricus superior

Plexus uretericus

Ureter (pars abdominalis and pars pelvica)

Nn. splanchnici pelvici (S2-S4)

Vesica urinaria

Gl. vesiculosa

**Plexus hypogastricus inferior

Plexus vesicalis

Prostata

——— Sympathetic preganglionic fibers

- - - - Sympathetic postganglionic fibers

——— Parasympathetic preganglionic fibers

- - - - Parasympathetic postganglionic fibers

**Minimal sympathetic preganglionic fibers traveling through the nn. splanchnici sacrales will synapse in the ganglia located in the plexus hypogastricus inferior.

B Schematic of innervation of the vesica urinaria and ureter.

Fig. 14.25 Innervation of the pelvic urinary organs
(From Gilroy AM et al. Atlas of Anatomy. 4th ed. 2020. Based on: Schuenke M, Schulte E, Schumacher U. THIEME Atlas of Anatomy. Internal Organs. Illustrations by Voll M and Wesker K. 3rd ed. New York: Thieme Medical Publishers; 2020.)

15 Pelvic Viscera

The pelvic cavity (cavitas pelvis) contains the male or female genital organs, the pelvic urinary organs, and the rectum. These organs normally reside in the pelvis minor, although when enlarged the vesica urinaria and uterus can extend into the cavitas abdominis.

15.1 Male Genital Structures

The male gonad, the testis, is located in the regio inguinalis and is discussed in Chapter 10. The seminal vesicle (glandula vesiculosa) and prostata are male accessory reproductive structures found in the pelvis (**Fig. 15.1**).

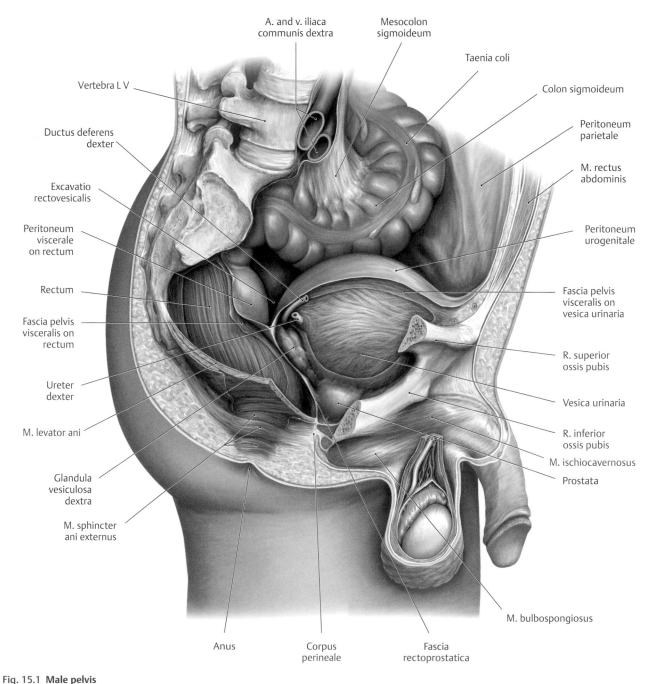

Fig. 15.1 Male pelvis
Parasagittal section, viewed from the right side. (From Gilroy AM et al. Atlas of Anatomy. 4th ed. 2020. Based on: Schuenke M, Schulte E, Schumacher U. THIEME Atlas of Anatomy. Internal Organs. Illustrations by Voll M and Wesker K. 3rd ed. New York: Thieme Medical Publishers; 2020.)

Seminal Vesicles (Glandula Vesiculosae)

The **seminal vesicles (glandulae vesiculosae)** are paired convoluted ducts that produce 70% of the seminal fluid (**Figs. 15.2** and **15.3**).

— They lie superior to the prostata, between the vesica urinaria and the rectum.
— The seminal vesicles are subperitoneal, located immediately below the peritoneum of the excavatio rectovesicalis.
— The duct of each vesicle joins with the ampulla of the ductus deferens to form the **ductus ejaculatorii**, which pierce the prostata and drain into the **pars prostatica urethrae**.
— The a. rectalis media and a. vesicalis inferior supply the vesicles. Veins of similar names accompany the arteries.
— Branches from the plexus pelvicus innervate the vesicles.

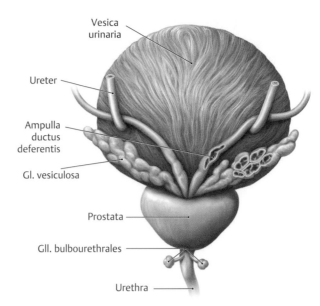

Fig. 15.2 Accessory sex glands
The vesica urinaria, prostata, gll. vesiculosae, and gll. bulbourethrales, posterior view. (From Schuenke M, Schulte E, Schumacher U. THIEME Atlas of Anatomy, Vol 2. Illustrations by Voll M and Wesker K. 3rd ed. New York: Thieme Publishers; 2020.)

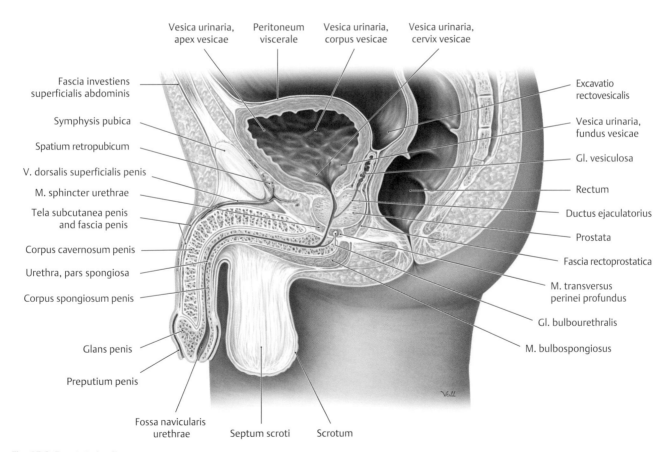

Fig. 15.3 Prostata in situ
Sagittal section through the male pelvis, left lateral view. (From Schuenke M, Schulte E, Schumacher U. THIEME Atlas of Anatomy, Vol 2. Illustrations by Voll M and Wesker K. 3rd ed. New York: Thieme Publishers; 2020.)

The Prostate (Prostata)

The **prostata** is an accessory reproductive gland that produces ~ 25% of the seminal fluid (**Fig. 15.4**; see also **Figs. 15.2** and **15.3**).

— The base, or superior surface, sits directly below the vesica urinaria. The apex points inferiorly and is in contact with the m. sphincter urethrae externus.

— It is posterior to the lower part of the symphysis pubica and anterior to the **septum rectovesicale**, which separates it from the rectum.

— The prostata surrounds the pars prostatica of the urethra. Secretions from prostatic glands drain into the urethra through numerous ductuli prostatici.

— A fibromuscular capsule surrounds the prostata. The capsula prostatica is separated from the outer fascia prostatae (derived from endopelvic fascia) by the plexus venosus prostaticus.

— **Ligg. puboprostatica**, anterior extensions of the arcus tendineus fasciae pelvis, attach the apex prostata (and cervix vesicae) to the os pubis (see **Fig. 15.17**). Posterior extensions of the arcus tendineus secure it to the os sacrum.

— The anatomic lobes of the prostata include the following:
  • A fibromuscular isthmus anterior to the urethra
  • Right and left lateral lobes that are subdivided into lobules

• The lower posterior lobule (sometimes referred to as the posterior lobe), which lies posterior to the urethra and inferior to the ductus ejaculatorii, is palpable by digital exam.

• A poorly defined middle lobe that sits above the lateral lobes between the urethra and ductus ejaculatorii and is in close contact with the cervix vesicae

— For clinical purposes, the prostata is divided into three major zones determined by their proximity to the urethra: **periurethral, central** (comparable to the anatomic middle lobe), and **peripheral.** A small **transition zone** consists of two lobes that account for approximately 5% of the glandular prostatic tissue (**Fig 15.5**).

— Aa. prostatica are usually branches of the aa. vesicales inferiores. Aa. rectalis media also contribute to the prostatic blood supply (see Section 14.6).

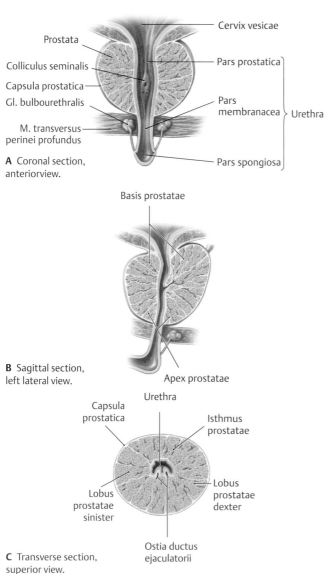

A Coronal section, anterior view.

B Sagittal section, left lateral view.

C Transverse section, superior view.

Fig. 15.4 Prostata
(From Schuenke M, Schulte E, Schumacher U. THIEME Atlas of Anatomy, Vol 2. Illustrations by Voll M and Wesker K. 3rd ed. New York: Thieme Publishers; 2020.)

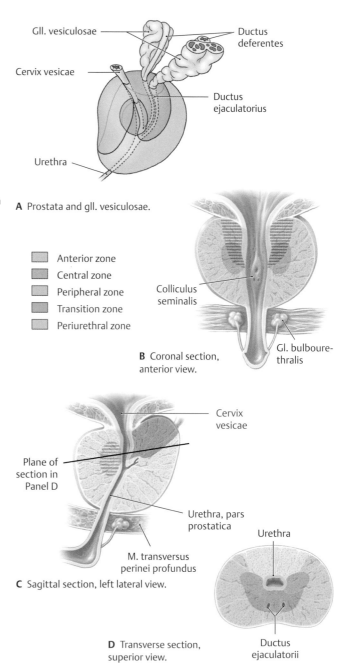

A Prostata and gll. vesiculosae.

Anterior zone
Central zone
Peripheral zone
Transition zone
Periurethral zone

B Coronal section, anterior view.

C Sagittal section, left lateral view.

D Transverse section, superior view.

Fig. 15.5 Clinical divisions of the prostata
(From Schuenke M, Schulte E, Schumacher U. THIEME Atlas of Anatomy, Vol 2. Illustrations by Voll M and Wesker K. 3rd ed. New York: Thieme Publishers; 2020.)

PROSTATECTOMY

Prostatectomy is the surgical removal of the prostata. Open radical prostatectomy involves removal of the prostata along with the seminal vesicles, ductus deferens, and nll. pelvici via a retropubic or perineal incision. Transurethral resection of the prostata (TURP) is performed using a cystoscope that is advanced through the urethra to resect the prostata. Nn. cavernosi carrying parasympathetic fibers that are responsible for penile erection run alongside the prostata and are particularly at risk during these procedures.

PROSTATIC CARCINOMA AND HYPERTROPHY

Prostatic carcinoma is one of the most common malignant tumors in older men, often growing at a subcapsular location (deep to the capsula prostatica) in the peripheral zone of the prostata. Unlike benign prostatic hypertrophy, which begins in the central part of the gland, prostatic carcinoma does not cause urinary outflow obstruction in its early stages. Being in the peripheral zone, the tumor is palpable as a firm mass through the anterior wall of the rectum during rectal examination. In certain prostate diseases, especially cancer, increased amounts of a protein, prostate-specific antigen or PSA, appear in the blood. This protein can be measured by a simple blood test.

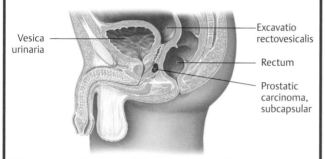

Vesica urinaria — Excavatio rectovesicalis — Rectum — Prostatic carcinoma, subcapsular

Most common site of prostatic carcinoma. (From Gilroy AM et al. Atlas of Anatomy. 4th ed. 2020. Based on: Schuenke M, Schulte E, Schumacher U. THIEME Atlas of Anatomy. Internal Organs. Illustrations by Voll M and Wesker K. 3rd ed. New York: Thieme Medical Publishers; 2020.)

— The plexus venosus prostaticus, continuous with the plexus venosus vesicalis of vesica urinaria, drains to vv. iliaca interna. The plexus venosus prostaticus also communicates with the plexus venosus vertebralis (see **Fig. 3.17**).
— The lymph vessels of the prostata follow venous pathways to the nll. iliaci interni.
— The plexus nervosus prostaticus is a derivative of the plexus hypogastricus inferior. The role of parasympathetic innervation is unclear, but sympathetic nerves cause the smooth muscle of the gland to contract, expelling prostatic secretion into the pars prostatica of the urethra during ejaculation.

15.2 Female Genital Structures

Female genital structures, which include the ovarium, tuba uterina, uterus, and vagina, are located in the middle of the pelvis between the vesica urinaria anteriorly and the rectum posteriorly (**Figs. 15.6** and **15.7**).

The Ovary (Ovarium)

The **ovary (ovarium)** is the female gonad, an ovoid structure that produces eggs and reproductive hormones and resides in the lateral wall of the pelvis (**Fig. 15.8**).
— The **lig. ovarii proprium** attaches the ovarium to the supralateral aspect of the uterus.
— The **lig. suspensorium ovarii** is a fold of peritoneum that encloses the ovarian vessels, lymphatics, and nerves as they pass over the pelvic brim to the ovarium.
— The **mesovarium** suspends the ovarium from the posterior part of the lig. latum uteri.
— The a. ovarica, a branch of the aorta abdominalis at L II, supplies the ovarium (see Section 14.6).
— Plexus pampiniformis, which may converge to form a single v. ovarica, drains the ovarium. The v. ovarica dextra is a direct tributary of the v. cava inferior; the v. ovarica sinistra is a tributary of the v. renalis sinistra.
— Lymphatic vessels follow the ovarian vessels superiorly to the nll. aortici laterales.
— Both the plexus nervosum ovaricus, which follows the ovarian vessels, and the plexus nervosum pelvicus, which follows the uterine vessels, innervate the ovarium.

The Uterine Tubes (Tubae Uterinae)

The **uterine tubes (tubae uterinae)** (tubae uterinae; fallopian tubes, oviducts), paired muscular tubes that extend laterally from the horns (supralateral corners) of the uterus, transmit ova from the ovary and sperm from the cavitas uteri (see **Fig. 15.8**).
— The tubae uterinae are the normal sites of fertilization and are also the most common sites of ectopic pregnancies (implantation of a fertilized ovum outside the uterus).
— The tuba uterina has four parts:
 1. The uterine (intramural) part, the segment that passes through the wall of the uterus
 2. The isthmus, the narrowest part
 3. The ampulla, the longest and widest part and normally the site of fertilization
 4. The infundibulum, the trumpet-shaped terminal part that is open to the cavitas peritonealis, with fingerlike fimbriae that surround the ovarium
— The tuba uterina is ensheathed in the upper edge of the lig. latum uteri, where it is supported by its mesosalpinx.
— The tuba uterina is supplied by the anastomosing a. ovarica and a. uterina and drained by accompanying veins.
— Lymph vessels follow the vv. ovaricae to the nll. aortici laterales.
— The ovarian and uterine plexuses innervate the tubae uterinae.

ECTOPIC PREGNANCY

Implantation of a fertilized ovum outside the uterus can occur anywhere, but the ampulla tubae uterinae is the most common site. Often the tube has been partially blocked by inflammation (salpingitis), preventing the blastocyst from completing its journey to the uterus. If not diagnosed early in the pregnancy, rupture of the tuba uterina with consequent hemorrhage into the cavitas peritonealis can result in a life-threatening situation for the mother. A ruptured ectopic pregnancy on the right side may be misdiagnosed as a ruptured appendix because both conditions irritate the peritoneum parietale and have similar presentations.

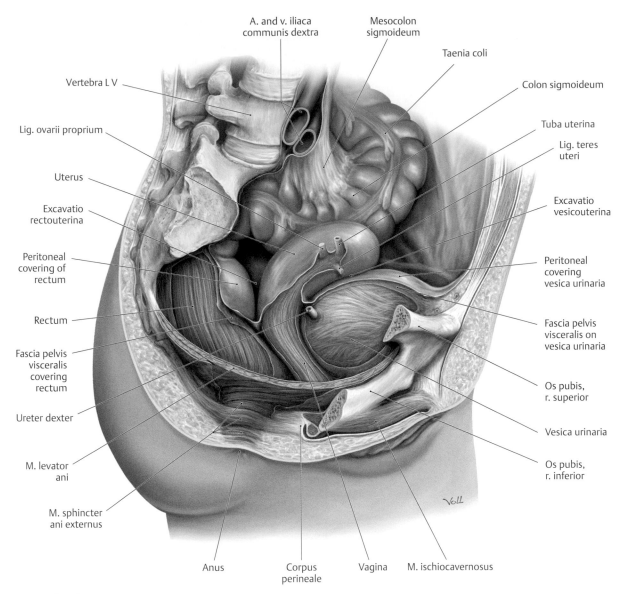

Fig. 15.6 Female pelvis
Parasagittal section, viewed from the right side. (From Gilroy AM et al. Atlas of Anatomy. 4th ed. 2020. Based on: Schuenke M, Schulte E, Schumacher U. THIEME Atlas of Anatomy. Internal Organs. Illustrations by Voll M and Wesker K. 3rd ed. New York: Thieme Medical Publishers; 2020.)

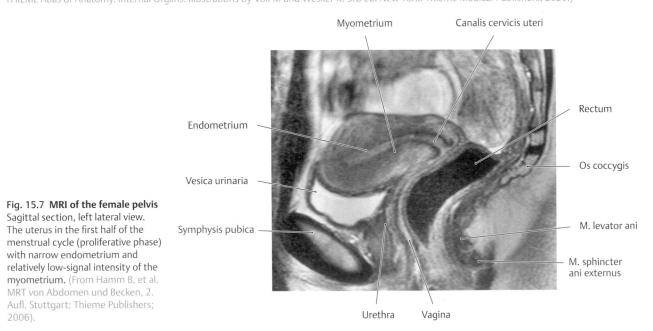

Fig. 15.7 MRI of the female pelvis
Sagittal section, left lateral view. The uterus in the first half of the menstrual cycle (proliferative phase) with narrow endometrium and relatively low-signal intensity of the myometrium. (From Hamm B, et al. MRT von Abdomen und Becken, 2. Aufl. Stuttgart: Thieme Publishers; 2006).

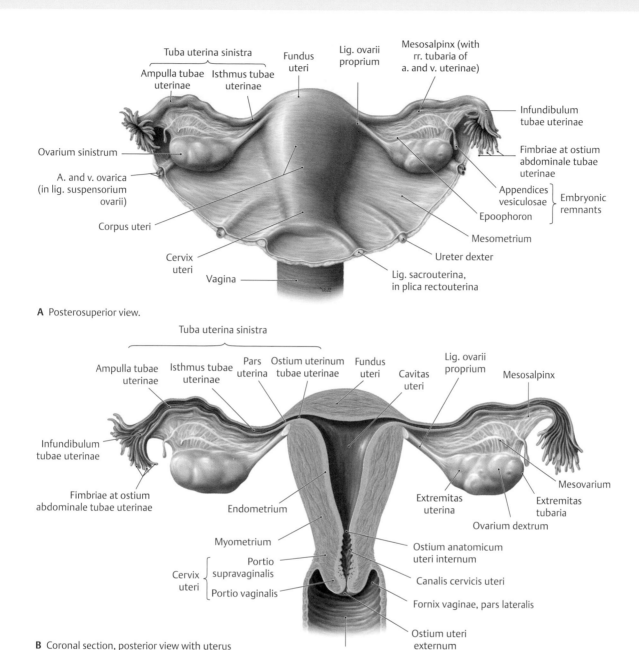

A Posterosuperior view.

B Coronal section, posterior view with uterus straightened. *Removed:* Mesometrium.

Fig. 15.8 Uterus, ovarium, and tubae uterinae
(From Gilroy AM et al. Atlas of Anatomy. 4th ed. 2020. Based on: Schuenke M, Schulte E, Schumacher U. THIEME Atlas of Anatomy. Internal Organs. Illustrations by Voll M and Wesker K. 3rd ed. New York: Thieme Medical Publishers; 2020.)

The Uterus

The **uterus** is a pear-shaped muscular organ located in the center of the pelvis, posterior to the vesica urinaria and anterior to the rectum. It is the site of implantation of the fertilized egg, subsequent development of the embryo, and parturition of the fetus.

— The uterus (see **Fig. 15.8**) has two parts:

1. The **corpus uteri** is the superior two thirds of the uterus and includes
   ○ the **fundus uteri**, the uppermost part above the openings of the tubae uterinae, and
   ○ the **isthmus uteri**, a narrow inferior segment that extends into the cervix uteri.
2. The **cervix uteri** is the narrow inferior third of the uterus and its least mobile part.
   ○ A portio supravaginalis cervicis sits above the vagina.
   ○ A portio vaginalis cervicis protrudes into the upper vagina and is surrounded by the fornices vaginae (upper recesses).

— The **cavitas uteri**, a narrow space within the corpus uteri,
  • communicates with the lumen of the tubae uterinae where they enter at the cornua uteri, and
  • extends inferiorly through the **ostium uteri internum** to the canalis cervicis uteri and terminates where the **ostium uteri externum** opens into the vagina.

> **BOX 15.4: DEVELOPMENTAL CORRELATION**
>
> **BICORNUATE UTERUS**
>
> The embryonic uterus is formed from the fusion of two paramesonephric ducts. When these ducts fail to fuse properly, a bicornuate uterus results in which the upper part of the uterus is bifurcated. The caudal part of the uterus is usually normal. Although a normal pregnancy is possible with this malformation, there is a greater risk of recurrent pregnancy loss, preterm birth, and malpresentation of the baby (e.g., the baby may be in a breech or transverse position).

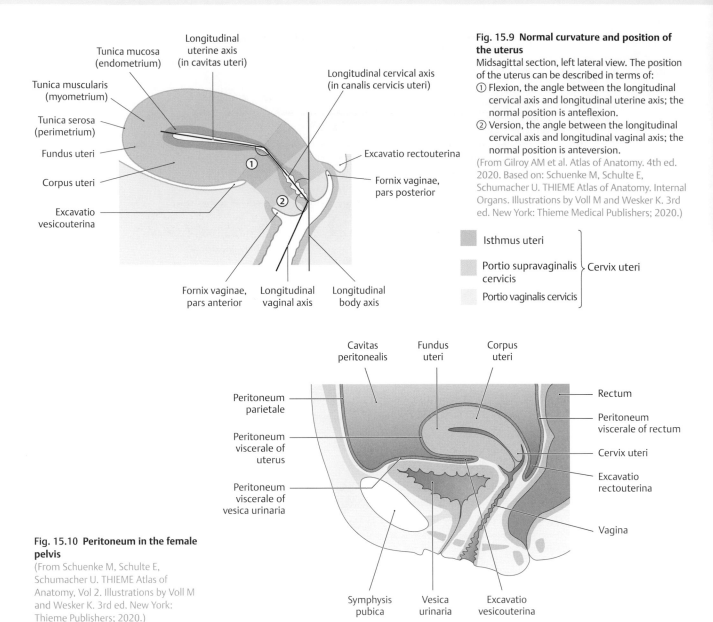

Fig. 15.9 **Normal curvature and position of the uterus**
Midsagittal section, left lateral view. The position of the uterus can be described in terms of:
① Flexion, the angle between the longitudinal cervical axis and longitudinal uterine axis; the normal position is anteflexion.
② Version, the angle between the longitudinal cervical axis and longitudinal vaginal axis; the normal position is anteversion.
(From Gilroy AM et al. Atlas of Anatomy. 4th ed. 2020. Based on: Schuenke M, Schulte E, Schumacher U. THIEME Atlas of Anatomy. Internal Organs. Illustrations by Voll M and Wesker K. 3rd ed. New York: Thieme Medical Publishers; 2020.)

Fig. 15.10 **Peritoneum in the female pelvis**
(From Schuenke M, Schulte E, Schumacher U. THIEME Atlas of Anatomy, Vol 2. Illustrations by Voll M and Wesker K. 3rd ed. New York: Thieme Publishers; 2020.)

— Although the corpus uteri is mobile, its position changes with the fullness of the vesica urinaria and rectum. Its normal position is anteflexed and anteverted (**Fig. 15.9**).
  - **Flexion** describes the angle between the long axis of the corpus uteri and the isthmus uteri and canalis cervicis uteri. In an anteflexed uterus, the long axis of the corpus uteri is tipped anteriorly; a **retroflexed** uterus is tipped posteriorly.
  - **Version** describes the angle between the cervix uteri and vagina. In an anteverted uterus, the axis of the cervix uteri is bent anteriorly; in a **retroverted** uterus, the cervix is bent posteriorly.
— Peritoneum covers the corpus uteri, extending as far inferiorly as the cervix uteri on its posterior surface. The uterus is flanked anteriorly by the excavatio vesicouterina and posteriorly by the excavatio rectouterina (**Fig. 15.10**).
— Uterine ligaments that arise from the corpus uteri include the lig. latum uteri and the lig. teres uteri (**Fig. 15.11**).
  - The **lig. latum uteri** is a double fold of peritoneum that extends laterally from each side of the uterus to the sidewalls of the pelvis. The parts of the lig. latum uteri (**Fig. 15.12**) are
    ○ the **mesosalpinx,** which ensheaths the uterine tube;
    ○ the **mesovarium,** a posterior extension, which suspends the ovarium; and
    ○ the **mesometrium,** which extends from the corpus uteri below the mesovarium to the sidewall of the pelvis.
  - The paired **ligg. teres uteri**, which originate near the fundus uteri from each side of the uterus, pass through the anulus inguinalis profundus, traverse the canalis inguinalis, and insert in the labia majora of the perineum.
— Uterine ligaments that arise from the cervix uteri include the ligg. transversa cervicis and the ligg. sacrouterina (**Fig. 15.13** and **15.14**).
  - The paired **lig. cardinale (lig. transversum cervicis)** are thickenings of fascia endopelvica that connect the cervix uteri to the pelvic sidewall. They are located at the base of the lig. latum uteri and transmit the uterine vessels.
  - The paired **lig. sacrouterinum** are thickenings of fascia endopelvica that connect the cervix uteri to the os sacrum

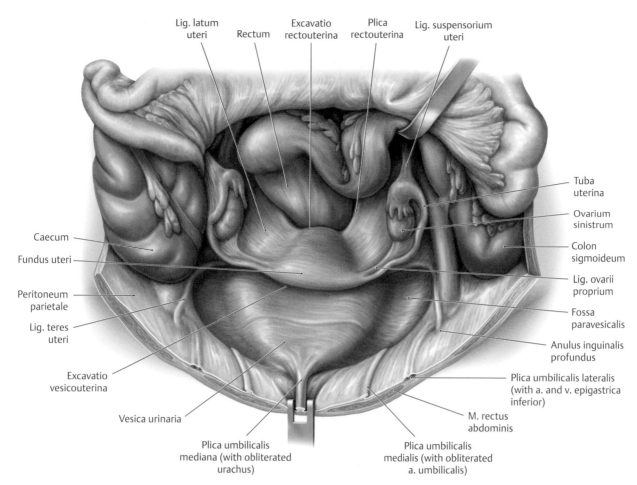

Fig. 15.11 Peritoneal relationships in the female pelvis
Pelvis minor, anterosuperior view. *Retracted:* Small intestine loops and colon (portions). (From Schuenke M, Schulte E, Schumacher U. THIEME Atlas of Anatomy, Vol 2. Illustrations by Voll M and Wesker K. 3rd ed. New York: Thieme Publishers; 2020.)

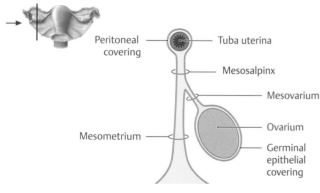

Fig. 15.12 Mesenteries of the lig. latum uteri
Sagittal section. The lig. latum uteri is a combination of the mesosalpinx, mesovarium, and mesometrium. (From Schuenke M, Schulte E, Schumacher U. THIEME Atlas of Anatomy, Vol 2. Illustrations by Voll M and Wesker K. 3rd ed. New York: Thieme Publishers; 2020.)

and help to maintain the anteverted position of the uterus.

— The a. uterina, the primary blood supply to the uterus (see Section 14.6), traverses the lig. cardinale and anastomoses superiorly with the a. ovarica and inferiorly with the a. vaginalis.

— A plexus venosus uterinus receives the vv. uterinae and drains to the v. iliaca interna.
— Lymphatic drainage of the uterus is complex but generally follows the vv. uterinae or the uterine ligaments (see Section 14.6).
  • The fundus uteri drains to nll. aortici laterales via the vv. ovaricae.
  • The supralateral part of the uterus drains to nll. inguinales superficiales via the lig. teres uteri.
  • The corpus uteri drains to nll. iliaci externi via the lig. latum uteri.
  • The cervix uteri drains to nll. iliaci interni and nll. sacrales via the lig. cardinale and lig. sacrouterinum.
— The plexus nervosus uterovaginalis, derived from the plexus hypogastricus inferior, innervates the uterus (see **Fig. 14.23**).

The Vagina

The **vagina** is a fibromuscular tube that extends from the cervix uteri to the ostium vaginae in the perineum (**Figs. 15.15** and **15.16**). It serves as the inferior part of the birth canal and the conduit for menstrual fluid, and it accommodates the penis during sexual intercourse.

— The vagina is posterior to the vesica urinaria and urethra and anterior to the rectum.

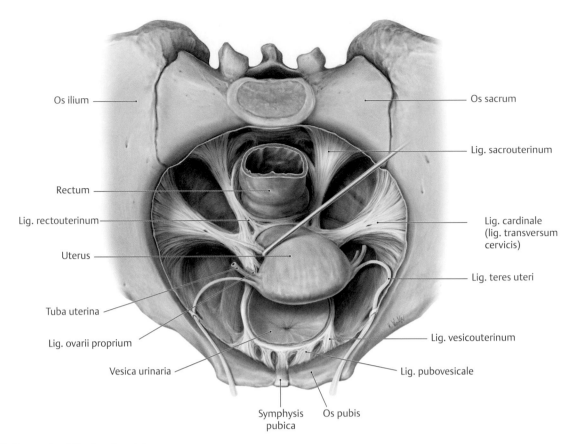

Fig. 15.13 Ligaments of the female pelvis
Superior view. *Removed:* Peritoneum, neurovasculature, and superior portion of vesica urinaria to demonstrate only the fascial condensations. Deep pelvic ligaments support the uterus within the cavitas pelvis and prevent uterine prolapse, the downward displacement of the uterus into the vagina. (From Gilroy AM et al. Atlas of Anatomy. 4th ed. 2020. Based on: Schuenke M, Schulte E, Schumacher U. THIEME Atlas of Anatomy. Internal Organs. Illustrations by Voll M and Wesker K. 3rd ed. New York: Thieme Medical Publishers; 2020.)

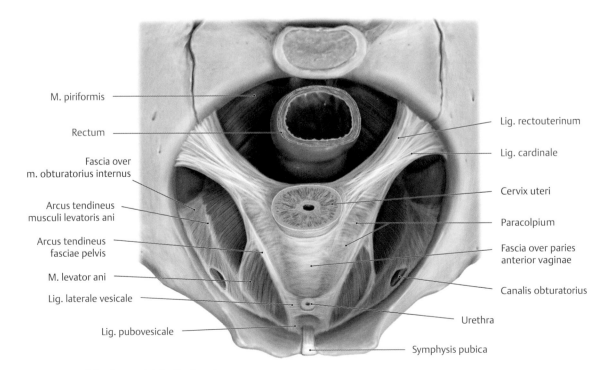

Fig. 15.14 Ligaments of the deep pelvis in the female
Superior view. Lig. sacrouterinum and paracolpium support and maintain the position of the cervix and vagina in the pelvis. (From Gilroy AM et al. Atlas of Anatomy. 4th ed. 2020. Based on: Schuenke M, Schulte E, Schumacher U. THIEME Atlas of Anatomy. Internal Organs. Illustrations by Voll M and Wesker K. 3rd ed. New York: Thieme Medical Publishers; 2020.)

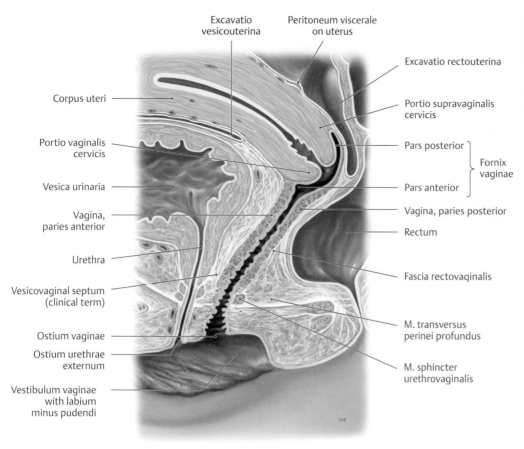

Excavatio vesicouterina

Peritoneum viscerale on uterus

Excavatio rectouterina

Corpus uteri

Portio supravaginalis cervicis

Portio vaginalis cervicis

Pars posterior ⎤
            ⎬ Fornix vaginae
Pars anterior ⎦

Vesica urinaria

Vagina, paries anterior

Vagina, paries posterior

Urethra

Rectum

Vesicovaginal septum (clinical term)

Fascia rectovaginalis

Ostium vaginae

Ostium urethrae externum

M. transversus perinei profundus

Vestibulum vaginae with labium minus pudendi

M. sphincter urethrovaginalis

Fig. 15.15 Vagina
Midsagittal section, left lateral view. (From Gilroy AM, MacPherson BR, Wikenheiser JC. Atlas of Anatomy. Illustrations by Voll M and Wesker K. 4th ed. New York: Thieme Publishers; 2020.)

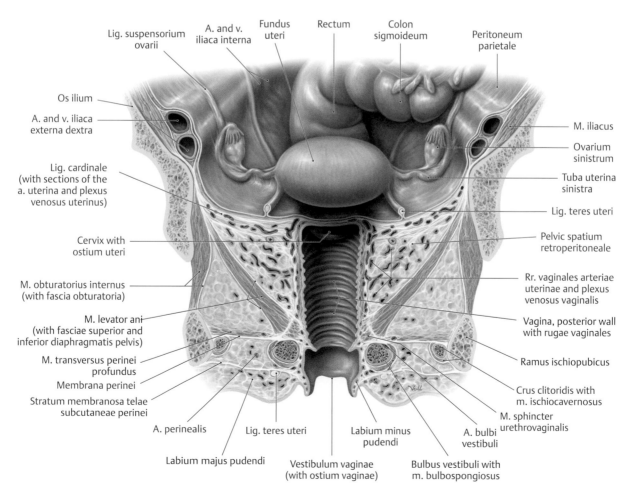

Lig. suspensorium ovarii

A. and v. iliaca interna

Fundus uteri

Rectum

Colon sigmoideum

Peritoneum parietale

Os ilium

A. and v. iliaca externa dextra

M. iliacus

Ovarium sinistrum

Lig. cardinale (with sections of the a. uterina and plexus venosus uterinus)

Tuba uterina sinistra

Lig. teres uteri

Cervix with ostium uteri

Pelvic spatium retroperitoneale

M. obturatorius internus (with fascia obturatoria)

Rr. vaginales arteriae uterinae and plexus venosus vaginalis

M. levator ani (with fasciae superior and inferior diaphragmatis pelvis)

Vagina, posterior wall with rugae vaginales

M. transversus perinei profundus

Ramus ischiopubicus

Membrana perinei

Stratum membranosa telae subcutaneae perinei

Crus clitoridis with m. ischiocavernosus

A. perinealis

Lig. teres uteri

Vestibulum vaginae (with ostium vaginae)

M. sphincter urethrovaginalis

Labium majus pudendi

Labium minus pudendi

A. bulbi vestibuli

Bulbus vestibuli with m. bulbospongiosus

Fig. 15.16 Female genital organs: Coronal section
Anterior view. (From Gilroy AM, MacPherson BR, Wikenheiser JC. Atlas of Anatomy. Illustrations by Voll M and Wesker K. 4th ed. New York: Thieme Publishers; 2020.)

- It is normally flattened with its anterior and posterior walls in contact.
- Connections to the os sacrum via the lig. sacrouterinum and to the arcus tendineus fasciae pelvis on the side wall of the pelvis via the **paracolpium** stabilize the vagina, especially during childbirth (see **Fig 15.14**).
- The **fornix vaginae**, which has anterior, lateral, and posterior parts, is a recess that surrounds the lower cervix as it protrudes into the upper vagina.
  • The pars posterior fornicis vaginae is in contact with the excavatio rectouterina, thereby providing access to the cavitas peritonealis. The pars anterior fornicis vaginae is shorter and lies against the posterior wall of the vesica urinaria.
- The a. iliaca interna supplies the vagina through its r. uterina, r. vaginalis, and r. pudenda interna (see Section 14.6).
- Veins of the vagina contribute to the plexus venosus uterovaginalis, which drains to the v. iliaca interna.
- Lymphatic vessels of the vagina drain to several groups of nodes.
  • The superior part of the vagina drains to nll. iliaci externi or nll. iliaci interni.
  • The inferior part of the vagina drains to nll. sacrales and nll. iliaci communes.
  • The vaginal orifice drains to nll. inguinales superficiales.
- The plexus nervosus uterovaginalis, an extension of the inferior hypogastric plexus, innervates the superior three fourths of the vagina (see **Fig. 14.23**).
- A deep perineal branch of n. pudendus, a branch of the plexus sacralis, innervates the lowest vaginal segment (see **Fig. 14.20**). This somatically innervated segment is the only part of the vagina that is sensitive to touch.

BOX 15.5: CLINICAL CORRELATION

CULDOCENTESIS

Culdocentesis is a procedure in which peritoneal fluid is extracted from the excavatio rectouterina by needle aspiration. The needle is advanced through the pars posterior fornicis vaginae. No fluid or a small amount of clear fluid is normal, but purulent fluid is suggestive of pelvic inflammatory disease (PID). The presence of blood is an indication for emergency surgery.

15.3   Pelvic Urinary Organs

The pelvic urinary organs include the distal ureters, the vesica urinaria, and the urethra.

The Ureters

Each ureter crosses over the brim of the pelvis at the bifurcation of the a. iliaca communis and descends along the lateral wall near the spina ischiadica. It runs anteriorly and enters the posterolateral wall of the vesica urinaria.

- In males, the ureter passes under the pelvic portion of the ductus deferens and enters the vesica urinaria lateral and superior to the free ends of the vesicles (**Fig. 15.17**; see also **Fig. 15.2**).
- In females, the ureter passes inferior to the aa. uterinae within the lig. cardinale, ~ 2 cm lateral to the portio vaginalis cervicis (**Fig. 15.18**).
- The most reliable blood supply to the pars pelvica ureteris is the a. uterina in females and the a. vesicalis inferior in males. Veins of similar names accompany the arteries.
- The pars pelvica ureteris derives its innervation from the plexus hypogastricus inferior. (**Fig. 14.25**).
- Visceral sensory fibers follow sympathetic nerves to levels T11–L2 of medulla spinalis; therefore, ureteric pain is usually felt in the ipsilateral inguinal region.

The Bladder (Vesica Urinaria)

The bladder (vesica urinaria) is a muscular reservoir for the temporary storage of urine. Although normally located in the pelvis minor, when full it may extend superiorly into the abdomen.

- It lies directly posterior to the symphysis pubica, separated from it by the spatium retropubicum. Posteriorly, it is related to the rectum in the male (see **Fig. 15.1**) and the upper vagina in the female (see **Fig. 15.6**).
- It is covered by peritoneum only on its superior surface.
- The vesica urinaria is tetrahedral with superior, posterior, and two inferolateral surfaces (**Fig. 15.19**). It has four parts:
  1. The **apex vesicae** points toward the symphysis pubica. The lig. umbilicale medium extends from the apex vesicae to the umbilicus.

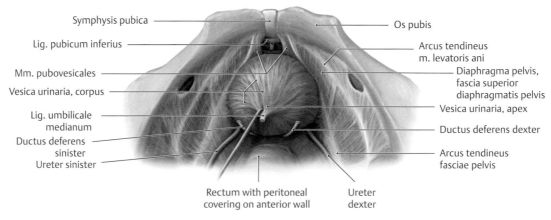

Symphysis pubica — Os pubis
Lig. pubicum inferius — Arcus tendineus m. levatoris ani
Mm. pubovesicales — Diaphragma pelvis, fascia superior diaphragmatis pelvis
Vesica urinaria, corpus — Vesica urinaria, apex
Lig. umbilicale medianum — Ductus deferens dexter
Ductus deferens sinister — Arcus tendineus fasciae pelvis
Ureter sinister
Rectum with peritoneal covering on anterior wall — Ureter dexter

Fig. 15.17 Ureter and vesica urinaria in the male pelvis
Superior view. (From Gilroy AM et al. Atlas of Anatomy. 4th ed. 2020. Based on: Schuenke M, Schulte E, Schumacher U. THIEME Atlas of Anatomy. Internal Organs. Illustrations by Voll M and Wesker K. 3rd ed. New York: Thieme Medical Publishers; 2020.)

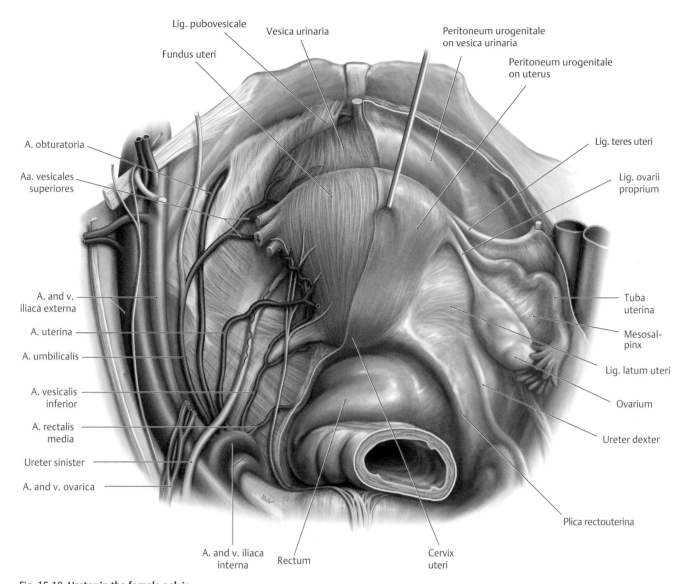

Fig. 15.18 Ureter in the female pelvis
Superior view. *Removed from right side:* Peritoneum and lig. latum uteri. (From Schuenke M, Schulte E, Schumacher U. THIEME Atlas of Anatomy, Vol 2. Illustrations by Voll M and Wesker K. 3rd ed. New York: Thieme Publishers; 2020.)

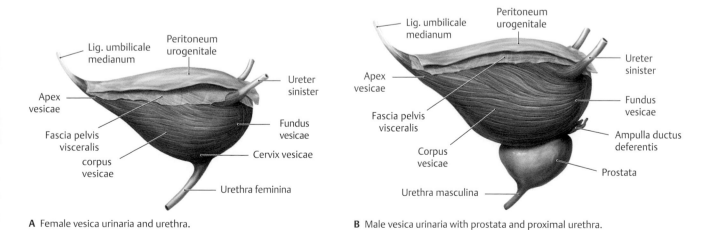

A Female vesica urinaria and urethra.

B Male vesica urinaria with prostata and proximal urethra.

Fig. 15.19 Structure of the vesica urinaria
Left lateral view. (From Schuenke M, Schulte E, Schumacher U. THIEME Atlas of Anatomy, Vol 2. Illustrations by Voll M and Wesker K. 3rd ed. New York: Thieme Publishers; 2020.)

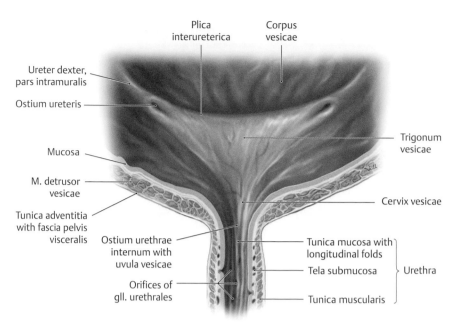

Plica interureterica

Corpus vesicae

Ureter dexter, pars intramuralis

Ostium ureteris

Mucosa

M. detrusor vesicae

Tunica adventitia with fascia pelvis visceralis

Ostium urethrae internum with uvula vesicae

Orifices of gll. urethrales

Trigonum vesicae

Cervix vesicae

Tunica mucosa with longitudinal folds

Tela submucosa

Tunica muscularis

Urethra

Fig. 15.20 Trigonum vesicae
Coronal section, anterior view. (From Gilroy AM et al. Atlas of Anatomy. 4th ed. 2020. Based on: Schuenke M, Schulte E, Schumacher U. THIEME Atlas of Anatomy. Internal Organs. Illustrations by Voll M and Wesker K. 3rd ed. New York: Thieme Medical Publishers; 2020.)

2. The **fundus vesicae** forms the bladder base, or posterior wall.
3. The **corpus vesicae** makes up most of the vesica urinaria.
4. The **cervix vesicae** is the lowest and least mobile region.
— The muscles of the vesica urinaria consist of the
  • **detrusor muscle (detrusor vesicae)** with stratum longitudinale internum and stratum longitudinale externum and middle stratum circulare, which are responsible for vesica urinaria emptying
  • **sphincter internus urethrae** in the cervix vesicae, which is responsible for bladder closure, and in the male contracts during ejaculation
— The cervix vesicae is firmly attached
  • to the os pubis by anterior extensions of the arcus tendineus fasciae pelvis, the **ligg. pubovesicales** in females, and ligg. puboprostatica in males. These provide an aponeurotic attachment for the paired **mm. pubovesicales** (see **Fig. 15.17**). These structures form an important vesicourethral suspension mechanism that suspends the cervix vesicae and ensures continence.
  • to the lateral pelvic walls by condensations of fascia endopelvica, the **ligg. laterales vesicae** (see **Fig.15.14**).
— The internal surface of the base of the vesica urinaria is marked by the **trigonum vesicae**, a smooth triangular region (**Fig. 15.20**). The corners of the triangle are formed posterolaterally by the slit-like openings of the ureter dexter and sinister and anteriorly by the ostium urethrae. The posterior circumference of the sphincter internum urethrae forms the morphological basis of the trigonum.
— The vesica urinaria is highly distensible and in most individuals may hold up to 600 to 800 mL (painfully), although micturition (urination) usually occurs at a much smaller volume. Normally, no urine remains in the vesica urinaria after voiding.
— The aa. vesicales superiores, with contributions from the aa. vesicales inferiores (in males) and aa. vaginae (in females), supply the vesica urinaria (see Section 14.6).
— The plexus venosus vesicalis surrounds the inferolateral surfaces of the vesica urinaria and drains to the vv. iliacae

internae. The plexus communicates with the plexus prostaticus in males, with the plexus uterovaginalis in females, and with the plexus venosus vertebralis in both sexes.
— Lymph from the vesica urinaria drains to nll. iliaci externi and nll. iliaci interni.
— The plexus nervosus vesicalis is a derivative of the plexus hypogastricus inferior (see **Fig. 14.25**).
  • Sympathetic stimulation relaxes the m. detrusor and contracts the sphincter internus urethrae, thus inhibiting micturition.
  • Parasympathetic nerves stimulate the m. detrusor to contract while inhibiting the sphincter internus urethrae, thereby facilitating micturition.
  • Afferent fibers carrying pain from the inferior vesica urinaria follow parasympathetic routes. Pain fibers from the superior vesica urinaria follow sympathetic routes.

The Urethra

The urethra is the muscular conduit for urine in the female and for urine and semen in the male. It extends from the ostium internum urethrae at the cervix vesicae to the ostium externum urethrae in the perineum.
— In males and females, the primary muscles of the urethra include the (**Fig. 15.21**)
  • **dilator urethrae**, which extends over the anterior circumference of the sphincter internus urethrae, through the ostium internum urethrae, and inferiorly along the anterior urethra. It shortens the urethra and widens the ostium internum urethrae, which initiates micturition.
  • **sphincter externus urethrae**, composed of smooth and striated layers, which is responsible for closure of the ostium internum urethrae.
— The urethra masculina extends 18 to 22 cm from the vesica urinaria to the tip of the glans penis (**Fig. 15.22**). The urethra masculina has four parts. Although all are mentioned here, the pars membranacea and pars spongiosa are located in the perineum and are discussed further in Chapter 16.

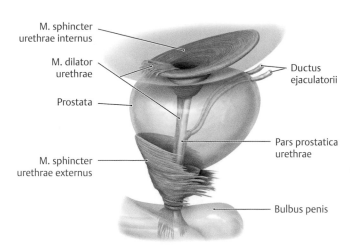

Fig. 15.21 Urethral sphincter mechanism in the male
Lateral view. (From Gilroy AM et al. Atlas of Anatomy. 4th ed. 2020. Based on: Schuenke M, Schulte E, Schumacher U. THIEME Atlas of Anatomy. Internal Organs. Illustrations by Voll M and Wesker K. 3rd ed. New York: Thieme Medical Publishers; 2020.)

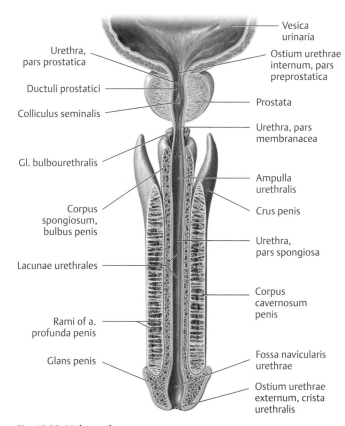

Fig. 15.22 Male urethra
Longitudinal section, anterior view. (From Gilroy AM et al. Atlas of Anatomy. 4th ed. 2020. Based on: Schuenke M, Schulte E, Schumacher U. THIEME Atlas of Anatomy. Internal Organs. Illustrations by Voll M and Wesker K. 3rd ed. New York: Thieme Medical Publishers; 2020.)

1. The **pars preprostatica** at the cervix vesicae contains the ostium urethrae internum. Sympathetic nerves of the plexus hypogastricus superior control closure of the **m. sphincter urethrae internus** during ejaculation.
2. The **pars prostatica** is surrounded by the prostata and characterized by

- the **crista urethralis**, a vertical ridge on the posterior wall that contains a central eminence, the **colliculus seminalis**; and
- ductus ejaculatorii that open onto the crista urethralis, and ductuli prostatici from the prostata that open into recesses on either side of the crista urethralis.

3. The **pars membranacea** passes through the membrana perinei in the regio urogenitalis and is surrounded by the m. sphincter urethrae externus.
4. The **pars spongiosa** passes through the corpus spongiosum, one of the vascular erectile bodies of the penis.

— The urethra feminina extends 4 cm from the ostium urethrae internum at the cervix vesicae to the ostium urethrae externum in the perineum (**Fig. 15.23**).
  - Within the pelvis it lies anterior to the vagina, forming an elevation within the anterior vaginal wall.
  - It passes through the hiatus genitalis of diaphragma pelvis, the m. sphincter urethrae externus (there is no organized sphincter urethrae internus), and the membrana perinei.
  - Paired ductus paraurethrales drain groups of **gll. paraurethrales** and open near the ostium urethrae externum.
  - In the perineum, the urethra opens within the vestibulum vaginae directly anterior to the ostium vaginae (see **Fig. 16.10**).

— Branches of the a. pudenda, as well as the a. vesicalis inferior in the male and a. vaginalis in the female, supply the urethra. In both sexes, a plexus venosus that accompanies the arteries drains the urethra.
— The urethra feminina and proximal parts of the urethra masculina (pars preprostatica, pars prostatica, and pars membranacea) drain to the nll. iliaci interni. The pars spongiosa of the urethra masculina (the pars perinei) drains to nll. inguinales profundi.
— Nerves to the urethra arise from the plexus nervosus prostaticus in the male and comparable plexus nervosus vesicalis in the female. Sympathetic nerves control the closure of the m. sphincter urethrae externus in males.
— Visceral sensory fibers from the pelvic urethra travel with nn. splanchnici pelvici; somatic sensory fibers from the perineal urethra travel with the n. pudendus.

BOX 15.6: CLINICAL CORRELATION

URETHRAL RUPTURE IN MALES
Fractures of the cingulum pelvicum may be accompanied by a rupture of the pars membranacea urethrae. This allows the extravasation (escape) of urine and blood into the spatium profundum perinei and superiorly through the hiatus genitalis to the subperitoneal spaces around the prostata and vesica urinaria. Rupture of the bulbous pars spongiosa may occur from a straddle injury in which there is a forceful blow to the perineum, or from the false passage of a transurethral catheter. In this case urine can leak into the spatium superficiale perinei, which is continuous with the scrotal sac, the space around the penis, and the space on the inferior anterior abdominal wall between the abdominal muscles and the membranous layer of the subcutaneous tissue. The attachment of the fascia perinei to the fascia lata (fascia enclosing the thigh muscles) prevents urine from spreading laterally into the thighs. Similarly, it is prevented from spreading into the regio analis by the attachment of the fascia to the fascia perinei profundus and membrana perinei.

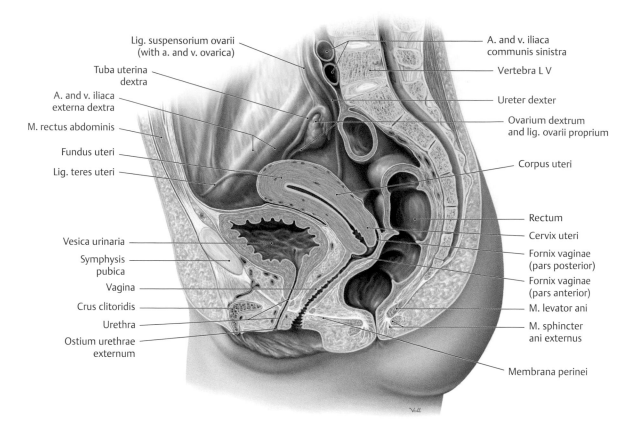

Fig. 15.23 Female urinary vesica urinaria and urethra
Midsagittal section of pelvis, viewed from the left side. Right hemipelvis.
(From Gilroy AM et al. Atlas of Anatomy. 4th ed. 2020. Based on: Schuenke M, Schulte E, Schumacher U. THIEME Atlas of Anatomy. Internal Organs. Illustrations by Voll M and Wesker K. 3rd ed. New York: Thieme Medical Publishers; 2020.)

15.4   The Rectum

The rectum is the continuation of the gastrointestinal tract in the pelvis and functions as a temporary storage site for fecal matter. It is continuous with the colon sigmoideum superiorly and the canalis analis inferiorly (**Figs. 15.24** and **15.25;** see Section 16.5).

— It lies anterior to the lower sacrum and coccyx and rests on the lig. anococcygeum of the pelvic floor.
— Anteriorly, the rectum is related to the vesica urinaria, seminal vesicles, and prostata in males and to the vagina in females. A septum rectovesicale or septum rectovaginale separates the rectum from these anterior structures.
— The rectum has no mesenterium. Its superior two thirds are retroperitoneal and form the posterior surface of the excavatio rectovesicalis and excavatio rectouterina. The distal third is subperitoneal.
— Unlike the colon, the rectum lacks taeniae coli, haustra, and appendices epiploicae.
— The rectum begins at the **rectosigmoid junction,** the point at which the taeniae coli disappear. At this junction, muscle fibers of the bands spread out evenly over the surface of the rectum. This junction usually occurs anterior to vertebra S III.
— The rectum terminates at the **junctio anorectalis** (its junction with the canalis analis), where it passes through the diaphragma pelvis adjacent to the tip of the os coccygis.

— The internal wall of the rectum has three **plica transversa recti**, one on the right and two on the left, which create flexurae laterales recti that are visible externally.
— The **ampulla recti**, the most distal segment of the rectum, stores accumulating fecal material until defecation and has an important role in fecal continence. It narrows abruptly as it joins with the canalis analis and passes through the diaphragma pelvis.
— The rectum has a dual blood supply:
  • The a. rectalis superior, the unpaired terminal branch of the a. mesenterica inferior, supplies the upper rectum (see Section 14.6).
  • A. rectalis media dextra and a. rectalis media sinistra, branches of the a. iliaca interna, supply the lower rectum.
— The vv. rectales drain a submucosal plexus venosus rectalis, which has internal and external (subcutaneous) components.
  • The external plexus communicates with other visceral venous plexuses in the pelvis.
  • The internal plexus communicates with branches from the aa. rectales (an arteriovenous anastomosis), forming a thickened vascular tissue (**plexus venosus rectalis inferior**) that surrounds the junctio anorectalis. This tissue forms prominent anal cushions in the left lateral, right anterolateral, and right posterolateral positions.

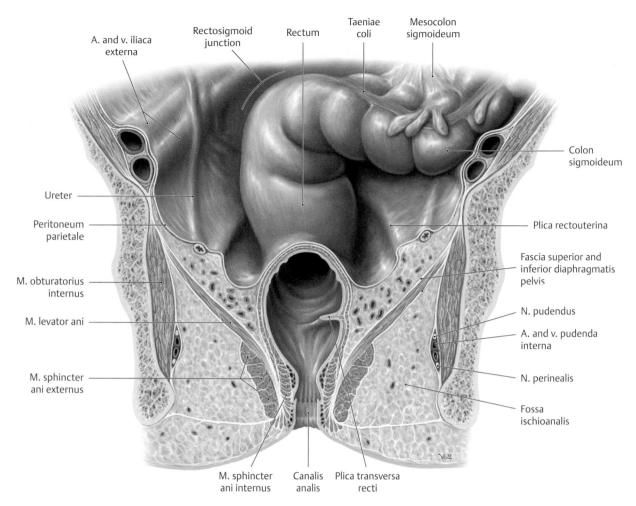

Fig. 15.24 Rectum in situ
Female pelvis, coronal section, anterior view. (From Gilroy AM et al. Atlas of Anatomy. 4th ed. 2020. Based on: Schuenke M, Schulte E, Schumacher U. THIEME Atlas of Anatomy. Internal Organs. Illustrations by Voll M and Wesker K. 3rd ed. New York: Thieme Medical Publishers; 2020.)

— Venous blood from the rectum drains into the portal and caval (systemic) venous systems (see Section 14.6).
  • A v. rectalis superior, which drains the upper rectum, is a tributary of the portal system via the v. mesenterica inferior.
  • The paired v. rectalis media and v. rectalis inferior that drain the lower rectum (and canalis analis) are tributaries of the v. cava inferior via the v. iliaca interna.
  • Communications between the v. rectalis superior, v. rectalis media, and v. rectalis inferior form clinically important portocaval anastomoses that enlarge in portal hypertension.
— Lymphatic drainage follows vascular pathways.
  • The upper rectum drains to nll. mesenterici inferiores along the course of the a. rectalis superior. It eventually drains to nll. lumbales, although some lymph may drain first to nll. sacrales.
  • The lower rectum drains primarily to nll. sacrales or directly to nll. iliaci interni.

— Sympathetic innervation to the rectum is carried by nn. splanchnici lumbales plexus hypogastricus, as well as by nerves of the plexus mesentericus inferior traveling along the a. rectalis superior (see **Fig. 14.22**).
— Parasympathetic innervation originates in nn. splanchnici pelvici, which are accompanied by visceral sensory fibers.

BOX 15.7: CLINICAL CORRELATION

RECTAL EXAMINATION
A rectal examination is performed by inserting a gloved, lubricated finger into the rectum, while the other hand is used to press on the lower abdomen or pelvic region. Palpable structures include the prostata, seminal vesicle, ampulla of the ductus deferens, vesica urinaria, uterus, cervix, and ovaries. Pathologic anomalies such as hemorrhoids, tumors, enlargements, and changes in consistency of the tissues can be felt. The tonicity of the anal sphincter, mediated by the n. pudendus (S2–S4), can also be assessed.

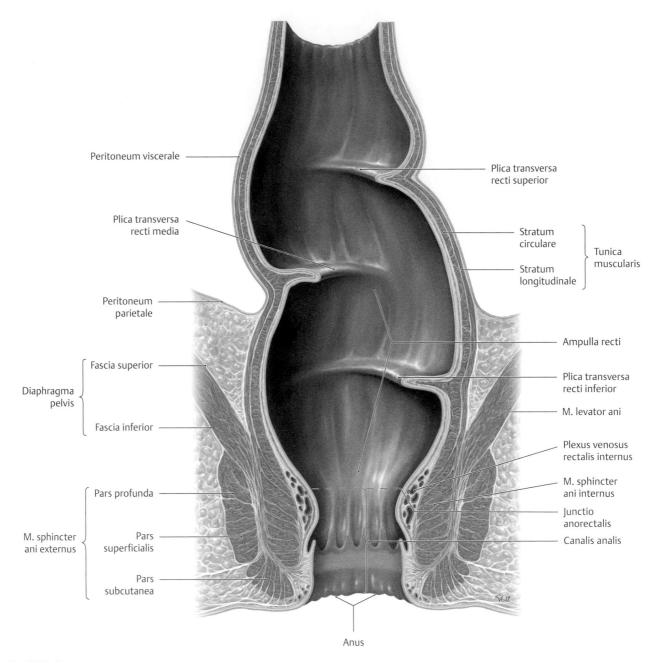

Fig. 15.25 Rectum
Coronal section, anterior view. (From Schuenke M, Schulte E, Schumacher U. THIEME Atlas of Anatomy, Vol 2. Illustrations by Voll M and Wesker K. 3rd ed. New York: Thieme Publishers; 2020.)

16 The Perineum

The perineum is the space inferior to the diaphragma pelvis, which is divided into a regio urogenitalis and a regio analis. The regio urogenitalis contains the male and female external genital structures, and the regio analis contains the canalis analis and anus.

16.1 Perineal Spaces

— The boundaries of the diamond-shaped perineum (**Figs. 16.1** and **16.2**; see also **Fig. 14.4**) are
   • the apertura pelvis inferior (symphysis pubica, rami ischiopubici, ligg. sacrotuberalia, and os coccygis), which forms the perimeter;
   • the lower parts of the m. obturator internus and their fasciae obturatoriae, which line the lateral walls;
   • the inferior surface of the diaphragma pelvis, which forms the roof; and
   • the skin of the perineum, which forms the floor.
— A line connecting the two tubera ischiadica separates the perineum into an anterior regio urogenitalis and a posterior regio analis
— The **membrana perinei**, a tough, fibrous sheet, stretches between the rr. ischiopubici, extending anteriorly almost to the symphysis pubica and posteriorly to the tubera ischiadica.
   • It separates the regio urogenitalis into the **spatium profundum perinei** and **spatium superficiale perinei.** (see **Fig. 14.3**).
   • It forms a platform for the attachment of the corpora cavernosa (which become engorged during arousal) of the external genitalia.
— The spatium superficiale perinei is a potential space bounded above by the membrana perinei and below by the **stratum membranosum perinei**, the extension of the stratum membranosum telae subcutaneae abdominis (Scarpa's fascia) on the abdominal wall.
   • In both sexes it contains
      ◦ the **m. bulbocavernosus**, **m. ischiocavernosus**, and **m. transversus perinei superficialis** (see Section 16.2) and
      ◦ the **deep perineal branches** of the a. pudenda interna and v. pudenda interna and n. pudendus.
   • In males (see Section 16.3) it also contains
      ◦ the **radix penis** and
      ◦ the proximal portion of the pars spongiosa urethrae.
   • In females (see Section 16.4) it also contains
      ◦ the **clitoris** and associated muscles,
      ◦ the **bulbus vestibuli** and
      ◦ the **gll. vestibulares majores**.
— The spatium profundum perinei is bounded inferiorly by the membrana perinei and superiorly by the inferior fascia of the diaphragma pelvis.
   • In both sexes it contains
      ◦ part of the urethra and inferior part of the **m. sphincter urethrae externus**.
      ◦ the anterior recesses of the **corpora adiposa fossae ischioanalis**, and
      ◦ neurovascular structures to the penis or clitoris.
   • In males it also contains
      ◦ the pars membranacea urethrae,
      ◦ the **gll. bulbourethrales**, and
      ◦ the **m. transversus perinei profundus**. (In females this is often replaced by smooth muscle.)
   • In females it also contains
      ◦ m. compressor urethrae, sphincter urethrovaginalis, and parts of the m. sphincter urethrae externus; and
      ◦ the proximal part of the urethra.

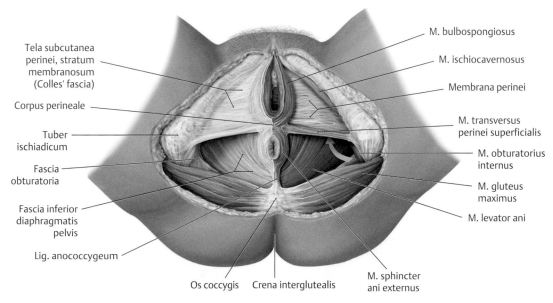

Fig. 16.1 Muscles and fascia of the female perineum
Lithotomy position, caudal (inferior) view. The *green arrow* is pointing forward to the recessus anterior of the fossa ischioanalis. (From Schuenke M, Schulte E, Schumacher U. THIEME Atlas of Anatomy, Vol 1. Illustrations by Voll M and Wesker K. 3rd ed. New York: Thieme Publishers; 2020.)

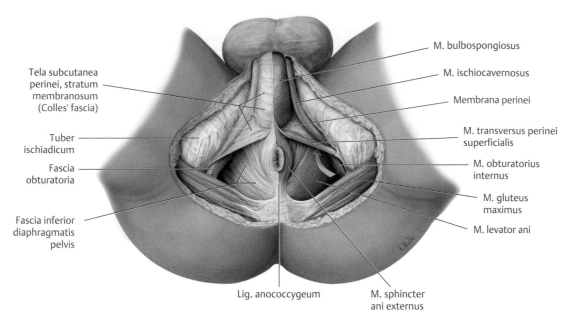

Tela subcutanea perinei, stratum membranosum (Colles' fascia)

Tuber ischiadicum

Fascia obturatoria

Fascia inferior diaphragmatis pelvis

M. bulbospongiosus

M. ischiocavernosus

Membrana perinei

M. transversus perinei superficialis

M. obturatorius internus

M. gluteus maximus

M. levator ani

Lig. anococcygeum

M. sphincter ani externus

Fig. 16.2 Muscles and fascia of the male perineum
Lithotomy position, caudal (inferior) view. The *green arrow* is pointing forward to the recessus anterior of the fossa ischioanalis. (From Schuenke M, Schulte E, Schumacher U. THIEME Atlas of Anatomy, Vol 1. Illustrations by Voll M and Wesker K. 3rd ed. New York: Thieme Publishers; 2020.)

16.2   Muscles of the Perineum

— Muscles of the perineum support the pelvic floor, surround the orifices of the urethra and anus, and assist in the erection of genital structures (**Table 16.1; Fig. 16.3**).
— The **perineal body (corpus perineale)** is an irregular subcutaneous mass of fibromuscular tissue formed by converging fibers of the m. levator ani, the m. transversus perinei profundus and m. bulbospongiosus, and the m. sphincter ani externus.
  • It lies between the rectum and bulbus penis in males and between the rectum and vagina in females.
  • It supports the diaphragma pelvis and viscera pelvis.
— **Perineal branches** of the a. pudenda interna supply muscles of the perineum. Venous blood drains to the v. pudenda interna and v. iliaca interna.
— The n. pudendus (S2–S4) innervates the muscles of the perineum.

BOX 16.1: CLINICAL CORRELATION

EPISIOTOMY
During vaginal delivery, pressure on the perineum risks tearing the perineal muscles. A clean incision through the posterior vaginal orifice into the corpus perineale, known as an episiotomy, is often performed to enlarge the opening and prevent damage to perineal muscles. A median, or midline, episiotomy extends only into the corpus perineale, but if further traumatic tearing occurs to extend the cut, it can damage the m. sphincter externus ani (resulting in fecal incontinence) or create an anovaginal fistula. Mediolateral episiotomies often replace the midline incisions. These extend laterally from the ostium vaginae to the m. transversus perinei superficialis, thus avoiding the corpus perineale and the possible sequelae from extensive tearing. However, while the more lateral incisions provide greater access, they are more difficult to repair.

BOX 16.2: CLINICAL CORRELATION

PROLAPSE OF PELVIC ORGANS
The diaphragma pelvis, pelvic ligaments, and corpus perineale provide important structural support for the pelvic viscera. Stretching or disruption of these tissues often occurs during childbirth and results in prolapse of the uterus into the vagina. A widening of the hiatus urogenitalis from an atrophic pelvic floor or a weakened corpus perineale can allow the bladder (cystocele), rectum (rectocele), or excavatio rectovesicalis (enterocele) to bulge into the vaginal wall.

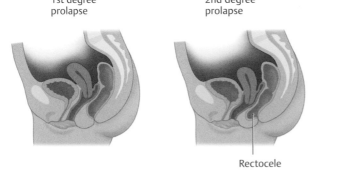

1st degree prolapse

2nd degree prolapse

3rd degree prolapse

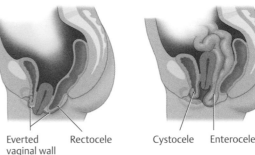

Rectocele

Everted vaginal wall

Rectocele

Cystocele   Enterocele

Table 16.1 Muscles of the Perineum

Muscle	Course	Innervation	Action
Spatium profundum perinei			
M. sphincter urethrae externus	Encircles the urethra (division of m. transversus perinei profundus). In males: ascends along apex of the prostata between collum vesicae and membrana perinei. In females: some fibers extend caudally from the sphincter to surround the lateral wall of the vagina as the *sphincter urethrovaginalis*. Other fibers curve posterolaterally from the sphincter to the ramus ossis ischii as the *m. compressor urethrae*.	N. pudendus (S2–S4)	Compresses urethra
M. transversus perinei profundus (typically replaced by smooth muscle in the female)	Extends from the ramus ossis ischii and tuber ischiadicum to the corpus perineale		Supports the corpus perineale and visceral channels through the pelvis floor
Spatium superficiale perinei			
M. bulbospongiosus	Runs anteriorly from the corpus perineale. In females: encloses the bulbus vestibuli and gl. vestibularis major, encircles the ostium vaginae, and attaches to the corpora cavernosa of the clitoris. In males: encircles the bulbus penis and corpora cavernosa and attaches to the raphe penis		In females: narrows the ostium vaginae, compresses the gll. vestibulares majores, and assists in erection of clitoris In males: compresses the bulbus penis to complete expulsion of urine/semen and assists in erection
M. ischiocavernosus	Covers the crus clitoridis (female) or penis (male), extending along the ramus ossis ischii		Compresses the crus clitoridis/crus penis and helps maintain erection
M. transversus perinei superficialis	Extends from the tuber ischiadicum to the corpus perineale anterior to the anus		Supports the corpus perineale and counters intrabdominal pressure
Regio analis			
M. sphincter ani externus	Encircles the anus from the corpus perineale to the lig. anococcygeum		Constricts the canalis analis, resists defecation

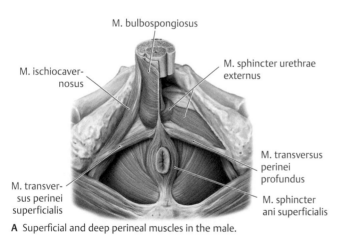

A Superficial and deep perineal muscles in the male.

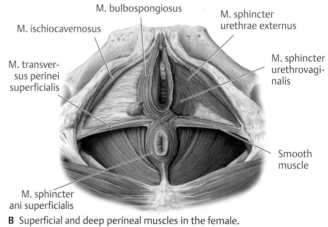

B Superficial and deep perineal muscles in the female.

Fig. 16.3 Muscles of the perineum
Inferior view. (From Gilroy AM et al. Atlas of Anatomy. 4th ed. 2020. Based on: Schuenke M, Schulte E, Schumacher U. THIEME Atlas of Anatomy. General Anatomy and Musculoskeletal System. Illustrations by Voll M and Wesker K. 3rd ed. New York: Thieme Medical Publishers; 2020.)

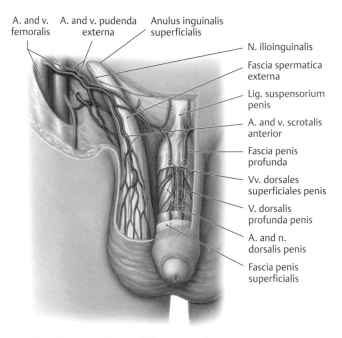

Fig. 16.4 Neurovasculature of the penis and scrotum
Anterior view. *Partially removed:* Skin and fascia. (From Schuenke M, Schulte E, Schumacher U. THIEME Atlas of Anatomy, Vol 1. Illustrations by Voll M and Wesker K. 3rd ed. New York: Thieme Publishers; 2020.)

16.3 Male Urogenital Triangle (Regio Urogenitalis)

The male regio urogenitalis contains the scrotum, penis, gll. bulbourethrales, mm. perinei, and associated neurovasculature.

The Scrotum

— The **scrotum** is a saccular extension of the anterior abdominal wall that encloses the testes and funiculus spermaticus (see Section 10.4).
— The subcutaneous layer of the skin over the scrotum is devoid of fat, but the **tunica dartos** that underlies the skin is continuous with the stratum membranosum telae subcutanei abdominis (Scarpa's fascia) and with the stratum membranosum telae subcutaneae perinei (Colles' fascia).
— An extension of tunica dartos divides the scrotum into right and left compartments and is visible externally as the **raphe scroti.**
— Scrotal branches of the a. pudenda interna and a. pudenda externa, and a. cremasterica from the a. epigastrica inferior supply the scrotum. Veins of similar names accompany the arteries (**Figs. 16.4** and **16.5**).
— Lymph from the scrotum drains to nll. inguinales superficiales. Recall that lymph from the contents within the scrotum (i.e., the testis and epididymis) drains directly to the nll. aortici laterales.
— Innervation of the scrotum (see **Fig. 14.21**) is supplied by
  • the n. ilioinguinalis and n. genitofemoralis (r. genitalis), which innervate the anterior scrotum, and
  • the n. pudendus and n. cutaneus femoris posterior of the thigh (sacral plexus), which innervate the posterior scrotum.

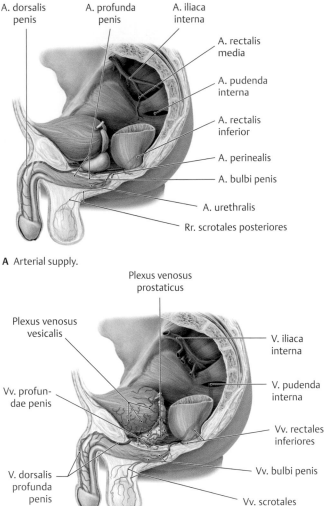

A Arterial supply.

B Venous drainage.

Fig. 16.5 Blood vessels of the male genitalia
Left lateral view. (From Schuenke M, Schulte E, Schumacher U. THIEME Atlas of Anatomy, Vol 1. Illustrations by Voll M and Wesker K. 3rd ed. New York: Thieme Publishers; 2020.)

The Penis

The **penis** serves both copulatory and urinary functions. It contains three cylindrical bodies of erectile tissue, one of which surrounds the pars spongiosa urethrae that transmits urine from the bladder during urination as well as semen during sexual intercourse (**Figs. 16.6** and **16.7**).
— The penis has three parts:
  1. The **radix penis**, the most proximal part, is attached to the membrana perinei and is covered by muscles. It is composed of
     ∘ right and left **crura** that are attached to the rami ischiopubici on either side and are covered by the mm. ischiocavernosi, and
     ∘ the **bulbus penis**, which is attached to the membrana perinei and covered by the m. bulbospongiosus. The pars spongiosa of the urethra enters on its dorsal surface.
  2. The **corpus penis**, pendulous and not covered by muscle, is made up of three cylindrical bodies of erectile tissue. A **tunica albuginea,** a dense fibrous coat, surrounds each

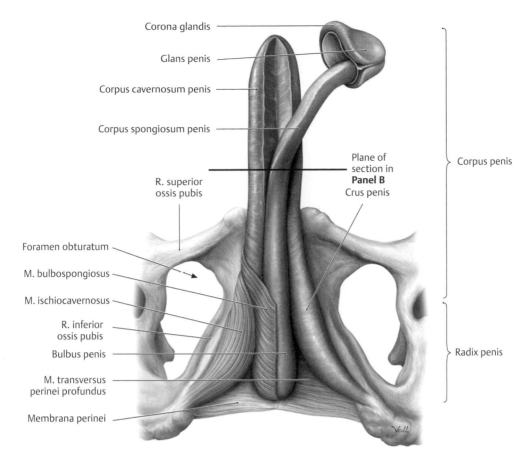

Corona glandis

Glans penis

Corpus cavernosum penis

Corpus spongiosum penis

Plane of section in **Panel B**
Crus penis

Corpus penis

R. superior ossis pubis

Foramen obturatum

M. bulbospongiosus

M. ischiocavernosus

R. inferior ossis pubis

Bulbus penis

M. transversus perinei profundus

Membrana perinei

Radix penis

A Inferior (ventral) view.

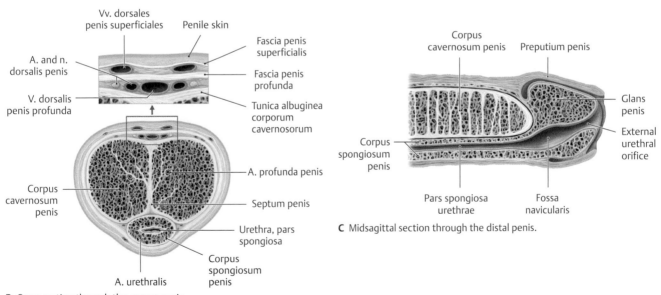

Vv. dorsales penis superficiales

Penile skin

A. and n. dorsalis penis

Fascia penis superficialis

Fascia penis profunda

V. dorsalis penis profunda

Tunica albuginea corporum cavernosorum

Corpus cavernosum penis

A. profunda penis

Septum penis

Urethra, pars spongiosa

Corpus spongiosum penis

A. urethralis

B Cross section through the corpus penis.

Corpus cavernosum penis

Preputium penis

Glans penis

External urethral orifice

Corpus spongiosum penis

Pars spongiosa urethrae

Fossa navicularis

C Midsagittal section through the distal penis.

Fig. 16.6 Penis
(From Schuenke M, Schulte E, Schumacher U. THIEME Atlas of Anatomy, Vol 1. Illustrations by Voll M and Wesker K. 3rd ed. New York: Thieme Publishers; 2020.)

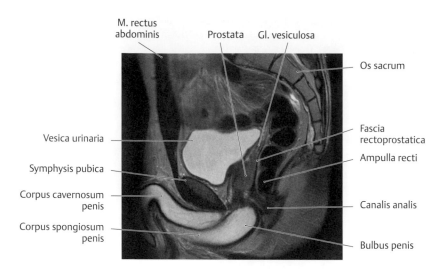

Fig. 16.7 MRI of the male pelvis
Sagittal section, left lateral view. (From Hamm B, et al. MRI Imaging of the Abdomen and Pelvis, 2nd ed. New York: Thieme Publishers; 2009.)

erectile body, and distally a **fascia penis profunda** (Buck's fascia) binds the three bodies together. The three erectile bodies include

- two **corpora cavernosa,** continuations of the crura, which lie side by side on the dorsum penis, and
- one **corpus spongiosum,** a continuation of the bulbus penis, which lies ventral to the two corpora cavernosa and is traversed by the penile urethra (pars spongiosa urethrae).

3. The **glans penis** (also known as the **glans**), an expansion of the distal end of the corpus spongiosum, is characterized by
  - the **corona glandis**, which overhangs the distal ends of the corpora cavernosa, and
  - a fusiform dilation of the spongy urethra, the **fossa navicularis urethrae**, which terminates at the **ostium urethrae externum** at its tip.

— The aa. pudendae externae supply the skin and subcutaneous tissue of the penis. Venous drainage of this tissue passes through the vv. dorsales superficiales penis, which drain to the vv. pudendae externae (see **Fig. 16.4**).

— Aa. pudendae internae supply the deep penile structures. Their branches (**Fig. 16.8;** see also **Fig. 16.6B**) include
  - the **a. bulbi penis**, which supplies the bulbus penis, the urethra within the bulb, and the gll. bulbourethrales;
  - the **a. dorsalis penis**, which runs between the fascia penis profunda and tunica albuginea to supply the penile fascia and skin and the glans; and
  - the **a. profunda penis**, which runs within the corpus cavernosum and gives off **aa. helicinae penis** that supply the erectile tissue and are responsible for engorgement of the corpora during erection.

— The erectile bodies are drained by plexus venosi that empty into the single **v. dorsalis profunda penis**, which passes under the symphysis pubica to join the plexus venosus prostaticus in the pelvis.

— Lymphatic drainage areas of the penis include
  - the erectile bodies of the penis, which drain to nll. iliaci interni;
  - the glans penis, which drains to nll. inguinales profundi; and
  - the urethra, which drains to nll. iliaci interni and nll. inguinales profundi.

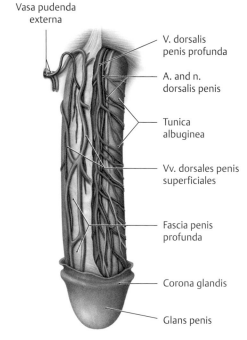

Fig. 16.8 Neurovasculature on the dorsum of the penis
Superior (dorsal) view. *Removed:* Skin. (From Schuenke M, Schulte E, Schumacher U. THIEME Atlas of Anatomy, Vol 1. Illustrations by Voll M and Wesker K. 3rd ed. New York: Thieme Publishers; 2020.)

— The glans of the penis is richly innervated by sensory fibers via the **n. dorsalis penis**, a branch of the n. pudendus. Sympathetic fibers from the plexus hypogastricus inferior are also carried along this route.

— Parasympathetic fibers carried by the nn. cavernosi derived from the plexus prostaticus innervate the aa. helicinae within the erectile tissue and are responsible for penile erection.

Glandulae Bulbourethrales

The gll. bulborethrales are paired mucus-secreting glands (see **Figs. 15.2** and **15.3**).

— They lie on either side of the urethra below the prostata surrounded by the m. sphincter urethrae.

— Their ducts open into the proximal part of the pars spongiosa urethrae.

— They are active during sexual arousal.

Erection, Emission, and Ejaculation

The sexual responses of **erection, emission,** and **ejaculation** involve sympathetic, parasympathetic, and somatic (via the n. pudendus) pathways.

— During erection
  • constriction of the aa. helicinae, normally maintained by sympathetic innervation, is inhibited by parasympathetic stimulation. As the arteries relax, the cavernous spaces within the erectile bodies dilate and become engorged;
  • contractions of the m. bulbocavernosus and m. ischiocavernosus, innervated by the n. pudendus, impede venous outflow and maintain the erection.
— During emission
  • parasympathetic stimulation mediates the secretion of seminal fluid from the gll. seminales, gll. bulborethrales, and prostata, and
  • sympathetic stimulation mediates emission (the movement of seminal fluid through the ducts) by initiating peristalsis of the ductus deferens and gll. seminales. This propels the seminal fluid into the pars prostatica urethrae, where additional fluid is added as the prostata contracts.
— During ejaculation
  • sympathetic stimulation constricts the m. sphincter urethrae internus, which prevents the seminal fluid from entering the vesica urinaria (retrograde ejaculation);
  • parasympathetic stimulation contracts the mm. urethrales; and
  • the n. pudendus contracts the m. bulbospongiosus.

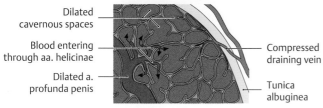

A Penis in cross-section showing blood vessels involved in erection (enlarged views in **B** and **C**).

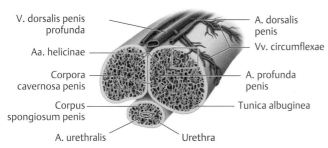

B Corpus cavernosum penis in the flaccid state.

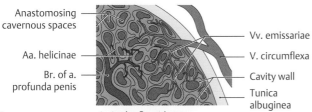

C Corpus cavernosum penis in the erect state.

Fig. 16.9 Mechanism of penile erection (after Lehnert)
(From Schuenke M, Schulte E, Schumacher U. THIEME Atlas of Anatomy, Vol 1. Illustrations by Voll M and Wesker K. 3rd ed. New York: Thieme Publishers; 2020.)

16.4 Female Urogenital Triangle (Regio Urogenitalis)

As in the perineum masculinum, the perineum femininum contains erectile bodies, secretory glands, and their associated neurovasculature. In addition, it contains paired folds of skin that surround the urethral and vaginal orifices. These external genitalia are known collectively as the **vulva** (**Figs. 16.10, 16.11, 16.12, 16.13**).
— **The mons pubis,** a superficial mound of fatty subcutaneous tissue that is continuous with the panniculus adiposus of the abdominal wall, lies anterior to the symphysis pubica and is continuous with the **labia majora.**
— **Labia majora,** bilateral folds of fatty subcutaneous tissue, flank the **pudendal cleft (rima pudendi),** the opening between the labia. The labia join anteriorly at the **commissura labiorum anterior** and posteriorly at the **commissura labiorum posterior**. Pigmented skin and coarse pubic hair cover the labia's outer surface; the inner surface is smooth and hairless.
— **Labia minora,** bilateral folds of hairless skin within the pudendal cleft, flank the vestibulum vaginae.
— The **vestibulum vaginae** is a space surrounded by the two labia minora. It contains the ostium externum urethrae and ostium vaginae and the openings of the ducts of the gll. vestibulares majores and gll. vestibulares minores.
— **Bulbi vestibuli** are paired masses of erectile tissue that lie deep to the labia minora and are covered by the mm. bulbospongiosi.
— **Gll. vestibulares majores** (Bartholin's glands), small glands that lie under the posterior end of the bulbi vestibuli, help to lubricate the vestibulum during sexual arousal.
— Small **gll. vestibulares minores** lie on each side of the vestibulum and secrete mucus to moisten the labia and vestibulum.
— The **clitoris,** a highly sensitive erectile organ, is located at the anterior junction of the paired labia minora (**Fig 16.12**).
  • Paired erectile bodies, the **corpora cavernosa,** make up the crura, which join to form the **corpus clitoridis**. The **preputium** (hood) covers the corpus.
  • The **glans** at the tip of the clitoris is its most sensitive part.
— The aa. pudendales externae supply the skin over the mons pubis and labia majora. Similar to those in the male, these superficial structures drain to the vv. pudendae externae.
— The aa. pudendae internae supply most of the external genitalia through branches that are similar to those in the male perineum (**Fig. 16.14A**).
  • The **aa. perineales** supply perineal muscles and labia minora.
  • The **aa. bulborum vestibuli** supply the bulbi vestibuli and gll. vestibulares majores.

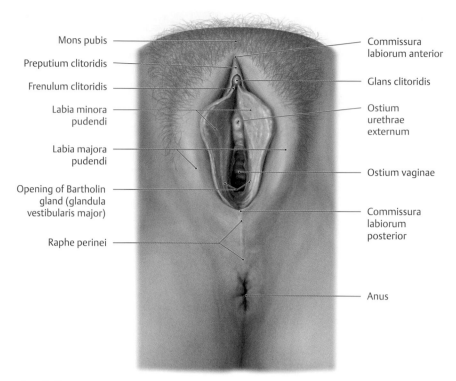

Mons pubis

Preputium clitoridis

Frenulum clitoridis

Labia minora pudendi

Labia majora pudendi

Opening of Bartholin gland (glandula vestibularis major)

Raphe perinei

Commissura labiorum anterior

Glans clitoridis

Ostium urethrae externum

Ostium vaginae

Commissura labiorum posterior

Anus

Fig. 16.10 Female external genitalia
Lithotomy position with labia minora separated. (From Schuenke M, Schulte E, Schumacher U. THIEME Atlas of Anatomy, Vol 1. Illustrations by Voll M and Wesker K. 3rd ed. New York: Thieme Publishers; 2020.)

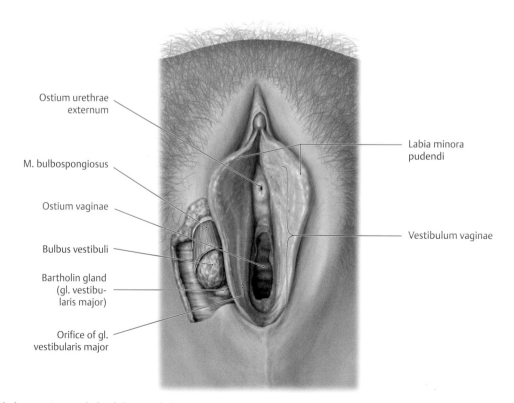

Ostium urethrae externum

M. bulbospongiosus

Ostium vaginae

Bulbus vestibuli

Bartholin gland (gl. vestibularis major)

Orifice of gl. vestibularis major

Labia minora pudendi

Vestibulum vaginae

Fig. 16.11 Vestibulum vaginae and glandulae vestibulares
Lithotomy position with labia separated. (From Schuenke M, Schulte E, Schumacher U. THIEME Atlas of Anatomy, Vol 1. Illustrations by Voll M and Wesker K. 3rd ed. New York: Thieme Publishers; 2020.)

Fig. 16.12 Erectile tissue in the female perineum

(From Gilroy AM et al. Atlas of Anatomy. 4th ed. 2020. Based on: Schuenke M, Schulte E, Schumacher U. THIEME Atlas of Anatomy. General Anatomy and Musculoskeletal System. Illustrations by Voll M and Wesker K. 3rd ed. New York: Thieme Medical Publishers; 2020.)

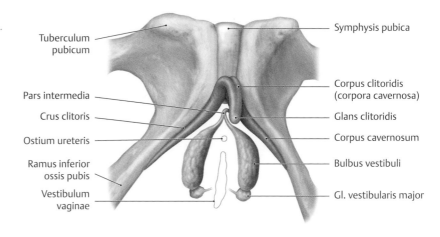

- Tuberculum pubicum
- Pars intermedia
- Crus clitoris
- Ostium ureteris
- Ramus inferior ossis pubis
- Vestibulum vaginae
- Symphysis pubica
- Corpus clitoridis (corpora cavernosa)
- Glans clitoridis
- Corpus cavernosum
- Bulbus vestibuli
- Gl. vestibularis major

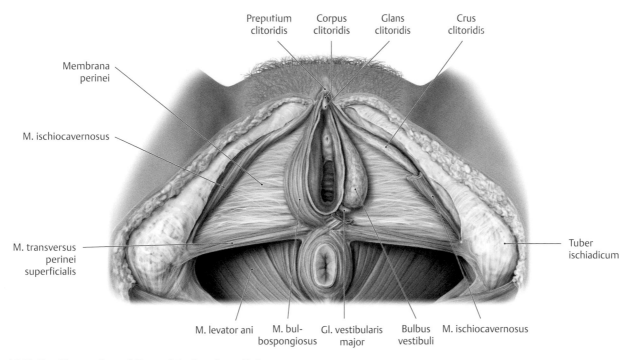

- Preputium clitoridis
- Corpus clitoridis
- Glans clitoridis
- Crus clitoridis
- Membrana perinei
- M. ischiocavernosus
- M. transversus perinei superficialis
- Tuber ischiadicum
- M. levator ani
- M. bulbospongiosus
- Gl. vestibularis major
- Bulbus vestibuli
- M. ischiocavernosus

Fig. 16.13 Erectile muscles and tissue of the female genitalia

Lithotomy position. *Removed:* Labia, skin, and membrana perinei. *Removed from left side:* M. ischiocavernosus and m. bulbospongiosus; gll. vestibulares majores (Bartholin's glands). (From Gilroy AM et al. Atlas of Anatomy. 4th ed. 2020. Based on: Schuenke M, Schulte E, Schumacher U. THIEME Atlas of Anatomy. General Anatomy and Musculoskeletal System. Illustrations by Voll M and Wesker K. 3rd ed. New York: Thieme Medical Publishers; 2020.)

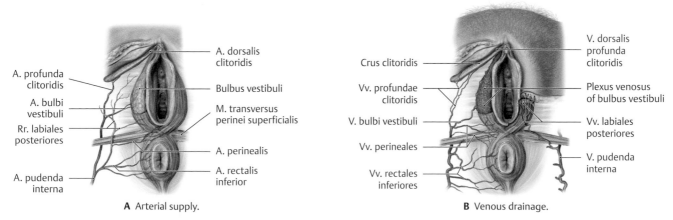

- A. profunda clitoridis
- A. bulbi vestibuli
- Rr. labiales posteriores
- A. pudenda interna
- A. dorsalis clitoridis
- Bulbus vestibuli
- M. transversus perinei superficialis
- A. perinealis
- A. rectalis inferior

A Arterial supply.

- Crus clitoridis
- Vv. profundae clitoridis
- V. bulbi vestibuli
- Vv. perineales
- Vv. rectales inferiores
- V. dorsalis profunda clitoridis
- Plexus venosus of bulbus vestibuli
- Vv. labiales posteriores
- V. pudenda interna

B Venous drainage.

Fig. 16.14 Blood vessels of the female external genitalia

Inferior view. (From Schuenke M, Schulte E, Schumacher U. THIEME Atlas of Anatomy, Vol 1. Illustrations by Voll M and Wesker K. 3rd ed. New York: Thieme Publishers; 2020.)

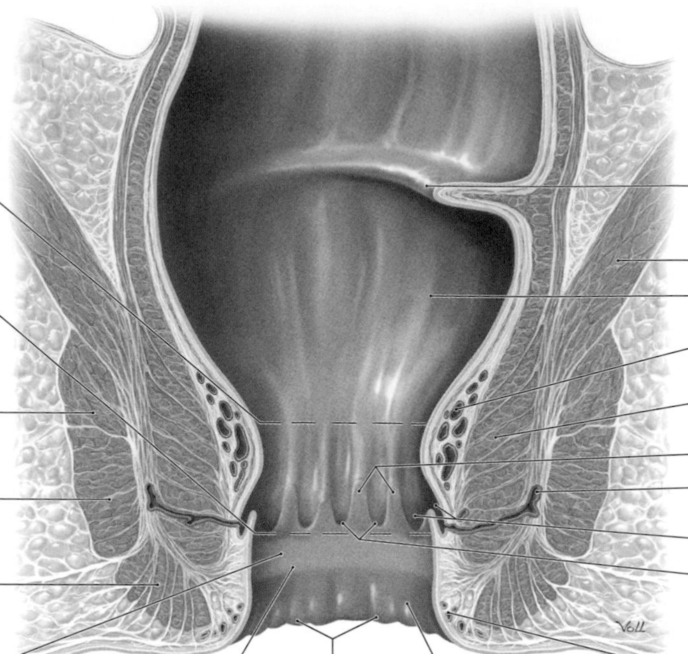

Junctio
anorectalis

Linea pectinata

Pars profunda

M. sphincter
ani externus

Pars
superficialis

Pars
subcutanea

Pecten analis
(white zone)

Linea
anocutanea

Anus

Perianal skin

Plica transversa
recti superior

M. levator ani

Ampulla recti

Plexus venosus
rectalis

M. sphincter
ani internus

Columnae anales

Anal (proctodeal)
gland

Sinus anales

Valvulae anales

Plexus venosus
subcutaneus

Fig. 16.15 Canalis analis
Coronal section, anterior view. (From Schuenke M, Schulte E, Schumacher U. THIEME Atlas of Anatomy, Vol 2. Illustrations by Voll M and Wesker K. 3rd ed. New York: Thieme Publishers; 2020.)

- The **aa. dorsales clitorides** supply the glans of the clitoris.
- The **aa. profundae clitoridis** supply the corpora cavernosa and are responsible for engorgement during arousal.
— Tributaries of the vv. pudendae internae drain most perineal structures and accompany the arteries. A single **v. dorsalis clitoridis profunda** drains the plexus venosus of the erectile tissue and passes under the symphysis pubica to join the plexus venosus in the pelvis (**Fig. 16.14B**).
— Most lymph from the perineum femininum drains to nll. inguinales superficiales. Exceptions include
  - the clitoris, bulbi vestibuli, and anterior labia, which drain to nll. inguinales profundi or nll. iliaci interni; and
  - the urethra, which drains to nll. sacrales or nll. iliaci interni.
— The right and left nn. pudendae are the primary nerves of the perineum (see **Fig. 14.20**). They supply
  - the **nn. perineales** to the ostium vaginae and superficial perineal muscles;
  - **nn. dorsales clitoridis** to deep perineal muscles and sensation from the clitoris, especially the glans; and
  - **nn. labiales posteriores** to the posterior vulva.
— Similar to the innervation of the male scrotum, the anterior vulva receives sensory innervation (see **Fig. 14.20**) from
  - the n. ilioinguinalis and n. genitalis from the n. genitofemoralis, which supply branches to the mons pubis and anterior labia; and
  - n. cutaneus femoris posterior, which supply the posterolateral vulva.
— Sympathetic fibers to the perineum travel with the plexus nervosus hypogastricus; parasympathetic fibers travel with nn. cavernosi of the plexus uterovaginalis. Both innervate the erectile tissue of the clitoris and bulbi vestibuli (**Fig.14.23**).

16.5   Anal Triangle (Regio Analis)

The anal triangle (regio analis) contains the canalis analis and fossae ischioanalis.

The Canalis Analis

The **canalis analis**, the terminal part of the gastrointestinal tract, controls fecal continence and the defecation response. It extends from the junctio anorectalis at the diaphragma pelvis to the **anus** (**Fig. 16.15**).
— The m. puborectalis forms a sling around the junctio anorectalis, pulling it anteriorly and creating the **flexura perinealis** (**Fig. 16.16**). From this angle the canalis analis descends inferiorly and posteriorly between the lig. anococcygeum (levator plate) and the perineal body (see **Fig. 16.1**).

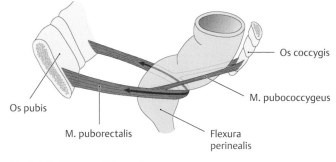

Os pubis

M. puborectalis

Os coccygis

M. pubococcygeus

Flexura
perinealis

Fig. 16.16 Closure of the rectum
Left lateral view.
The m. puborectalis acts as a muscular sling that kinks the junctio anorectalis. It functions in the maintenance of fecal continence. (From Gilroy AM et al. Atlas of Anatomy. 4th ed. 2020. Based on: Schuenke M, Schulte E, Schumacher U. THIEME Atlas of Anatomy. Internal Organs. Illustrations by Voll M and Wesker K. 3rd ed. New York: Thieme Medical Publishers; 2020.)

— Two sphincters surround the canalis analis:
  1. The **m. sphincter ani internus** is a thickening of the circular muscular layer that surrounds the upper part of the canalis analis.
     ○ It is an involuntary sphincter.
     ○ It remains contracted via sympathetic innervation except in response to distension of the ampulla recti. Parasympathetic innervation relaxes the sphincter.
  2. The **m. sphincter ani externus** is a broad band of muscle that extends anteriorly to merge with the corpus perineale, posteriorly to attach to the os coccygis (through the lig. anococcygeum), and superiorly to merge with the m. puborectalis of the pelvic floor (see also **Figs. 15.1, 16.1, 16.2**). Although it is described as having deep, superficial, and subcutaneous parts, they are functionally, and often anatomically, indistinct.
     ○ It is a voluntary sphincter.
     ○ The n. rectus inferior, a branch of the n. pudendus, innervates this sphincter.
— The inner surface of the canalis analis is characterized by
  • **anal columns (columnae anales)**, vertical ridges formed by underlying branches of the superior rectal vessels;
  • **anal valves (valvulae anales)** that connect the inferior edges of the anal columns; and
  • **anal sinuses (sinus anales)**, recesses at the base of the anal columns that secrete mucus to facilitate defecation.
— The **linea pectinata** is an irregular ridge at the base of the anal columns.
  • It divides the canalis analis into a superior part derived from the endoderm of the embryonic hindgut and an inferior part derived from the embryonic ectoderm.
  • It divides the canalis analis in its blood supply, lymphatic drainage, and innervation.
— Below the linea pectinata, a smooth lining devoid of glands and hair, the **pecten analis**, extends down to the **linea anocutanea**, or sulcus intersphinctericus.
— Below the linea anocutanea, the canalis analis is lined by hair-bearing skin that is continuous with **perianal skin** that surrounds the anus.
— Above the linea pectinata the neurovasculature of the canalis analis is similar to that of the distal gastrointestinal tract (see Section 14.6).
  • It receives its blood supply from the a. rectalis superior, a branch of the a. mesenterica inferior.
  • The plexus venosus rectalis drains through the v. rectalis superior into the portal venous system.
  • Lymph drains to the nll. iliaci interni.
  • Visceral innervation is transmitted via plexus nervosum rectalis to the plexus hypogastricus inferior.
     ○ Sympathetic stimulation maintains the tone of the sphincter.
     ○ Parasympathetic innervation relaxes the sphincter and stimulates peristalsis of the rectum.
     ○ Visceral sensory fibers travel with nn. splanchnici pelvici (parasympathetic) and convey only sensation of stretching (no sensitivity to pain).
— Below the linea pectinata, the neurovasculature of the canalis analis is similar to that of the perineum (see Section 14.6).
  • It receives its blood supply from the **a. rectalis inferior dextra** and **a. rectalis inferior sinistra**, branches of the aa. pudendae internae.

• The plexus venosus rectalis drains into **vv. rectales inferiores**, which in turn drain to vv. iliacae internae of the venae cavae.
• Lymph drains to nll. inginales superficiales.
• Somatic innervation is transmitted via the **n. rectalis inferior**, a branch of the n. pudendus.
  ○ Somatic efferent fibers stimulate contraction of the m. sphincter ani externus.
  ○ Somatic afferent fibers transmit pain, touch, and temperature.

BOX 16.4: CLINICAL CORRELATION

HEMORRHOIDS

External hemorrhoids are thrombosed veins of the external plexus venosus anorectalis, commonly associated with pregnancy or chronic constipation. They lie below the linea pectinata and are covered by skin. Because they are somatically innervated, they are more painful than internal hemorrhoids.

Internal hemorrhoids contain dilated veins of the internal plexus venosus anorectalis. With a breakdown of the tunica muscularis, these vascular cushions prolapse into the anal canal and may become ulcerated. Because they lie above the linea pectinata and are viscerally innervated, these hemorrhoids are painless. They are generally not associated with portal hypertension, but bleeding is characteristically bright red due to the arteriovenous anastomoses between the venous plexus and branches of the aa. rectales.

BOX 16.5: CLINICAL CORRELATION

ANAL FISSURES

Anal fissures are tears in the mucosa around the anus (usually in the posterior midline) that are caused by the passing of hard or large stools. Because they are below the linea pectinata and innervated by the nn. recti inferiores, these lesions are painful. Most anal fissures heal spontaneously within a few weeks if care is taken to prevent constipation. Perianal abscesses that develop from the fissures can spread into the adjacent fossae ischioanales.

Defecation and Continence

The opening (defecation) and closing (continence) of the canalis analis is controlled by a complex apparatus that involves muscular, vascular, and neural components.
— The sphincter internus ani, under visceromotor control, is responsible for 70% of fecal continence. Sympathetic stimulation allows it to maintain a constant constriction of the canalis analis until it relaxes in response to a rise in intra-rectal pressure.
— The m. sphincter ani externus and m. puborectalis of the levator ani, under somatomotor control, constrict the canalis analis and maintain the anorectal angle, respectively. Voluntary relaxation during defecation results in widening of the canalis analis and straightening of the m. puborectalis sling.
— The vascular part of the continence apparatus involves the hemorrhoidal plexus, a permanently distended cavernous body within the submucosa, which forms circular cushions above the anal columns (**Fig. 16.17**). When filled with blood (supplied by the a. rectalis superior) these cushions serve as

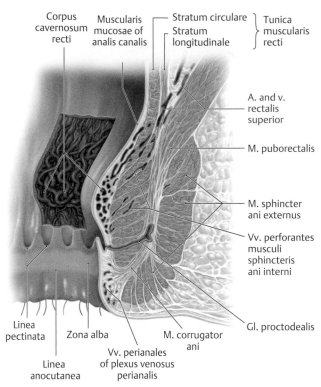

A Longitudinal section of the canalis analis with the hemorrhoidal plexus windowed.

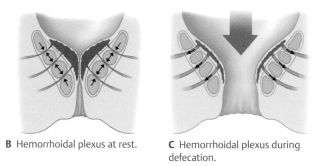

B Hemorrhoidal plexus at rest.

C Hemorrhoidal plexus during defecation.

Fig. 16.17 Structure of the vascular continence mechanism
(From Schuenke M, Schulte E, Schumacher U. THIEME Atlas of Anatomy, Vol 2. Illustrations by Voll M and Wesker K. 3rd ed. New York: Thieme Publishers; 2020.)

an effective continence mechanism that ensures liquid- and gas-tight closure. The sustained contraction of the muscular sphincter apparatus inhibits venous drainage, but when the sphincter relaxes during defecation, blood is allowed to drain via arteriovenous anastomoses to the v. mesenterica inferior (to the portal system) and vv. rectales mediae and vv. rectales inferiores (to the systemic system).

— The neural component of this mechanism involves (see **Fig. 14.22**)
  • somatic motor nerves primarily via the n. pudendus (S2–S4) to the m. sphincter ani externus and m. puborectalis, and somatic sensory nerves via nn. rectales inferiores from the anus and perianal skin.
  • visceral motor (parasympathetic) nerves via nn. splanchnici pelvici to the m. sphincter ani internus in the plexus rectalis and visceral sensory nerves from the wall of the rectum.

Fossae Ischioanales and Canalis Pudendalis

— The fossae ischioanales are paired wedge-shaped spaces on either side of the canalis analis bounded by the diaphragma pelvis superiorly and the skin of the regio analis inferiorly (see **Fig. 15.24**).
  • Fat and loose connective tissue, strengthened by strong fibrous bands, fill the fossae. These tissues support the canalis analis but can be displaced readily when the canalis analis distends with feces.
  • The a. rectalis inferior, v. rectalis inferior, and n. rectalis inferior, branches of the a. pudenda and v. pudenda and n. pudendus, traverse the fossae.
  • The fossae ischioanales extend anteriorly into the regio urogenitalis superior to the membrana perinei.
— The canalis pudendalis is a passageway formed by the splitting of the fascia of the m. obturatorius internus on the lateral wall of the fossa ischioanalis.
  • The a. pudenda interna and v. pudenda interna and the n. pudendus enter the canal after exiting the foramen ischiadicum minus and giving off rami rectales inferiores.

17 Clinical Imaging Basics of the Pelvis and Perineum

Radiography of the pelvis is used in the evaluation of trauma patients and for a quick first-line assessment of the hip joints. If greater detail of the soft tissues is required, magnetic resonance imaging (MRI) is the next step. For evaluation of pelvic contents in female patients, ultrasound provides superb images quickly and inexpensively and without exposing the gonads to radiation. Therefore, ultrasound is very useful in emergent situations (e.g., acute pelvic pain). MRI also shows excellent detail of the pelvis, but because it takes longer to acquire the images, it is less useful in emergencies (**Table 17.1**).

In children, ultrasound can also be valuable in evaluation of the hips. The developing skeleton is only partially ossified, thus making portions of it invisible on x-rays (**Fig. 17.1**). To assess the art. coxae, such as for developmental dysplasia of the hip (DDH), ultrasound is used to assess the position of the cartilaginous femoral head (caput femoris; **Fig 17.2**).

Standard radiographic views of the bony pelvis include an anteroposterior (AP) projection showing both artt. coxarum (**Fig. 17.3**). In patients with pelvic fractures, different obliquities are often used to assess alignment. There are several approaches to imaging the contents of the pelvis. As in the abdomen, computed tomography (CT) is often used with oral or intravenous contrast to enhance the pelvic organs (**Fig. 17.4**), but in non-emergent conditions, MRI provides the best anatomic detail (**Fig. 17.5**). In comparison, ultrasound offers less detail, but because it is safer and faster, it is usually the first choice for imaging female pelvic organs (**Figs. 17.6** and **17.7**).

Table 17.1 Suitability of Imaging Modalities for the Pelvis

Modality	Clinical Uses
Radiographs (x-rays)	Used primarily to evaluate the pelvic bones
CT (computed tomography)	Provides excellent anatomic detail, but at the expense of radiation
MRI (magnetic resonance imaging)	Ideal for evaluation of the pelvic bones and surrounding muscles and soft tissues; also useful as an adjunct to ultrasound for the female pelvis
Ultrasound	The primary imaging modality for evaluation of the female pelvis, specifically the uterus and ovaries; in males, the mainstay of imaging of the scrotum and testicles

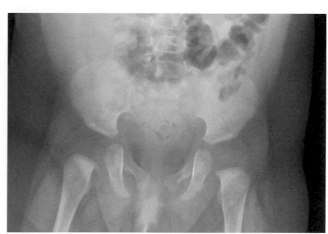

A Infant.

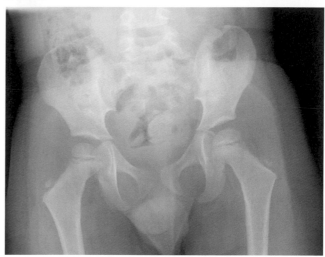

B School-age child.

Fig. 17.1 Frontal radiographs of the pelvis illustrating the developmental ossification of the skeleton
Note how the caput femoris and pelvic growth plates progressively ossifiy with age and thus become visible as bone by radiography. Compare to the fully grown adult pelvis in 17.3. (Courtesy of Joseph Makris, MD, Baystate Medical Center.)

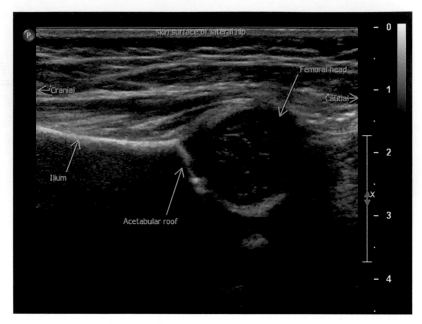

Fig. 17.2 Infant hip ultrasound
The probe is positioned at the lateral aspect of the infant's hip sagittally. The cartilaginous (has not ossified yet) caput femoris is well seen by ultrasound due to the water component of the growing epiphyseal cartilage. The shape of the developing acetabulum and the position of the caput femoris relative to the acetabulum are evaluated for signs of developmental dysplasia. (Courtesy of Joseph Makris, MD, Baystate Medical Center.)

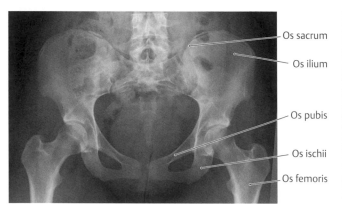

Fig. 17.3 Radiograph of the pelvis in an adult
Anterior view.
Note that the rounded femoral heads (capita femora) sit uniformly in each acetabulum, and the artt. sacroiliacae and symphysis pubica are sharply seen. The lower part of the os sacrum is partially obscured by gas and stool in the rectum (irregular dark and light gray shapes in the mid-pelvis). The cristae iliacae can be traced along their edges to the acetabulum and into the os ischii and symphysis pubica. The edges of the bones should curve smoothly and be sharply defined. (Courtesy of Joseph Makris, MD, Baystate Medical Center.)

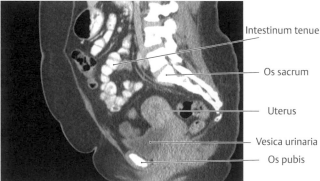

Fig. 17.4 CT of the female pelvis
Left lateral view.
This CT reconstruction, shown in the "soft tissue window," highlights the relationships of the pelvic organs. Oral contrast causes the bowel to appear white; intravenous contrast enhances the vascularized soft tissues (*light gray*). The urine-filled vesica urinaria has a water density of dark gray. The uterus is enhanced by the intravenous contrast and is easily seen against the vesica urinaria anteriorly and fat superiorly. The endometrium is barely seen within the uterus. It is difficult to precisely define the plane between the uterus and the adjacent rectum. (Courtesy of Joseph Makris, MD, Baystste Medical Center.)

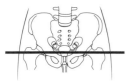

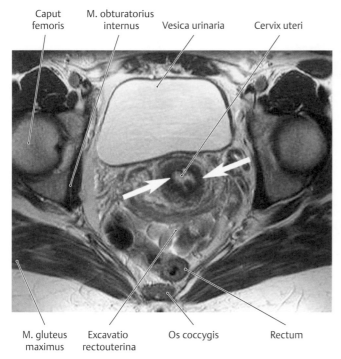

Caput femoris M. obturatorius internus Vesica urinaria Cervix uteri

M. gluteus maximus Excavatio rectouterina Os coccygis Rectum

Fig. 17.5 MRI of the female pelvis
Transverse section through the level of the cervix uteri.
In this MRI sequence, fluid is white, muscle is black, and other soft tissues are gray. Soft tissue detail seen on MRI is superior to that seen on CT and ultrasound. Note the dark *(black)* cervical stroma *(arrows)* that surrounds the white fluid in the canalis cervicis uteri. Because MRI is very sensitive in differentiating tissue types, it is easy to distinguish the pelvic organs from each other and from the adjacent bowel. The bright fat planes between structures provide good contrast. (From Hamm B, et al. MRI Imaging of the Abdomen and Pelvis, 2nd ed. New York: Thieme Publishers; 2009.)

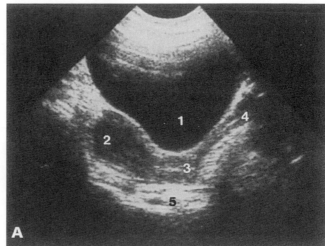

A Midsagittal (longitudinal) section.

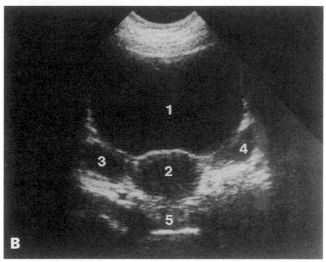

B Transverse section.

Fig. 17.6 Transabdominal ultrasound of the uterus and ovaries
With transabdominal imaging of the pelvis, the ultrasound probe is placed on the lower abdominal wall anterior to the vesica urinaria. A full bladder provides an acoustic "window" to better visualize the uterus and related structures. (Patients are required to drink plenty of fluid prior to the exam.) The urine in the vesica urinaria is anechoic *(black)*. The muscular and vascular structure of the uterus and follicular and vascular structure of the ovaries make these structures hypoechoic *(dark gray)*. The ovaries should appear relatively symmetric in size and shape. *1,* urine-filled vesica urinaria; *2,* uterus; *3,* cervix uteri; *4,* vagina; *5,* rectum. (From Gunderman R. Essential Radiology, 3rd ed. New York: Thieme Publishers; 2014.)

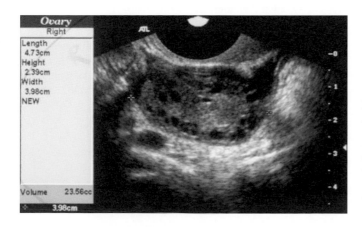

Fig. 17.7 Transvaginal ultrasound of the right ovarum
An empty vesica urinaria (patient is asked to urinate immediately before the exam) positions the uterus and associated structures for optimal visualization. The tip of the ultrasound probe is positioned directly against the cervix uteri and pointed toward the side of interest until the ovary is found. The close proximity of the tip of the ultrasound probe to the pelvic structures provides significantly improved image detail over transabdominal images. This patient has enlarged ovaries due to polycystic ovarian syndrome. Note the detail of the numerous small ovarian follicles (*black,* since they are fluid filled). (From Gunderman R. Essential Radiology, 3rd ed. New York: Thieme Publishers; 2014)

Unit V   Review Questions: Pelvis and Perineum

1. After a prolonged labor, Janice delivered a healthy 9 lb 8 oz baby boy through a normal vaginal birth, although the delivery required an episiotomy to prevent tearing of the perineum. During the procedure, her m. sphincter externus ani and some fibers of the m. puborectalis were cut. As a medical student who understands the role of these muscles, Janice is concerned about her ability to maintain fecal continence. Relaxation of these muscles
   A. straightens the flexura perinealis of the junctio anorectalis
   B. allows venous drainage from the vascular cushions of the hemorrhoid plexus
   C. widens the canalis analis
   D. would result from damage to the nn. rectales inferiores, branches of the nn. pudendae
   E. all of the above

2. Which one of the following statements best describes the muscles of the pelvis?
   A. The m. obturatorius internus leaves the pelvis through the foramen ischiadicum majus.
   B. The m. levator ani is composed of the m. pubococcygeus, m. puborectalis, and m. iliococcygeus.
   C. The diaphragma pelvis is a sling of muscle that separates the pelvis minor from the pelvis major.
   D. The m. piriformis forms the lateral wall of the pelvis.
   E. The m. coccygeus attaches to the lig. sacrotuberale.

3. Typically, the posterior division of the a. iliaca interna supplies
   A. structures of the perineum
   B. muscles of the medial thigh
   C. meninges of the radices spinales sacrales
   D. uterus and tubae uterinae
   E. prostata

4. The components of the nn. splanchnici pelvici are most similar to the components of the
   A. nn. splanchnici lumbales
   B. nn. splanchnici sacrales
   C. n. pudendus
   D. n. vagus
   E. nn. hypogastrici

5. Carcinoma of the prostata can metastasize to bone and the brain through its connections with the plexus venosus vertebralis. Which other structures communicate with this plexus venosus?
   A. Breast
   B. Medulla spinalis
   C. Mm. intercostales
   D. Oesophagus
   E. All of the above

6. Although branches of the a. uterina anastomose extensively throughout the pelvis, the main stem of the vessel travels within the
   A. lig. ovarii proprium
   B. lig. cardinale
   C. lig. uterosacrale
   D. lig. suspensorium ovarii
   E. lig. teres uteri

7. Which of the following statements accurately describes the relations of the ureter?
   A. It is crossed anteriorly by the gonadal vessels on the posterior abdominal wall.
   B. It crosses the brim of the pelvis at the bifurcation of the a. iliaca communis.
   C. In females it passes under the a. uterina ~ 2 cm lateral to the cervix uteri.
   D. It enters the vesica urinaria at the posterolateral aspect of the trigonum vesicae.
   E. All of the above

8. During a routine physical exam on a male patient, you test the integrity of the m. sphincter ani externus. What spinal cord segments are involved in this?
   A. T12–L1
   B. L2–L4
   C. L4–L5
   D. S1–S2
   E. S2–S4

9. The fascia perinei superficialis is continuous with the
   A. membrana perinei
   B. tunica dartos
   C. fascia penis profunda
   D. tunica albuginea penis
   E. fascia endopelvica

10. The boundary of the apertura superior pelvis
    A. provides the attachment site for the diaphragma pelvis
    B. includes the cristae iliacae
    C. includes the r. ischii
    D. is crossed by the a. ovarica and a. testicularis
    E. separates the cavity of the cavitas pelvis from the cavitas abdominis

11. Several years after delivering twin boys, a woman experienced mild uterine prolapse and urinary incontinence. Her gynecologist was able to confirm that the angle of her lig. anococcygeum had changed, suggesting a laxity in her pelvic floor muscles. Which muscles insert on the lig. anococcygeum?
    A. M. coccygeus
    B. M. iliococcygeus
    C. M. piriformis
    D. M. transversus perinei profundus
    E. M. obturatorius internus

12. Tumors that metastasize via the bloodstream often form metastases in the first capillary bed that the cells reach after they enter the bloodstream. Based on their venous drainage, tumors in which of the following locations are likely to reach the lung before they reach the liver?
A. Colon ascendens
B. Colon sigmoideum
C. Pancreas
D. Superior (proximal) rectum
E. Inferior (distal) rectum

13. Which one of the following structures passes through the hiatus urogenitalis?
A. Ductus deferens
B. Nn. cavernosi
C. Lig. teres uteri
D. N. obturatorius
E. A. iliaca externa

14. A 44-year-old woman undergoes a total hysterectomy for painful fibroids. The ovaries will not be removed during the procedure. Which of the following ligaments must be preserved?
A. Lig. suspensorium ovarii
B. Lig. ovarii
C. Lig. uterosacrale
D. Lig. transversum cervicis
E. Lig. teres uteri

15. Which of the following statements best describes the cervix uteri?
A. In a normally anteflexed uterus, the cervix is tilted posteriorly.
B. Fornices vaginae surround its portio supravaginalis.
C. It is the attachment site for the lig. teres uteri.
D. It makes up the inferior third of the uterus.
E. It communicates with the cavitas uteri through the ostium uteri.

16. A 53-year-old man had an aortic aneurysm that extended through his bifurcatio aortae into his aa. iliacae communes. During the open repair, the surgeon opened the vessels longitudinally and fixed a synthetic graft to the walls of the vessels above and below the aneurysm. Following surgery, the man experienced retrograde ejaculation because of damage to nerves that innervated his m. sphincter urethrae internus. Which nerves were damaged?
A. Sympathetic nerves of the plexus nervosus hypogastricus superior
B. Parasympathetic nerves of the plexus nervosus hypogastricus superior
C. Somatic nerves of the plexus sacralis
D. Nn. splanchnici pelvici
E. Truncus sympathicus

17. You are treating a 34-year-old woman for hemorrhoids. Although she does not complain of pain, the hemorrhoids protrude into her canalis analis and are becoming ulcerated. There is no evidence of portal hypertension, but blood from the ulcers is bright red. Based on her brief history, what can you surmise about her condition?
A. The prolapsed tissue contains the dilated veins of the plexus venosus rectalis externus.
B. The hemorrhoids originate from below the linea pectinata.

C. The dilated veins in the hemorrhoids drain to the vv. rectales inferiores.
D. The dilated veins communicate with the aa. rectales to form an arteriovenous hemorrhoidal plexus.
E. All of the above

18. During a robotic prostatectomy on a 41-year-old man, the nn. cavernosi were inadvertently damaged. What symptoms would you expect in this patient?
A. Loss of tone in his m. sphincter ani externus
B. Urinary incontinence
C. Inability to ejaculate
D. Inability to form an erection
E. Loss of sensation at the tip of the penis

19. Structures that pass through the foramen ischiadicum majus include the
A. m. obturator internus
B. m. coccygeus
C. m. iliopsoas
D. m. piriformis
E. n. obturatorius

20. The arcus tendineus fasciae pelvis
A. is a condensation of fascia endopelvica
B. includes the lig. recti laterale
C. supports the viscera pelvis
D. provides an attachment site for the diaphragma pelvis
E. All of the above

21. Structures that drain (directly or indirectly) into the nll. inguinales profundi include the
A. glans penis
B. perianal skin
C. supralateral part of the uterus via the lig. teres uteri
D. scrotum
E. All of the above

22. During the national championships an Olympic gymnast fell backward off the balance beam, fracturing the tip of her os coccygis and subluxing (dislocating) her art. sacroiliaca. The team physician was concerned about damage to her plexus sacralis and its branches that exit the pelvis. Nerves of the plexus sacralis pass through the
A. foramina sacralia posteriora
B. canalis obturatorius
C. foramen ischiadicum minus
D. anulus inguinalis superficialis
E. anulus inguinalis profundus

23. A young, pregnant woman in her third trimester was alarmed when she experienced a sharp pain in the anterior part of her labia majora when she stood up. Her obstetrician assured her that this was a common problem in late pregnancy and was most likely caused by
A. stretching of the lig. teres uteri
B. tightening of the lig. inguinale
C. pressure on the n. obturatorius
D. irritation of the r. perinei of the n. pudendus
E. stretching of the n. iliohypogastricus

24. A vascular surgeon is repairing an aneurysm of the bifurcatio aortae that extends along the a. iliaca communis dextra to its division into a. iliaca interna and a. iliaca externa. What structure does the surgeon encounter that is at risk as it crosses over the pelvic brim at this distal end of the aneurysm?
   A. Ureter
   B. A. testicularis
   C. Truncus lumbosacralis
   D. N. ischiadicus
   E. Ductus deferens

25. Similar to other sections of the intestinum crassum, the rectum is characterized by
   A. taeniae coli
   B. haustra coli
   C. a mesenterium
   D. appendices epiploicae
   E. None of the above

26. Which of the following are found within the spatium superficiale perinei?
   A. Gll. bulbourethrales
   B. M. sphincter urethrae externus
   C. M. bulbospongiosus
   D. Anterior extension of corpus adiposum fossae ischioanalis
   E. N. rectalis inferior

27. The pars spongiosa urethrae masculinae
   A. passes through the corpus spongiosum penis
   B. is surrounded by the m. sphincter internus urethrae
   C. is surrounded by the m. sphincter externus urethrae
   D. is characterized by a vertical ridge, the crista urethralis, on its posterior wall
   E. contains openings for the ductus ejaculatorii

28. Similar to the penis in the male, the clitoris is formed by highly sensitive erectile tissue. Which of the following structures is composed of erectile tissue but does not form part of the clitoris?
   A. Corpora cavernosa
   B. Bulbi vestibuli
   C. Gll. vestibulares majores
   D. Preputium
   E. Glans

29. During a routine physical, which included a digital rectal exam, your physician discovered a firm nodule on your prostate, suggesting prostate carcinoma. This was confirmed in subsequent blood tests that revealed increased levels of prostate specific antigen (PSA). Prostate carcinoma is
   A. a common and non-malignant disease of older men
   B. usually found in the peripheral zone
   C. usually found in the largely glandular anterior lobe
   D. a disease of the periurethral zone, causing urethral obstruction in the early stages
   E. also known as benign prostatic hypertrophy

30. What imaging modality is best for routine evaluation of a developing fetus?
   A. CT
   B. Ultrasound
   C. X-rays
   D. MRI

31. A 24-year-old male has acute onset of severe scrotal pain. You suspect that he may have testicular torsion (twisting of the funiculus spermaticus and testicle, restricting blood to the testicle) and send the patient for an emergent ultrasound of his scrotum to confirm your suspicion. What feature of ultrasound imaging is useful for assessing blood flow to the testicles?
   A. Low cost
   B. Lack of ionizing radiation
   C. Real-time color and spectral Doppler imaging
   D. Ultrasound waves travel best through water

Answers and Explanations

1. **E.** All are correct (Section 16.5).
   A. Contraction of the muscles maintains the flexure, relaxation of the muscles straightens it.
   B. Contraction of the muscular sphincter apparatus inhibits the venous drainage of the vascular cushions. They drain when the sphincters relax during defecation.
   C. The function of the external canalis analis is to widen the canalis analis during defecation.
   D. The nn. anales inferiores maintain the tone of the m. sphincter externus ani and m. puborectalis. Denervaton of these muscles would result in their relaxation.

2. **B.** The m. levator ani is composed of the m. pubococcygeus, m. puborectalis, and m. iliococcygeus (Section 14.3).
   A. The m. obturatorius internus covers the sidewall of the pelvis and perineum. Its tendon passes from the perineum to the regio glutealis through the foramen ischiadicum minus.
   C. The diaphragma pelvis separates the pelvis major from the perineum, which lies below it.
   D. The m. piriformis forms the posterior muscular wall of the pelvis.
   E. The m. coccygeus attaches to the lig. sacrospinale along its entire length.

3. **C.** The posterior division supplies parietal branches to the posterior abdominal wall, some gluteal muscles, and the meninges of the sacral spinal roots (Section 14.6).
   A. The a. pudenda interna, a branch of the anterior division of the a. iliaca interna, supplies most structures of the perineum.
   B. The a. obturatoria, a branch of the anterior division of the a. iliaca interna, supplies muscles of the medial thigh.
   D. The a. uterina, a branch of the anterior division of the a. iliaca interna, supplies the uterus and tubae uterinae.
   E. The aa. prostaticae, usually branches of the aa. vesicales inferiorae, are derived from the anterior division of the a. iliaca interna.

4. **D.** The nn. splanchnici pelvici represent the sacral component of the parasympathetic system; the n. vagus represents the cranial component of the parasympathetic system (Section 14.6).
   A. Nn. splanchnici lumbales arise from the truncus sympatheticus lumbalis and carry postganglionic sympathetic fibers.
   B. Nn. splanchnici sacrales arise from the truncus sympatheticus sacralis and carry postganglionic sympathetic fibers.

C. The n. pudendus arises from the plexus sacralis and carries somatic sensory and motor fibers.

E. Nn. hypogastrici derive from the plexus hypogastricus superior carrying postganglionic sympathetic fibers to the plexus pelvicus.

5. **E.** The vertebral venous system is a tributary of the azygos system. The breast, mm. intercostales, and oesophagus drain via vv. intercostales to the azygos system, and the medulla spinalis drains directly into the plexus venosus vertebralis (Section 15.1 and Unit III, Thorax).

A. Blood from the breast drains to vv. intercostales and the azygos system, which communicates with the plexus venosus vertebralis. B through D are also correct (E).

B. The veins of the medulla spinalis drain to the plexus venosus vertebralis. A, C, and D are also correct (E).

C. The vv. intercostales that drain mm. intercostales terminate in the azygos system, which also receives the plexus venosus vertebralis. A, B, and D are also correct (E).

D. Veins of the lower oesophagus drain to the portal system, but in the thorax vv. oesophageales drain to the azygos system, which also receives the plexus venosus vertebralis. A through C are also correct (E).

6. **B.** The a. uterina and v. uterina travel within the lig. cardinale at the base of the lig. latum uteri (Section 15.2).

A. The lig. ovarii proprium connects the ovarium to the uterus and does not contain any major vessels.

C. The lig. uterosacrale is a thickening of endopelvic fascia that connects the cervix uteri to the os sacrum. It does not contain any major vessels.

D. The lig. suspensorium ovarii is a fold of peritoneum that contains the ovarian vessels as they cross over the pelvic brim.

E. The lig. teres uteri extends from the uterus through the canalis inguinalis to the labia majora. Although it is accompanied by small vessels, it does not contain any major arteries.

7. **E.** All are correct (Section 15.3).

A. The gonadal vessels cross anterior to the ureter as it descends along the posterior abdominal wall. B through D are also correct (E).

B. The bifurcation of the a. iliaca communis is a useful landmark for locating the ureter as it crosses the pelvic brim. A, C, and D are also correct (E).

C. The ureter passes under the a. uterina lateral to the cervix uteri and therefore is at risk of injury during a hysterectomy. A, B, and D are also correct (E).

D. The ureteral openings posterolaterally and the urethral opening in the anterior midline define the apexes of the trigone. A through C are also correct (E).

8. **E.** The n. pudendus (S2–S4) provides motor innervation to the m. sphincter externus (Sections 14.6 and 15.4).

A. T12–L1 nerve roots contribute to the n. subcostalis, n. iliohypogastricus, and n. ilioinguinalis, which innervate muscles of the anterior abdominal wall.

B. The L2–L4 nerve roots form the n. femoralis and n. obturatorius, which innervate muscles of the anterior and medial thigh.

C. Nerves from L4–L5 spinal cord segments form the truncus lumbosacralis, which joins the plexus sacralis to innervate muscles of the lower limb.

D. S1–S2 nerve roots contribute to the plexus sacralis, which innervates muscles of the lower limb.

9. **B.** The fascia perinei superficialis is continuous with the tunica dartos that lines the scrotum and with Scarpa's fascia (stratum membranosum telae subcutaneae abdominis; Section 16.1).

A. The membrana perinei is a fibrous sheet that forms the roof of the spatium superficiale perinei.

C. Fascia penis profunda is a fibrous layer that binds the three erectile bodies of the penis.

D. Each of the three erectile bodies of the penis is surrounded by the dense, fibrous tunica albuginea.

E. Fascia endopelvica is the loose connective tissue matrix that fills the spatia infraperitonealia of the pelvis.

10. **E.** The apertura pelvis superior separates the pelvis minor from the pelvis major. The cavitas pelvis is the lower part of the cavitas abdominalis and contains abdominal viscera (Section 14.1).

A. The diaphragma pelvis attaches to the r. pubicus superior, arcus tendineus m. levator ani, and lig. sacrospinale.

B. The cristae iliacae form the upper boundary of the pelvis major. The apertura pelvis superior forms its lower boundary.

C. The ramus ischii forms part of the apertura pelvis inferior but not the apertura pelvis superior.

D. The aa. ovaricae cross the apertura pelvis superior, but the aa. testiculares pass along the brim of the pelvis (apertura pelvis superior) to the anulus inguinalis profundus, where they enter the canalis inguinalis as part of the funiculus spermaticus.

11. **B.** The lig. anococcygeum (also known as the levator plate) is a midline raphe between the anus and os coccygis that serves as the insertion for the m. pubococcygeus and m. iliococcygeus (Section 14.3).

A. The m. coccygeus inserts on the spina ischiadica.

C. The m. piriformis inserts on the trochanter major of the femur.

D. Mm. transversi perinei profundi insert on the vagina (or prostata) and corpus perineale.

E. The m. obturatorius internus inserts on the trochanter major of the femur.

12. **E.** The vv. rectales inferiores drain through the caval system (via the v. iliaca interna and v. cava inferior) back to the heart and pulmonary circulation. All other choices are tributaries of the portal system, which drains through the liver before returning to the heart (Sections 11.2 and 15.4).

A. Veins of the colon ascendens are tributaries of the portal system. Therefore, blood passes through the liver before returning to the heart and pulmonary circulation.

B. Veins of the colon sigmoideum, and all parts of the gastrointestinal tract, are tributaries of the portal system. Therefore, blood passes through the liver before returning to the heart and pulmonary circulation.

C. Veins of the pancreas are tributaries of the portal system. Therefore, blood from the pancreas drains through the liver before returning to the heart and pulmonary circulation.

D. The v. rectalis superior that drains the superior rectum is a tributary of the portal system. Therefore, this blood passes through the liver before returning to the heart and pulmonary circulation.

13. **B.** The nn. cavernosi carry parasympathetic innervation from the plexus pelvicus to the perineum by passing through the hiatus urogenitalis (Section 14.6).

    A. The ductus deferens passes through the anulus inguinalis profundus and canalis inguinalis of the male.

    C. The lig. teres uteri traverses the canalis inguinalis terminates in the labia majora.

    D. The nervus obturatorius passes through the canalis obturatorius into the medial thigh.

    E. The a. iliaca externa passes below the lig. inguinale into the anterior thigh.

14. **A.** The lig. suspensorium contains the ovarian vessels and is removed only during the removal of the ovarium (Section 15.2).

    B. The lig. ovarii attaches the ovarium to the uterus and must be ligated to extract the uterus.

    C. The lig. uterosacrale connects the cervix uteri to the os sacrum.

    D. The lig. transversum cervicis contains the aa. uterinae, which are ligated during a hysterectomy.

    E. The lig. teres uteri passes through the canalis inguinalis and connects the uterus to the labia majora.

15. **D.** The uterus comprises a body that forms the superior two thirds and a cervix that forms the inferior one third (Section 15.2).

    A. In an anteflexed uterus, the cervix is tilted anteriorly.

    B. The portio vaginalis cervicis is surrounded by the fornices vaginae.

    C. The lig. teres uteri arises from the upper part of the uterus.

    E. The cervix communicates with the corpus uteri through the ostium uteri.

16. **A.** The plexus hypogastricus superior, a plexus nervosus sympathicus, drapes over the bifurcatio aortae as it enters the pelvis. It is frequently cut during surgery for the repair of an aneurysm at the location. The sympathetic nerves stimulate closure of the m. sphincter urethrae internus during ejaculation, preventing the retrograde flow of seminal fluid into the vesica urinaria. Damage to these nerves can result in retrograde ejaculation (Sections 14.6 and 16.3).

    B. The plexus hypogastricus superior is a plexus nervosus sympathicus derived from the plexus intermesentericus and nn. splanchnici lumbales.

    C. Somatic nerves do not stimulate visceral responses such as closure of the sphincter.

    D. Nn. splanchnici pelvici do not innervate the m. sphincter urethrae internus.

    E. The paired trunci sympathici run along the corpora vertebrae on either side and would not be damaged in this procedure.

17. **D.** The submucosal plexus venosus of the regio anorectalis communicates with rami of the aa. rectales in an arteriovenous anastomosis, creating a thickened vascular tissue known as the hemorrhoidal plexus. As a result of these anastomoses, bleeding from the plexus venosus rectalis internus appears bright red (Section 15.4).

    A. Prolapsed internal hemorrhoids contain the dilated veins of the plexus venosus rectalis internus and are painless.

External hemorrhoids, containing the plexus venosus rectalis externus, are covered by skin and sensitive to pain.

    B. External hemorrhoids that occur below the linea pectinata are somatically innervated and therefore very painful, but internal hemorrhoids are viscerally innervated and painless.

    C. Veins of painless internal hemorrhoids lie above the linea pectinata and therefore drain to the v. rectalis superior, a tributary of the portal system.

    E. A, B, and C are incorrect.

18. **D.** The nn. cavernosi carry parasympathetic nerves that are responsible for engorgement of the erectile tissue of the penis (Sections 14.6 and 16.3).

    A. The m. sphincter ani externus is innervated by the n. pudendus, a branch of the plexus sacralis.

    B. The m. sphincter urethrae externus that regulates urinary continence is innervated by the n. pudendus, a branch of the plexus sacralis.

    C. Ejaculation is a sympathetically mediated response. The nn. cavernosi carry parasympathetic nerves from the plexus hypogastricus inferior.

    E. The n. pudendus carries sensation from perineal structures such as the tip of the penis.

19. **D.** The m. piriformis passes through the foramen ischiadicum majus to insert on the trochanter of the femur (Section 14.3).

    A. The tendon of the m. obturatorius internus passes through the foramen ischiadicum minus from the perineum to the regio glutealis.

    B. The m. coccygeus lies along the lig. sacrospinale and forms the lower border of the foramen ischiadicum majus.

    C. The m. iliopsoas passes under the lig. inguinale into the thigh.

    E. The n. obturatorius passes along the sidewall of the pelvis and through the canalis obturatorius into the thigh.

20. **C.** The arcus tendineus fasciae pelvis is a thickening of the membranous fascia on the floor of the pelvis where visceral and parietal fascial layers meet. It provides support for viscera pelvis (Section 14.4).

    A. The arcus tendineus fasciae pelvis is a thickening of the membranous fascia, which lines the pelvic walls and viscera. Fascia endopelvica is a loose connective tissue layer that fills the subperitoneal spaces.

    B. The ligg. rectales laterales, like the ligg. vesiculares laterales, are supporting columns of fascia endopelvica that connect the viscera to the pelvic walls.

    D. The arcus tendineus levatoris ani, a condensation of the fascia over the m. obturatorius internus, is the attachment site for the levator ani part of the diaphragma pelvis.

    E. A, B, and D are incorrect.

21. **E.** The nll. inguinales superficiales and nll. inguinales profundi drain most structures of the perineum, including the glans penis, perianal skin, and scrotum. The supralateral parts of the uterus drain along the lig. teres uteri (which terminate in the labia majora) to nll. inguinales superficiales. These nodes drain to the nll. inguinales profundi (Section 14.6).

    A. Lymph from the glans penis drains to nll. inguinales profundi. B through D are also correct (E).

B. Lymph from perianal skin, like all skin of the perineum, drains to nll. inguinales superficiales, which drain to nll. inguinales profundi. A, C, and D are also correct (E).

C. Lymph from the supralateral parts of the uterus drain along the lig. teres uteri (which terminate in the labia majora) to nll. inguinales superficiales. These nodes drain to the nll. inguinales profundi. A, B, and D are also correct (E).

D. Lymph from the scrotum drains to nll. inguinales superficiales, which drain to nll. inguinales profundi. A through C are also correct (E).

22. **C.** Most nerves of the plexus sacralis pass through the foramen ischiadicum majus to innervate muscles of the gluteal region and lower limb (Section 14.6).
A. Only rami posteriores of nn. spinales sacrales pass through the foramina sacralia posteriores. The plexus sacralis is formed by rami anteriores of nn. spinales sacrales.
B. The n. obturatorius, which passes through the canalis obturatorius, is a branch of the plexus lumbalis.
D. The n. ilioinguinalis and n. genitofemoralis, which pass through the anulus inguinalis superficialis, are branches of the plexus lumbalis.
E. The n. genitofemoralis, a branch of the plexus lumbalis, passes through the anulus inguinalis profundus.

23. **A.** The lig. teres uteri originates on the superior aspect of the anterolateral uterus and inserts in the labia majora. As the uterus enlarges and stretches the ligament, pain is felt in the labia (Section 15.2).
B. During late pregnancy pelvic ligaments are more relaxed in preparation for the passage of the child through the birth canal.
C. Pressure on the n. obturatorius would be felt on the medial thigh.
D. The anterior part of the labia majora is innervated by the labial branches of the n. genitofemoralis, not the n. pudendus.
E. The n. iliohypogastricus innervates the skin above the crista pubica and does not extend inferiorly to the labia.

24. **A.** The ureter crosses the pelvic brim at the bifurcation of the a. iliaca communis into the a. iliaca interna and a. iliaca externa (Section 15.3).
B. The a. testicularis does not cross the pelvic brim but enters the anulus inguinalis profundus.
C. The truncus lumbosacralis crosses the pelvic brim posterior to the a. iliaca communis and v. iliaca communis and anterior to the art. sacroiliaca. It enters the pelvis to join the plexus sacralis.
D. The n. ischiadicus passes through the foramen ischiadicum majus and does not cross the pelvic brim.
E. The ductus deferens courses around the a. epigastrica inferior and v. epigastrica inferior and over the distal end of the a. iliaca externa and v. iliaca externa to descend into the pelvis.

25. **E.** The rectum is devoid of taeniae coli, haustra coli, a mesenterium, and appendices epiploicae (Section 15.4).
A. The taeniae coli of the intestinum crassum converge to form a uniform layer surrounding the rectum.
B. The haustra coli of the intestinum crassum disappear at the rectosigmoid junction.

C. The rectum has no mesenterium. The upper rectum is covered anteriorly by peritoneum, but the lower rectum lies in the spatium infraperitoneale.
D. Appendices epipolicae are not present in the rectum.

26. **C.** The m. bulbospongiosus is found within the spatium superficiale perinei (Section 16.1).
A. The gll. bulbourethrales are found in the spatium profundum perinei.
B. The m. sphincter urethrae externus is located in the spatium profundum perinei.
D. The anterior extensions of the corpus adiposum fossae ischioanalis are found in the spatium profundum perinei.
E. The n. rectalis inferior is found in the regio analis, not the spatium profundum perinei or the spatium superficiale perinei of the regio urogenitalis.

27. **A.** The pars spongiosa urethrae passes through the bulbus and corpus spongiosum penis (Section 15.3).
B. The sphincter internus urethrae surrounds the pars intramuralis urethrae at the cervix vesicae.
C. Part of the sphincter externus urethrae surrounds the pars membranacea urethrae.
D. The crista urethralis is a feature of the pars prostatica urethrae.
E. Ductus ejaculatorii open into the pars prostatica urethrae on the crista urethralis.

28. **B.** The bulbi vestibuli are masses of erectile tissue that lie deep to the labia minora. Unlike in the male, where the bulbus and corpus spongiosum forms part of the penis, the bulbi vestibuli do not form part of the clitoris (Section 16.4).
A. The paired corpora cavernosa converge to form the corpus clitoridis.
C. Gll. vestibulares majores, which lie deep to the bulbi vestibuli, are not part of the clitoris and are not composed of erectile tissue.
D. The preputium is a part of the clitoris that forms a hood over the body.
E. The glans is the highly sensitive tip of the clitoris.

29. **B.** Prostate tumors most often grow deep to the capsula prostata in the peripheral zone.
A. Prostatic carcinoma is a common disease of older men but can metastasize via the plexus venosus vertebralis to the bony pelvis, columna vertebralis, skull, and brain, and via other venous routes, to the heart and lungs.
C. The anterior lobe, or isthmus, is fibromuscular and not a common site of carcinoma.
D. Although prostate carcinoma may eventually invade the periurethral zone, it generally does not cause urethral obstruction in the early stages.
E. Benign prostatic hypertrophy results from proliferation of the epithelial and stromal tissues, particularly of the periurethral zone, and is unrelated to carcinoma.

30. **B.** Ultrasound is the optimal imaging tool for fetal evaluation due to its lack of ionizing radiation and relative low cost. Additionally, the fluid-filled amniotic sac provides an excellent acoustic window.
A. A developing fetus is particularly vulnerable to the potential deleterious effects of radiation and thus CT is contraindicated in fetal evaluation.

C. X-rays would also expose the fetus to radiation, although at a lower dose than CT. Additionally, a radiograph would show only limited detail of the developing fetal skeleton, and would not be sufficient in this setting.

D. MRI is safe for fetal imaging and provides excellent anatomic detail. However, it is expensive, less available, and requires very long scan times, making it impractical for use in routine or screening fetal evaluation. MRI is used as a supplement to ultrasound for further evaluation of fetal and maternal abnormalities detected at screening ultrasound.

31. C. Doppler ultrasound can detect motion and is excellent for assessment of blood flow. The use of Doppler ultrasound is an important step in the evaluation of acute scrotal pain as it can be obtained very quickly and provides excellent imaging detail of the testes and scrotal contents. Testicular torsion is a surgical emergency, and rapid diagnosis and treatment are key to preventing infarction and subsequent loss of the testicle.

A. The relative low cost of ultrasound contributes to its high availability, but is not related to blood flow assessment.

B. Lack of radiation makes ultrasound particularly well suited for imaging the gonads but is not related to blood flow assessment.

D. Ultrasound waves do travel well through water/fluid but since the testicles are located in the scrotum, this is not a critical factor. Transabdominal imaging of the uterus on the other hand, requires a full bladder to be used as an acoustic "window."

Unit VI   Upper Limb

18 Overview of the Upper Limb

The upper limb is designed for mobility and dexterity. Actions at the shoulder and elbow joints (art. glenohumeralis and art. cubiti) that allow positioning of the limb complement fine movements of the hands and fingers. Some stability is sacrificed for this extensive mobility, particularly in the shoulder, which makes the upper limb vulnerable to injury.

18.1 General Features

— In the anatomic position, the upper limbs hang vertically with the elbow joint pointing posteriorly and the palm of the hand facing anteriorly.
— The major regions of the upper limb **(Fig. 18.1)** are
   • the **shoulder region,** which includes the **regio pectoralis, regio scapularis, regio deltoidea,** and **regio cervicalis lateralis** and overlies the **cingulum pectorale;**
   • the **regio axillaris,** the armpit;
   • the **regio brachialis,** between the shoulder and elbow (cubitus);
   • the **regio cubitalis,** at the elbow;
   • the **forearm (antebrachial region, regio antebrachialis),** between the elbow and wrist (cubitus and carpus);
   • the **regio carpalis,** at the wrist; and
   • the **hand (manus),** which has palmar and dorsal surfaces.
— Movements at joints of the upper limb include
   • **flexion,** bending in a direction that narrows the distance between ventral surfaces, as represented in the embryo (in the upper limb, ventral surfaces can be interpreted as anterior surfaces, but in the lower limb, due to rotation of the limbs during development, some ventral surfaces have rotated to the posterior surface);

   • **extension,** bending, or straightening in the direction that is opposite that of flexion;
   • **abduction,** movement away from a central axis;
   • **adduction,** movement toward a central axis;
   • **external (lateral) rotation,** outward rotation around a longitudinal axis;
   • **internal (medial) rotation,** inward rotation around a longitudinal axis;
   • **circumduction,** circular motion around the point of articulation;
   • **supination,** turning the palm up;
   • **pronation,** turning the palm down;
   • **radial** or **ulnar deviation,** angling the wrist toward the radius or ulnar side (also abduction or adduction of the wrist); and
   • **opposition,** movement of the thumb or 5th digit to oppose the other fingers.
— Muscles of the upper limb are categorized as
   • **intrinsic muscles,** whose origin and insertion are near the joint (e.g., intrinsic muscles of the hand originate and insert on bones of the wrist and hand), and
   • **extrinsic muscles,** whose origin is distant from the area of movement but insert near the joint via a long tendon (e.g., forearm muscles that flex the fingers are extrinsic muscles of the hand).
      ◦ The tendons of extrinsic muscles are often referred to as **long flexor (or extensor) tendons.**
      ◦ **Synovial tendon sheaths,** which surround tendons of extrinsic muscles at the wrist and fingers, provide a lubricated surface that facilitates movement of these tendons across the joint.

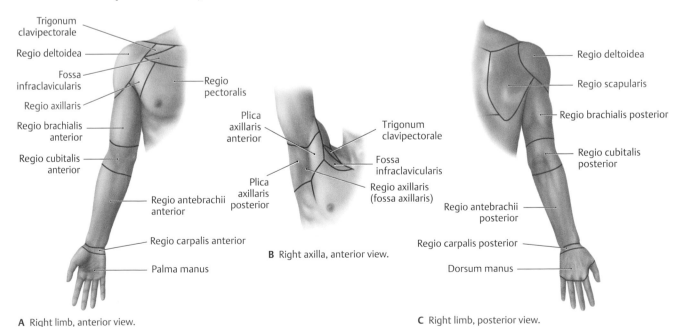

A Right limb, anterior view.

B Right axilla, anterior view.

C Right limb, posterior view.

Fig. 18.1 Regions of the upper limb
(From Schuenke M, Schulte E, Schumacher U. THIEME Atlas of Anatomy, Vol 1. Illustrations by Voll M and Wesker K. 3rd ed. New York: Thieme Publishers; 2020.)

18.2   Bones of the Upper Limb

Bones of the upper limb include the clavicula and scapula that make up the cingulum pectorale, the humerus of the arm, the radius and ulna of the forearm, the carpal bones of the wrist, and the metacarpal bones and phalanges of the hand (**Fig. 18.2**).

— The cingulum pectorale attaches the arm to the trunk (**Fig. 18.3**).

— The **clavicula** is an S-shaped bone that forms the anterior part of the cingulum pectorale (**Fig. 18.4**).

  • It articulates with the incisura clavicularis of the manubrium medially and the acromion of the scapula laterally.

  • It is palpable along its entire length.

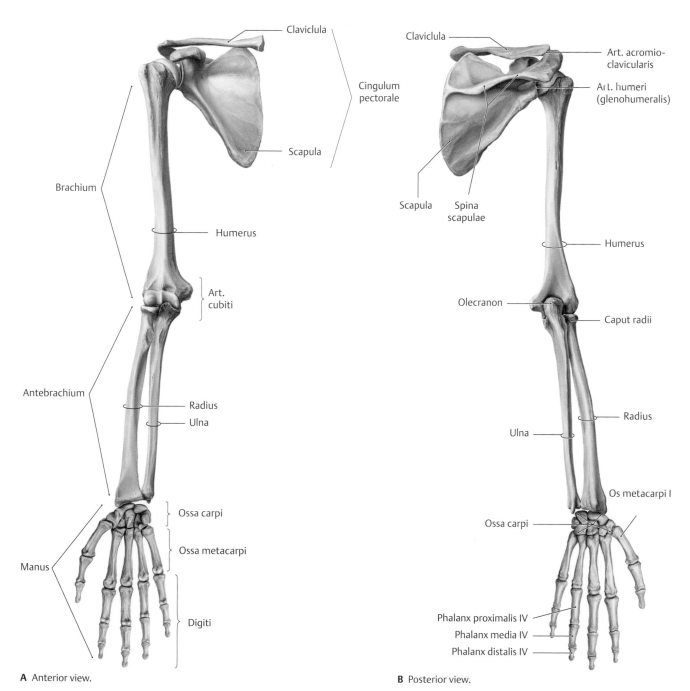

A Anterior view.

B Posterior view.

Fig. 18.2 Skeleton of the upper limb
Right limb. The upper limb is subdivided into three regions: arm, forearm, and hand. The cingulum pectorale (clavicula and scapula) joins the upper limb to the thorax at the art. sternoclavicularis. (From Schuenke M, Schulte E, Schumacher U. THIEME Atlas of Anatomy, Vol 1. Illustrations by Voll M and Wesker K. 3rd ed. New York: Thieme Publishers; 2020.)

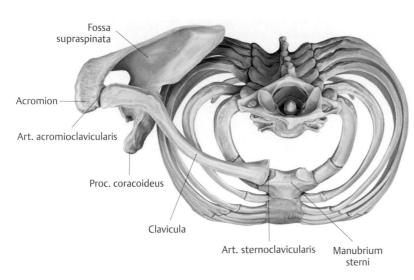

— The **scapula** is a flat triangular bone that forms the posterior part of the cingulum pectorale **(Fig. 18.5)**.
- It overlies the 2nd to 7th ribs on the posterior thoracic wall.
- It has a margo medialis, margo lateralis, and margo superior and an angulus superior and angulus inferior.
- Laterally, a shallow depression, the **cavitas glenoidalis**, articulates with the humerus.
- A narrow **collum scapulae** separates the cavitas glenoidalis from the large body of the scapula.
- A **fossa subscapularis** lies on the anterior surface against the rib cage.
- The **spina scapulae** on the posterior surface separates the **fossa supraspinata** and **fossa infraspinata.** Laterally, the spine expands to form the **acromion.**
- A **proc. coracoideus** extends anteriorly and superiorly over the cavitas glenoidalis.

Fig. 18.3 Cingulum pectorale in situ
Right shoulder, superior view. (From Gilroy AM et al. Atlas of Anatomy. 4th ed. 2020. Based on: Schuenke M, Schulte E, Schumacher U. THIEME Atlas of Anatomy. General Anatomy and Musculoskeletal System. Illustrations by Voll M and Wesker K. 3rd ed. New York: Thieme Medical Publishers; 2020.)

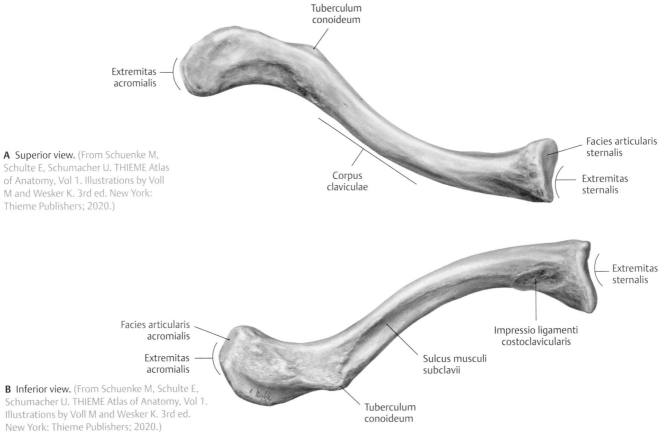

A Superior view. (From Schuenke M, Schulte E, Schumacher U. THIEME Atlas of Anatomy, Vol 1. Illustrations by Voll M and Wesker K. 3rd ed. New York: Thieme Publishers; 2020.)

B Inferior view. (From Schuenke M, Schulte E, Schumacher U. THIEME Atlas of Anatomy, Vol 1. Illustrations by Voll M and Wesker K. 3rd ed. New York: Thieme Publishers; 2020.)

Fig. 18.4 Clavicula
Right clavicle.

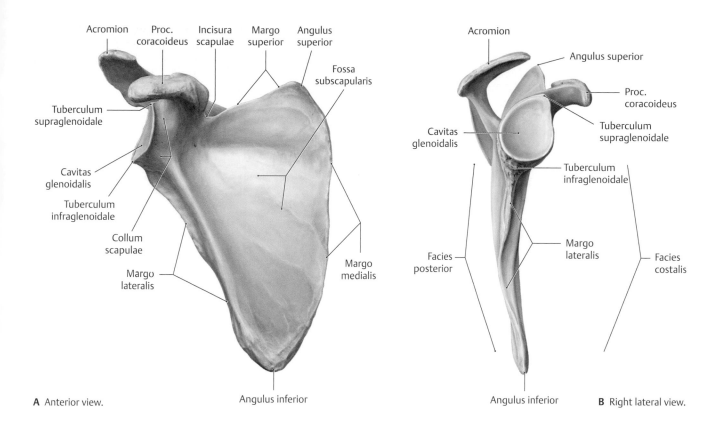

A Anterior view.

B Right lateral view.

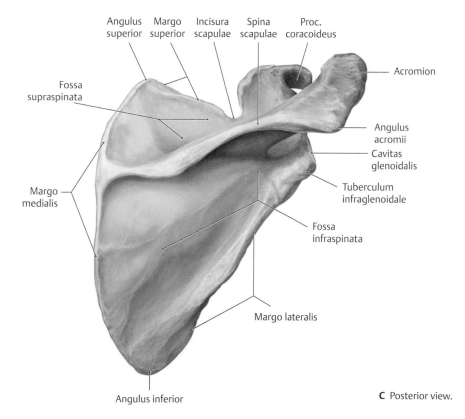

C Posterior view.

Fig. 18.5 Scapula
Right scapula. (From Schuenke M, Schulte E, Schumacher U. THIEME Atlas of Anatomy, Vol 1. Illustrations by Voll M and Wesker K. 3rd ed. New York: Thieme Publishers; 2020.)

— The **humerus** is the long bone of the arm (**Fig. 18.6**).
  • Proximally, the **caput humeri** articulates with the cavitas glenoidalis of the scapula.
  • Anteriorly, a **sulcus intertubercularis** separates the **tuberculum majus** and **tuberculum minus.**
  • A **collum anatomicum** separates the head from the tuberculum majus and tuberculum minus. The **collum chirurgicum** is the narrow part of the shaft immediately distal to the head and tubercles.

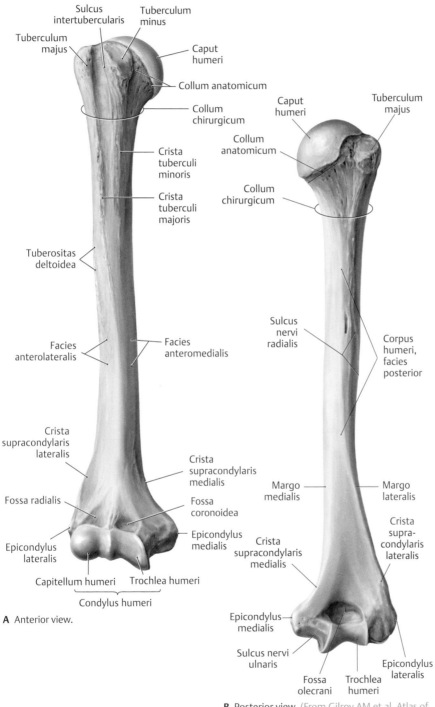

A Anterior view.

B Posterior view. (From Gilroy AM et al. Atlas of Anatomy. 4th ed. 2020. Based on: Schuenke M, Schulte E, Schumacher U. THIEME Atlas of Anatomy. General Anatomy and Musculoskeletal System. Illustrations by Voll M and Wesker K. 3rd ed. New York: Thieme Medical Publishers; 2020.)

Fig. 18.6 Humerus
Humerus dexter. The caput humeri articulates with the scapula at the art. humeri. The capitulum and trochlea humeri articulate with the radius and ulna, respectively, at the art. cubiti.

BOX 18.2: CLINICAL CORRELATION

HUMERAL FRACTURES
Fractures of the proximal humerus are very common and occur predominantly in older patients who sustain a fall onto the outstretched arm or directly onto the shoulder. Three main types are distinguished.

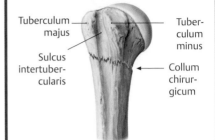

A Extra-articular fracture.

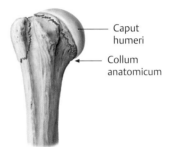

B Intra-articular fracture.

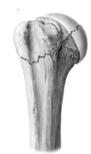

C Comminuted fracture.
(From Gilroy AM et al. Atlas of Anatomy. 4th ed. 2020. Based on: Schuenke M, Schulte E, Schumacher U. THIEME Atlas of Anatomy. General Anatomy and Musculoskeletal System. Illustrations by Voll M and Wesker K. 3rd ed. New York: Thieme Medical Publishers; 2020.)

Extra-articular fractures and intra-articular fractures are often accompanied by injuries of the blood vessels that supply the caput humeri (a. circumflexa anterior humeri and a. circumflexa humeri), with an associated risk of post-traumatic avascular necrosis.

Fractures of the collum chirurgicum can damage the n. axillaris and fractures of the humeral shaft (corpus humeri) and distal humerus are frequently associated with damage to the n. radialis.

- A **tuberositas deltoidea** on the midshaft is a site for attachment of the m. deltoideus.
- A **sulcus nervi radialis** runs obliquely around the posterior and lateral surfaces.
- Distally, the humerus articulates with the radius at the **capitulum humeri** and with the ulna at the **trochlea humeri.**
- A large **epicondylus medialis** and smaller **epicondylus lateralis** are attachment sites for muscles.
- A **sulcus nervi ulnaris** separates the epicondyluis medialis and trochlea
- The **ulna** is the medial bone of the forearm (**Fig. 18.7**).
  - A C-shaped **incisura trochlearis**, formed by the **olecranon** posteriorly and the **proc. coronoideus** anteriorly, articulates with the trochlea humeri.
  - The ulna articulates with the radius at the **incisura radialis.**
  - A **membrana interossea antebrachii** joins the shafts of the radius and ulna.

- An **proc. stylodius ulnae** projects from its distal end.
- The **radius** is the lateral bone of the forearm (see **Fig. 18.7**).
  - A round **caput radii** articulates with the humerus and ulna and sits on top of a narrow **collum radii.**
  - A **tuberositas radii** on the anterior surface provides attachments for the m. biceps brachii.
  - Distally, the radius is triangular in cross section with a flattened anterior surface.
  - The radius articulates with the ulna proximally at the elbow and distally at the wrist. The membrana interossea attaches the radius to the corpus ulnae
  - A **proc. styloideus radii** projects from the distal end and extends farther than the proc. styloideus ulnae.
  - The radius articulates with ossa carpi at the wrist.

BOX 18.3: CLINICAL CORRELATION

COLLES' FRACTURES

A Colles' fracture, a transverse fracture through the distal 2 cm of the radius, is the most common forearm fracture and results from a fall on an outstretched hand. The distal segment of bone is displaced dorsally and proximally, and with shortening of the radius, the proc. styloideus appears proximal to the proc. styloideus ulnae. The resulting appearance is referred to as the "dinner fork" deformity.

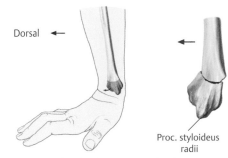

(From Gilroy AM et al. Atlas of Anatomy. 4th ed. 2020. Based on: Schuenke M, Schulte E, Schumacher U. THIEME Atlas of Anatomy. General Anatomy and Musculoskeletal System. Illustrations by Voll M and Wesker K. 3rd ed. New York: Thieme Medical Publishers; 2020.))

- The **ossa carpi** consist of eight short bones that are arranged in two curved rows at the wrist (**Figs. 18.8** and **18.9**). From lateral to medial, they are
  - in the proximal row, the **os scaphoideum, os lunatum, os triquetrum,** and **os pisiforme;** and,
  - in the distal row, the **os trapezium, os trapezoideum, os capitatum,** and **os hamatum.**

BOX 18.4: CLINICAL CORRELATION

LUNATE DISLOCATION

The os lunatum is the most commonly displaced of the ossa carpi. Normally located in the floor of the canalis carpi, a displaced bone moves toward the palmar surface and can compress structures of the canalis carpi.

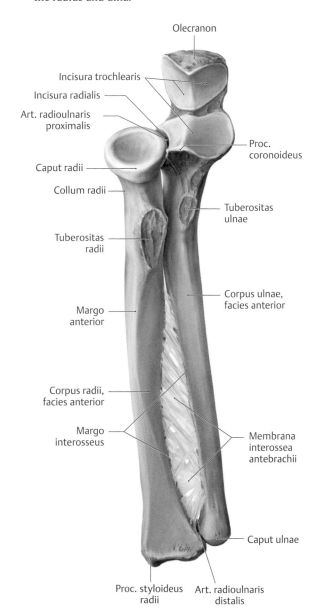

Olecranon

Incisura trochlearis

Incisura radialis

Art. radioulnaris proximalis

Caput radii

Collum radii

Tuberositas radii

Margo anterior

Corpus radii, facies anterior

Margo interosseus

Proc. coronoideus

Tuberositas ulnae

Corpus ulnae, facies anterior

Membrana interossea antebrachii

Caput ulnae

Proc. styloideus radii

Art. radioulnaris distalis

Fig. 18.7 Radius and ulna

Right forearm, anterosuperior view. (From Schuenke M, Schulte E, Schumacher U. THIEME Atlas of Anatomy, Vol 1. Illustrations by Voll M and Wesker K. 3rd ed. New York: Thieme Publishers; 2020.)

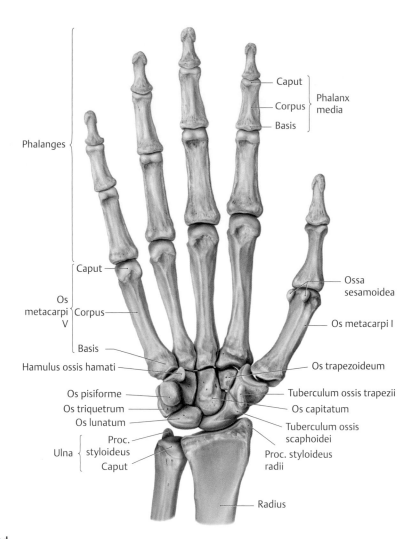

Fig. 18.8 Bones of the hand
Right hand, palmar view. (From Schuenke M, Schulte E, Schumacher U. THIEME Atlas of Anatomy, Vol 1. Illustrations by Voll M and Wesker K. 3rd ed. New York: Thieme Publishers; 2020.)

BOX 18.5: CLINICAL CORRELATION

SCAPHOID FRACTURES
Scaphoid fractures are the most common carpal bone fractures, generally occurring at the narrow waist between the proximal and distal poles. Because the blood supply to the bone is transmitted via the distal segment, fractures at the waist (**A**, right scaphoid, *red line*; **B**, *white arrow*) can compromise the supply to the proximal segment, often resulting in nonunion and avascular necrosis.

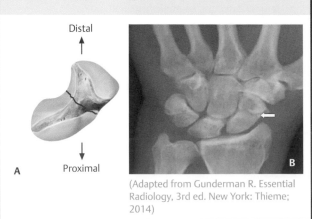

(Adapted from Gunderman R. Essential Radiology, 3rd ed. New York: Thieme; 2014)

— The **ossa metacarpi** consist of five long bones that form the hand.
  • Proximally, their **bases** articulate with the ossa carpi.
  • Distally, the **caput ossis metacarpi**, the knuckles of the hand, articulate with the phalanges proximales.
— The **phalanges** are small long bones that form the fingers.
  • They are designated as proximal, middle, and distal in each finger except in the thumb, which has only a proximal and a distal phalanx.
— Fingers and their corresponding ossa metacarpi and phalanges are designated as 1st through 5th, with the thumb as the 1st digit and the little finger as the 5th digit.

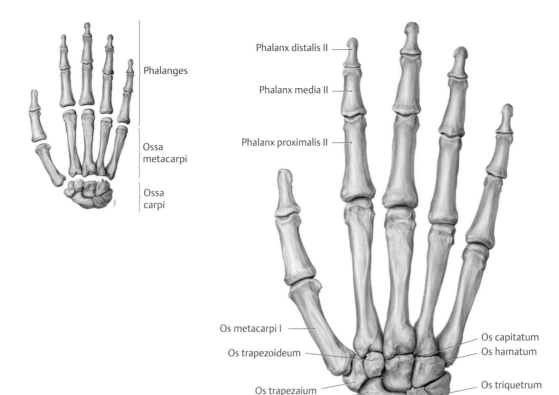

Fig. 18.9 Bones of the hand
Right hand, dorsal view. (From Schuenke M, Schulte E, Schumacher U. THIEME Atlas of Anatomy, Vol 1. Illustrations by Voll M and Wesker K. 3rd ed. New York: Thieme Publishers; 2020.)

18.3 Fascia and Compartments of the Upper Limb

— Deep fascia snugly encloses muscles of the upper limb. It is continuous over the pectoral girdle (cingulum pectorale), the axilla, and the upper limb but has regional designations.
  • **Fascia pectoralis** invests the m. pectoralis major.
  • **Fascia clavipectoralis** invests the m. subclavius and m. pectoralis minor.
  • **Fascia axillaris** forms the floor of the **axilla.**
  • **Fascia brachii** invests muscles of the arm.
  • **Fascia antebrachii** invests muscles of the forearm and extends onto the wrist as transverse thickened bands, the **retinaculum musculorum flexorum** and **retinaculum musculorum extensorum.**
  • Fascia of the hand is continuous over the dorsum and palm, but in the center of the palm it forms a thickened fibrous sheet, the **aponeurosis palmaris**.
  • **Digital fibrous sheaths** (**vaginae fibrosae digitorum manus**), extensions of the aponeurosis palmaris onto the fingers, surround the flexor tendons.
— Septa intermuscularia arising from the deep fascia attach to the bones of the arm, forearm, and hand, separating the limb musculature into discrete compartments. The muscles within each compartment usually share a similar function, innervation, and blood supply. The compartments of the upper limb (see **Figs. 19.38** and **19.39**) are
  • the **anterior** and **posterior compartments** of the arm;
  • the **anterior** and **posterior compartments** of the forearm; and
  • the **thenar, hypothenar, central, adductor,** and **interosseous compartments** of the palm of the hand.

18.4 Neurovasculature of the Upper Limb

Arteries of the Upper Limb

— The **a. subclavia** and its branches supply structures in the neck, part of the thoracic wall, and the entire upper limb (**Fig. 18.10**).
  • The a. subclavia dextra is a branch of the truncus brachiocephalicus, which arises from the arcus aortae. The a. subclavia sinistra arises directly from the arcus aortae.

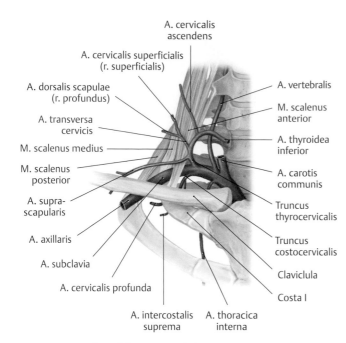

A. cervicalis ascendens

A. cervicalis superficialis (r. superficialis)

A. dorsalis scapulae (r. profundus)

A. transversa cervicis

M. scalenus medius

M. scalenus posterior

A. supra-scapularis

A. axillaris

A. subclavia

A. cervicalis profunda

A. intercostalis suprema

A. thoracica interna

A. vertebralis

M. scalenus anterior

A. thyroidea inferior

A. carotis communis

Truncus thyrocervicalis

Truncus costocervicalis

Claviclula

Costa I

Fig. 18.10 Branches of the arteria subclavia
Right side, anterior view. (From Schuenke M, Schulte E, Schumacher U. THIEME Atlas of Anatomy, Vol 1. Illustrations by Voll M and Wesker K. 3rd ed. New York: Thieme Publishers; 2020.)

- The aa. subclaviae enter the neck through the apertura thoracis superior, pass laterally toward the shoulder, and terminate as they pass over the 1st rib.
- The subclavian artery branches that supply the neck and thoracic wall (discussed further in Section 17.3) include
  ○ the **a. vertebralis**;
  ○ the a. thoracica interna; and
  ○ the **truncus thyrocervicalis**, whose branches are the **a. suprascapularis, a. cervicalis ascendens, a. thyroidea inferior,** and **a. transversa colli**.
- The branches of the truncus thyrocervicalis that supply muscles and skin of the scapular region include
  ○ the a. transversa colli and the **a. dorsalis scapulae** and
  ○ the a. suprascapularis.
— The **a. axillaris**, the continuation of the a. subclavia, begins at the lateral edge of the 1st rib and terminates at the lateral border of the axilla (the lower border of the m. teres major).
— Within the axilla, the **m. pectoralis minor** muscle lies anterior to the middle third of the a. axillaris, thus dividing the artery into three segments. The origins of the branches of the a. axillaris show considerable variation but generally are described as arising from its proximal, middle, or distal thirds **(Fig. 18.11)**.
  - The proximal third has one branch:
    ○ The **a. thoracica superior** supplies the muscles of the first intercostal space.
  - The middle third has two branches:
    ○ The **a. thoracoacromialis** divides into r. deltoideus, r. pectoralis, r. clavicularis, and r. acromialis.
    ○ The **a. thoracica lateralis** supplies the lateral thoracic wall, including the m. serratus anterior and the breast.

- The distal third has three branches:
  ○ The **a. subscapularis** further divides into the **a. thoracodorsalis**, supplying the m. latissimus dorsi, and a **a. circumflexa scapulae**, supplying muscles of the scapula.
  ○ The **a. circumflexa humeri anterior**.
  ○ The **a. circumflexa humeri posterior**. These circumflex arteries encircle the humeral neck to supply the deltoid region.
— A **scapular arcade**, formed by the anastomoses of the a. dorsalis scapulae and a. suprascapularis from the a. subclavia, and the a. circumflexa scapulae and a. thoracodorsalis from the a. axillaris, provide an important collateral circulation to the scapular region when the a. axillaris is injured or ligated **(Fig. 18.12)**.
— The **a. brachialis**, the continuation of the a. axillaris, begins at the lateral border of the axilla (the lower margin of the tendon of the m. teres major), runs superficially along the medial border of the **m. teres major**, and terminates at its bifurcation in the fossa cubitalis (anterior elbow region). Its branches (see **Fig. 18.11**) include
  - the **a. profunda brachii**, which arises proximally, descends on the posterior surface of the humerus, and supplies muscles of the posterior arm; its branches, a. collateralis media and a. collateralis radialis communicate with the a. radialis via the a. recurrens radialis and a. interossea recurrens.
  - the **a. collateralis ulnaris superior** and **a. collateralis ulnaris inferior**, distal branches, which anastomose with the a. profunda brachii and a. ulnaris of the forearm to supply the art. cubiti.
  - the **a. radialis** and **a. ulnaris**, the terminal branches of the a. brachialis, which supply the forearm and hand.
— The arterial anastomosis around the elbow allows the ligation of the brachial artery distal to the origin of the deep artery of the arm without compromising the blood supply to the elbow region.
— The a. ulnaris originates in the fossa cubitalis, descends along the medial side of the forearm, and crosses through a narrow space at the wrist, the **canalis ulnaris**. It terminates as the **arcus palmaris superficialis**. The major branches of the a. ulnaris in the forearm (see **Fig. 18.11**) are
  - the **a. recurrens ulnaris**, which anastomoses with aa. collaterales ulnares to supply the art. cubiti, and
  - the **a. interossea communis**, which arises in the proximal forearm and branches into **a. interossea posterior** and **a. interossea anterior**. These interosseous branches descend on either side of the membrana interossea and supply the anterior and posterior muscle compartments of the forearm.
— The a. radialis, the smaller lateral branch of the a. brachialis, descends from the fossa cubitalis along the lateral side of the forearm to the wrist. It crosses the wrist through the **anatomic snuffbox** on the dorsal side, pierces the muscles between the 1st and 2nd digits, and enters the palm of the hand, where it ends as the **arcus palmaris profundus**. Its branches (see **Fig. 18.11**) include
  - the **a. recurrens radialis**, which anastomoses with collateral branches of the a. profunda brachii to supply the art. cubiti, and
  - the **r. carpalis palmaris** and **r. carpalis dorsalis**, which anastomose with branches of the a. ulnaris in the wrist and hand.

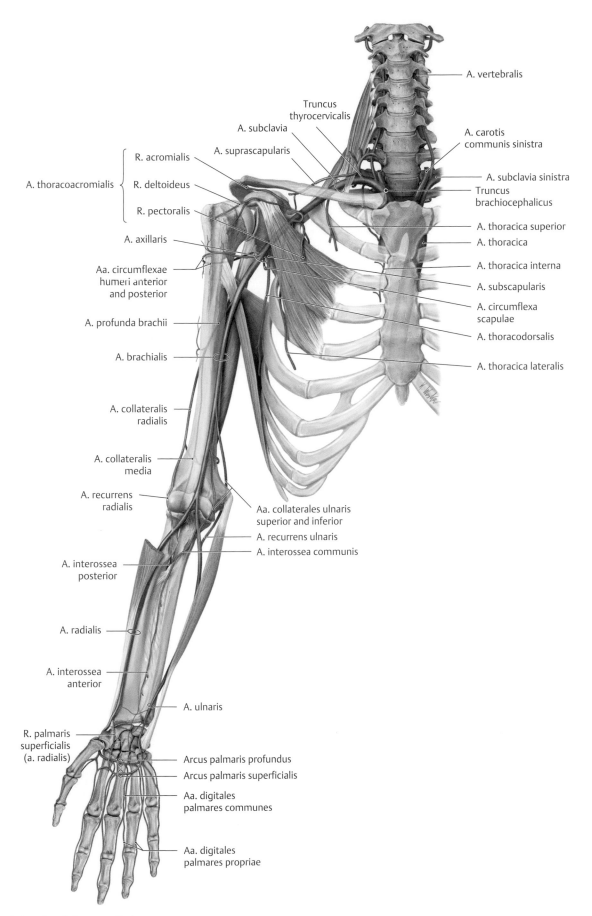

Fig. 18.11 Arteries of the upper limb
Right limb, anterior view. (From Gilroy AM et al. Atlas of Anatomy. 4th ed. 2020. Based on: Schuenke M, Schulte E, Schumacher U. THIEME Atlas of Anatomy. General Anatomy and Musculoskeletal System. Illustrations by Voll M and Wesker K. 3rd ed. New York: Thieme Medical Publishers; 2020.)

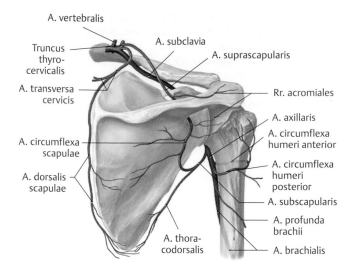

A. vertebralis

Truncus thyro-cervicalis

A. transversa cervicis

A. circumflexa scapulae

A. dorsalis scapulae

A. subclavia

A. suprascapularis

Rr. acromiales

A. axillaris

A. circumflexa humeri anterior

A. circumflexa humeri posterior

A. subscapularis

A. profunda brachii

A. thora-codorsalis

A. brachialis

Fig. 18.12 Scapular arcade
Right side, posterior view. (From Schuenke M, Schulte E, Schumacher U. THIEME Atlas of Anatomy, Vol 1. Illustrations by Voll M and Wesker K. 3rd ed. New York: Thieme Publishers; 2020.)

— Arteries of the wrist and hand (**Fig. 18.13**) include
- **palmar** and **dorsal carpal networks,** which form by contributions from the a. radialis, a. ulnaris, and a. interossea anterior and a. interossea posterior;
- an **arcus palmaris profundus** formed largely by the a. radialis that gives rise to
  ∘ the **a. princeps pollicis,** which follows the ulnar surface of the 1st metacarpal to the base of the thumb, where it divides into two digital branches
  ∘ the **a. radialis indicis,** which can arise from the a. princeps pollicis or a. radialis and courses along the radial side of the index finger
  ∘ three **aa. palmares metacarpales,** which anastomose with the common palmar digital arteries;
- an **arcus palmaris superficialis** formed largely by the a. ulnaris, which anastomoses with the a. palmaris profundus via an r. palmaris profundus, and gives rise to
  ∘ three **aa. digitales palmares communes,** which divide into paired **aa. digitales palmares propriae** that run along the sides of the 2nd to 4th digits;
- a **dorsal carpal arch,** formed from the dorsal carpal network (rete carpale dorsale), which gives rise to three **aa. metacarpeae dorsales** that branch into **aa. digitales dorsales manus** that run on the dorsal sides of the 2nd to 4th digits; and
- a **1st dorsal metacarpal artery,** which arises directly from the radial artery.

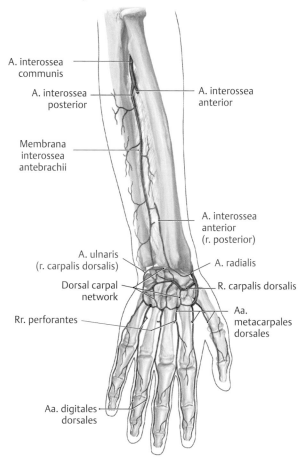

A. interossea recurrens

A. interossea posterior

A. interossea anterior

A. radialis

A. interossea communis

A. ulnaris

Membrana interossea antebrachii

Rr. carpales palmares (to palmar carpal network)

Arcus palmaris profundus

Aa. palmares metacarpales

A. princeps pollicis

Arcus palmaris superficialis

Rr. perforantes

Aa. digitales palmares propriae

Aa. digitales palmares communes

A. radialis indicis

Aa. digitales palmares

A Anterior (palmar) view.

A. interossea communis

A. interossea posterior

A. interossea anterior

Membrana interossea antebrachii

A. interossea anterior (r. posterior)

A. ulnaris (r. carpalis dorsalis)

Dorsal carpal network

Rr. perforantes

A. radialis

R. carpalis dorsalis

Aa. metacarpales dorsales

Aa. digitales dorsales

B Posterior (dorsal) view.

Fig. 18.13 Arteries of the forearm and hand
Right limb. The a. ulnaris and a. radialis are interconnected by the arcus palmaris superficialis and arcus palmaris profundus, the rr. perforantes, and the dorsal carpal network. (From Gilroy AM et al. Atlas of Anatomy. 4th ed. 2020. Based on: Schuenke M, Schulte E, Schumacher U. THIEME Atlas of Anatomy. General Anatomy and Musculoskeletal System. Illustrations by Voll M and Wesker K. 3rd ed. New York: Thieme Medical Publishers; 2020.)

Veins of the Upper Limb

— Veins of the limbs, similar to veins of the trunk, are more variable than the arteries, and they often form anastomoses that surround the arteries they accompany. Veins of the limbs have unidirectional valves that prevent pooling of blood in the extremities and facilitate the movement of blood back to the heart. The limbs have both deep and superficial veins.

— Deep veins accompany the major arteries and their branches and have similar names (**Fig. 18.14**).

  • In the distal limb, the deep veins, referred to as **accompanying veins** (venae comitantes), are paired and surround the artery. Proximally, the pairs merge to form a single vessel.

  • The **v. axillaris** drains the shoulder, arm, forearm, and hand and receives additional contributions from
    ◦ the lateral chest wall, including the breast, and
    ◦ the v. thoracoepigastrica of the anterolateral abdominal wall.

  • The **v. subclavia**, the continuation of the v. axillaris, begins at the lateral edge of the 1st rib and receives the venous drainage from the scapular region.

— The superficial veins are found in the subcutaneous tissue and drain into the deep venous system via **vv. perforantes** (connecting) (**Fig. 18.15**).

  • The **rete venosum dorsale manus** on the dorsum of the hand drains into two large superficial veins, the **v. cephalica** and **v. basilica**

  • The **v. cephalica** originates on the lateral side of the dorsum of the hand and ascends on the lateral side of the forearm and arm. In the shoulder, it passes through the **sulcus deltoideopectoralis** (formed by the borders of the m. deltoideus and m. pectoralis major) before emptying into the v. axillaris.

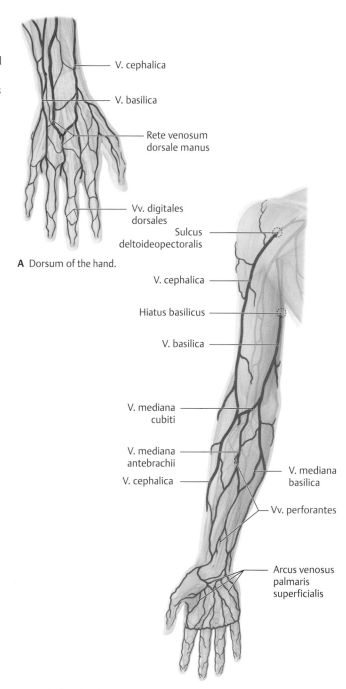

A Dorsum of the hand.

B Anterior view.

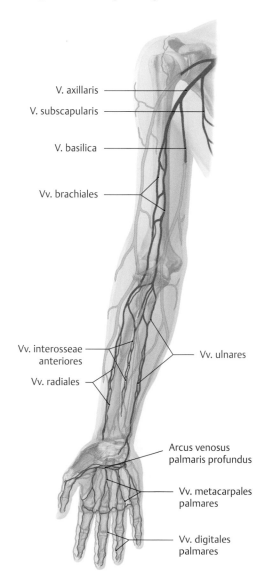

Fig. 18.14 Deep veins of the upper limb
Right limb, anterior view. (From Schuenke M, Schulte E, Schumacher U. THIEME Atlas of Anatomy, Vol 1. Illustrations by Voll M and Wesker K. 3rd ed. New York: Thieme Publishers; 2020.)

Fig. 18.15 Superficial veins of the upper limb
Right limb. (From Schuenke M, Schulte E, Schumacher U. THIEME Atlas of Anatomy, Vol 1. Illustrations by Voll M and Wesker K. 3rd ed. New York: Thieme Publishers; 2020.)

- The **v. basilica** arises on the medial side of the dorsum of the hand and runs posteromedially to pass anterior to the epicondylus medialis of the humerus. In the arm, it pierces the fascia brachii (at the **hiatus basilicus**) and joins the paired **vv. brachiales profundus** to form the v. axillaris.
- The **v. mediana cubiti** connects the v. cephalica and v. basilica anterior to the fossa cubitalis.
- The **v. mediana antebrachii** arises from the venous network of the palm, ascends on the anterior forearm, and terminates in the v. basilica or v. mediana cubiti.

Lymphatic Drainage of the Upper Limb

Lymphatic vessels of the upper limb drain toward the axilla. They usually accompany the veins of the superficial system (v. cephalica and v. basilica), although there are numerous connections between the deep and superficial drainages.

— Axillary lymph node groups, each containing four to seven large nodes (nll. axillares), are described in relation to the m. pectoralis minor (**Fig. 18.16**).
- The lower axillary group lies lateral and deep to the pectoralis minor.
    - **Nll. axillares pectorales** on the anterior wall of the axilla drain the anterior thoracic wall, including the breast (75% of lymph from the breast drains to nll. axillares).
    - **Nll. axillares subscapulares** along the plica axillaris posterior drain the posterior thoracic wall and scapular region.
    - **Nll. brachiales** lie medial and posterior to the v. axillaris and receive lymphatic vessels that accompany the v. basilica and the deep veins of the arm.
    - **Nll. axillares centrales** lie deep to the m. pectoralis minor and receive lymph from the nll. axillares pectorales, nll. axillares subscapulares, and nll. axillares laterales.
- The middle axillary group lies on the surface of the m. pectoralis minor.
    - **Nll. interpectorales** lie between the m. pectoralis major and m. pectoralis minor and drain to the nll. axillares apicales.
- The upper axillary group lies medial to the m. pectoralis minor.
    - **Nll. axillares apicales** lie along the v. axillaris adjacent to the first part of the a. axillaris in the apex of the axilla. They receive lymph from the nll. axillares centrales as well as from lymphatic vessels traveling along the v. cephalica.

— Apical lymph vessels unite to form the trunci lymphatici subclavii, which usually drain to the truncus lymphaticus dexter and the ductus thoracicus (left lymphatic duct).

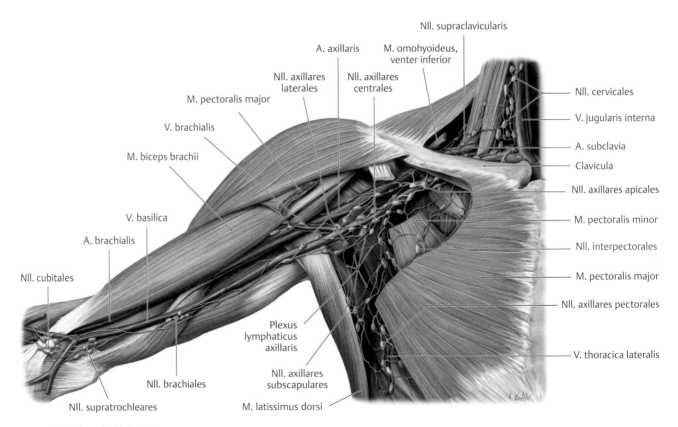

Fig. 18.16 Nodi lymphoidei axillares
Anterior view. (From Schuenke M, Schulte E, Schumacher U. THIEME Atlas of Anatomy, Vol 1. Illustrations by Voll M and Wesker K. 3rd ed. New York: Thieme Publishers; 2020.)

Nerves of the Upper Limb: The Plexus Brachialis

The upper limb is innervated almost entirely by the nerves of the **brachial plexus (plexus brachialis)**, which originates from the lower cervical and upper thoracic spinal cord **(Table 18.1; Figs. 18.17, 18.18, 18.19, 18.20, 18.21)**. (One exception, the n. intercostobrachialis, formed by the anterior rami of T1 and T2, is sensory to the medial arm but is not part of the plexus.)

— Roots of the plexus brachialis emerge from the columna vertebralis between the m. scalenus anterior and m. scalenus medius (interscalene groove) in the neck.

— Formation of the plexus begins in the neck **(pars supraclavicularis),** where it accompanies the a. subclavia, and continues into the axilla **(pars infraclavicularis)**, where it accompanies the a. axillaris.

— The roots, trunks, and divisions of the plexus are **supraclavicular** (above the clavicula); the cords (fasciculi) form at the level of the clavicula, and their branches are **infraclavicular** (below the clavicula).

— **Fig. 18.17** shows the architecture of the plexus brachialis.

• Rr. anteriores of nn. spinales C5–T1 form five **roots.**

  ◦ Within the plexus, upper roots form nerves that innervate muscles of the proximal limb; lower roots form nerves that innervate muscles of the distal limb.

  ◦ The terms **pre-fixed** or **post-fixed plexus** indicate that the plexus includes rr. anteriores from one spinal level above (C4) or below (T2) the normal levels, respectively.

• Roots C5 to T1 combine to form three **trunks:**
  1. C5 and C6 form the **truncus superior**.
  2. C7 forms the **truncus medius**.
  3. C8 and T1 form the **truncus inferior**.

• Anterior and posterior divisions (divisiones anteriores and posteriores) (components of the rr. anteriores of all nn. spinales), which are bundled together in the roots and trunks of the plexus, separate to form three **cords:**
  1. Anterior divisions of the truncus superior and truncus medius (C5–C7) form the **fasciculus lateralis**.
  2. Anterior divisions of the lower trunk (C8–T1) form the **fasciculus medialis**.
  3. Posterior divisions of all trunks (C5–T1) form the **fasciculus posterior**.

The three cords divide to form the five **nn. terminales** of the plexus.

  ◦ Fasciculus medialis and fasciculus lateralis form the **n. musculocutaneus, n. medianus,** and **n. ulnaris,** which innervate the anterior muscles of the arm and forearm, and all muscles of the palm.

  ◦ The fasciculus posterior forms the **n. axillaris** and **n. radialis,** which innervate muscles of the scapular and deltoid regions and posterior muscles of the arm and forearm.

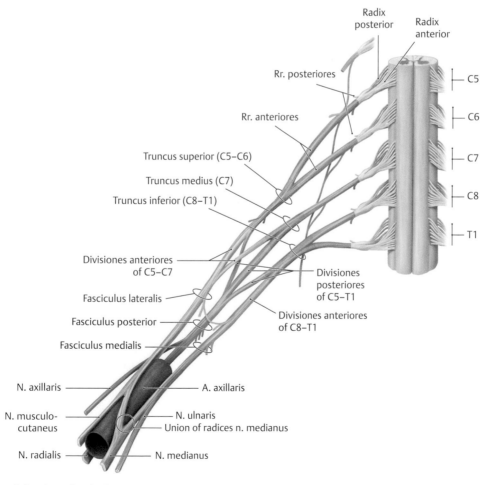

Fig. 18.17 Structure of the plexus brachialis
Right side, anterior view. (From Schuenke M, Schulte E, Schumacher U. THIEME Atlas of Anatomy, Vol 1. Illustrations by Voll M and Wesker K. 3rd ed. New York: Thieme Publishers; 2020.)

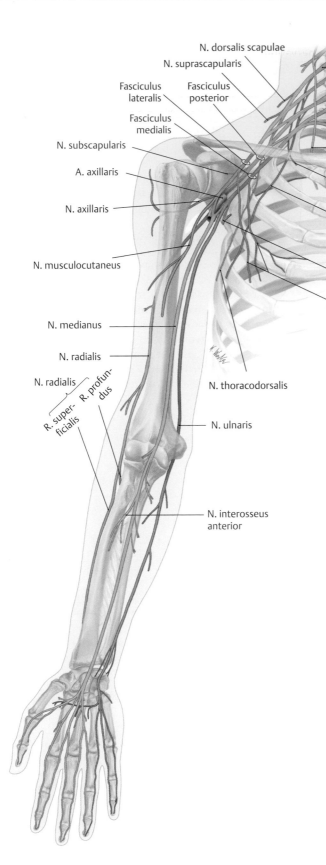

N. dorsalis scapulae

N. suprascapularis

Fasciculus lateralis

Fasciculus posterior

Fasciculus medialis

N. subscapularis

A. axillaris

N. axillaris

N. musculocutaneus

N. medianus

N. radialis

N. radialis

R. superficialis

R. profundus

N. thoracodorsalis

N. ulnaris

N. interosseus anterior

C5

T1

N. phrenicus

N. subclavius

N. thoracicus longus

N. cutaneus brachii medialis

Nn. pectorales medialis and lateralis

Fig. 18.18 Plexus brachialis
Right side, anterior view. *(See table 18.1 for explanation of color coding.)* (From Gilroy AM et al. Atlas of Anatomy. 4th ed. 2020. Based on: Schuenke M, Schulte E, Schumacher U. THIEME Atlas of Anatomy. General Anatomy and Musculoskeletal System. Illustrations by Voll M and Wesker K. 3rd ed. New York: Thieme Medical Publishers; 2020.)

BOX 18.6: CLINICAL CORRELATION

ROOT- AND TRUNK-LEVEL INJURIES

Injuries to the proximal segments of the plexus brachialis, involving the avulsion of the roots or stretching or compression of the trunks, have classic presentations that represent the distribution of the affected nerves. Nerves derived from the upper plexus innervate muscles of the proximal limb, while nerves derived from the lower plexus innervate muscles of the distal limb.

Upper plexus injuries (Erb-Duchenne palsy) involve the C5 and C6 roots or the truncus superior and are usually caused by trauma that forcefully separates the head and shoulder. The resulting deformity includes an adducted shoulder and medially rotated limb that is extended at the elbow.

Injuries of the lower plexus (Klumpke's palsy) are far less common than those of the upper plexus, but a violent upward pull of the limb can avulse the C8 and T1 roots or damage the truncus inferior. This affects the intrinsic muscles of the hand and can create a "claw hand" deformity. Because C8 and T1 are the superiormost contributions to the truncus sympathicus, avulsion of these nerve roots can also affect the sympathetic innervation in the head. The manifestation of this is known as Horner's syndrome (see Section 28.1).

Table 18.1 Nerves of the Plexus Brachialis

Nerve			Level	Area of Innervation
Pars supraclavicularis				
Direct branches from the rr. anteriores or plexus brachialis				
●	N. dorsalis scapulae		C4–C5	M. levator scapulae, mm. rhomboideus major and minor
	N. suprascapularis		C4–C6	M. supraspinatus, m. infraspinatus
	N. subclavius		C5–C6	M. subclavius
	N. thoracicus longus		C5–C7	M. serratus anterior
Pars infraclavicularis				
Short and long branches from the fasciculi plexus brachialis				
● **Fasciculus lateralis**	N. pectoralis lateralis		C5–C7	M. pectoralis major
	N. musculocutaneus			Mm. coracobrachialis, biceps brachii, brachialis; skin of lateral forearm
●	N. medianus	R. lateralis	C6–C7	Mm. pronator teres, flexor radialis carpi, m. palmaris longus, flexor superficialis digitorum, pronator quadratus, flexor longus pollicis, flexor profundus digitorum (radial half), abductor brevis pollicis, flexor brevis pollicis (caput superficiale), m. opponens pollicis, 1st and 2nd mm. lumbricales manus; skin of radial half of palm and palmar surface and distal dorsal segment of 2nd and 3rd digits and half of 4th digit
Fasciculus medialis		R. medialis	C8–T1	
●	N. pectoralis medialis			Mm. pectoralis major and minor
	N. cutaneus antebrachii medialis			Skin of medial forearm
	N. cutaneus brachii medialis		T1	Skin of medial arm
	N. ulnaris		C7–T1	Mm. flexor, flexor profundus digitorum (ulnar half), m. palmaris brevis, abductor digiti minimi, flexor digiti minimi, m. opponens digiti minimi manus, 3rd and 4th mm. lumbricales manus, mm. interossei, adductor pollicis, flexor brevis pollicis (caput profundum); skin of ulnar half of the dorsum and palm of the hand, dorsum and palmar surface of the 5th digit and half of the 4th digit
● **Fasciculus posterior**	N. subscapularis superior		C5–C6	M. subscapularis (upper part)
	N. thoracodorsalis		C6–C8	M. latissimus dorsi
	N. subscapularis inferior		C5–C6	M. subscapularis (lower part), m. teres major
	N. axillaris			M. deltoideus, m. teres minor; skin of lower deltoid region
	N. radialis		C5–T1	Muscles of posterior arm and forearm; skin of posterior and inferolateral arm, posterior forearm, radial half of dorsum of hand, dorsum of 1st, 2nd, 3rd digits and half of 4th digit

— The n. musculocutaneus (C5–C7) pierces and innervates the m. coracobrachialis of the arm as it leaves the axilla and then descends within the anterior compartment of the arm between the m. biceps brachii and m. brachialis.
  • In the arm, its **muscular branches** innervate the muscles of the anterior compartment, the m. biceps brachii and m. brachialis.
  • It enters the forearm at the lateral edge of the fossa cubitalis as the **n. cutaneus antebrachii lateralis** to supply the skin of the lateral forearm.

BOX 18.7: CLINICAL CORRELATION

MUSCULOCUTANEOUS NERVE INJURY

The n. musculocutaneus is protected on the medial side of the arm, and isolated injuries are uncommon, but they would affect the m. coracobrachialis, m. biceps brachii, and m. brachialis. Flexion and supination at the elbow would be weakened but not absent because the m. brachioradialis and m. supinator, which are innervated by the n. radialis, also provide those movements.

— The n. medianus (C6–T1) is formed by contributions from the fasciculus medialis and fasciculus lateralis.
- In the arm, the n. medianus descends with the brachial vessels, medial to the m. biceps brachii, but it does not innervate any arm muscles.
- In the forearm, it travels deep within the anterior compartment but becomes superficial at the wrist before passing through the canalis carpi into the hand. It innervates most muscles in the anterior forearm (except the m. flexor carpi ulnaris and the medial half of the m. flexor digitorum profundus).
  - Its largest branch in the forearm is the **n. interosseus antebrachii anterior**.
  - **A palmar branch** arises distally and crosses the wrist superficial to the canalis carpi to supply the skin of the palm.
- In the hand, the n. medianus has motor and sensory functions.
  - A thenar muscular branch, the **n. recurrens,** innervates most muscles of the thenar compartment (intrinsic muscles of the thumb).
  - **Rr. digitales palmares** innervate the lateral two mm. lumbricales (intrinsic muscles of the central compartment) and the skin of the 1st through 3rd fingers and lateral half of the 4th finger.
— The n. ulnaris [(C7) C8, T1] is a branch of the fasciculus medialis.
- In the arm, it descends on the medial side with the a. brachialis. At the mid-arm, it pierces the septum intermusculare to enter the posterior compartment. It crosses the art. cubiti behind the epicondylus medialis, where it is subcutaneous and vulnerable to injury. It does not innervate any muscles in the arm.
- In the forearm, it runs deep to the flexor muscles but becomes superficial just proximal to the wrist.

BOX 18.8: CLINICAL CORRELATION

MEDIAN NERVE INJURY

Injury at the distal humerus is often caused by a supracondylar fracture and results in
- loss of sensation in the palm and palmar surface of the lateral three and a half digits,
- loss of flexion of the 1st to 3rd digits,
- positive "bottle sign" due to loss of thumb abduction (with proximal nerve lesion)
- weakened flexion of the 4th and 5th digits,
- loss of thenar opposition,
- loss of pronation,
- an "ape hand" produced by flattening of the thenar eminence, and
- the "hand of benediction" produced by flexing the hand in a fist (the 2nd and 3rd digits remain partly extended).

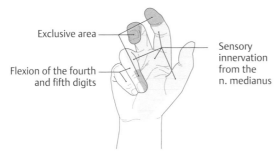

Exclusive area — Sensory innervation from the n. medianus — Flexion of the fourth and fifth digits

A "Hand of benediction" following a proximal median nerve injury.

In a healthy hand, the thumb can be abducted to fully grasp a cylindrical object — With a proximal median nerve lesion, the thumb cannot be fully abducted

B Positive "bottle sign" due to loss or weakness of finger flexion and thumb abduction.

(From Schuenke M, Schulte E, Schumacher U. THIEME Atlas of Anatomy, Vol 1. Illustrations by Voll M and Wesker K. 3rd ed. New York: Thieme Publishers; 2020.)

BOX 18.9: CLINICAL CORRELATION

ULNAR NERVE INJURY

The n. ulnaris may be injured at the elbow by a fracture of the epicondylus medialis, compressed in the fossa cubitalis between the two heads of the m. flexor carpi ulnaris, or compressed in the canalis ulnaris at the wrist. These injuries result in the following:
- Paresthesia of the palmar and dorsal side of the medial hand and the medial one and a half digits
- Loss of thumb adduction
- Hyperextension of the artt. metacarpophalangeae
- Loss of extension of artt. interphalangeae
- Weakened adduction and flexion of the wrist (for lesions at the elbow)
- Inability to form a fist due to "claw hand" deformity

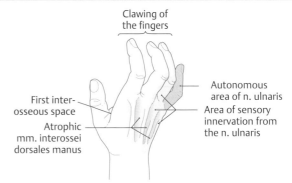

Clawing of the fingers — First interosseous space — Atrophic mm. interossei dorsales manus — Autonomous area of n. ulnaris — Area of sensory innervation from the n. ulnaris

A "Claw hand" deformity with hollowing of interosseous spaces (due to atrophy of mm. interossei dorsales manus).

Strong adduction of the thumb in the healthy hand — The thumb is flexed at the art. interphalangea, signifying an ulnar nerve lesion

B Positive "Froment sign" indicating palsy of the m. adductor pollicis.

(From Schuenke M, Schulte E, Schumacher U. THIEME Atlas of Anatomy, Vol 1. Illustrations by Voll M and Wesker K. 3rd ed. New York: Thieme Publishers; 2020.)

○ Its **rr. musculares** innervate the flexors on the medial side (m. flexor carpi ulnaris and medial half of the m. flexor digitorum profundus).

○ **Palmar** and **dorsal cutaneous nerves** arise in the wrist but are distributed to the skin of the medial half of the hand, proximal parts of the 5th digit, and medial half of the 4th digit.

• It crosses the wrist with the a. ulnaris within a narrow space, the **canalis ulnaris**, where it splits into deep and superficial branches.

○ Its **r. profundus** supplies most of the intrinsic muscles of the palm (except the m. adductor pollicis, half of the m. flexor pollicis brevis, and mm. lumbricales I and II).

○ Its **r. superficialis** innervates a small superficial muscle of the palm (m. palmaris brevis) and contributes to sensory innervation of the 4th and 5th digits.

— The n. axillaris (C5–C6), a branch of the fasciculus posterior, passes to the posterior shoulder region with the a. circumflexa humeri posterior and v. circumflexa humeri posterior.

• In the shoulder region, it innervates m. scapularis and m. deltoideus and skin of the deltoid region.

BOX 18.10: CLINICAL CORRELATION

AXILLARY NERVE INJURY
The n. axillaris is most vulnerable as it courses around the neck of the humerus and can be injured by fractures at the collum chirurgicum humeri or dislocation of the art. glenohumeralis. Denervation of the deltoid results in substantial functional weakness of shoulder movements and other effects, including

• Weakened flexion and extension at the shoulder joint
• Inability to abduct the shoulder even to the horizontal position
• Loss of sensation over the deltoid region
• A flattened shoulder contour

— The n. radialis (C5–T1) forms from the fasciculus posterior.

• In the arm, it runs posteriorly around the humerus in the sulcus nervi radialis with the a. profunda brachii and descends within the posterior compartment.

○ Its **rr. musculares** innervate all of the muscles of the posterior arm, the m. triceps brachii and m. anconeus.

○ Its sensory branches of the arm include the **n. cutaneus brachii posterior** and **n. cutaneus brachii lateralis inferior.**

○ An **n. cutaneus antebrachii posterior** arises in the arm but innervates skin over the posterior forearm.

• In the cubital region, it passes through the septum intermusculare brachii laterale into the anterior compartment, where it runs anterior to the epicondylus medialis. As it enters the proximal forearm, it splits into deep and superficial branches.

○ The r. profundus becomes the **n. interosseus posterior** as it circles around the radius into the posterior forearm compartment. It innervates all muscles of this compartment.

○ The **r. superficialis nervi radialis** descends along the lateral forearm to the wrist.

• In the hand, the n. radialis has no motor branches.

○ At the wrist, the r. superficialis nervi radialis runs posteriorly to innervate the skin on the dorsum of the hand and proximal segments of the 1st through 3rd digits and half of the 4th digit.

BOX 18.11: CLINICAL CORRELATION

RADIAL NERVE INJURY
The n. radialis is most vulnerable to injury from a midhumeral fracture where the nerve courses along the sulcus n. radialis. Because branches to the m. triceps brachii are usually proximal to the injury, elbow flexion is unaffected. Other effects include the following:

• Loss of wrist extension
• Loss of extension at the artt. metacarpophalangeae
• Weakened pronation
• Flexed wrist and fingers producing the "wrist drop" position

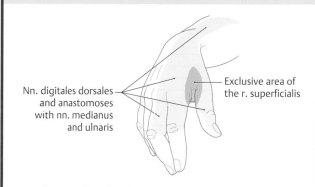

Nn. digitales dorsales and anastomoses with nn. medianus and ulnaris

Exclusive area of the r. superficialis

"Wrist drop" resulting from loss of wrist extensors.
(From Schuenke M, Schulte E, Schumacher U. THIEME Atlas of Anatomy, Vol 1. Illustrations by Voll M and Wesker K. 3rd ed. New York: Thieme Publishers; 2020.)

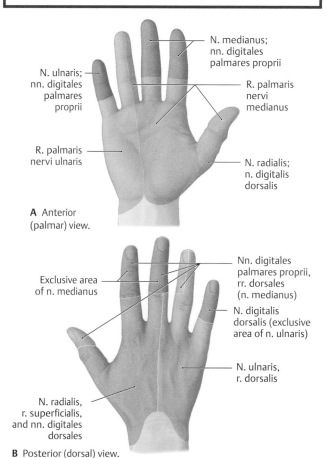

N. ulnaris; nn. digitales palmares proprii

N. medianus; nn. digitales palmares proprii

R. palmaris nervi medianus

R. palmaris nervi ulnaris

N. radialis; n. digitalis dorsalis

A Anterior (palmar) view.

Exclusive area of n. medianus

Nn. digitales palmares proprii, rr. dorsales (n. medianus)

N. digitalis dorsalis (exclusive area of n. ulnaris)

N. ulnaris, r. dorsalis

N. radialis, r. superficialis, and nn. digitales dorsales

B Posterior (dorsal) view.

Fig. 18.19 Sensory innervation of the hand
Right hand. Extensive overlap exists between adjacent areas. Exclusive nerve territories indicated with darker shading. (From Schuenke M, Schulte E, Schumacher U. THIEME Atlas of Anatomy, Vol 1. Illustrations by Voll M and Wesker K. 3rd ed. New York: Thieme Publishers; 2020.)

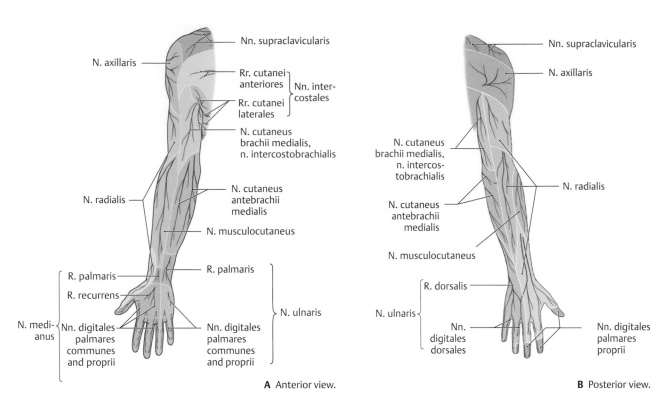

A Anterior view.

B Posterior view.

Fig. 18.20 Cutaneous innervation of the upper limb
(From Schuenke M, Schulte E, Schumacher U. THIEME Atlas of Anatomy, Vol 1. Illustrations by Voll M and Wesker K. 3rd ed. New York: Thieme Publishers; 2020.)

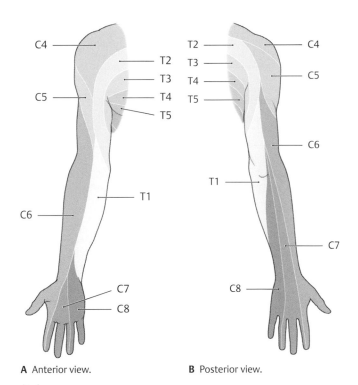

A Anterior view.

B Posterior view.

Fig. 18.21 Dermatomes of the upper limb
(From Schuenke M, Schulte E, Schumacher U. THIEME Atlas of Anatomy, Vol 1. Illustrations by Voll M and Wesker K. 3rd ed. New York: Thieme Publishers; 2020.)

19   Functional Anatomy of the Upper Limb

The upper limb is characterized by its wide range of movement and fine motor ability. Coordinated movements at the pectoral girdle, as well as the shoulder, art. cubitus, art. radioulnaris, and art. radiocarpalis, position the hand for performing work as vital as eating and as complicated as playing a violin.

Schematics of upper limb muscles accompany the muscle tables (origin, attachment, innervation, and action) in the appropriate chapter sections. To see the muscles in situ, view the gallery of topographic images in Section 14.7 at the end of this chapter.

19.1   The Pectoral Girdle (Cingulum Pectorale)

The **pectoral girdle (cingulum pectorale)**, formed by the clavicula and scapula, attaches the upper limb to the trunk (**Fig. 19.1**). The clavicula, acting as a strut, holds the scapula and humerus away from the trunk, allowing the free range of motion necessary for upper limb function.

Joints of the Pectoral Girdle

The joints of the pectoral girdle include articulations of the clavicula with the sternum and scapula, and a nonosseous joint that permits gliding movement between muscles of the trunk and scapula.

— The **art. sternoclavicularis** is a strong but highly mobile synovial joint between the sternal end of the clavicula and the manubrium sterni and cartilago costalis I (**Fig. 19.2**).
  • It is the only bony articulation between the upper limb and the trunk.
  • A discus articularis separates the articulating surfaces.
  • **Lig. sternoclaviculare anterius, lig. sternoclaviculare posterius, lig. costoclaviculare,** and **lig. interclaviculare** strengthen the joint.
  • The joint allows the clavicula to elevate and rotate in conjunction with limb movements.
— The **art. acromioclavicularis** is a plane type of synovial joint between the acromion of the scapula and acromial end of the clavicula (**Fig. 19.3**).
  • A discus articularis separates the articulating surfaces.
  • A **lig. acromioclaviculare** supports the joint superiorly.
  • The **lig. coracoclaviculare**, an extrinsic ligament (distant from the joint), strengthens the joint by anchoring the clavicula to the proc. coracoideus. Its two parts are the **lig. conoideum** and **lig. trapezoideum.**
— The **art. scapulothoracica** is not a bony articulation but a functional relationship between the m. serratus anterior and m. subscapularis that allows the scapula to glide and pivot on the chest wall (**Fig. 19.4**).

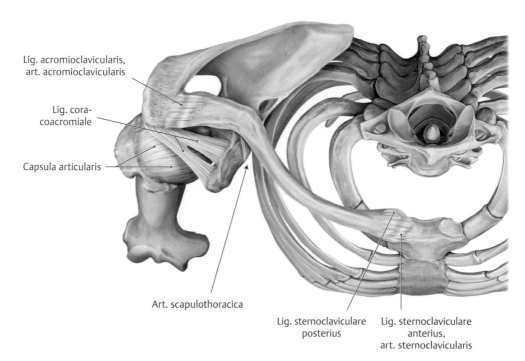

Lig. acromioclavicularis, art. acromioclavicularis

Lig. cora-coacromiale

Capsula articularis

Art. scapulothoracica

Lig. sternoclaviculare posterius

Lig. sternoclaviculare anterius, art. sternoclavicularis

Fig. 19.1 Joints of the shoulder girdle
Right side, superior view. (From Schuenke M, Schulte E, Schumacher U. THIEME Atlas of Anatomy, Vol 1. Illustrations by Voll M and Wesker K. 3rd ed. New York: Thieme Publishers; 2020.)

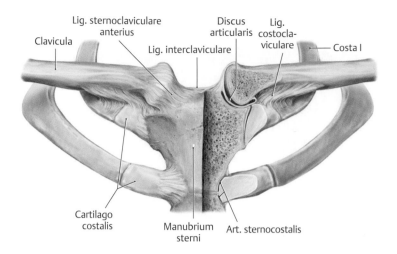

Fig. 19.2 Articulatio sternoclavicularis
Anterior view with sternum coronally sectioned *(left)*.
Note: A fibrocartilaginous discus articularis compensates for the mismatch of surfaces between the two saddle-shaped articular facets of the clavicula and the manubrium. (From Schuenke M, Schulte E, Schumacher U. THIEME Atlas of Anatomy, Vol 1. Illustrations by Voll M and Wesker K. 3rd ed. New York: Thieme Publishers; 2020.)

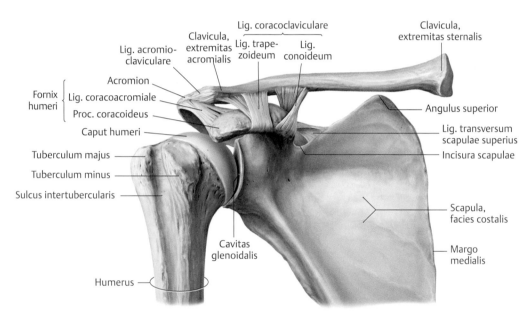

Fig. 19.3 Articulatio acromioclavicularis
Anterior view. The art. acromioclavicularis is a plane joint. Because the articulating surfaces are flat, they must be held in place by strong ligaments, greatly limiting the mobility of the joint. (From Schuenke M, Schulte E, Schumacher U. THIEME Atlas of Anatomy, Vol 1. Illustrations by Voll M and Wesker K. 3rd ed. New York: Thieme Publishers; 2020.)

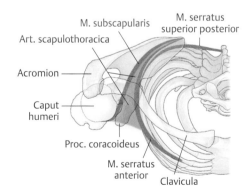

Fig. 19.4 Articulatio scapulothoracica
Right side, superior view. In all movements of the shoulder girdle, the scapula glides on a curved surface of loose connective tissue between the m. serratus anterior and the m. subscapularis. This surface can be considered an art. scapulothoracica. (From Schuenke M, Schulte E, Schumacher U. THIEME Atlas of Anatomy, Vol 1. Illustrations by Voll M and Wesker K. 3rd ed. New York: Thieme Publishers; 2020.)

Muscles of the Pectoral Girdle

Muscles of the pectoral girdle attach the upper limb to the trunk and move and stabilize the pectoral girdle in response to movements of the art. glenohumeralis at the shoulder **(Table 19.1)**.

— Anterior muscles of the pectoral girdle, which lie on the anterior and lateral thoracic wall,
  • include the **m. subclavius, m. pectoralis minor,** and **m. serratus anterior,** and
  • are anchored to the ribs, as well as to the bones of the pectoral girdle.
— Posterior muscles of the pectoral girdle, which are part of the superficial muscular layer of the back,
  • include the **m. trapezius, m. levator scapulae, m. rhomboideus major,** and **m. rhomboideus minor**, and
  • arise from cervical and thoracic vertebrae and insert on the scapula.
— Movements of the pectoral girdle and the muscles that provide them are listed in **Table 19.2.**

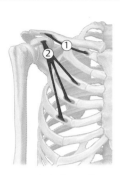

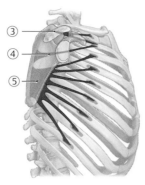

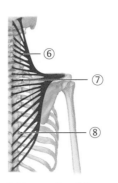

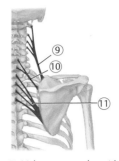

A M. subclavius and m. pectoralis minor, right, anterior view.

B M. serratus anterior, right lateral view.

C M. trapezius, right posterior view.

D M. levator scapulae with mm. rhomboidei major and minor, right posterior view.

(From Schuenke M, Schulte E, Schumacher U. THIEME Atlas of Anatomy, Vol 1. Illustrations by Voll M and Wesker K. 3rd ed. New York: Thieme Publishers; 2020.)

Table 19.1 Pectoral Girdle Muscles

Muscle		Origin	Insertion	Innervation	Action
① M. subclavius		Costa I	Clavicula (inferior surface)	N. subclavius (C5, C6)	Steadies the clavicula in the art. sternoclavicularis
② M. pectoralis minor		Costae III to V	Proc. coracoideus	N. pectoralis medialis (C8, T1)	Protracts and depresses scapula, causing angulus inferior to move posteromedially; rotates cavitas glenoidalis inferiorly; assists in respiration
M. serratus anterior	③ Pars superior	Costae I and II	Scapula (facies costalis and posterior of angulus superior)	N. thoracicus longus (C5–C7)	Pars superior: protracts scapula; lowers the raised arm
	④ Pars divergens	Costa II	Scapula (facies costalis of margo medialis)		Entire muscle: draws scapula laterally forward; elevates costae when shoulder is fixed
	⑤ Pars convergens	Costae III to IX or X	Scapula (facies costalis of margo medialis and facies costalis and posterior of angulus inferior)		Pars convergens: rotates angulus inferior scapulae laterally forward (allows elevation of arm above 90 degrees)
M. trapezius	⑥ Pars descendens	Os occipitale; procc. spinosi of C I–C VII	Clavicula (lateral one third)	N. accessorius (CN XI); C3–C4 of plexus cervicalis	Elevates scapula obliquely upward; rotates cavitas glenoidalis superiorly and rotates inferior angle laterally; tilts head to same side and rotates it to opposite
	⑦ Pars transversa	Aponeurosis at procc. spinosi T I–T IV	Acromion		Retracts scapula medially
	⑧ Pars ascendens	Procc. spinosi of T V–T XII	Spina scapulae		Depresses scapula and draws it medially downward
					Entire muscle: steadies scapula on thorax
⑨ M. levator scapulae		Procc. transversi of C I–C IV	Angulus superior scapulae	N. dorsalis scapulae and nn. cervicales (C3, C4)	Elevates and medially rotates inferior angle of scapula; inclines neck to same side
⑩ M. rhomboideus minor		Procc. spinosi of C VI, C VII,	Margo medialis scapulae above (minor) and below (major) spina scapulae	N. dorsalis scapulae (C4, C5)	Steadies scapula; retracts and medially rotates inferior angle of scapula
⑪ M. rhomboideus major		Procc. spinosi of vertebrae T I -T IV			

Abbreviation: CN, n. cranialis.

BOX 19.1: CLINICAL CORRELATION

LONG THORACIC NERVE INJURY
The n. thoracicus longus arises from the C5–C7 roots of the plexus brachialis. Its superficial course along the medial wall of the axilla puts it at risk of injury during regional surgeries such as axillary node dissection. Nerve damage results in the inability of the m. serratus anterior to laterally rotate the scapula, which is necessary to abduct the arm above the horizontal plane. The m. serratus anterior is also unable to support the scapula against the thoracic wall, which creates a "winged" scapula, especially noticeable when the subject presses the outstretched arm against a hard surface.

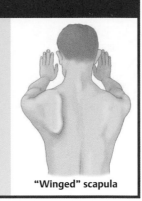

"Winged" scapula

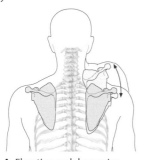

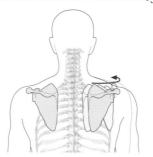

A Elevation and depression during elevation and depression of the shoulder girdle.

B Abduction and adduction during protraction and retraction of the shoulder girdle.

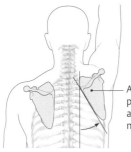

Antero-posterior axis of motion

C Lateral rotation of the inferior angle during abduction or elevation of the arm.

(From Schuenke M, Schulte E, Schumacher U. THIEME Atlas of Anatomy, Vol 1. Illustrations by Voll M and Wesker K. 3rd ed. New York: Thieme Publishers; 2020.)

Table 19.2 Movements of the Pectoral Girdle

Action	Primary Muscles
Elevation	M. trapezius (pars descendens)
	M. levator scapulae
Depression	M. pectoralis minor
	M. trapezius (pars ascendens)
Protraction	M. pectoralis minor
	M. serratus anterior
Retraction	M. trapezius (pars transversa)
	M. rhomboideus minor
	M. rhomboideus major
Lateral rotation	M. serratus anterior (inferior part)
	M. trapezius (pars descendens)
Medial rotation	M. levator scapulae
	M. rhomboideus minor
	M. rhomboideus major

19.2   The Shoulder Region

The shoulder region includes the axilla, a passageway for neurovascular structures between the trunk and upper limb, and the art. humeri, the largest joint of the upper limb. Muscles of the pectoral, scapular, and deltoid regions support the joint.

The Axilla

The **axilla (fossa axillaris)** is a four-sided pyramidally shaped region between the upper parts of the arm and lateral thoracic wall (**Fig. 19.5;** see also **Fig. 18.1**).
— Its boundaries are
 • the **cervicoaxillary canal,** the narrow space between the clavicula and 1st rib, which forms the apex;
 • the axillary fascia and axillary skin between the upper arm and the lateral thoracic wall, which form the base, or floor;
 • the m. pectoralis major and m. pectoralis minor, which form the anterior axillary wall (the lower edge of the pectoralis major forms a prominent ridge called the **anterior axillary fold**);

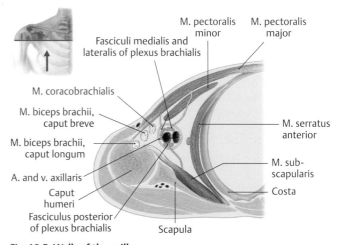

M. pectoralis minor
M. pectoralis major
Fasciculi medialis and lateralis of plexus brachialis
M. coracobrachialis
M. biceps brachii, caput breve
M. biceps brachii, caput longum
A. and v. axillaris
Caput humeri
Fasciculus posterior of plexus brachialis
Scapula
M. serratus anterior
M. sub-scapularis
Costa

Fig. 19.5 Walls of the axilla
Right side, inferior view. (From Schuenke M, Schulte E, Schumacher U. THIEME Atlas of Anatomy, Vol 1. Illustrations by Voll M and Wesker K. 3rd ed. New York: Thieme Publishers; 2020.)

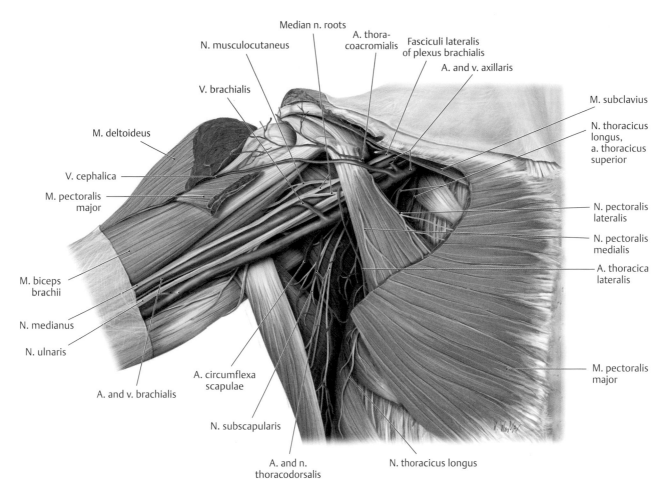

Fig. 19.6 Dissection of the axilla

Right shoulder, anterior view. *Removed*: M. pectoralis major and clavipectoral fascia. (From Schuenke M, Schulte E, Schumacher U. THIEME Atlas of Anatomy, Vol 1. Illustrations by Voll M and Wesker K. 3rd ed. New York: Thieme Publishers; 2020.)

- the m. subscapularis, m. latissimus dorsi, and m. teres major, which form the posterior axillary wall (the lower edge of the m. latissimus dorsi and m. teres major form a prominent ridge called the **posterior axillary fold**); and the lateral thoracic wall and the humerus of the arm, which form the medial and lateral walls, respectively.
- The contents of the axilla (**Fig. 19.6**), which are embedded in axillary fat, include
  - the a. axillaris and its branches,
  - the v. axillaris and its tributaries,
  - nll. axillaris and vessels, and
  - the cords and terminal nerves of the plexus brachialis.
- An extension of the fascia of the neck forms a sleevelike **axillary sheath** that encloses the axillary vessels and the brachial plexus.

The Glenohumeral (Shoulder) Joint

The **art. humeri (glenohumeralis)** is a ball-and-socket type of synovial joint between the shallow cavitas glenoidalis of the scapula and the large caput humeri (**Fig. 19.7**).

- The **labrum glenoidale**, a rim of fibrocartilage attached to the cavitas glenoidalis, deepens the articular surface.
- A fibrous capsule lined by a membrana synovialis surrounds the joint (**Fig. 19.8**). Although relatively lax and thin posteriorly, the capsule is reinforced
  - anteriorly by the **lig. glenohumerale superius, lig. glenohumerale medius,** and **lig. glenohumerale inferius** and
  - superiorly by the **lig. coracohumerale,** which extends from the proc. coracoideus to the tuberculum majus and tuberculum minus. This ligament stabilizes the tendon of the m. biceps brachii before it passes through the sulcus intertubercularis.
- The **lig. coracoacromiale** between the coracoid process and acromion prevents superior dislocation of the humerus.
- A membrana synovialis lines the joint space (cavitas synovialis) (**Fig. 19.9**).
  - It forms a tubular sheath around the tendon of the m. biceps brachii as the tendon passes through the joint space.
  - The cavitas synovialis communicates with a bursa under the subscapularis tendon (bursa subtendinea m. subscapularis).

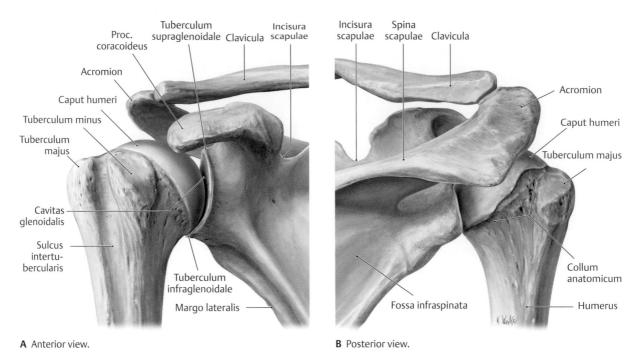

A Anterior view.

B Posterior view.

Fig. 19.7 Articulatio humeri (glenohumeralis): bony elements
Right shoulder, anterior view. (From Schuenke M, Schulte E, Schumacher U. THIEME Atlas of Anatomy, Vol 1. Illustrations by Voll M and Wesker K. 3rd ed. New York: Thieme Publishers; 2020.)

— Three large bursae are associated with the art. humeri **(Fig. 19.10)**:

1. Anteriorly, the **bursa subtendinea m. subscapularis,** which lies between the tendon of the m. subscapularis and the neck of the scapula, communicates with the cavitas synovialis of the joint.

2. Superiorly, the **bursa subacromialis** lies under the lig. coracoacromiale and above the supraspinatus tendon and art. humeri capsule.

3. Laterally, the **bursa subdeltoidea** lies deep to the m. deltoideus and above the subscapularis tendon. It communicates with the bursa subacromialis.

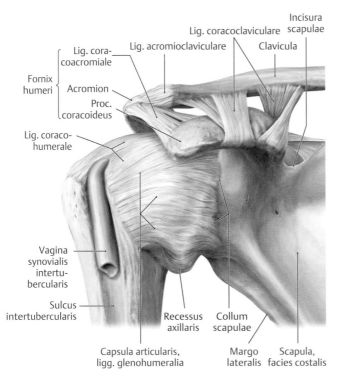

Fig. 19.8 Articulatio humeri (glenohumeralis): capsule and ligaments
Right shoulder, anterior view. (From Schuenke M, Schulte E, Schumacher U. THIEME Atlas of Anatomy, Vol 1. Illustrations by Voll M and Wesker K. 3rd ed. New York: Thieme Publishers; 2020.)

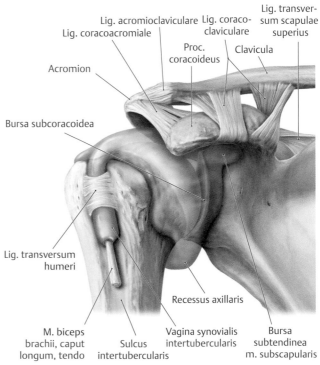

Fig. 19.9 Articulatio humeri (glenohumeralis) cavity
Right shoulder, anterior view. (From Schuenke M, Schulte E, Schumacher U. THIEME Atlas of Anatomy, Vol 1. Illustrations by Voll M and Wesker K. 3rd ed. New York: Thieme Publishers; 2020.)

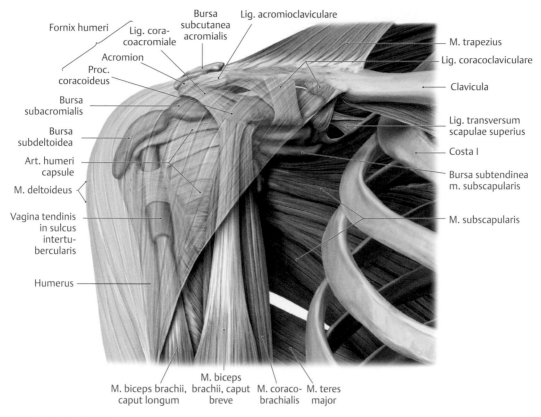

Fig. 19.10 Bursae of the shoulder region
Right shoulder, anterior view. (From Schuenke M, Schulte E, Schumacher U. THIEME Atlas of Anatomy, Vol 1. Illustrations by Voll M and Wesker K. 3rd ed. New York: Thieme Publishers; 2020.)

BOX 19.2: CLINICAL CORRELATION

GLENOHUMERAL DISLOCATION

The art. humeri is the most mobile but least stable joint of the body and dislocations are frequent. Rotator cuff muscles provide the greatest stability, supporting the joint anteriorly, posteriorly, and superiorly, but inferior support is lacking. The fornix humeri, coracohumeral ligament, and capsular glenohumeral ligaments add further support. The majority of dislocations (90%) occur inferiorly, although most are labeled "anterior" dislocations based on the position of the displaced caput humerale relative to the glenoid. These injuries can damage the n. axillaris and lead to a flattened shoulder profile. Posterior dislocations are rare and most often associated with seizures or electrocutions.

Muscles of the Shoulder Region

Muscles that cross the art. humeri stabilize the caput humeri in the cavitas glenoidalis and assist in movements of the arm (**Tables 19.3** and **19.4**).

— Two muscles of the trunk, the **m. pectoralis major** and **m. latissimus dorsi,** extend from the axial skeleton to the humerus and together provide strong adduction and medial rotation of the arm.
  • The m. pectoralis major is a strong flexor of the arm.
  • The m. latissimus dorsi is a strong extensor of the arm.
— Scapulohumeral muscles attach the humerus to the scapula and provide stability for the art. humeri.

• The **m. deltoideus,** which forms the rounded contour of the shoulder, abducts, flexes, and extends the arm.
• The **m. teres major** adducts and internally rotates the arm.
• The **m. supraspinatus** initiates abduction of the arm and assists the deltoid in the first 15 degrees of movement.
• The **m. infraspinatus** externally rotates the arm.
• The **m. teres minor** externally rotates the arm.
• The **m. subscapularis** on the anterior surface of the scapula internally rotates the arm.
— A musculotendinous **rotator cuff** around the art. humeri includes four of the scapulohumeral muscles, which are the important dynamic stabilizers of the joint.
  • The rotator cuff muscles include the **m. supraspinatus, m. infraspinatus, m. teres minor,** and **m. subscapularis**.
  • Their tendons insert on, and reinforce, the fibrous capsule of the joint, forming a supportive cuff around the anterior, posterior, and superior aspects of the joint.
— A few muscles of the arm cross the art. humeri and support its movements (see **Table 19.6**).
  • The tendon of the long head of the **m. biceps brachii** passes through the intertubercular groove of the humerus and enters the capsula articularis, where it is ensheathed by the synovial layer of the capsule. It prevents dislocation of the humerus during abduction and flexion.
  • The short head of the m. biceps brachii and the **m. coracobrachialis** cross the joint anteriorly and assist in flexion of the arm.
  • The long head of the **m. triceps brachii** crosses the joint posteriorly and assists in adduction and extension.
— Movements at the art. humeri and the muscles that provide them are listed in **Table 19.5**.

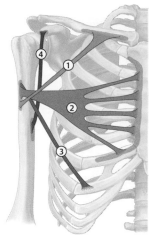

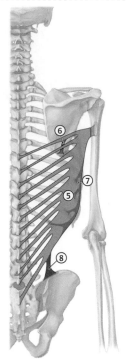

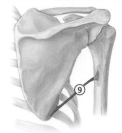

A M. pectoralis major and m. coracobrachialis, right side, anterior view.

(From Schuenke M, Schulte E, Schumacher U. THIEME Atlas of Anatomy, Vol 1. Illustrations by Voll M and Wesker K. 3rd ed. New York: Thieme Publishers; 2020.)

C M. teres major, right side, posterior view.

B M. latissimus dorsi, right side, posterior view.

Table 19.3 Shoulder Muscles

Muscle		Origin	Insertion	Innervation	Action
M. pectoralis major	① Pars clavicularis	Clavicula (medial half)	Humerus (crista tuberculi majus)	Nn. pectorales mediales and laterales (C5–T1)	Entire muscle: adduction, internal rotation
	② Pars sternocostalis	Sternum and cartilagines costales 1–6			Pars clavicularis and pars sternocostalis: flexion; assist in respiration when shoulder is fixed
	③ Pars abdominalis	Vagina musculi recti abdominis (lamina anterior)			
④ M. coracobrachialis		Scapula (proc. coracoideus)	Humerus (in line with crista tuberculi minoris)	N. musculocutaneous (C5–C7)	Flexion, adduction, internal rotation
M. latissimus dorsi	⑤ Pars vertebralis	Procc. spinosi of T VII–T XII; fascia thoracolumbalis	Crista tuberculi minoris (angulus anterior)	N. thoracodorsalis (C6–C8)	Internal rotation, adduction, extension, respiration ("cough muscle")
	⑥ Pars scapularis	Angulus inferior scapulae			
	⑦ Pars costalis	Costa IX–XII			
	⑧ Pars iliaca	Crista iliaca (posterior one third)			
⑨ M. teres major		Angulus inferior scapulae	Crista tuberculi minoris (angulus anterior)	Lower subscapular n. (C5, C6)	Internal rotation, adduction, extension

---

BOX 19.3: CLINICAL CORRELATION

ROTATOR CUFF TEARS
Rotator cuff tears can occur at any age but are most common in the older patient and usually involve the m. supraspinatus tendo. Degenerative changes, calcification, and chronic inflammation from repetitive use (baseball pitchers are a good example) can cause the tendon to fray and rupture. When the bursa subacromialis and bursa subdeltoidea tear in conjunction with the ruptured tendon, they become continuous with the cavity of the art. humeri **(Fig. 19.11)**.

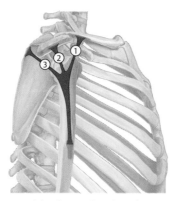

A M. deltoideus, right side, right lateral view.

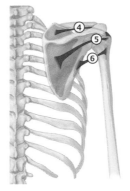

B Rotator cuff (m. supraspinatus, m. infraspinatus, and m. teres minor), right shoulder, posterior view.

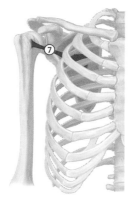

C Rotator cuff (m. subscapularis), right shoulder, anterior view.

(From Schuenke M, Schulte E, Schumacher U. THIEME Atlas of Anatomy, Vol 1. Illustrations by Voll M and Wesker K. 3rd ed. New York: Thieme Publishers; 2020.)

Table 19.4 Musculus Deltoideus and Rotator Cuff Muscles

Muscle		Origin	Insertion	Innervation	Action
M. deltoideus	① Pars clavicularis	Lateral one third of clavicula	Humerus (tuberositas deltoidea)	N. axillaris (C5, C6)	Flexion, internal rotation, adduction
	② Pars acromialis	Acromion			Abduction
	③ Pars spinalis	Spina scapularis			Extension, external rotation, adduction
④ M. supraspinatus	Scapula	Fossa supraspinata	Tuberculum majus humeri	N. suprascapularis (C5, C6)	Initiates abduction
⑤ M. infraspinatus		Fossa infraspinata			External rotation
⑥ M. teres minor		Margo lateralis		N. axillaris (C5, C6)	External rotation, weak adduction
⑦ M. subscapularis		Fossa subscapularis	Tuberculum minus humeri	Upper and lower nn. subscapulares (C5, C6)	Internal rotation

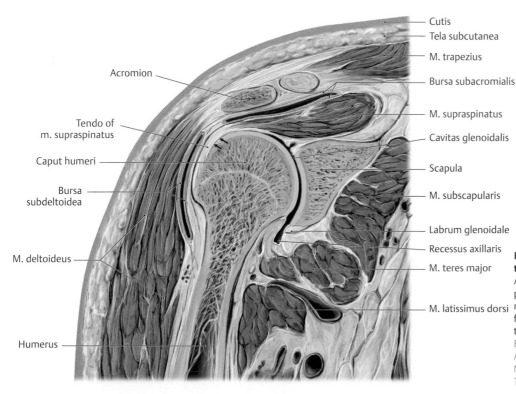

Cutis
Tela subcutanea
M. trapezius
Bursa subacromialis
M. supraspinatus
Cavitas glenoidalis
Scapula
M. subscapularis
Labrum glenoidale
Recessus axillaris
M. teres major
M. latissimus dorsi

Acromion
Tendo of m. supraspinatus
Caput humeri
Bursa subdeltoidea
M. deltoideus
Humerus

Fig. 19.11 Coronal section through the right shoulder Anterior view. The *arrows* are pointing at the tendon of m. supraspinatus, which is frequently injured in a "rotator cuff tear." (From Schuenke M, Schulte E, Schumacher U. THIEME Atlas of Anatomy, Vol 1. Illustrations by Voll M and Wesker K. 3rd ed. New York: Thieme Publishers; 2020.)

Table 19.5 Movements at the Articulatio Humeri (Glenohumeralis)

Action	Primary Muscles
Flexion	M. deltoideus (pars clavicularis) M. pectoralis major (pars clavicularis and pars sternocostalis) M. coracobrachialis M. biceps brachii (caput breve)
Extension	M. deltoideus (pars spinalis) M. latissimus dorsi M. teres major M. triceps brachii (caput longum)
Abduction	M. deltoideus (pars acromialis) M. supraspinatus
Adduction	M. deltoideus (pars clavicularis and pars spinalis) M. pectoralis major M. latissimus dorsi M. teres major M. triceps brachii (caput longum)
Internal rotation	M. deltoideus (pars clavicularis) M. pectoralis major (pars clavicularis) M. latissimus dorsi M. teres major M. subscapularis
External rotation	M. deltoideus (pars spinalis) M. infraspinatus M. teres minor

(From Schuenke M, Schulte E, Schumacher U. THIEME Atlas of Anatomy, Vol 1. Illustrations by Voll M and Wesker K. 3rd ed. New York: Thieme Publishers; 2020.)

A Flexion.

B Extension.

C Abduction.

D Adduction.

E Internal rotation.

F External rotation.

Spaces of the Posterior Shoulder Region

Spaces formed between muscles of the shoulder and the scapula allow nerves and vessels to pass between the axilla and the posterior scapular and humeral regions (**Fig. 19.12**).

— The **incisura scapulae,** limited superiorly by the lig. transversum scapulae superius, lies deep to the m. supraspinatus. The n. suprascapularis passes below the ligament, and the a. suprascapularis and v. suprascapularis pass above it.

— The **quadrangular space,** bounded laterally by the long head of m. triceps, medially by the humerus, inferiorly by the m. teres major, and superiorly by the m. teres minor, transmits the a. circumflexa humeri posterior and n. axillaris.

— The **triangular space,** bounded by the long head of m. triceps and m. teres major and m. teres minor, transmits the a. circumflexa scapula and v. circumflexa scapula.

— The **triceps hiatus,** between the long and lateral heads of m. triceps and below m. teres major, transmits the n. radialis and a. profunda brachii and v. profunda brachii.

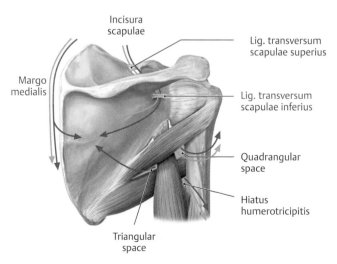

A Schematic. The course of arteries and nerves through the spaces are shown by *red* and *yellow arrows*. (From Gilroy AM, MacPherson BR, Wikenheiser JC. Atlas of Anatomy. Illustrations by Voll M and Wesker K. 4th ed. New York: Thieme Publishers; 2020.)

Fig. 19.12 Spaces of the posterior shoulder region
Right shoulder, posterior view.

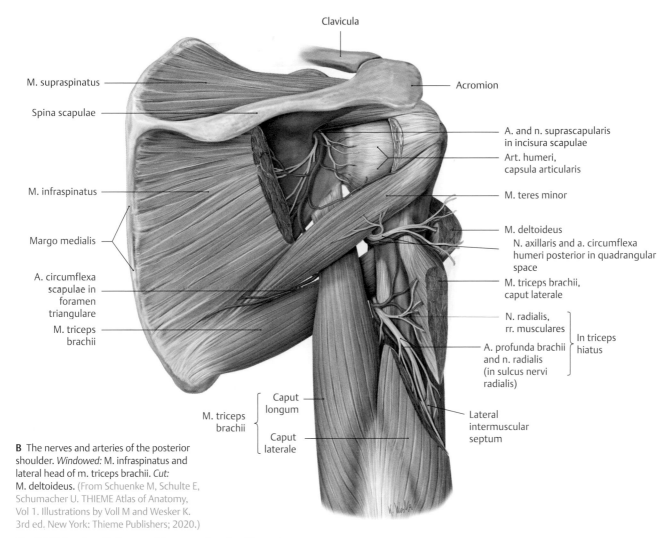

Clavicula

M. supraspinatus

Spina scapulae

Acromion

A. and n. suprascapularis
in incisura scapulae

Art. humeri,
capsula articularis

M. infraspinatus

M. teres minor

Margo medialis

M. deltoideus

N. axillaris and a. circumflexa
humeri posterior in quadrangular
space

A. circumflexa
scapulae in
foramen
triangulare

M. triceps
brachii

M. triceps brachii,
caput laterale

N. radialis,
rr. musculares

In triceps
hiatus

A. profunda brachii
and n. radialis
(in sulcus nervi
radialis)

Caput
longum

M. triceps
brachii

Caput
laterale

Lateral
intermuscular
septum

B The nerves and arteries of the posterior
shoulder. *Windowed:* M. infraspinatus and
lateral head of m. triceps brachii. *Cut:*
M. deltoideus. (From Schuenke M, Schulte E,
Schumacher U. THIEME Atlas of Anatomy,
Vol 1. Illustrations by Voll M and Wesker K.
3rd ed. New York: Thieme Publishers; 2020.)

Fig. 19.12 (*continued*) **Spaces of the posterior shoulder region**

19.3 The Arm and Cubital Region

The arm (brachial region) extends from the shoulder to the elbow
and contains the humerus and muscles of the arm. The cubital
region contains the fossa cubitalis and art. cubiti.

Muscles of the Arm

Muscles of the arm move the shoulder and art. cubiti. Fascia brachialis that surrounds the arm divides these muscles into anterior
and posterior compartments (**Table 19.6**).

– The anterior compartment contains
  • muscles that flex the art. humeri and art. cubiti and
    supinate the art. radioulnaris,
  • the n. musculocutaneus, and
  • the a. brachialis and v. brachialis.
– The posterior compartment contains
  • muscles that extend the art. humeri and art. cubiti,
  • the n. radialis, and
  • the a. profunda brachii and v. profunda brachii.
– The n. medianus and n. ulnaris descend along the medial side
  of the arm between the anterior and posterior compartments
  but do not innervate muscles of the arm.

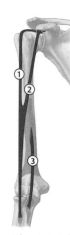
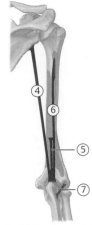
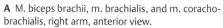

A M. biceps brachii, m. brachialis, and m. coracho-brachialis, right arm, anterior view.

B M. triceps brachii and m. anconeus, right arm, posterior view.

(From Gilroy AM et al. Atlas of Anatomy. 4th ed. 2020. Based on: Schuenke M, Schulte E, Schumacher U. THIEME Atlas of Anatomy. General Anatomy and Musculoskeletal System. Illustrations by Voll M and Wesker K. 3rd ed. New York: Thieme Medical Publishers; 2020.)

Table 19.6 Musculi Brachii, Anterior and Posterior Compartments

Muscle	Origin	Insertion	Innervation	Action
Anterior Compartment				
M. biceps brachii ① Caput longum	Tuberculum supraglenoi-dale scapulae	Tuberositas radii and aponeurosis bicipitalis	N. musculocutaneus (C5, C6)	Art. cubiti: flexion; supination*
② Caput breve	Proc. coracoideus scapulae			Art. humeri: flexion; stabilization of caput humeri during m. deltoideus contraction; abduction and internal rotation of the humerus
③ M. brachialis	Humerus (distal half of anterior surface)	Tuberositas ulnae and aponeurosis bicipitalis	N. musculocutaneus (C5–C6) and n. radialis (C7, minor)	Flexion at the art. cubiti
Posterior compartment				
M. triceps brachii ④ Caput longum	Tuberculum supraglenoi-dale scapulae	Olecranon ulnae	N. radialis (C6–C8)	Art. cubiti: extension
⑤ Caput mediale	Posterior humerus, distal to sulcus radialis; septum intermuscularis medialis septum			Art. humeri, caput longum: extension and adduction
⑥ Caput laterale	Posterior humerus, proximal to sulcus radialis; septum intermuscularis lateralis			
⑦ M. anconeus	Epicondylus lateralis humeri (variance: posterior joint capsule)	Olecranon ulnae (radial surface)		Extends the elbow and tightens its joint

*Note: When the elbow is flexed, the m. biceps brachii acts as a powerful supinator because the lever arm is almost perpendicular to the axis of pronation/supination.

The Fossa Cubitalis

The **fossa cubitalis** is a shallow depression anterior to the art. cubiti (**Fig. 19.13**).
— Its boundaries are,
  • medially, the m. pronator teres;
  • laterally, the m. brachioradialis; and
  • superiorly, a line that connects the epicondylus medialis humeri and epicondylus lateralis humeri.
— The fossa cubitalis contains

• the tendon of the m. biceps brachii,
• the a. brachialis and v. brachialis,
• the proximal part of a. radialis and v. radialis and a. ulnaris and v. ulnaris, and
• the n. medianus and n. radialis and the r. cutaneus of the n. musculocutaneus (n. cutaneus antebrachii lateralis).
— The **aponeurosis musculi bicipitis brachii**, a fascial extension of the m. biceps brachii, forms the root of the fossa, and the v. mediana cubiti crosses the fossa superficially.

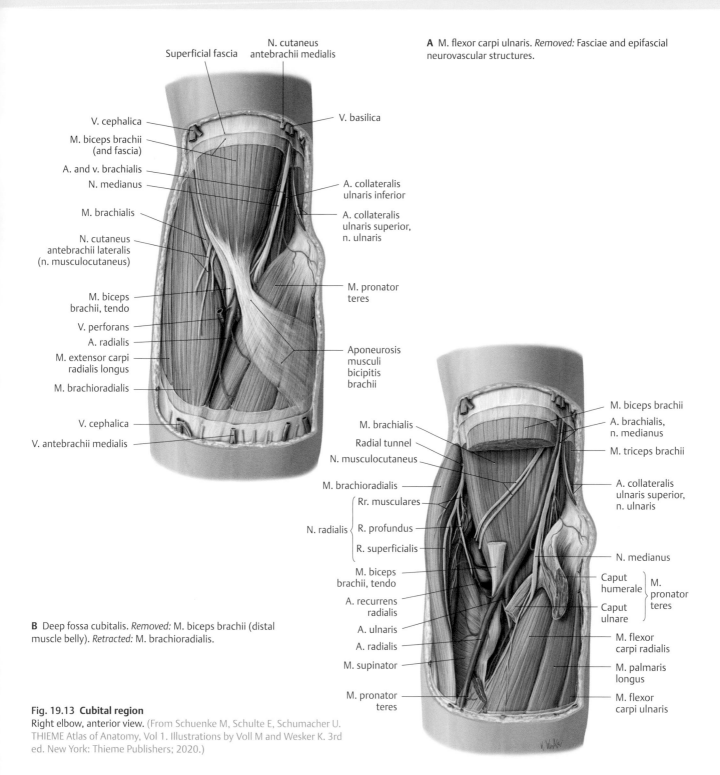

A M. flexor carpi ulnaris. *Removed:* Fasciae and epifascial neurovascular structures.

B Deep fossa cubitalis. *Removed:* M. biceps brachii (distal muscle belly). *Retracted:* M. brachioradialis.

Fig. 19.13 Cubital region
Right elbow, anterior view. (From Schuenke M, Schulte E, Schumacher U. THIEME Atlas of Anatomy, Vol 1. Illustrations by Voll M and Wesker K. 3rd ed. New York: Thieme Publishers; 2020.)

The Elbow Joint (Art. Cubiti)

The elbow joint (art. cubiti) is made up of three separate synovial joints contained within a single capsula articularis (**Figs. 19.14 and 19.15**).

— The hinge-type **art. humeroulnaris** is an articulation between the trochlea humeri and the incisura trochlearis of the ulna.
  • The **lig. collaterale ulnare**, which supports the joint medially, connects the proc. coronoideus and olecranon with the epicondylus medialis humeri.
— The hinge-type **art. humeroradialis** is an articulation between the capitulum humeri and the caput radii.

• The **lig. collaterale radiale**, which supports the joint laterally, extends from the epicondylus lateralis humeri to the **lig. anulare radii** of the radius that encircles the radial neck.
— The art. radioulnaris proximalis, the articulation between the caput radii and the incisura radialis of the ulna, is discussed further with the art. radioulnaris of the forearm.
— Movements at the art. humeroulnaris and art. humeroradialis and the muscles that provide them are listed in **Table 19.7.**

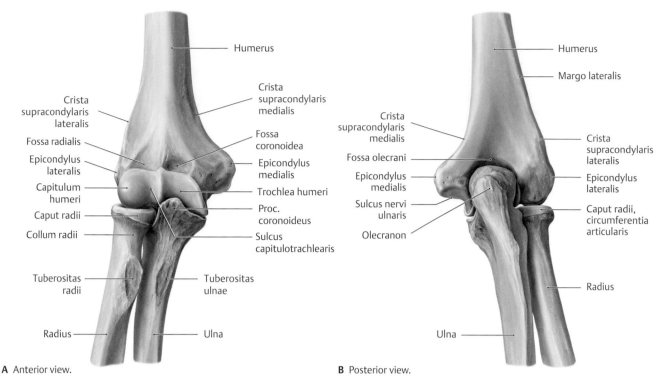

A Anterior view.   **B** Posterior view.

Fig. 19.14 Articulatio cubiti, capsula articularis
Right elbow in extension. The elbow consists of three articulations: the art. humeroulnaris, art. humeroradialis, and art. radioulnaris proximalis. (From Schuenke M, Schulte E, Schumacher U. THIEME Atlas of Anatomy, Vol 1. Illustrations by Voll M and Wesker K. 3rd ed. New York: Thieme Publishers; 2020.)

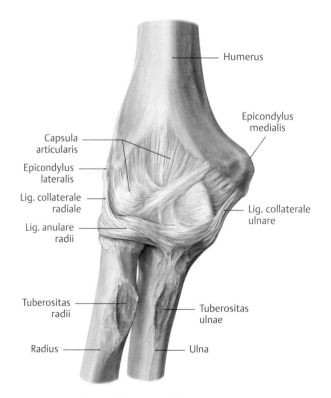

Fig. 19.15 Capsula articularis of the elbow
Right elbow in extension, anterior view. (From Schuenke M, Schulte E, Schumacher U. THIEME Atlas of Anatomy, Vol 1. Illustrations by Voll M and Wesker K. 3rd ed. New York: Thieme Publishers; 2020.)

Table 19.7 Movements at the Articulatio Humeroulnaris and Articulatio Humeroradialis

Action	Primary Muscles
Flexion	M. biceps brachii
	M. brachialis
	M. brachioradialis
Extension	M. triceps brachii

19.4   The Forearm

The forearm (antebrachial region) extends from the elbow to the wrist and contains the radius and ulna and the muscles of the forearm.

Artt. Radioulnares

The artt. radioulnares connect the bones of the forearm proximally at the elbow and distally at the wrist. Movement at these joints allows rotation of the distal radius around the ulna, causing supination (palm up) and pronation (palm down) of the hand (**Figs. 19.16** and **19.17**). These movements and the muscles of the arm and forearm that provide them are listed in **Table 19.8.**

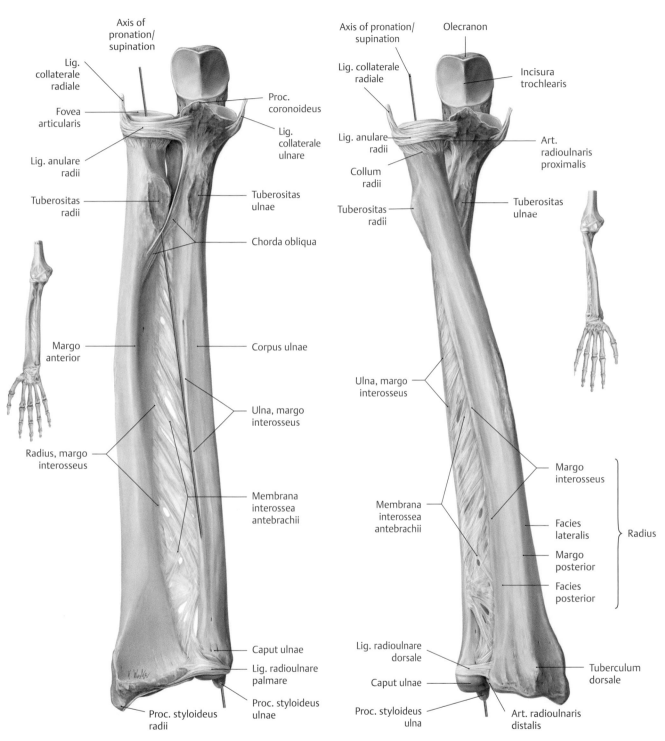

Fig. 19.16 Forearm in supination
Right forearm, anterior view. (From Schuenke M, Schulte E, Schumacher U. THIEME Atlas of Anatomy, Vol 1. Illustrations by Voll M and Wesker K. 3rd ed. New York: Thieme Publishers; 2020.)

Fig. 19.17 Forearm in pronation
Right forearm, anterior view. (From Schuenke M, Schulte E, Schumacher U. THIEME Atlas of Anatomy, Vol 1. Illustrations by Voll M and Wesker K. 3rd ed. New York: Thieme Publishers; 2020.)

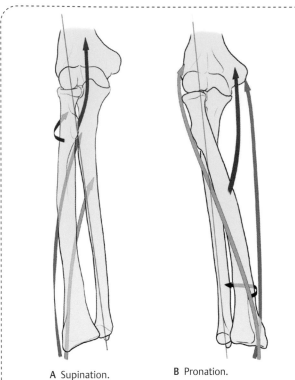

A Supination.   B Pronation.

(From Gilroy AM et al. Atlas of Anatomy. 4th ed. 2020. Based on: Schuenke M, Schulte E, Schumacher U. THIEME Atlas of Anatomy. General Anatomy and Musculoskeletal System. Illustrations by Voll M and Wesker K. 3rd ed. New York: Thieme Medical Publishers; 2020.)

Table 19.8 Movements at the Articulationes Radioulnares

Action	Primary Muscles
Supination	M. supinator
	M. biceps brachii
Pronation	M. pronator teres
	M. pronator quadratus

— The **art. radioulnaris proximalis** is a synovial joint that allows rotation of the caput radii within the cuff formed by the lig. anulare and the incisura radialis of the ulna. This articulation is contained within the capsula articularis of the art. cubiti.
— The **art. radioulnaris distalis** has an L-shaped capsula articularis with a triangular discus articularis that separates the art. radioulnaris from the cavity of the art. carpi. It is supported by palmar and dorsal radioulnar ligaments.
— A **membrana interossea** connects the shafts of the radius and ulna and transfers energy absorbed by the distal radius to the proximal ulna.

Muscles of the Forearm

Muscles of the forearm move joints of the elbow, wrist, and hand. Most forearm flexors and extensors have long tendons that cross the wrist and extend into the fingers. Septa intermusculares and the membrana interossea create anterior and posterior muscular compartments.

BOX 19.4: CLINICAL CORRELATION

SUBLUXATION OF THE RADIAL HEAD (NURSEMAID'S ELBOW)
A common and painful injury of small children occurs when the arm is jerked upward with the forearm pronated, tearing the anular ligament from its loose attachment on the radial neck. As the immature radial head slips out of the socket, the ligament may become trapped between the radial head and the capitulum of the humerus. Supinating the forearm and flexing the elbow usually returns the radial head to the normal position.

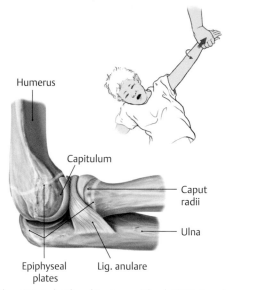

Humerus

Capitulum

Caput radii

Ulna

Epiphyseal plates   Lig. anulare

(From Gilroy AM et al. Atlas of Anatomy. 4th ed. 2020. Based on: Schuenke M, Schulte E, Schumacher U. THIEME Atlas of Anatomy. General Anatomy and Musculoskeletal System. Illustrations by Voll M and Wesker K. 3rd ed. New York: Thieme Medical Publishers; 2020.)

BOX 19.5: CLINICAL CORRELATION

LATERAL EPICONDYLITIS ("TENNIS ELBOW")
Repetitive use of the forearm extensors can inflame the attachment of the common extensor tendon at the epicondylus lateralis (lateral epicondylitis). Pain is focused over the tendon insertion but radiates along the extensor forearm and is exacerbated by stretching of the extensor tendons by pronation and wrist flexion.

— The compartimentum antebrachii anterius (**Table 19.9**) contains
  • muscles that flex and pronate joints of the elbow, wrist, and hand;
  • the n. medianus and n. ulnaris; and
  • the a. ulnaris and v. ulnaris and a. interossea anterior and v. interossea anterior.
— The compartimentum antebrachii posterius (**Table 19.10**) contains
  • muscles that extend joints of the elbow, wrist, and hand and supinate the art. radioulnaris (one muscle, m. brachioradialis, passes anterior to the elbow and therefore acts as a flexor, instead of an extensor of this joint);
  • the n. radialis; and
  • the a. radialis and v. radialis and a. interossea posterior and v. interossea posterior.

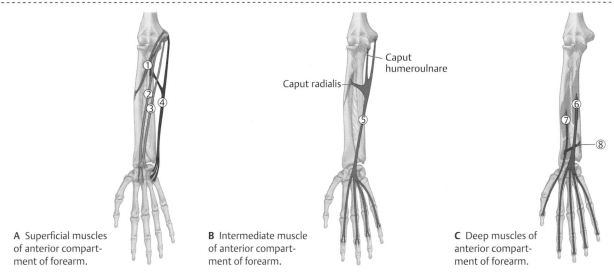

A Superficial muscles of anterior compartment of forearm.

B Intermediate muscle of anterior compartment of forearm.

C Deep muscles of anterior compartment of forearm.

(From Gilroy AM et al. Atlas of Anatomy. 4th ed. 2020. Based on: Schuenke M, Schulte E, Schumacher U. THIEME Atlas of Anatomy. General Anatomy and Musculoskeletal System. Illustrations by Voll M and Wesker K. 3rd ed. New York: Thieme Medical Publishers; 2020.)

Table 19.9 Forearm Muscles: Anterior Compartment

Muscle	Origin	Insertion	Innervation	Action
Superficial muscles				
① M. pronator teres	Caput humerale: epicondylus medialis humeri Caput ulnare: proc. coronoideus ulnae	Lateral radius (distal to m. supinator insertion)	N. medianus (C6, C7)	Elbow: weak flexion Forearm: pronation
② M. flexor carpi radialis	Epicondylus medialis humeri	Base of os metacarpale II (variance: basis of os metacarpale III)		Wrist: flexion and abduction (radial deviation) of hand
③ M. palmaris longus		Aponeurosis palmaris	N. medianus (C7, C8)	Elbow: weak flexion Wrist: flexion tightens palmar aponeurosis
④ M. flexor carpi ulnaris	Caput humerale: epicondylus medialis humeri Caput ulnare: olecranon	Os pisiforme; hamulus ossis hamati; basis of os metacarpale V	N. ulnaris (C7–T1)	Wrist: flexion and adduction (ulnar deviation) of hand
Intermediate muscles				
⑤ M. flexor digitorum superficialis	Caput humeroulnare: epicondylus medialis humeri and proc. coronoideus ulnae Caput radiale: upper half of margo anterior radii	Sides of phalanges mediales of digiti II–V	N. medianus (C8, T1)	Elbow: weak flexion Wrist, MCP, and PIP joints of 2nd to 5th digits: flexion
Deep muscles				
⑥ M. flexor digitorum profundus	Ulna (proximal two thirds of flexor surface) and membrana interossea antebrachii	Phalanges distales of digiti II–V (palmar surface)	N. medianus (C8, T1) radial half of 2nd and 3rd digits; N. ulnaris (C8, T1) ulnar half of 4th and 5th digits	Wrist, MCP, PIP, and DIP of 2nd to 5th digits: flexion
⑦ M. flexor pollicis longus	Radius (midanterior surface) and adjacent membrana interossea antebrachii	Phalanx distalis pollicis (palmar surface)	N. medianus (C8, T1)	Wrist: flexion and abduction (radial deviation) of hand Carpometacarpal of thumb: flexion MCP and IP of thumb: flexion
⑧ M. pronator quadratus	Distal quarter of ulna (anterior surface)	Distal quarter of radius (anterior surface)		Hand: pronation Distal radioulnar joint: stabilization

Abbreviations: DIP, distal interphalangeal; IP, interphalangeal; MCP, metacarpophalangeal; PIP, proximal interphalangeal.

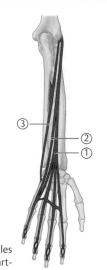
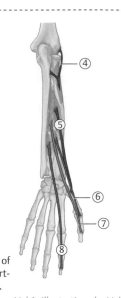
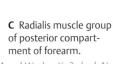

A Superficial muscles of posterior compartment of forearm.

B Deep muscles of posterior compartment of forearm.

C Radialis muscle group of posterior compartment of forearm.

(From Schuenke M, Schulte E, Schumacher U. THIEME Atlas of Anatomy, Vol 1. Illustrations by Voll M and Wesker K. 3rd ed. New York: Thieme Publishers; 2020).

Table 19.10 Forearm Muscles: Posterior Compartment

Muscle	Origin	Insertion	Innervation	Action
Superficial muscles				
① M. extensor digitorum	Common head (epicondylus lateralis humeri)	Dorsal digital expansion of digiti II–V	N. radialis (C7, C8)	Wrist: extension MCP, PIP, and DIP of 2nd to 5th digits: extension
② M. extensor digiti minimi		Dorsal digital expansion of digitus V		Wrist: extension, ulnar abduction of hand MCP, PIP, and DIP of 5th digit: extension of 5th digit
③ M. extensor carpi ulnaris	Common head (epicondylus lateralis humeri) Caput ulnare (facies dorsalis)	Os metacarpale V (base)		Wrist: extension, adduction (ulnar deviation) of hand
Deep muscles				
④ M. supinator	Olecranon, epicondylus lateralis humeri, lig. collaterale radiale, lig. anulare radii	Radius (between tuberositas radii and insertion of m. pronator teres)	N. radialis (C6, C7)	Art. radioulnaris: supination
⑤ M. abductor pollicis longus	Radius and ulna (dorsal surfaces, interosseous membrane)	Os metacarpale I	N. radialis (C7, C8)	Art. radioulnaris: abduction of the hand Art. carpometacarpalis pollicis: abduction
⑥ M. extensor pollicis brevis	Radius (posterior surface) and membrana interossea antebrachii	Base of phalanx proximalis pollicis		Art. radioulnaris: abduction (radial deviation) of hand Art. carpometacarpalis pollicis and MCP of thumb: extension
⑦ M. extensor pollicis longus	Ulna (posterior surface) and membrana interossea antebrachii	Base of phalanx distalis pollicis		Wrist: extension and abduction (radial deviation) of hand Art. carpometacarpalis pollicis: adduction MCP and IP of thumb: extension
⑧ M. extensor indicis	Ulna (posterior surface) and membrana interossea antebrachii	Posterior digital extension of digitus II		Wrist: extension MCP, PIP, and DIP of 2nd digit: extension
Radialis muscles				
⑨ M. brachioradialis	Distal humerus (distal surface), septum intermusculare laterale	Proc. styloideus radii	N. radialis (C5, C6)	Elbow: flexion Forearm: semipronation
⑩ M. extensor carpi radialis longus	Crista supraconylaris lateralis humeri, septum intermusculare laterale	Os metacarpale II (base)	N. radialis (C6, C7)	Elbow: weak flexion Wrist: extension and abduction
⑪ M. extensor carpi radialis brevis	Epicondylus lateralis humeri	Os metacarpale III (base)	N. radialis (C7, C8)	

Abbreviations: DIP, distal interphalangeal; IP, interphalangeal; MCP, metacarpophalangeal; PIP, proximal interphalangeal.

19.5 The Wrist

The wrist, the narrow space between the forearm and hand, contains the ossa carpi and the tendons of forearm muscles that move the wrist and fingers.

Joints of the Carpal Region

The carpal region is made up of the eight ossa carpi that articulate with the radius proximally and the ossa metacarpi distally (**Fig. 19.18**). The ulna is not a component of the wrist joint. Movements at the wrist joints and the muscles that provide them are listed in **Table 19.11**.

— The wrist, or **art. radiocarpalis**, is a condyloid type of joint between the distal radius and discus articularis of the art. radioulnaris distalis and the os scaphoideum and os lunatum in the proximal carpal row.
  • **Lig. radiocarpale palmare** and **lig. radiocarpale dorsale, ligg. ulnocarpale,** and **lig. collaterale radiale** and **lig. collaterale ulnare,** considered extrinsic ligaments of the joint, are interwoven with the fibrous capsule and function to stabilize the joint (**Fig. 19.19**).
  • A capsula articularis attaches proximally to the radius and ulna and distally to the bones of the proximal carpal row.

— **Intercarpal joints** are formed between the ossa carpi within each row; the **art. mediocarpalis** is the articulation between the bones of the proximal and distal carpal rows.
  • **Interosseous ligaments** between individual ossa carpi are intrinsic ligaments that limit excess movement and provide stability for these articulations. They also divide the joint space into compartments (**Fig. 19.20**).
  • A single articular cavity encloses the intercarpal and carpometacarpal joints and is separate from the articular cavity of the wrist joint.
  • Movements at these joints augment movements at the radiocarpal joint.

— The **ulnocarpal complex,** also known as the triangular fibrocartilage complex, supports the medial side of the wrist. It's a combination of an discus articularis and ligaments that connect the distal ulna, the art. radioulnaris, and the proximal carpal row (**Fig. 19.20**).
  • The complex includes the **discus ulnocarpalis**, lig. radiocarpale dorsale and lig. radiocarpale palmare, ligg. ulnocarpalia (lig. ulnolunatum and lig. ulnotriquetrum), **meniscus ulnocarpalis**, and lig. radiocarpale dorsale (lig. radiotriquetrum).

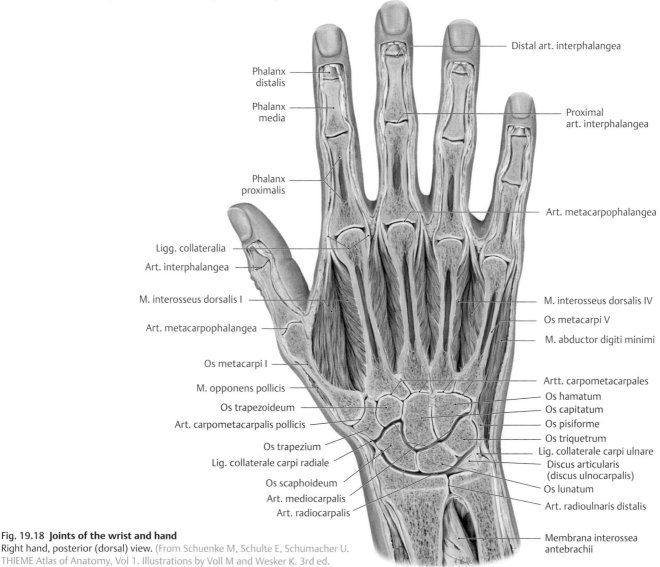

Fig. 19.18 Joints of the wrist and hand
Right hand, posterior (dorsal) view. (From Schuenke M, Schulte E, Schumacher U. THIEME Atlas of Anatomy, Vol 1. Illustrations by Voll M and Wesker K. 3rd ed. New York: Thieme Publishers; 2020.)

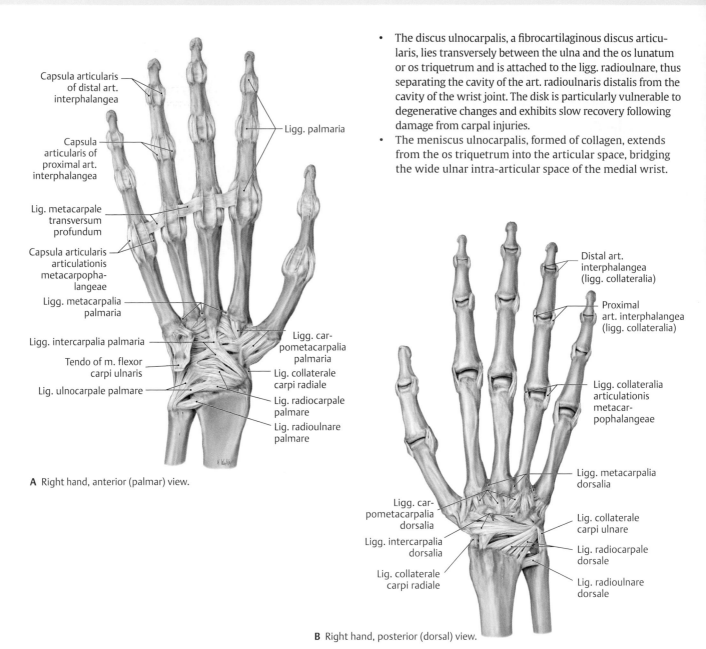

- The discus ulnocarpalis, a fibrocartilaginous discus articularis, lies transversely between the ulna and the os lunatum or os triquetrum and is attached to the ligg. radioulnare, thus separating the cavity of the art. radioulnaris distalis from the cavity of the wrist joint. The disk is particularly vulnerable to degenerative changes and exhibits slow recovery following damage from carpal injuries.
- The meniscus ulnocarpalis, formed of collagen, extends from the os triquetrum into the articular space, bridging the wide ulnar intra-articular space of the medial wrist.

Capsula articularis of distal art. interphalangea

Capsula articularis of proximal art. interphalangea

Lig. metacarpale transversum profundum

Capsula articularis articulationis metacarpophalangeae

Ligg. metacarpalia palmaria

Ligg. intercarpalia palmaria

Tendo of m. flexor carpi ulnaris

Lig. ulnocarpale palmare

Ligg. palmaria

Ligg. carpometacarpalia palmaria

Lig. collaterale carpi radiale

Lig. radiocarpale palmare

Lig. radioulnare palmare

A Right hand, anterior (palmar) view.

Distal art. interphalangea (ligg. collateralia)

Proximal art. interphalangea (ligg. collateralia)

Ligg. collateralia articulationis metacarpophalangeae

Ligg. metacarpalia dorsalia

Ligg. carpometacarpalia dorsalia

Ligg. intercarpalia dorsalia

Lig. collaterale carpi radiale

Lig. collaterale carpi ulnare

Lig. radiocarpale dorsale

Lig. radioulnare dorsale

B Right hand, posterior (dorsal) view.

Fig. 19.19 Ligaments of the hand and wrist
(From Gilroy AM et al. Atlas of Anatomy. 4th ed. 2020. Based on: Schuenke M, Schulte E, Schumacher U. THIEME Atlas of Anatomy. General Anatomy and Musculoskeletal System. Illustrations by Voll M and Wesker K. 3rd ed. New York: Thieme Medical Publishers; 2020.)

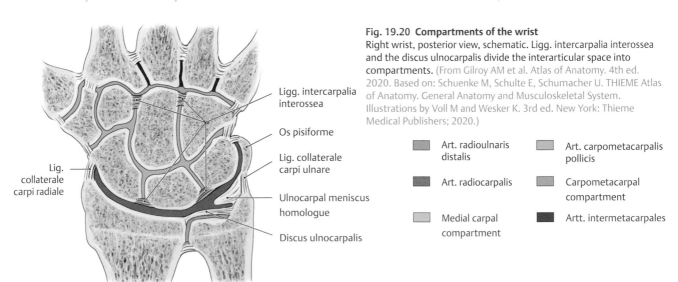

Ligg. intercarpalia interossea

Os pisiforme

Lig. collaterale carpi ulnare

Ulnocarpal meniscus homologue

Discus ulnocarpalis

Lig. collaterale carpi radiale

Fig. 19.20 Compartments of the wrist
Right wrist, posterior view, schematic. Ligg. intercarpalia interossea and the discus ulnocarpalis divide the interarticular space into compartments. (From Gilroy AM et al. Atlas of Anatomy. 4th ed. 2020. Based on: Schuenke M, Schulte E, Schumacher U. THIEME Atlas of Anatomy. General Anatomy and Musculoskeletal System. Illustrations by Voll M and Wesker K. 3rd ed. New York: Thieme Medical Publishers; 2020.)

Art. radioulnaris distalis

Art. radiocarpalis

Medial carpal compartment

Art. carpometacarpalis pollicis

Carpometacarpal compartment

Artt. intermetacarpales

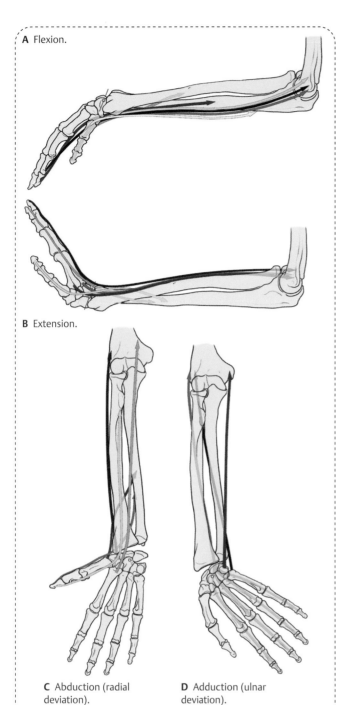

A Flexion.

B Extension.

C Abduction (radial deviation).

D Adduction (ulnar deviation).

(From Schuenke M, Schulte E, Schumacher U. THIEME Atlas of Anatomy, Vol 1. Illustrations by Voll M and Wesker K. 3rd ed. New York: Thieme Publishers; 2020.)

Table 19.11 Movements at the Wrist Joints

Action	Primary Muscles
Flexion	M. flexor carpi radialis
	M. flexor carpi ulnaris
Extension	M. extensor carpi radialis longus
	M. extensor carpi radialis brevis
	M. extensor carpi ulnaris
Abduction (radial deviation)	M. flexor carpi radialis
	M. flexor carpi radialis longus
	M. extensor carpi radialis brevis
Adduction (ulnar deviation)	M. flexor carpi ulnaris
	M. extensor carpi ulnaris

Spaces of the Wrist

Neurovascular structures and the long tendons of the forearm muscles pass between the forearm and hand through narrow spaces that are usually defined by fascial thickenings.

— The **canalis carpi** is a fascio-osseous space on the anterior wrist.
  • Ossa carpi form the floor and sides; the retinaculum musculorum flexorum forms the roof (**Fig. 19.21**).
  • The tendons of m. flexor pollicis longus, m. flexor digitorum superficialis, and m. flexor digitorum profundus and n. medianus pass through the tunnel (**Figs.19.22** and **19.23**).
  • **A common flexor synovial tendon sheath** encloses the flexor tendons as they pass through the carpal tunnel.
  • The lig. carpi palmare and retinaculum musculorum flexorum prevent bowing of the flexor tendons as they cross the wrist.
— The **canalis ulnaris** (Guyon's canal) is a narrow passageway on the medial side of the anterior wrist (**Figs. 19.23, 19.24, 19.25**).

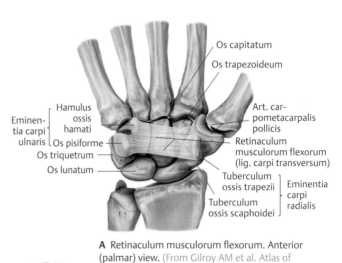

A Retinaculum musculorum flexorum. Anterior (palmar) view. (From Gilroy AM et al. Atlas of Anatomy. 4th ed. 2020. Based on: Schuenke M, Schulte E, Schumacher U. THIEME Atlas of Anatomy. General Anatomy and Musculoskeletal System. Illustrations by Voll M and Wesker K. 3rd ed. New York: Thieme Medical Publishers; 2020.)

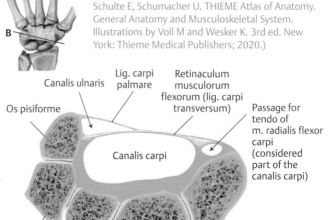

B Transverse section, proximal view. (From Schuenke M, Schulte E, Schumacher U. THIEME Atlas of Anatomy, Vol 1. Illustrations by Voll M and Wesker K. 3rd ed. New York: Thieme Publishers; 2020.)

Fig. 19.21 Ligaments and bony boundaries of the canalis carpi Right hand.

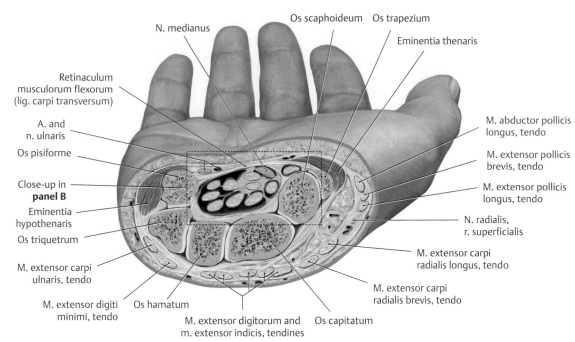

A Cross section through the right wrist.

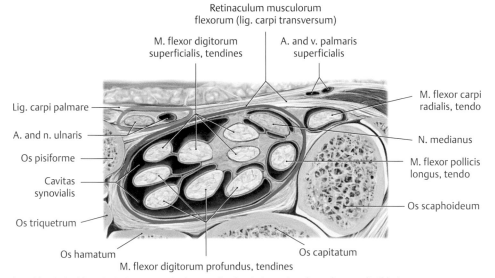

B Blowup of area enclosed by *dashed lines* in **A**. Structures in the canalis ulnaris (*green*) and canalis carpalis (*blue*).

Fig. 19.22 Contents within the canalis carpi

Right hand, proximal view. The tight fit of sensitive neurovascular structures with closely apposed, frequently moving tendons in the canalis carpi often causes problems (carpal tunnel syndrome) when any of the structures swell or degenerate. (From Schuenke M, Schulte E, Schumacher U. THIEME Atlas of Anatomy, Vol 1. Illustrations by Voll M and Wesker K. 3rd ed. New York: Thieme Publishers; 2020.)

BOX 19.6: CLINICAL CORRELATION

CARPAL TUNNEL SYNDROME

The canalis carpi, defined by inflexible fibrous and osseous boundaries, can be compromised by the swelling of its contents, infiltration of fluid from inflammation or infection, protrusion of a dislocated os carpale, or pressure from an external source. The n. medianus is most sensitive to the increased pressure, and signs of carpal tunnel syndrome reflect the nerve's distribution. These include tingling or numbness on the palmar surface of the lateral three and a half digits and weakness and eventual atrophy of the mm. thenares. The r. cutaneus palmaris of n. medianus arises proximal to the canal and passes over the retinaculum musculorum flexorum, so sensation of the palm remains intact.

BOX 19.7: CLINICAL CORRELATION

ULNAR NERVE COMPRESSION

Compression of the n. ulnaris at the wrist affects the innervation of most intrinsic hand muscles. When the patient attempts to form a fist, it results in a deformity known as a "claw hand"—the artt. metacarpophalangeales are hyperextended due to the loss of the mm. interossei, and the artt. interphalangeales are flexed (see **Box 18.9**).

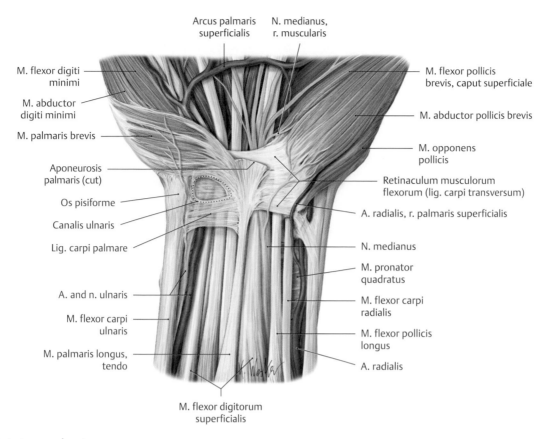

Fig. 19.23 Anterior carpal region
Right hand, anterior (palmar) view. Canalis ulnaris and deep palm. Canalis carpalis with retinaculum musculorum flexorum transparent. (From Gilroy AM et al. Atlas of Anatomy. 4th ed. 2020. Based on: Schuenke M, Schulte E, Schumacher U. THIEME Atlas of Anatomy. General Anatomy and Musculoskeletal System. Illustrations by Voll M and Wesker K. 3rd ed. New York: Thieme Medical Publishers; 2020.)

- The retinaculum musculorum flexorum forms the floor, and the **lig. carpi palmare** forms the roof. The os pisiforme and os hamatum form the medial and lateral borders, respectively.
- The a. ulnaris and n. ulnaris pass through the tunnel into the palm of the hand.
— The **anatomic snuffbox** is a small triangular depression on the radial side of the back of the wrist (**Fig. 19.25**).
  - Tendons of the m. extensor pollicis longus, m. extensor pollicis brevis, and m. abductor pollicis longus form the borders. The os scaphoideum and os trapezium form its floor.
  - The a. radialis passes through the snuffbox.
  - The v. cephalica and r. superficialis of n. radialis cross the snuffbox superficially.
— Six small **dorsal compartments** (designated as 1st through 6th) form on the posterior surface of the wrist (**Table 19.12; Fig. 19.26**).
  - The retinaculum musculorum extensorum forms their roof, and the dorsal surfaces of the distal radius and ulna form their floor.
  - Extensor tendons of forearm muscles pass through the compartments onto the dorsum of the hand.
  - **Vaginae tendinum carpales dorsales** enclose the extensor tendons as they pass through the dorsal compartments.

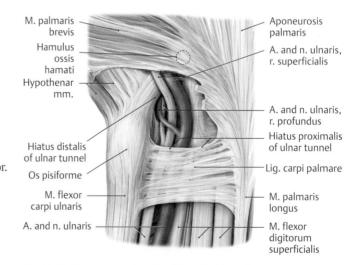

Fig. 19.24 Apertures and walls of the ulnar tunnel
Right hand, anterior (palmar) view. (From Schuenke M, Schulte E, Schumacher U. THIEME Atlas of Anatomy, Vol 1. Illustrations by Voll M and Wesker K. 3rd ed. New York: Thieme Publishers; 2020.)

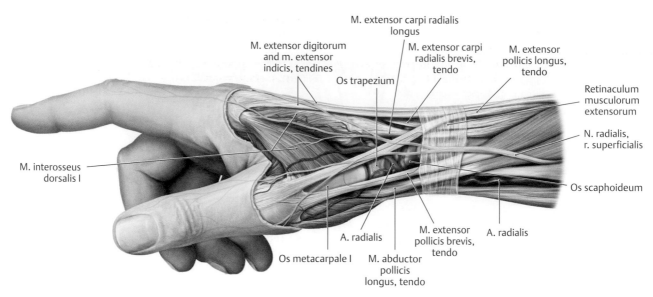

Fig. 19.25 Anatomic snuffbox
Right hand, radial view. The three-sided "anatomic snuffbox" *(shaded light yellow)* is bounded by the tendons of insertion of the m. abductor pollicis longus and the m. extensor pollicis brevis and m. extensor pollicis longus. (From Schuenke M, Schulte E, Schumacher U. THIEME Atlas of Anatomy, Vol 1. Illustrations by Voll M and Wesker K. 3rd ed. New York: Thieme Publishers; 2020.)

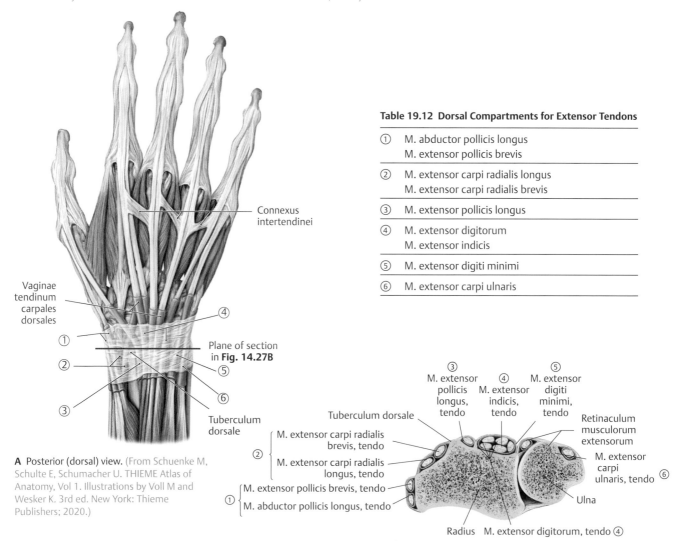

Table 19.12 Dorsal Compartments for Extensor Tendons

①	M. abductor pollicis longus M. extensor pollicis brevis
②	M. extensor carpi radialis longus M. extensor carpi radialis brevis
③	M. extensor pollicis longus
④	M. extensor digitorum M. extensor indicis
⑤	M. extensor digiti minimi
⑥	M. extensor carpi ulnaris

A Posterior (dorsal) view. (From Schuenke M, Schulte E, Schumacher U. THIEME Atlas of Anatomy, Vol 1. Illustrations by Voll M and Wesker K. 3rd ed. New York: Thieme Publishers; 2020.)

Fig. 19.26 Retinaculum musculorum extensorum and dorsal compartments
Right hand.

B Proximal view of section indicated in **A**. (From Gilroy AM et al. Atlas of Anatomy. 4th ed. 2020. Based on: Schuenke M, Schulte E, Schumacher U. THIEME Atlas of Anatomy. General Anatomy and Musculoskeletal System. Illustrations by Voll M and Wesker K. 3rd ed. New York: Thieme Medical Publishers; 2020.)

19.6 The Hand

The muscles and joints of the hand create a flexible tool that is adept at fine motor movements. The ability to grasp objects by positioning the thumb in opposition to the other fingers is a feature that is unique to humans and apes.

Joints of the Hand and Fingers

Joints of the hand and fingers are the articulations between the ossa carpi distales and proximal end of the ossa metacarpi of the palms, the distal end of the ossa metacarpi and the phalanges proximales, and between the phalanges proximales, phalanges mediales, and phalanges distales of each digit (see **Fig. 19.18**). Movements at these joints and the muscles of the forearm and hand that provide them are listed in **Tables 19.13** and **19.14.**

— **Artt. carpometacarpales** are the synovial joints between the distal row of ossa carpi and the ossa metacarpi.
  • Little or no movement occurs at the plane-type joints of the 2nd, 3rd, and 4th digits.
  • The joint of the 5th digit between the metacarpus and the os hamatum is moderately mobile.

• The saddle-type joint between the metacarpus of the thumb and the os trapezium in the distal carpal row allows movement in all directions, which is essential for thumb opposition (**Fig. 19.27**).
— **Artt. metacarpophalangeae (MCP)** are condyloid synovial joints between the heads of the ossa metacarpi and bases of the phalanges proximales.
  • Movement in two planes, flexion-extension and abduction-adduction, occurs in digits 2 through 5.
  • Only flexion and extension occur at the MCP joint of the thumb.
— **Artt. interphalangeae (IP)** are hinge-type synovial joints between phalanges.
  • Digits 2 through 4 have artt. interphalangeae proximales (PIP) and artt. interphalangeae distales (DIP).
  • The thumb has only a single IP joint.
  • IP joints permit only flexion and extension.
— MCP and IP joints are surrounded by a capsula fibrosa and supported by ligg. collateralia mediales and laterales.

Table 19.13 Movements at the Joints of the Fingers (Digits 2 through 5)

Action	Primary Muscles
Flexion at MCP	Mm. lumbricales Mm. interossei M. flexor digiti minimi (only 5th digit)
Flexion at DIP	M. flexor digitorum superficialis Mm. lumbricales
Flexion at PIP	M. flexor digitorum profundus M. flexor digitorum superficialis
Extension at MCP	M. extensor digitorum M. extensor indicis (only 2nd digit) M. extensor digiti minimi (only 5th digit)
Extension at DIP and PIP	Mm. lumbricales Mm. interossei
Abduction at MCP	Mm. interossei dorsales M. abductor digiti minimi (only 5th digit)
Adduction	Mm. interossei palmares (digits 2, 4, and 5 only)
Opposition	M. opponens digiti minimi (only 5th digit)

Abbreviations: DIP, distal interphalangeal; MCP, metacarpophalangeal; PIP, proximal interphalangeal.

(From Schuenke M, Schulte E, Schumacher U. THIEME Atlas of Anatomy, Vol 1. Illustrations by Voll M and Wesker K. 3rd ed. New York: Thieme Publishers; 2020.)

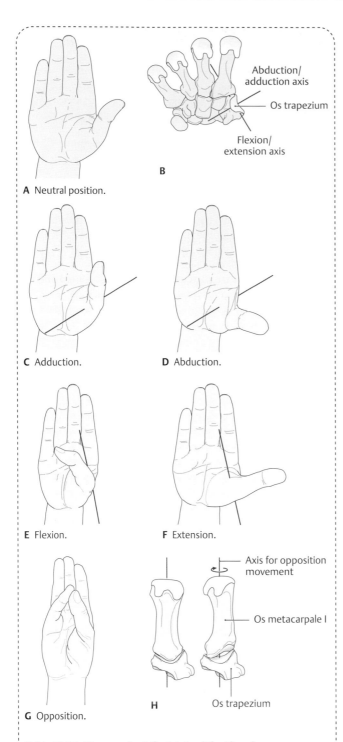

A Neutral position.

Abduction/
adduction axis

Os trapezium

Flexion/
extension axis

B

C Adduction.

D Abduction.

E Flexion.

F Extension.

G Opposition.

Axis for opposition
movement

Os metacarpale I

Os trapezium

H

Table 19.14 Movements at the Joints of the Thumb

Action	Primary Muscles
Flexion	M. flexor pollicis longus M. flexor pollicis brevis
Extension	M. extensor pollicis longus M. extensor pollicis brevis
Abduction	M. abductor pollicis longus M. abductor pollicis brevis
Adduction	M. adductor pollicis
Opposition	M. opponens pollicis

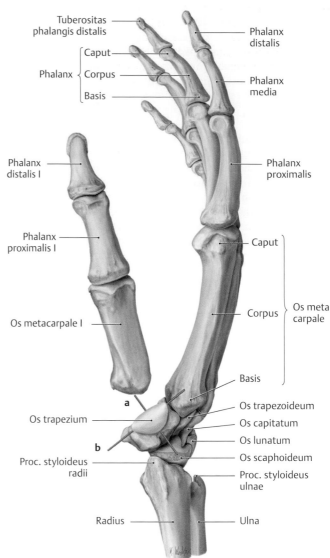

Tuberositas
phalangis distalis

Phalanx
distalis

Caput

Phalanx   Corpus

Basis

Phalanx
media

Phalanx
distalis I

Phalanx
proximalis

Phalanx
proximalis I

Caput

Os metacarpale I

Corpus   Os meta
carpale

Basis

a

Os trapezium

Os trapezoideum

Os capitatum

b

Os lunatum

Os scaphoideum

Proc. styloideus
radii

Proc. styloideus
ulnae

Radius

Ulna

Fig. 19.27 Articulatio carpometacarpalis pollicis
Radial view. The os metacarpale I has been moved slightly distally to expose the articular surface of the os trapezium. Two cardinal axes of motion are shown here: *a*, abduction/adduction; and *b*, flexion/extension.
(From Schuenke M, Schulte E, Schumacher U. THIEME Atlas of Anatomy, Vol 1. Illustrations by Voll M and Wesker K. 3rd ed. New York: Thieme Publishers; 2020.)

The Palm of the Hand and Fingers

— The palm of the hand has the following surface anatomy (**Fig. 19.28**):
  • The skin is thickened, firmly attached to the underlying fascia, and supplied with numerous sweat glands.
  • A central concavity separates an **eminentia thenaris** at the base of the thumb from an **eminentia hypothenaris** at the base of the 5th digit.
  • Longitudinal and transverse **flexion creases** form where the skin is tightly bound to the fascia palmaris.

— Deep fascia over the central palm forms a tough, thickened aponeurosis palmaris (**Fig. 19.29**), which
  • firmly adheres to the skin of the palm,
  • is continuous proximally with the retinaculum musculorum flexorum and m. palmaris longus muscle, and
  • is continuous distally with a **lig. metacarpale transversum** and the four digital fibrous sheaths of the fingers that surround the long flexor tendons and their synovial digital tendon sheaths.

— The aponeurosis palmaris and fascia palmaris profunda divide the palm into five muscular compartments (**Tables 19.15, 19.16, 19.17**):
  1. The **thenar compartment,** which contains thenar muscles that abduct, flex, and oppose the thumb.
  2. The **central compartment,** which contains forearm flexor tendons that flex the fingers and lumbricals that flex and extend joints of the fingers.
  3. The **hypothenar compartment,** which contains hypothenar muscles that flex, abduct, and oppose the 5th digit.
  4. The **adductor compartment,** which contains the m. adductor pollicis that adducts the thumb.
  5. The interosseous **compartment,** which contains mm. interossei that abduct and adduct the fingers.

— **Thenar** and **midpalmar spaces** are potential spaces deep within the palm between the long flexor tendons and the fascia over the deep palmar muscles. The midpalmar space is

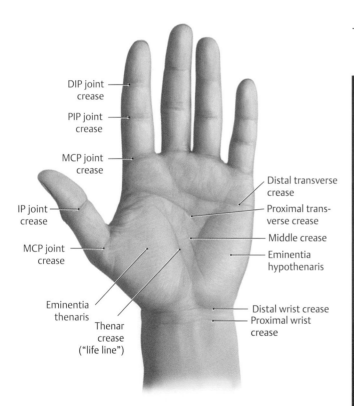

Fig. 19.28 Surface anatomy of the palm of the hand
Left hand. DIP, distal interphalangeal; IP, interphalangeal; MCP, metacarpophalangeal; PIP, proximal interphalangeal. (From Schuenke M, Schulte E, Schumacher U. THIEME Atlas of Anatomy, Vol 1. Illustrations by Voll M and Wesker K. 3rd ed. New York: Thieme Publishers; 2020.)

Labels on figure:
DIP joint crease
PIP joint crease
MCP joint crease
IP joint crease
MCP joint crease
Eminentia thenaris
Thenar crease ("life line")
Distal transverse crease
Proximal transverse crease
Middle crease
Eminentia hypothenaris
Distal wrist crease
Proximal wrist crease

BOX 19.8: CLINICAL CORRELATION

DUPUYTREN'S DISEASE
Dupuytren's disease is the progressive fibrosis and contracture of the longitudinal bands of the palmar fascia to the 4th and 5th digits, causing flexion of these fingers. It presents as painless nodular thickenings that progress to raised ridges on the palm. Surgical excision is usually required to release the bands.

continuous with the anterior forearm compartment through the canalis carpi.

— On the palmar surface of the fingers
  • tendons of the m. flexor digitorum superficialis split into two bands that insert on the phalanx media,
  • tendons of m. flexor digitorum profundus pass between the bands of the m. flexor digitorum superficialis to insert on the phalanges distales, and
  • **synovial tendon sheaths** (**vaginae synoviales**) surround the flexor tendons as they enter the **fibrous tendon sheaths** of the fingers (**Fig. 19.30**).
    ◦ The digital vagina synovialis of the 5th digit normally communicates with the common flexor sheath at the wrist.
    ◦ The vagina synovialis of the thumb extends into the wrist and may communicate with the sheath of the 5th digit and with the common vagina synovialis.
    ◦ The vagina synovialis of the 2nd, 3rd, and 4th digits usually remain independent from the common vagina synovialis and other digital vagina synovialis.

— Muscles of the forearm and intrinsic muscles of the hand move the joints of the hand and fingers (see **Tables 19.13** and **19.14**).

BOX 19.9: CLINICAL CORRELATION

TENDON SHEATH COMMUNICATION
The digital tendon sheath of the thumb is continuous with the carpal tendon sheath of the m. flexor pollicis longus. The remaining fingers show variable communication with the carpal tendon sheaths (**A** is the most common variation). Infections within the tendon sheaths from puncture wounds of the fingers can track proximally to communicating spaces of the hand.

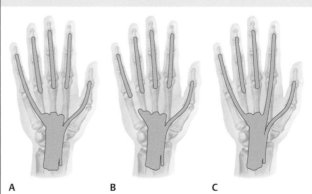

A   B   C

(From Gilroy AM et al. Atlas of Anatomy. 4th ed. 2020. Based on: Schuenke M, Schulte E, Schumacher U. THIEME Atlas of Anatomy. General Anatomy and Musculoskeletal System. Illustrations by Voll M and Wesker K. 3rd ed. New York: Thieme Medical Publishers; 2020.)

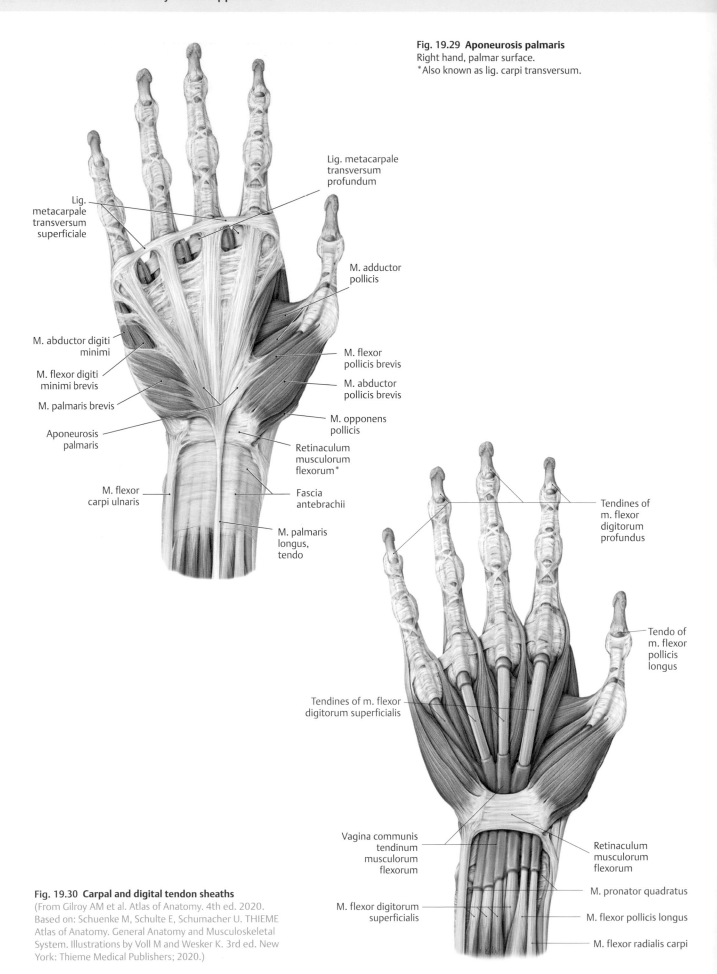

Fig. 19.29 Aponeurosis palmaris
Right hand, palmar surface.
*Also known as lig. carpi transversum.

Lig. metacarpale transversum profundum

Lig. metacarpale transversum superficiale

M. adductor pollicis

M. abductor digiti minimi

M. flexor pollicis brevis

M. flexor digiti minimi brevis

M. abductor pollicis brevis

M. palmaris brevis

M. opponens pollicis

Aponeurosis palmaris

Retinaculum musculorum flexorum*

M. flexor carpi ulnaris

Fascia antebrachii

M. palmaris longus, tendo

Tendines of m. flexor digitorum profundus

Tendo of m. flexor pollicis longus

Tendines of m. flexor digitorum superficialis

Vagina communis tendinum musculorum flexorum

Retinaculum musculorum flexorum

M. pronator quadratus

M. flexor digitorum superficialis

M. flexor pollicis longus

M. flexor radialis carpi

Fig. 19.30 Carpal and digital tendon sheaths
(From Gilroy AM et al. Atlas of Anatomy. 4th ed. 2020.
Based on: Schuenke M, Schulte E, Schumacher U. THIEME
Atlas of Anatomy. General Anatomy and Musculoskeletal
System. Illustrations by Voll M and Wesker K. 3rd ed. New
York: Thieme Medical Publishers; 2020.)

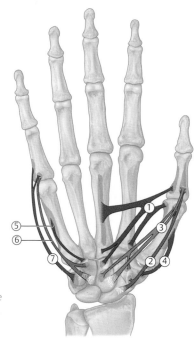

Thenar and hypothenar muscles, right hand, anterior (palmar) view. (From Schuenke M, Schulte E, Schumacher U. THIEME Atlas of Anatomy, Vol 1. Illustrations by Voll M and Wesker K. 3rd ed. New York: Thieme Publishers; 2020.)

Table 19.15 Thenar Muscles

Muscle	Origin	Insertion	Innervation	Action
① M. adductor pollicis	Caput transversum: os metacarpi III (palmar surface)	Pollex (basis phalangis proximalis I) via the ulnar os sesamoideum	N. ulnaris (C8, T1)	CMC joint of thumb: adduction
	Caput obliquum: os capitatum, bases ossium metacarpi II and III			MCP joint of thumb: flexion
② M. abductor pollicis brevis	Ossa scaphoideum and trapezium, retinaculum musculorum flexorum	Pollex (basis phalangis proximalis I) via the radial os sesamoideum	N. medianus (C8, T1)	CMC joint of thumb: abduction
③ M. flexor pollicis brevis	Caput superficiale: retinaculum musculorum flexorum		Caput superficiale: n. medianus (C8, T1)	CMC joint of thumb: flexion
	Caput profundum: os capitatum, os trapezium		Caput profundum: n. ulnaris (C8, T1)	
④ M. opponens pollicis	Os trapezium	Os metacarpi I (radial border)	N. medianus (C8, T1)	CMC joint of thumb: opposition

Abbreviations: CMC, carpometacarpal; MCP, metacarpophalangeal.

Table 19.16 Hypothenar Muscles

Muscle	Origin	Insertion	Innervation	Action
⑤ M. opponens digiti minimi	Hamulus ossis hamati, retinaculum flexorum	Os metacarpi V (ulnar border)	N. ulnaris (C8, T1)	Draws os metacarpi in palmar direction (opposition)
⑥ M. flexor digiti minimi brevis		Basis phalangis proximalis V		MCP joint of little finger: flexion
⑦ M. abductor digiti minimi	Os pisiforme	Phalanx proximalis V (ulnar base) and dorsal digital expansion of digitus minimus		MCP joint of little finger: flexion and abduction of little finger. PIP and DIP joints of little finger: extension
M. palmaris brevis	Aponeurosis palmaris (ulnar border)	Cutis hypothenaris		Tightens the aponeurosis palmaris (protective function)

Abbreviations: DIP, distal interphalangeal; MCP, metacarpophalangeal; PIP, proximal interphalangeal.

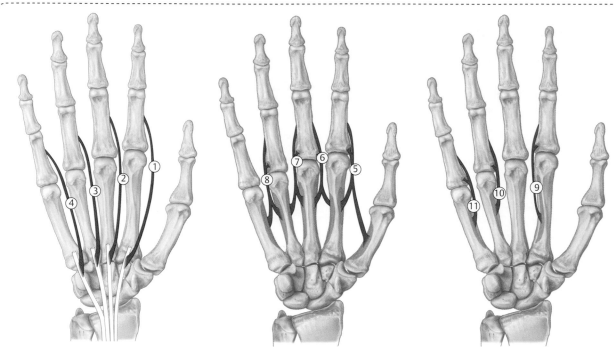

A Mm. lumbricales, right hand, palmar view.

B Mm. interossei dorsales, right hand, palmar view.

C Mm. interossei palmares, right hand, palmar view.

((From Gilroy AM et al. Atlas of Anatomy. 4th ed. 2020. Based on: Schuenke M, Schulte E, Schumacher U. THIEME Atlas of Anatomy. General Anatomy and Musculoskeletal System. Illustrations by Voll M and Wesker K. 3rd ed. New York: Thieme Medical Publishers; 2020.)

Table 19.17 Metacarpal Muscles

Muscle Group	Muscle	Origin	Insertion	Innervation	Action
Mm. lumbricales	① 1st	Tendons of m. flexor digitorum profundus (radial sides)	Digitus II (dde)	N. medianus (C8–T1)	Digiti II to V: • MCP joints: flexion • Proximal and distal IP joints: extension
	② 2nd		Digitus III (dde)		
	③ 3rd	Tendons of m. flexor digitorum profundus (bipennate from medial and lateral sides)	Digitus IV (dde)	N. ulnaris (C8–T1)	
	④ 4th		Digitus V (dde)		
Mm. interossei dorsales	⑤ 1st	Ossa metacarpi I and II (adjacent sides, two heads)	Digitus II (dde) Phalanx proximalis III (radial side)		Digiti II to IV: • MCP joints: flexion • Proximal and distal IP joints: extension and abduction from 3rd digit
	⑥ 2nd	Ossa metacarpi II and III (adjacent sides, two heads)	Digitus III (dde) Phalanx proximalis III (radial side)		
	⑦ 3rd	Ossa metacarpi III and IV (adjacent sides, two heads)	Digitus III (dde) Phalanx proximalis III (ulnar side)		
	⑧ 4th	Ossa metacarpi IV and V (adjacent sides, two heads)	Digitus IV (dde) Phalanx proximalis IV (ulnar side)		
Mm. interossei palmares	⑨ 1st	Os metacarpi II (ulnar side)	Digitus II (dde) Basis phalangis proximalis II (base)		Digiti II, IV, and V: • MCP joints: flexion • Proximal and distal IP joints: extension and adduction toward 3rd digit
	⑩ 2nd	Os metacarpi IV (radial side)	Digitus IV (dde) Basis phalangis proximalis IV (base)		
	⑪ 3rd	Os metacarpi V (radial side)	Digitus V (dde) Basis phalangis proximalis V (base)		

Abbreviations: dde, dorsal digital expansion; IP, interphalangeal; MCP, metacarpophalangeal.

The Dorsum of the Hand and Fingers

— The dorsum of the hand has the following surface anatomy (**Fig. 19.31**):
  - The skin is thin and loose.
  - A prominent superficial dorsal venous network (rete venosum dorsale manus) gives rise to the v. cephalica and v. basilica.

  The heads of the ossa metacarpi of the 2nd through 5th digits form distinct "knuckles" when the hand is flexed into a fist.
  - The extensor tendons fan out from the wrist to the fingers.

— On the dorsum of the fingers, the long extensor tendons (of the posterior forearm compartment) flatten to form a **dorsal digital expansion** (extensor expansion, extensor hood), a triangular tendinous aponeurosis (**Fig. 19.32**). The dorsal digital expansion
  - forms a hood that wraps around the sides of the distal metacarpus and proximal phalanx and holds the extensor tendon in place;
  - inserts onto the middle and distal phalanges via a **central slip (tractus intermedius)** and paired **lateral bands (tractus lateralis)**; and
  - is reinforced by the mm. lumbricales and mm. interossei of the palm, which connect to the lateral bands and assist in extension of the interphalangeal joints of the fingers.

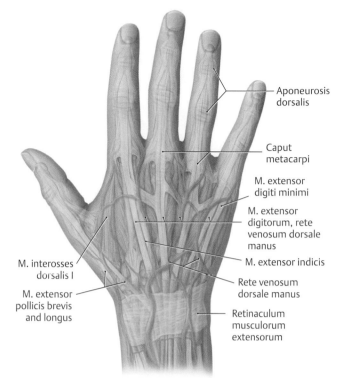

Fig. 19.31 Surface anatomy of the dorsum of the hand
Right hand.

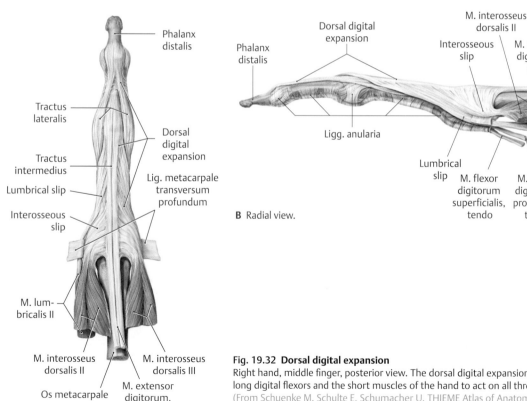

A Posterior view.

B Radial view.

Fig. 19.32 Dorsal digital expansion
Right hand, middle finger, posterior view. The dorsal digital expansion permits the long digital flexors and the short muscles of the hand to act on all three finger joints.
(From Schuenke M, Schulte E, Schumacher U. THIEME Atlas of Anatomy, Vol 1.
Illustrations by Voll M and Wesker K. 3rd ed. New York: Thieme Publishers; 2020.)

19.7   Topographic Views of Upper Limb Musculature

Shoulder and Arm

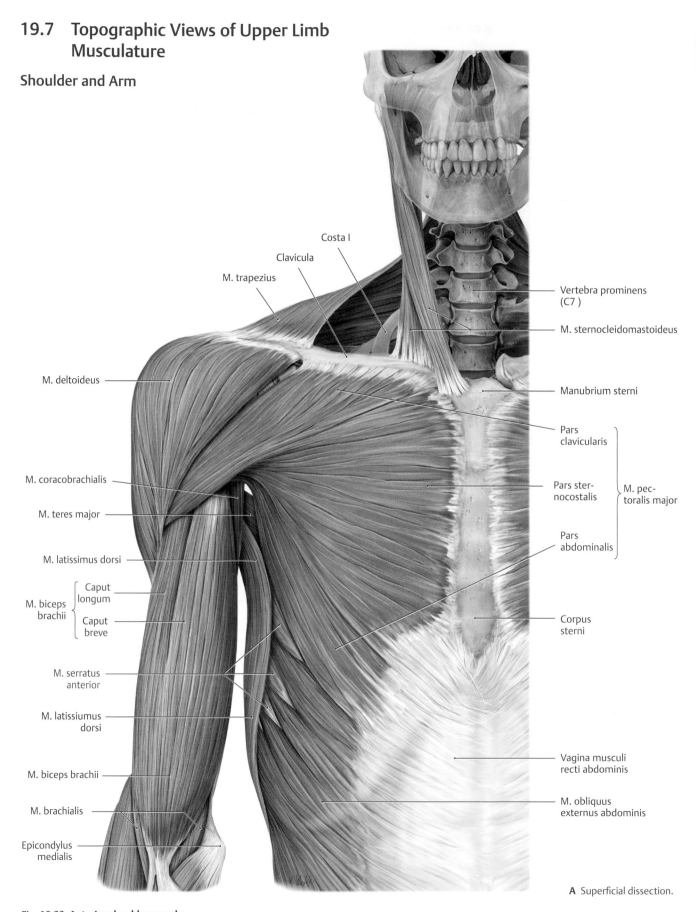

Costa I

Clavicula

M. trapezius

Vertebra prominens (C7)

M. sternocleidomastoideus

M. deltoideus

Manubrium sterni

Pars clavicularis

M. coracobrachialis

Pars sternocostalis

M. pectoralis major

M. teres major

Pars abdominalis

M. latissimus dorsi

M. biceps brachii { Caput longum / Caput breve

Corpus sterni

M. serratus anterior

M. latissiumus dorsi

Vagina musculi recti abdominis

M. biceps brachii

M. obliquus externus abdominis

M. brachialis

Epicondylus medialis

A Superficial dissection.

Fig. 19.33 Anterior shoulder muscles
Right side, anterior view. (From Schuenke M, Schulte E, Schumacher U. THIEME Atlas of Anatomy, Vol 1. Illustrations by Voll M and Wesker K. 3rd ed. New York: Thieme Publishers; 2020.)

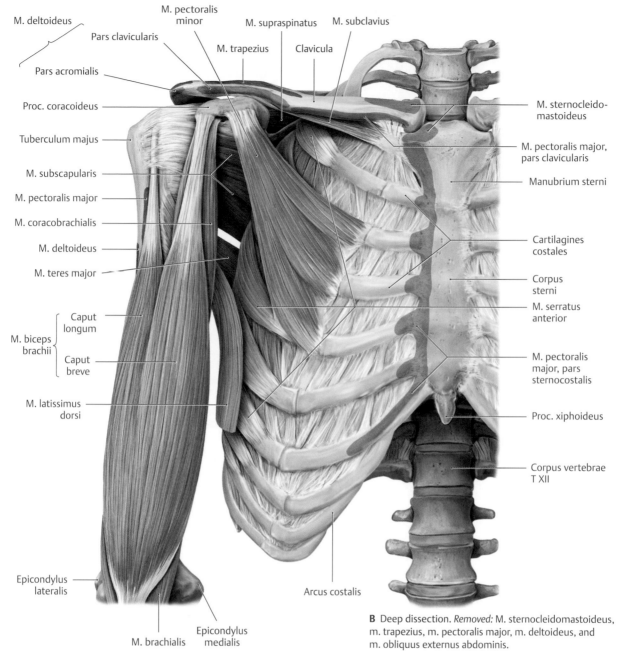

M. deltoideus

Pars clavicularis

M. pectoralis minor

M. supraspinatus

M. subclavius

Pars acromialis

M. trapezius

Clavicula

Proc. coracoideus

Tuberculum majus

M. subscapularis

M. pectoralis major

M. coracobrachialis

M. deltoideus

M. teres major

M. biceps brachii { Caput longum / Caput breve }

M. latissimus dorsi

Epicondylus lateralis

M. brachialis

Epicondylus medialis

M. sternocleido-mastoideus

M. pectoralis major, pars clavicularis

Manubrium sterni

Cartilagines costales

Corpus sterni

M. serratus anterior

M. pectoralis major, pars sternocostalis

Proc. xiphoideus

Corpus vertebrae T XII

Arcus costalis

B Deep dissection. *Removed:* M. sternocleidomastoideus, m. trapezius, m. pectoralis major, m. deltoideus, and m. obliquus externus abdominis.

Fig. 19.33 (*continued*) **Anterior shoulder muscles**

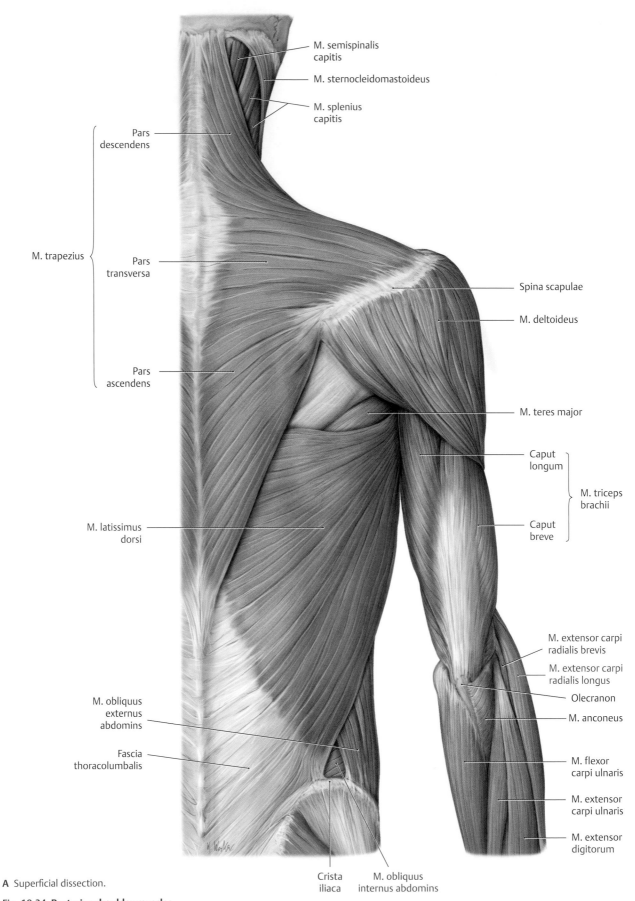

A Superficial dissection.

Fig. 19.34 Posterior shoulder muscles
Right side, posterior view. (From Schuenke M, Schulte E, Schumacher U. THIEME Atlas of Anatomy, Vol 1. Illustrations by Voll M and Wesker K. 3rd ed. New York: Thieme Publishers; 2020.)

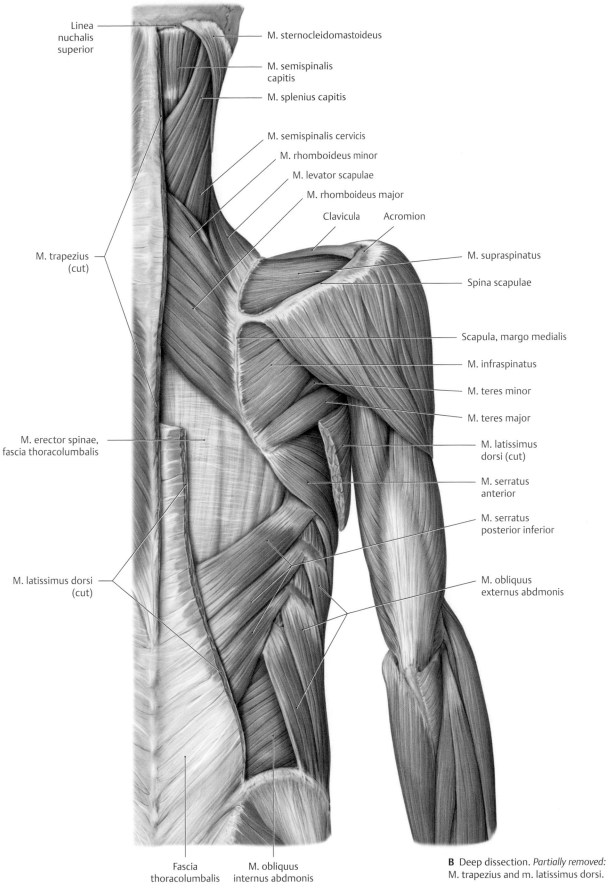

Linea nuchalis superior

M. sternocleidomastoideus

M. semispinalis capitis

M. splenius capitis

M. semispinalis cervicis

M. rhomboideus minor

M. levator scapulae

M. rhomboideus major

Clavicula

Acromion

M. supraspinatus

Spina scapulae

M. trapezius (cut)

Scapula, margo medialis

M. infraspinatus

M. teres minor

M. teres major

M. erector spinae, fascia thoracolumbalis

M. latissimus dorsi (cut)

M. serratus anterior

M. serratus posterior inferior

M. latissimus dorsi (cut)

M. obliquus externus abdmonis

Fascia thoracolumbalis

M. obliquus internus abdmonis

B Deep dissection. *Partially removed:* M. trapezius and m. latissimus dorsi.

Fig. 19.34 (*continued*) **Posterior shoulder muscles**

Forearm and Wrist

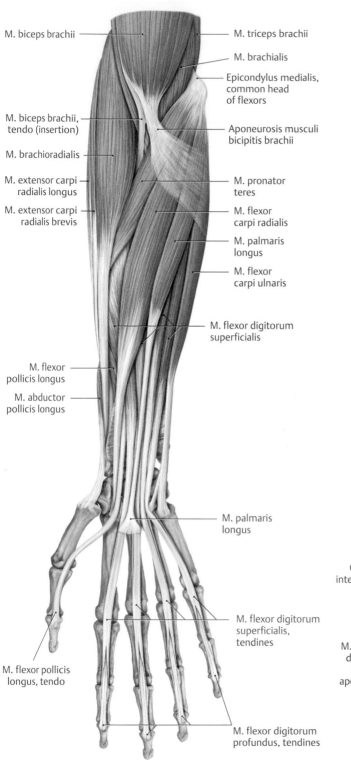

M. biceps brachii

M. triceps brachii

M. brachialis

Epicondylus medialis, common head of flexors

M. biceps brachii, tendo (insertion)

Aponeurosis musculi bicipitis brachii

M. brachioradialis

M. extensor carpi radialis longus

M. pronator teres

M. extensor carpi radialis brevis

M. flexor carpi radialis

M. palmaris longus

M. flexor carpi ulnaris

M. flexor digitorum superficialis

M. flexor pollicis longus

M. abductor pollicis longus

M. palmaris longus

M. flexor digitorum superficialis, tendines

M. flexor pollicis longus, tendo

M. flexor digitorum profundus, tendines

Fig. 19.35 Anterior forearm muscles
Right forearm, anterior view.
Superficial flexors and radialis group. (From Schuenke M, Schulte E, Schumacher U. THIEME Atlas of Anatomy, Vol 1. Illustrations by Voll M and Wesker K. 3rd ed. New York: Thieme Publishers; 2020.)

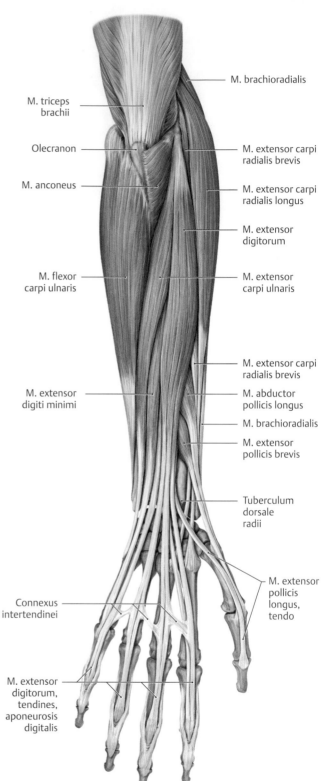

M. brachioradialis

M. triceps brachii

Olecranon

M. anconeus

M. flexor carpi ulnaris

M. extensor carpi radialis brevis

M. extensor carpi radialis longus

M. extensor digitorum

M. extensor carpi ulnaris

M. extensor digiti minimi

M. extensor carpi radialis brevis

M. abductor pollicis longus

M. brachioradialis

M. extensor pollicis brevis

Tuberculum dorsale radii

M. extensor pollicis longus, tendo

Connexus intertendinei

M. extensor digitorum, tendines, aponeurosis digitalis

Fig. 19.36 Posterior forearm muscles
Right forearm, posterior view.
Superficial extensors and radialis group. (From Schuenke M, Schulte E, Schumacher U. THIEME Atlas of Anatomy, Vol 1. Illustrations by Voll M and Wesker K. 3rd ed. New York: Thieme Publishers; 2020.)

Hand

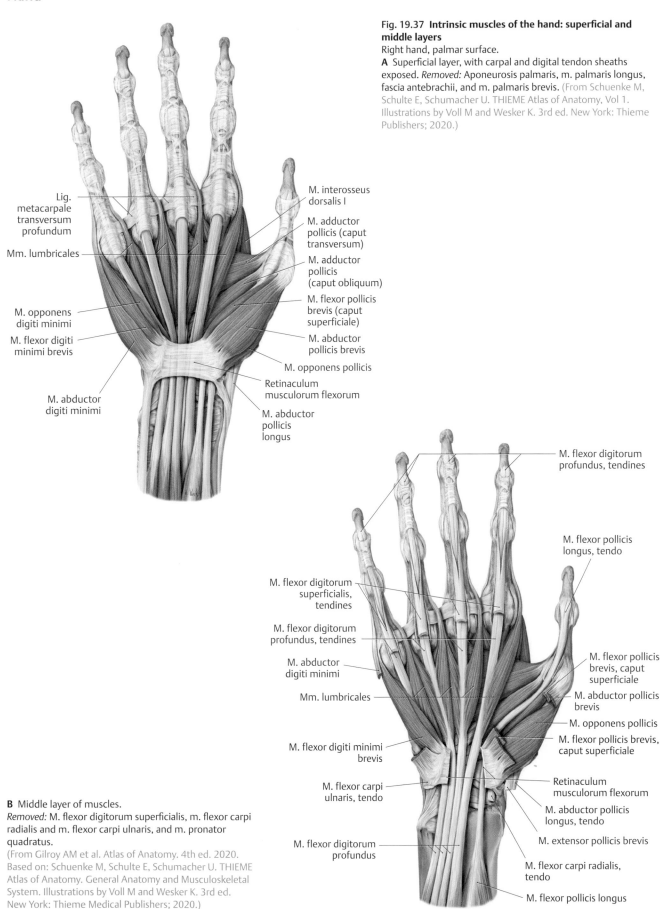

Fig. 19.37 Intrinsic muscles of the hand: superficial and middle layers
Right hand, palmar surface.
A Superficial layer, with carpal and digital tendon sheaths exposed. *Removed:* Aponeurosis palmaris, m. palmaris longus, fascia antebrachii, and m. palmaris brevis. (From Schuenke M, Schulte E, Schumacher U. THIEME Atlas of Anatomy, Vol 1. Illustrations by Voll M and Wesker K. 3rd ed. New York: Thieme Publishers; 2020.)

Lig. metacarpale transversum profundum

Mm. lumbricales

M. opponens digiti minimi

M. flexor digiti minimi brevis

M. abductor digiti minimi

M. interosseus dorsalis I

M. adductor pollicis (caput transversum)

M. adductor pollicis (caput obliquum)

M. flexor pollicis brevis (caput superficiale)

M. abductor pollicis brevis

M. opponens pollicis

Retinaculum musculorum flexorum

M. abductor pollicis longus

M. flexor digitorum profundus, tendines

M. flexor pollicis longus, tendo

M. flexor digitorum superficialis, tendines

M. flexor digitorum profundus, tendines

M. abductor digiti minimi

Mm. lumbricales

M. flexor digiti minimi brevis

M. flexor carpi ulnaris, tendo

M. flexor digitorum profundus

M. flexor pollicis brevis, caput superficiale

M. abductor pollicis brevis

M. opponens pollicis

M. flexor pollicis brevis, caput superficiale

Retinaculum musculorum flexorum

M. abductor pollicis longus, tendo

M. extensor pollicis brevis

M. flexor carpi radialis, tendo

M. flexor pollicis longus

B Middle layer of muscles.
Removed: M. flexor digitorum superficialis, m. flexor carpi radialis and m. flexor carpi ulnaris, and m. pronator quadratus.
(From Gilroy AM et al. Atlas of Anatomy. 4th ed. 2020. Based on: Schuenke M, Schulte E, Schumacher U. THIEME Atlas of Anatomy. General Anatomy and Musculoskeletal System. Illustrations by Voll M and Wesker K. 3rd ed. New York: Thieme Medical Publishers; 2020.)

Compartments of the Arm and Forearm

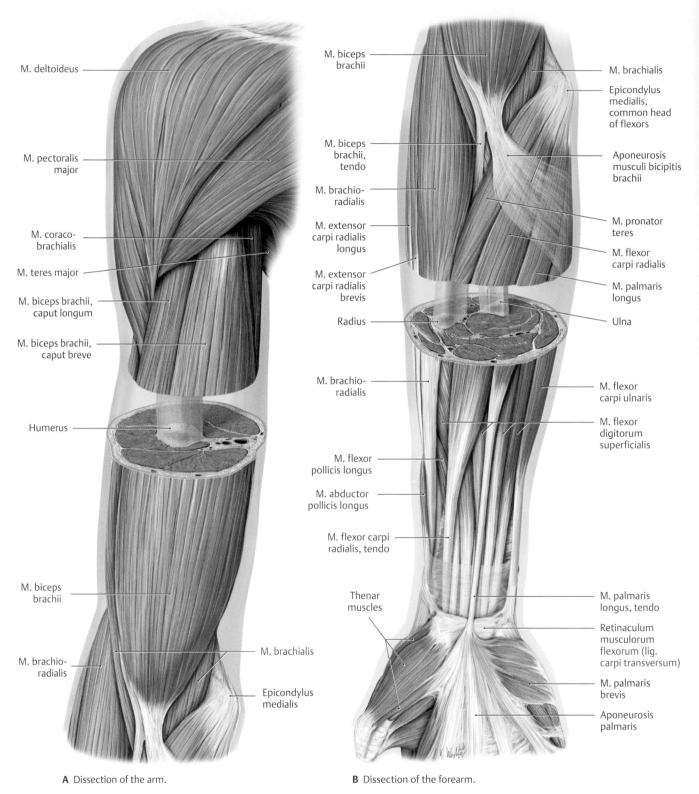

A Dissection of the arm.

B Dissection of the forearm.

Fig. 19.38 Windowed dissection
Right limb, anterior view. (From Schuenke M, Schulte E, Schumacher U. THIEME Atlas of Anatomy, Vol 1. Illustrations by Voll M and Wesker K. 3rd ed. New York: Thieme Publishers; 2020.)

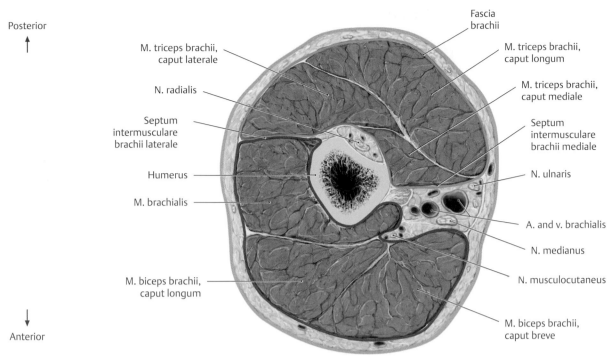

Posterior

N. radialis

M. triceps brachii, caput laterale

Fascia brachii

M. triceps brachii, caput longum

M. triceps brachii, caput mediale

Septum intermusculare brachii laterale

Septum intermusculare brachii mediale

Humerus

N. ulnaris

M. brachialis

A. and v. brachialis

N. medianus

N. musculocutaneus

M. biceps brachii, caput longum

M. biceps brachii, caput breve

Anterior

A Arm (plane of section in **Fig. 19.38A**).

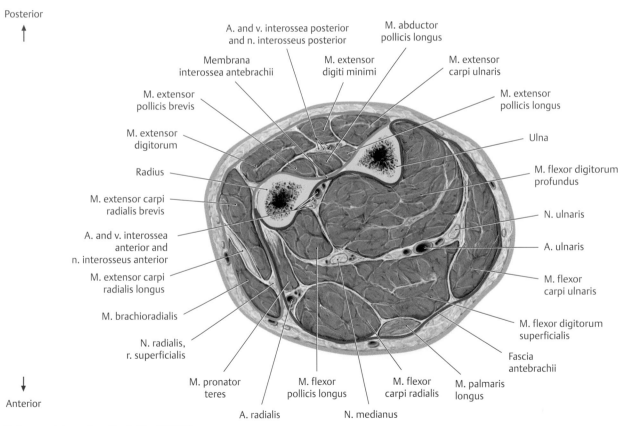

Posterior

A. and v. interossea posterior and n. interosseus posterior

M. abductor pollicis longus

Membrana interossea antebrachii

M. extensor digiti minimi

M. extensor carpi ulnaris

M. extensor pollicis brevis

M. extensor pollicis longus

M. extensor digitorum

Ulna

Radius

M. flexor digitorum profundus

M. extensor carpi radialis brevis

N. ulnaris

A. and v. interossea anterior and n. interosseus anterior

A. ulnaris

M. extensor carpi radialis longus

M. flexor carpi ulnaris

M. brachioradialis

M. flexor digitorum superficialis

N. radialis, r. superficialis

Fascia antebrachii

M. pronator teres

M. flexor pollicis longus

M. flexor carpi radialis

M. palmaris longus

Anterior

A. radialis

N. medianus

B Forearm (plane of section in **Fig. 19.38B**).

Fig. 19.39 Transverse sections
Right limb, proximal (superior) view.
The anterior compartment is outlined in *pink* and the posterior compartment in *green*. (From Schuenke M, Schulte E, Schumacher U. THIEME Atlas of Anatomy, Vol 1. Illustrations by Voll M and Wesker K. 3rd ed. New York: Thieme Publishers; 2020.)

20 Clinical Imaging Basics of the Upper Limb

Radiographs are always the first imaging choice in evaluation of bones and joints in the setting of trauma or pain (**Table 20.1**). Radiographs, or x-rays, are highly sensitive for the detection of fractures and misalignment of joints.

Computed tomography (CT) provides significantly more detail of bone and is sometimes helpful for seeing subtle nondisplaced fractures, especially in older adults with decreased bone mass. The superior soft tissue contrast of magnetic resonance imaging (MRI) makes it the ideal imaging method for evaluation of the soft tissue components of joints.

Ultrasound has the benefit of real time imaging and is good for seeing superficial tissues, but its utility decreases substantially in larger patients. Ultrasound can also be very useful for image-guided procedures such as joint aspirations and joint injections. Additionally, in small children ultrasound can be useful for the anatomic evaluation of cartilaginous growth plates, especially in the growing elbow (see **Table 20.1**).

Since a radiograph is a summation shadow, all bones need to be evaluated in at least two projections (orthogonal) and all joints should be evaluated in at least three projections. The orthogonal view allows evaluation of the position of structures that may be overlapping in a single projection (**Fig. 20.1**). When viewing a bone x-ray, the cortical edge should be smooth along its entire length, and the trabecular pattern of the bone should be uniform throughout. Joints should be evaluated for even spacing, smoothness of the reticular surface, and alignment of the joint itself (**Fig.20.2**).

Table 20.1 Suitability of Imaging Modalities for the Upper Limb

Modality	Clinical Uses
Radiographs (x-rays)	Primarily used to evaluate the bones and alignment of joints
CT (computed tomography)	Usually reserved as a troubleshooting tool to evaluate for subtle nondisplaced fractures
MRI (magnetic resonance imaging)	One of the most important imaging modalities for the evaluation of joints, specifically the non-osseous components of the joint—cartilage, ligaments, tendons, and muscles
Ultrasound	Limited role in evaluation of superficial soft tissue abnormalities, and for guidance of interventional procedures involving the joints. In children, ultrasound plays a larger role in diagnosis of joint disorders and for evaluation of cartilaginous growth plates.

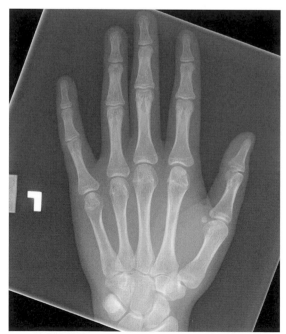

A Anteroposterior (AP) view of the hand appears normal, even the 5th digit.

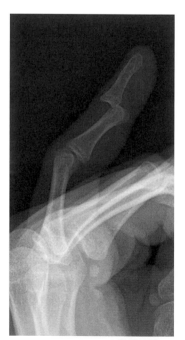

B Coned down (magnified) view of the 5th digit *(arrow)* shows that the distal phalanx is dislocated and positioned dorsally. This is not seen on the frontal projection since there is no lateral displacement of the bone, and the ends of the bones at the DIP joint line up in the AP summation shadow.

Fig. 20.1 Radiograph of the hand demonstrating the importance of orthogonal views
(Courtesy of Joseph Makris, MD, Baystate Medical Center.)

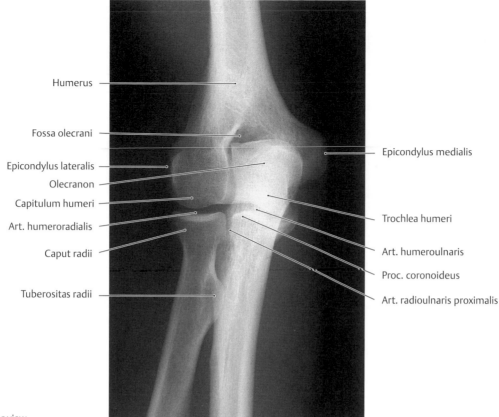

Humerus

Fossa olecrani

Epicondylus lateralis

Olecranon

Capitulum humeri

Art. humeroradialis

Caput radii

Tuberositas radii

Epicondylus medialis

Trochlea humeri

Art. humeroulnaris

Proc. coronoideus

Art. radioulnaris proximalis

A Anteroposterior view.

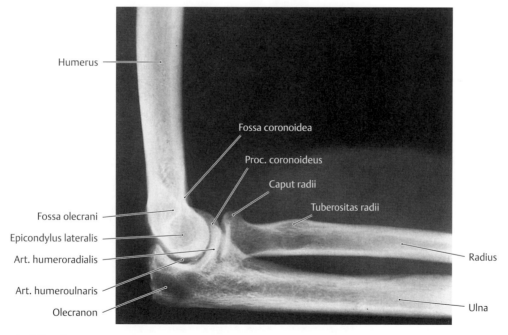

Humerus

Fossa coronoidea

Proc. coronoideus

Caput radii

Tuberositas radii

Fossa olecrani

Epicondylus lateralis

Art. humeroradialis

Art. humeroulnaris

Olecranon

Radius

Ulna

B Lateral view.

Fig. 20.2 Radiograph of the elbow
(From Moeller TB, Reif E. Pocket Atlas of Sectional Anatomy, Vol 3, 2nd ed. New York: Thieme Publishers; 2017.)

While x-rays are best for evaluating bones after trauma for fractures, MRI is the best choice for imaging soft tissues around the joints and for evaluation of the bone marrow (**Figs. 20.3** and **20.4**). Infiltration of the bone marrow from cancer or infection (osteomyelitis) can be invisible on x-rays early in the disease and still very subtle even as the disease progresses. MRI on the other hand is very sensitive for even the earliest changes in bone marrow and is essential for initial imaging and surveillance of these processes (**Fig. 20.5**). MRI is also helpful in assessing the extent of disease

and adjacent soft tissue involvement, evaluation for metastases, surgical planning, disease staging, and monitoring effectiveness of therapy.

MRI arthrography involves injecting contrast material into a joint prior to MR imaging to better evaluate the key soft tissue components of the joint, such as the labrum, ligaments, and articular cartilage (**Fig. 20.6**). The joint injection procedure itself is usually performed with imaging guidance using ultrasound or fluoroscopy.

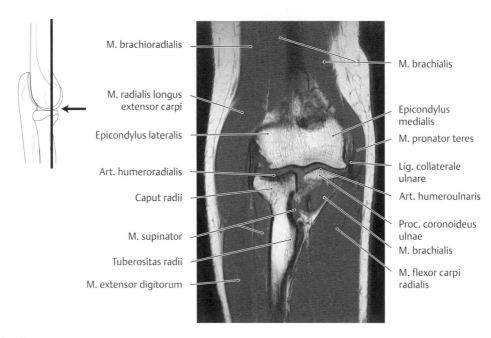

Fig. 20.3 MRI of the elbow
Coronal section.
In this sequence, fat is *white* (the fat in the bone marrow causes the bones to be a *very light gray/white* as well). Muscles are *dark gray* and ligaments and cortical bone are *black*.
The utility of MRI is the ability to see the ligaments, tendons, muscles, and cartilage. A muscle tear, tendon rupture, or ligamentous tear is invisible on an x-ray, but well demonstrated on MRI. (From Moeller TB, Reif E. Pocket Atlas of Sectional Anatomy, Vol 3, 2nd ed. New York: Thieme Publishers; 2017.)

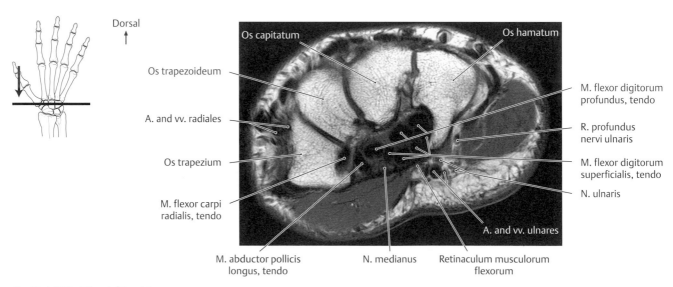

Fig. 20.4 MRI of the right wrist
Transverse (axial) section, distal view.
In this sequence, fat is *white,* muscles are *dark gray,* and nerves and tendons are *black*. Note the detail of the tendons and nerves crossing the wrist through the sulcus carpi. (From Moeller TB, Reif E. Pocket Atlas of Sectional Anatomy, Vol 3, 2nd ed. New York: Thieme Publishers; 2017.)

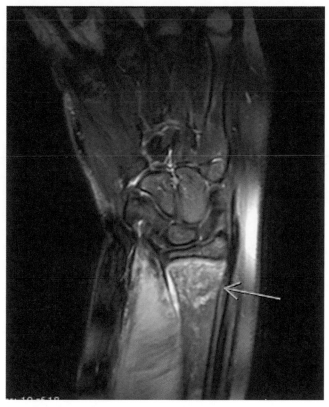

Fig. 20.5 Osteomyelitis
Coronal MRI of the right wrist in a teenager with pain, swelling, fever, and elevated white blood cell count. In this sequence, normal bone marrow should be uniformly dark. Note the patchy bright *(whiter)* areas in the distal radial metaphysis indicative of osteomyelitis in this patient *(arrow)*. (Courtesy of Joseph Makris, MD, Baystate Medical Center.)

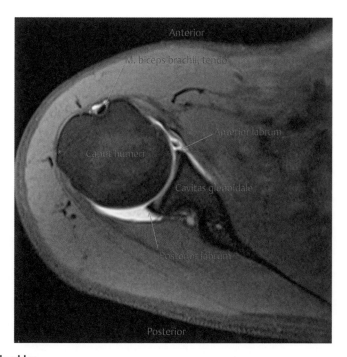

Fig. 20.6 MRI arthrogram of the shoulder
Axial image of a normal right shoulder at the level of the mid joint. The MRI was performed after contrast was injected directly into the joint space. The contrast fluid (white on this image) distends the joint capsule and outlines the articular cartilage, labrum, and ligaments, increasing sensitivity for evaluation of injuries to these structures. (Courtesy of Joseph Makris, MD, Baystate Medical Center.)

Unit VI   Review Questions: Upper Limb

1. A patient complains of tingling and pain in the upper arm. Upon further examination and additional tests, you determine that the a. axillaris has been occluded by atherosclerosis. The patient, however, still has a radial pulse at the wrist. Which of the following arteries could provide a collateral circulation around the occlusion?
   A. A. suprascapularis and a. circumflexa scapulae
   B. A. suprascapularis and a. thoracica lateralis
   C. A. circumflexa humeri posterior and a. circumflexa humeri anterior
   D. A. thoracica superior and a. thoracica lateralis
   E. A. intercostales posteriores and a. thoracica lateralis

2. The arcus palmaris profundus of the hand is formed mainly by the
   A. a. ulnaris
   B. a. radialis
   C. a. brachialis
   D. aa. digitales palmares
   E. aa. metacarpales palmares

3. Each cord of the plexus brachialis
   A. contains nerve fibers from C5 to T1 levels of the medulla spinalis
   B. is formed from the junction of one anterior and one posterior division
   C. gives a branch to the n. medianus
   D. lies within the axilla
   E. gives rise to a n. subscapularis (upper, middle, and lower)

4. Nerves often pair with arteries to travel as neurovascular bundles. Which of the following is *not* an accurate pairing?
   A. N. axillaris and a. circumflexa humeri posterior
   B. N. medianus and a. brachialis
   C. N. musculocutaneus and a. circumflexa scapulae
   D. N. radialis and a. profunda brachii
   E. N. thoracicus longus and a. thoracica lateralis

5. During a radical mastectomy on a 50-year-old woman, the surgeon does a careful but thorough axillary node dissection. What nerve lies along the medial wall of the axilla and is particularly vulnerable during this procedure?
   A. R. lateralis of n. intercostalis posterior
   B. N. musculocutaneus
   C. N. pectoralis lateralis
   D. N. thoracicus longus
   E. N. dorsalis scapulae

6. One of your patients ruptured the tendon of the caput longum of the m. biceps brachii. Although he is bothered by the unattractive bulge that formed in his anterior arm, he is surprised to find that he has lost little flexor strength. You confirm that the m. brachialis has greater leverage at the joint and therefore is the more powerful flexor of the elbow. Where does the m. brachialis insert?
   A. Tuberositas radii
   B. Tuberositas ulnae
   C. Epicondylus medialis
   D. Aponeurosis bicipitalis
   E. Olecranon

7. Which part(s) of the m. triceps brachii crosses/cross the art. glenohumeralis?
   A. Caput mediale
   B. Caput laterale
   C. Caput longum
   D. Caput laterale and caput mediale
   E. Caput laterale and caput longum

8. Structures that pass through the quadrangular space of the upper limb include the
   A. n. radialis
   B. n. suprascapularis
   C. a. circumflexa humeri posterior
   D. a. circumflexa humeri anterior
   E. a. profunda brachii

9. Which of the following bones articulates with the radius at the wrist?
   A. Os pisiforme
   B. Os hamatum
   C. Os capitatum
   D. Os trapezium
   E. Os scaphoideum

10. The retinaculum musculorum flexorum
    A. forms the floor of the canalis ulnaris
    B. forms the roof of the canalis carpalis
    C. is continuous with the aponeurosis palmaris
    D. is continuous with the m. palmaris longus
    E. All of the above

11. As a second-year resident doing a pediatric surgery rotation, you set up an arterial line on a 6-year-old girl prior to surgery. You choose the a. radialis of her left (nondominant) hand. Because you know that the procedure can result in occlusion of the artery, you verify that the collateral circulation to the hand is patent. The a. radialis
    A. forms the arcus palmaris superficialis
    B. passes superficial to the anatomic snuffbox
    C. supplies the muscles of the posterior compartment through its a. interossea posterior
    D. supplies the a. princeps pollicis
    E. lies medial to the tendon of m. flexor carpi radialis in the wrist

12. During your first training session as a phlebotomist, you are relieved to find that your "patient" is a 24-year-old weight lifter whose superficial veins stand out dramatically against his overdeveloped muscles. Superficial veins of the upper limb
  A. include a v. basilica that runs in the sulcus deltopectoralis
  B. include a v. cephalica that joins the vv. brachiales in the arm
  C. drain into the veins of the deep venous system via vv. perforantes
  D. course with the arteries as paired accompanying veins
  E. have bidirectional valves that allow flow in either direction

13. An injury to the lower plexus brachialis (Klumpke's palsy) would affect
  A. sensation in the nail bed of the 5th digit
  B. abduction of the 2nd through 5th digits
  C. adduction of the thumb
  D. adduction of the wrist
  E. All of the above

14. While moonlighting in the emergency department one night, you treat a 14-year-old gang member who was stabbed in the supraclavicular region of the neck 2 cm above the middle third of the clavicula. A chest x-ray confirms that he has a pneumothorax. What other structure could be injured in this area?
  A. N. axillaris
  B. M. pectoralis minor
  C. A. subscapularis
  D. Fasciculus posterior of the plexus brachialis
  E. V. cephalica

15. The m. serratus anterior
  A. forms a scapulothoracic joint with the mm. intercostales externi
  B. is innervated by a branch of the posterior cord
  C. elevates the scapula off the thoracic wall
  D. rotates the scapula laterally during abduction of the arm above the horizontal plane
  E. originates from the fossa subscapularis

16. A professional rodeo cowboy fell off his horse and fractured his humerus at the collum anatomicum and the tuberculum minor. Which of the following muscles inserts on this tuberculum?
  A. M. supraspinatus
  B. M. infraspinatus
  C. M. subscapularis
  D. M. coracobrachialis
  E. M. teres major

17. Damage to which nerve would most affect elbow flexion?
  A. N. radialis
  B. N. ulnaris
  C. N. medianus
  D. N. musculocutaneus
  E. N. axillaris

18. At a neighborhood block party several children engage in a tug-of-war. Suddenly, Jason, a 5-year-old boy, hugs his right elbow and cries out in pain. The inconsolable child is eventually taken to the local clinic, where the pediatrician recognizes that Jason has subluxed (partially dislocated) his caput radii. By gently supinating the flexed arm, the doctor restores it to its normal position. Which of the following is true regarding the art. radioulnaris proximalis?
  A. The caput radii rotates within the lig. annulare.
  B. It includes a hinge-type joint between the caput radii and capitulum humeri.
  C. The m. biceps brachii pronates the joint.
  D. A discus articularis separates the radius and ulna.
  E. The subluxation of the caput radii results from a tear of the lig. collaterale radiale.

19. On your first day of shadowing in your preceptor's office, you are asked to get some baseline information on the patients. You start by taking their pulse. The a. radialis is easiest to palpate in the wrist where it lies immediately lateral to the tendon of the
  A. m. flexor carpi radialis
  B. m. flexor digitorum
  C. m. flexor pollicis longus
  D. m. palmaris longus
  E. m. extensor carpi radialis

20. You examine a 14-year-old girl in the emergency department. She has a puncture wound from a dog bite in the flesh over the middle phalanx of her 5th digit. The incident occurred 2 days ago, and the finger is inflamed and likely infected. What are your thoughts regarding possible spread of the infection via the vagina synovialis?
  A. It will spread into the superficial space on the dorsum of the hand.
  B. It will spread to the common flexor sheath in the wrist.
  C. It will spread to the adjacent finger.
  D. It will remain confined to the sheath of the infected finger.
  E. A and B are correct.

21. The a. axillaris
  A. begins at the lateral border of the costa I
  B. lies anterior to the v. axillaris
  C. ends by dividing into a. brachialis and a. profunda brachii
  D. passes through the axilla between the m. pectoralis major and m. pectoralis minor
  E. branches include the truncus thyrocervicalis

22. Nll. axillares that lie medial to the m. pectoralis minor include
  A. nll. pectorales
  B. nll. humerales
  C. nll. apicales
  D. nll. centrales
  E. nll. subscapulares

23. The C4 ramus anterior is a component of
  A. the pre-fixed plexus
  B. the upper trunk
  C. the fasciculus posterior
  D. the n. axillaris
  E. All of the above

24. A young man suffered a crushing injury to his right arm, fracturing his humerus at midshaft and damaging the nerve that runs in the posterior compartment. What functional loss would you expect from this injury?
   A. Inability to extend the elbow
   B. Inability to supinate the hand
   C. Inability to abduct the thumb
   D. Inability to extend the wrist
   E. All of the above

25. One of your orthopedic colleagues introduces you, an anatomist, to his patient, a famous baseball pitcher, who suffers from chronic rotator cuff pain. He asks you to demonstrate the rotator cuff on a cadaver specimen and explain the anatomy of this type of injury. You tell him the following:
   A. Tendons of the rotator cuff muscles insert onto the capsula articularis of the art. glenohumeralis.
   B. The m. supraspinatus tendo passes through the subacromial space between the art. glenohumeralis and the coracoacromial arch.
   C. An abnormal communication between the bursa subacromialis and art. glenohumeralis cavity can result from rupture of the m. supraspinatus tendo.
   D. Rupture of the m. supraspinatus tendo will impair the patient's ability to initiate abduction of the arm.
   E. All of the above

26. Which of the following muscles has no attachment on the humerus?
   A. M. deltoideus
   B. M. coracobrachialis
   C. M. flexor digitorum superficialis
   D. M. pronator teres
   E. M. biceps brachii

27. Which muscle provides strong adduction of the art. glenohumeralis?
   A. M. teres minor
   B. M. pectoralis major
   C. M. pectoralis minor
   D. Caput breve of the m. biceps brachii
   E. M. subscapularis

28. A young woman riding a 10-speed bicycle accidentally engaged the front brake, was thrown over the handlebars, and landed on her outstretched hands. In the emergency department, imaging of the elbow revealed a subtle fracture of the collum radii that allowed proximal movement of the radius relative to the ulna, which also suggested a tear in the membrana interossea. Which movements were most impaired by this injury?
   A. Flexion of the wrist
   B. Extension of the elbow
   C. Extension of the digits
   D. Abduction of the thumb
   E. Adduction of the thumb

29. An elderly man had injured his wrist in a fall and is now experiencing tingling in his fingers and a weakened grip. A lateral X-ray of the wrist shows that his os lunatum has dislocated and is pressing on the structures within the canalis carpi. Which of the following structures pass through the canalis carpi?

   A. A. ulnaris
   B. A. radialis
   C. M. flexor carpi radialis
   D. M. flexor pollicis longus
   E. M. palmaris longus

30. In the anatomy lab you are fascinated by the deep dissection of the hand because as an amateur violinist you appreciate that the intrinsic muscles of the palm are important for the fine movements of the hand. Which of the following is true for both the mm. lumbricales and the mm. interossei?
   A. All are innervated by the n. medianus.
   B. All are innervated by the n. ulnaris.
   C. They flex the artt. metacarpophalangeae.
   D. They arise from the tendons of the m. flexor digitorum profundus.
   E. They abduct or adduct the fingers.

31. Your 7-year-old nephew suffered a distal clavicular fracture after falling from a tree. Which of the following structures would likely be disrupted with this type of injury?
   A. Ligg. interclaviculare
   B. Lig. coracohumerale
   C. Art. acromioclavicularis
   D. Art. scapulothoracica
   E. Lig. coracoacromiale

32. Your grandmother tripped on the stairs and landed on her outstretch arms. In the emergency department an initial physical exam strongly indicated a fractured os scaphoideum. What part of the exam suggested this diagnosis?
   A. Pain over palmar surface of the wrist
   B. Pain over the ulnar styloid process
   C. Displacement of the radial styloid process
   D. Pain in the anatomic snuffbox
   E. Inability to oppose the thumb

33. Deep fascia of the limbs forms discrete compartments of muscles that usually share similar functions and innervations. The effects of trauma are often limited to the contents of a single compartment. Muscles effected by trauma to the anterior forearm compartment would include
   A. m. brachioradialis
   B. m. pronator teres
   C. m. supinator
   D. m. abductor pollicis longus
   E. m. extensor carpi ulnaris

34. As a pediatric orthopedist, you've created some simple and fun shortcuts for diagnosing nerve injuries to the hand in children. Which of the following activities would selectively test the indicated nerve?
   A. "Thumbs up" sign (extending the thumb away from the fist): n. medianus
   B. "OK" sign (forming a circle with the 1st and 2nd digits): n. radialis
   C. "Peace" sign (separating the 2nd and 3rd digits while extended): n. ulnaris
   D. All the above
   E. None of the above

35. A young woman is seen in the local clinic following a fall she suffered while hiking. She has severe pain and swelling of her left elbow but a lateral x-ray confirms that there is no fracture. You suspect a soft tissue injury. What additional imaging modality would you choose to confirm this?
　A. Frontal x-ray
　B. MRI
　C. CT
　D. Ultrasound

36. You convinced your boyfriend to help you move some boxes of books out of your basement. During the move he felt a sharp pain in his neck that remained throughout the following day. His physician recommended an MRI of his neck, which revealed a rupture of his m. scalenus medius caused by the strain of steadying his trunk as he lifted the heavy boxes. In addition, he demonstrated a "winged" scapula, indicating that there was significant damage to his long thoracic nerve, which passes through the m. scalenus medius before descending into the neck and axilla. Which activity would be affected by injury to the long thoracic nerve?
　A. Adducting his arm to touch the elbow of the opposite side
　B. Internally rotating the arm to touch the back of his waist
　C. Externally rotating his arm to throw a baseball
　D. Flexing his arm directly forward
　E. Abducting his arm above his head

Answers and Explanations

1. **A.** The suprascapular and transverse cervical branches of the a. subclavia and the thoracodorsal and circumflex scapular branches of the distal segment of the a. axillaris participate in a scapular arcade that provides a collateral circulation that would circumvent the occlusion (Section 18.4).
　B. The a. thoracica lateralis does not supply the scapula, nor does it anastomose with the a. suprascapularis.
　C. The a. circumflexa humeri posterior and a. circumflexa humeri anterior anastomose around the neck of the humerus but do not anastomose with arteries proximal to the occlusion.
　D. Neither the a. thoracica superior nor the a. thoracica lateralis supplies the scapular region.
　E. Aa. intercostales posteriores supply the medial scapular region, but they do not anastomose with the a. thoracica lateralis.

2. **B.** The arcus palmaris profundus is formed mainly by the a. radialis (Section 18.4).
　A. The a. ulnaris forms the arcus palmaris superficialis.
　C. The a. brachialis begins at the lateral border of the axilla and terminates in the fossa cubitalis.
　D. The common palmar digital arteries are branches of the superficial palmar arch in the palm of the hand.
　E. The aa. metacarpales palmares arise from the deep palmar arch in the palm of the hand.

3. **D.** Each cord of the plexus brachialis lies within the axilla (Section 18.4).

　A. The fasciculus posterior contains fibers from C5 to T1; the fasciculus medialis contains fibers from C8 and T1; the fasciculus lateralis contains fibers from C5 to C7.
　B. The posterior divisions form the fasciculus posterior; only anterior divisions form the fasciculus medialis and fasciculus lateralis.
　C. The n. medianus is formed from the fasciculus medialis and fasciculus lateralis.
　E. The nn. subscapulares arise from the fasciculus posterior.

4. **C.** The n. musculocutaneus passes from the axilla to pierce the m. coracobrachialis of the anterior arm. The a. circumflexa scapulae passes through the triangular space into the scapular region (Section 19.2).
　A. The a. axillaris and a. circumflexa humeri posterior pass through the quadrangular space to the deltoid region.
　B. The n. medianus and a. brachialis descend on the medial side of the m. biceps brachii and enter the fossa cubitalis.
　D. The n. radialis and a. profunda brachii wind around the posterior humerus through the triceps hiatus.
　E. The n. thoracicus longus and a. thoracica lateralis descend on the medial wall of the axilla to supply the m. serratus anterior.

5. **D.** The n. thoracicus longus runs superficial to, and innervates, the m. serratus anterior, which forms the medial wall of the axilla. Injury to this nerve can result in a "winged" scapula (Section 19.1).
　A. In the axilla the nn. intercostales run deep to the m. serratus anterior and mm. intercostales externi and are not vulnerable to injury.
　B. The n. msuculocutaneus leaves the axilla just inferior to the art. glenohumeralis where it enters the m. coracobrachialis.
　C. The n. pectoralis lateralis passes anteriorly to penetrate the m. pectoralis major.
　E. The n. dorsalis scapulae descends posteriorly from the upper roots of the plexus to innervate the m. levator scapulae and m. rhomboideus.

6. **B.** The m. brachialis inserts on the tuberositas ulnae of the ulna (Section 19.3).
　A. The m. biceps brachii inserts on the tuberositas radii.
　C. The proc. coronoideus forms the anterior lip of the incisura trochlearis of the ulna and is the origin of the caput ulnare of the m. pronator teres.
　D. The aponeurosis bicipitalis is a fascial extension of the m. biceps brachii.
　E. The olecranon of the ulna forms the posterior prominence of the elbow and is the insertion for the m. triceps brachii and m. anconeus.

7. **C.** The caput longum of the m. triceps brachii crosses the art. glenohumeralis to attach to the tuberculum infraglenoidale, where it contributes to extension of the joint (Section 19.2).
　A. The caput mediale arises from the medial aspect of the humeral shaft. It joins with the caput laterale and caput longum to insert on the olecranon of the ulna.
　B. The caput laterale arises from the lateral aspect of the humeral shaft. It joins with the caput mediale and caput longum to insert on the olecranon of the ulna.

D. The caput mediale and caput laterale arise from the humeral shaft and cross only the art. cubiti.

E. The caput laterale arises from the shaft of the humerus and crosses the art. cubiti. The caput longum originates on the tuberculum infraglenoidale of the scapula and crosses the art. glenohumerale and art. cubiti.

8. C. The a. circumflexa humeri posterior and the n. axillaris pass through the quadrangular space (Section 19.2).

A. The n. radialis passes through the triceps hiatus.

B. The n. suprascapularis passes through the incisura scapularis.

D. The a. circumflexa humeri anterior runs horizontally beneath the m. coracobrachialis and the caput breve of the m. biceps brachii to encircle the collum humeri.

E. The a. profunda brachii passes through the triceps hiatus with the n. radialis.

9. E. The radius articulates distally with the os scaphoideum and os lunatum of the wrist (Section 19.5).

A. The os pisiforme on the medial side of the wrist articulates with the os triquetrum.

B. The os hamatum articulates with the os capitatum, os lunatum, os triquetrum, and ossa metacarpi IV and V.

C. The os capitatum articulates with the os hamatum, os trapezoideum, os scaphoideum, os lunatum, and os metacarpale III.

D. The os trapezium articulates with the os trapezoideum, os scaphoideum, and os metacarpale I.

10. E. The retinaculum musculorum flexorum forms the roof of the canalis carpi and floor of the canalis ulnaris. As a thickening of the deep fascia of the palm, it is continuous with the aponeurosis palmaris, m. palmaris longus, lig. metacarpale transversum, and fibrous digital sheaths (Sections 19.5 and 19.6).

A. The retinaculum musculorum flexorum forms the floor of the canalis ulnaris; the palmar carpal ligament form its roof. B through D are also correct (E).

B. The canalis carpi is a fascio-osseous tunnel. Ossa carpalia form the floor and sides; the retinaculum musculorum flexorum forms the roof. A, C, and D are also correct (E).

C. The retinaculum musculorum flexorum is continuous with the tough aponeurosis palmaris of the hand. A, B, and D are also correct (E).

D. The m. palmaris longus passes over the canalis carpi and inserts on the retinaculum musculorum flexorum and aponeurosis palmaris. A through C are also correct (E).

11. D. The a. princeps pollicis arises from the a. radialis at the base of the os metacarpale I and divides into two aa. digitales of the thumb (Section 18.4).

A. The a. ulnaris forms the arcus palmaris superficialis. The a. radialis forms the arcus palmaris profundus.

B. The a. radialis courses along the floor of the anatomic snuffbox.

C. The a. interossea posterior, which supplies muscles of the posterior forearm compartment, arises from the a. interossea communis, a branch of the a. ulnaris on the fossa cubitalis.

E. The a. radialis lies lateral to the tendon of the m. flexor carpi radialis at the wrist.

12. C. The veins of the superficial venous system drain into the deep veins via vv. perforantes (Section 18.4).

A. The v. cephalica courses along the deltopectoral groove before terminating in the v. axillaris.

B. The v. basilica joins with the paired vv. brachiales to form the v. axillaris.

D. Veins of the deep venous system travel with the arteries as paired accompanying veins. There is no superficial arterial system that accompanies the superficial veins.

E. Veins of the limbs have unidirectional valves that prevent pooling of blood and facilitate flow back toward the heart.

13. E. The n. ulnaris arises from the lower part of the plexus. Its r. cutaneus dorsalis in the hand supplies the palmar and dorsal surfaces of the 4th (half) and 5th digits, and its deep branch supplies the mm. interossei dorsales that abduct the fingers and the m. adductor pollicis that adducts the thumb. It also innervates the m. flexor carpi ulnaris that assists in adduction of the wrist (Section 18.4).

A. The ulnar nerve's (C8–T1) dorsal cutaneous branch in the hand supplies the palmar and dorsal surfaces of the 4th (half) and 5th digits. B through D are also correct (E).

B. The ulnar nerve's (C8–T1) deep branch in the hand supplies the dorsal interossei muscles that abduct the fingers. A, C, and D are also correct (E).

C. The ulnar nerve's (C8–T1) deep branch in the hand supplies the m. adductor pollicis that adducts the thumb. A, B, and D are also correct (E).

D. The n. ulnaris (C8–T1) innervates the m. flexor carpi ulnaris that assists the m. extensor carpi ulnaris (n. radialis) in adduction of the wrist. A through C are also correct (E).

14. D. The fasciculus posterior is part of the pars supraclavicularis of the plexus brachialis plexus and could be injured in the area (Section 18.4).

A. The terminal nerves of the plexus brachialis form below the clavicula. Although damage to the pars supraclavicularis could affect the n. axillaris, the stab wound would not directly damage the nerve itself.

B. The m. pectoralis minor attaches to the proc. coracoideus, which lies below the middle part of the clavicula.

C. The a. subscapularis is a branch of the distal part of the a. axillaris, which is infraclavicular.

E. The v. cephalica drains into the v. axillaris below the clavicula and most likely would not be affected by this injury.

15. D. The m. serratus anterior pulls the inferior angle of the scapula laterally when the art. glenohumeralis is abducted above the horizontal plane (Section 19.1).

A. The scapulothoracic joint is a functional relationship between the m. serratus anterior and m. subscapularis.

B. The n. thoracicus longus, which innervates the m. serratus anterior, arises directly from the C5–C7 roots of the plexus brachialis.

C. The m. serratus anterior supports the scapula against the thoracic wall. Denervation of the muscle allows the scapula to lift away from the thoracic wall, a condition known as a "winged" scapula.

E. The m. serratus anterior inserts on the entire medial border of the scapula.

16. C. The m. subscapularis inserts on the tuberculum minus humeri and capsula fibrosa of art. glenohumeralis (Section 19.2).

A. The m. supraspinatus inserts on the tuberculum majus humeri.

B. The m. infraspinatus inserts on the tuberculum majus humeri.

D. The m. coracobrachialis inserts on the shaft of the middle part of the humerus.

E. The m. teres major inserts on the crest that extends inferiorly from the tuberculum minus.

17. **D.** The n. musculocutaneus innervates the m. biceps brachii and mm. brachiales, the primary flexors of the elbow. There would also be loss of sensation to the skin of the lateral forearm (Sections 19.2 and 19.3).

A. Damage to the n. radialis results in wrist drop and loss of sensation to the dorsum of the hand and the proximal segments of the 1st through 3rd digits and half of the 4th digit.

B. Damage to the n. ulnaris may cause paresthesia (numbness and tingling) in the forearm, 4th and 5th fingers, or paralysis of most of the intrinsic muscles of the hand (so-called claw hand deformity).

C. Damage to the n. medianus above the fossa cubitalis will cause the inability to flex the art. interphalangeae proximalis of the 1st to 3rd digits and the inability to flex the art. interphalangeae distalis of the 2nd and 3rd digits. This results in "benediction hand" (2nd and 3rd finger are partially extended) when trying to form a fist. It also causes the inability to flex the terminal phalanx of the thumb (due to damage of m. flexor pollicis longus) and loss of sensation over the lateral aspect of the hand.

E. Damage to the n. axillaris causes paralysis of the m. deltoideus, resulting in weakened flexion and extension of the shoulder and the inability to abduct the arm above the horizontal.

18. **A.** The lig. anulare forms a circular cuff around the caput radii that allows the bone to rotate in the joint (Section 19.4).

B. The hinge-type joint between the radius and capitulum of the humerus is the art. humeroradialis.

C. The m. biceps brachii inserts on the tuberositas radii and, therefore, supinates the joint when contracted.

D. In the art. radioulnaris proximalis the radius articulates at the incisura radialis of the ulna. A discus articularis separates the radius and ulna in the art. radioulnaris distalis.

E. Subluxation of the caput radii results from a laxity of the lig. anulare.

19. **A.** The a. radialis descends on the lateral side of the forearm and at the wrist lies immediately lateral to the tendon of the m. flexor carpi radialis (Section 19.5).

B. The tendons of the m. flexor digitorum superficialis lie in the middle of the wrist, medial to the a. radialis.

C. The tendon of the m. flexor pollicis longus lies lateral to the n. medianus and medial to the tendon of the m. flexor carpi radialis and to the a. radialis

D. The m. palmaris longus runs superficial to the retinaculum musculorum flexorum and medial to the m. flexor pollicis longus.

E. The a. radialis lies medial (palmar) to the m. extensor carpi radialis tendon.

20. **B.** The vagina synovialis of the 5th digit normally communicates with the common vagina synovialis (Section 19.6).

A. The vagina synovialis of the 5th digit communicates with the common vagina synovialis and with that of the thumb, but it does not normally communicate with the superficial space on the dorsum of the hand.

C. The vagina synovialis of the 2nd, 3rd, and 4th digits do not normally communicate with any other tendon sheaths. It is unlikely the infection will spread to these fingers.

D. Although the infection may remain confined to the infected finger, the vagina synovialis of the 5th digit communicates with that of the thumb and with the common tendon sheath. Therefore, the concern is that it will spread via this route to the thumb, wrist, and forearm.

E. The vagina synovialis of the 5th digit normally communicates with the common flexor sheath at the wrist but not with the superficial space on the dorsum of the hand.

21. **A.** The a. subclavia continues as the a. axillaris at the lateral border of the costa I (Section 18.4).

B. The a. axillaris lies posterior to the v. axillaris.

C. The a. brachialis is a continuation of the a. axillaris in the axilla. The a. profunda brachii is one of the branches of the a. brachialis.

D. The a. axillaris passes through the axilla posterior to the m. pectoralis minor.

E. The truncus thyrocervicalis is a branch of the a. subclavia

22. **C.** The nll. apicales are the nodes of the upper infraclavicular group. These lie medial to the m. pectoralis minor along the v. axillaris and adjacent to the proximal part of the a. axillaris (Section 18.4).

A. Nll. pectorales are part of the nll. axillares that lies lateral to the m. pectoralis minor.

B. Nll. interpectorales are part of the middle axillary group that lies between the m. pectoralis major and m. pectoralis minor.

D. Nll. centrales are part of the lower axillary group that lies deep to m. pectoralis minor.

E. The subscapular nodes are part of the lower axillary group that lies along the posterior axillary fold.

23. **A.** The plexus brachialis contains the rami anteriores of C5 to T1. A prefixed plexus also contains the C4 ramus anterior (Section 18.4).

B. The upper trunk contains C5 and C6 rami anteriores.

C. The fasciculus posterior contains the rami anteriores of C5 to T1.

D. The n. axillaris contains the rami anteriores of C5 and C6.

E. B, C, and D are incorrect.

24. **D.** Damage to the n. radialis from a midhumeral fracture results in loss of innervation to the m. extensor carpi radialis and m. extensor carpi ulnaris (Sections 18.4 and 19.4).

A. The branches of the n. radialis to the m. triceps brachii arise high in the arm, so a midhumeral lesion of the nerve would not affect the function of this muscle.

B. The n. radialis innervates only one of the muscles that supinate the hand, the m. supinator. The m. biceps brachii, also a supinator, is innervated by the n. musculocutaneus.

C. Abduction of the thumb is weakened by damage to the n. radialis.

E. A, B, and C are incorrect.

25.   E. All of the rotator cuff muscles insert on the capsula fibrosa of the art. glenohumeralis. The m. supraspinatus, the most frequently involved in rotator cuff tears, passes through the narrow subacromial space and, with repetitive use, becomes frayed. Rupture of the tendon allows the overlying bursa to communicate with the cavitas articularis and impairs the initial phase of abduction. Later phases of abduction remain intact through the action of the m. deltoideus (Section 19.2).

A. The tendons of the rotator cuff muscles insert on, and reinforce, the capsula fibrosa of the joint. B through D are also correct (E).

B. The tendon of m. supraspinatus and bursa subacromialis pass through the narrow subacromial space between the capsule of the shoulder joint and the coracoacromial arch. A, C, and D are also correct (E).

C. The tendo of m. supraspinatus separates the bursa subacromialis and bursa subdeltoidea from the joint cavity. With rupture of the tendon, a communication between the bursae and joint cavity may result. A, B, and D are also correct (E).

D. The m. deltoideus is the primary abductor of the art. glenohumeralis, but the m. supraspinatus assists in the first 15 degrees of abduction. A through C are also correct (E).

26.   E. The two heads of the m. biceps brachii originate on the tuberculum supraglenoidale and proc. coracoideus of the scapula and insert on the tuberositas radii (Sections 19.2 and 19.3).

A. The m. deltoideus originates along the spina scapulae and clavicula and inserts on the tuberositas deltoidea of the humerus.

B. The m. coracobrachialis originates on the proc. coracoideus of the scapula and inserts on the shaft of the humerus.

C. The m. flexor digitorum superficialis originates on the epicondylus medialis of the humerus and upper part of the radius and inserts on the middle phalanx of the 2nd through 4th digits.

D. The m. pronator teres originates on the epicondylus medialis of the humerus and proc. coronoideus of the ulna and inserts on the lateral radius.

27.   B. The broad origin of the m. pectoralis major on the anterior trunk wall allows it to strongly adduct the arm (Section 19.2).

A. As part of the rotator cuff, the m. teres minor supports the head of the humerus in the art. glenohumeralis. It also weakly adducts and laterally rotates the arm.

C. The m. pectoralis minor draws the scapula forward and down, causing the scapula to rotate medially.

D. The caput breve of the m. biceps brachii provides some flexion, abduction, and internal rotation of the art. glenohumeralis.

E. The m. subscapularis supports the head of the humerus in the art. glenohumeralis and medially rotates the arm.

28.   D. The function of the m. abductor pollicis, the primary abductor of the thumb, would be greatly impaired because it originates on the membrana interossea (Section 19.4).

A. The m. flexor carpi radialis and m. flexor carpi ulnaris originate from the epicondylus medialis humeri and olecranon of the ulna and would be unaffected by this injury.

B. The m. triceps brachii, which extends the elbow, inserts on the olecranon. It would not be impaired by this injury.

C. The m. extensor digitorum originates from the humerus and ulna and would be unaffected by this injury.

E. The adductor of the thumb, m. adductor pollicis, attaches to the os metacarpale II and III and the os capitatum. It would not be affected by this injury.

29.   D. The m. flexor pollicis longus passes through the canalis carpi with the m. flexor digitorum superficialis, m. flexor digitorum profundus, and n. medianus (Section 19.5).

A. The a. ulnaris and n. ulnaris pass through the canalis ulnaris at the wrist.

B. At the wrist the a. radialis turns dorsally to run through the floor of the anatomic snuffbox.

C. The m. flexor carpi radialis crosses the wrist lateral to the canalis carpi and inserts on the base of the os metacarpale II.

E. The m. palmaris longus passes superficial to the retinaculum musculorum flexorum to insert into the aponeurosis palmaris.

30.   C. The mm. interossei and mm. lumbricales flex the artt. metacarpophalangeae and extend the artt. interphalangeae (Section 19.6).

A. Only the lateral two mm. lumbricales are innervated by the n. medianus. The medial mm. lumbricales and all of the mm. interossei are innervated by the n. ulnaris.

B. The n. ulnaris innervates all of the mm. interossei and the medial two mm. lumbricales. The lateral two mm. lumbricales are innervated by the n. medianus.

D. Only the mm. lumbricales arise from the flexor tendons. The mm. interossei arise from the shafts of the metacarpal bones.

E. The mm. interossei palmares adduct the fingers, the mm. interossei dorsales abduct the fingers. The mm. lumbricales have no effect on these movements.

31.   C. Distal clavicular fractures often disrupt the art. acromioclavicularis and the ligg. coracoacromiale (Sections 18.2 and 19.1).

A. Ligg. interclaviculare connect the medial ends of the claviculae to the sternum and are less likely to be disrupted by a distal fracture.

B. The ligg. coracohumerale are part of the art. humeri capsule and not at risk with this type of injury.

D. The art. scapulothoracica is a functional relationship between the m. serratus anterior and m. subscapularis and not at risk in clavicular fractures.

E. The lig. coracoacromiale is part of the fornix humeri, which protects the art. humeri and is unlikely to be injured in this case.

32.   D. The os scaphoideum is most easily palpated in the anatomic snuffbox, where it forms the floor of this space. Pain in this region is indicative of a fractured os scaphoideum (Section 19.5).

A. Pain over the palmar surface of the wrist would suggest a carpal fracture but not definitively indicate the os scaphoideum.

B. The ulna lies on the medial side of the wrist, the os scaphoideum is on the lateral side.

C. Displacement of the radius would suggest a fracture or rupture of some of the radial ligaments but would not be diagnostic of a scaphoid fracture.

E. Although movement of the thumb would likely be painful, the ability to oppose the thumb would remain intact since the m. oppponens pollicis does not attach to the os scaphoideum.

33. **B.** The m. pronator teres is located in the superficial layer of the anterior forearm compartment.
   A. The m. brachioradialis is a muscle of the posterior forearm compartment.
   C. The m. supinator is a muscle of the posterior forearm compartment.
   D. The m. abductor pollicis longus is a muscle of the posterior forearm compartment.
   E. The m. extensor carpi ulnaris is a muscle of the posterior forearm compartment.

34. **C.** The "peace" sign tests the ability of the mm. interossei dorsales, innervated by the n. ulnaris, to abduct the 2nd digit (Section 19.6).
   A. A "thumbs up" sign requires extension of the thumb, performed by the m. extensor pollicis longus and brevis, which are innervated by the n. radialis.
   B. The "OK" sign tests the ability of the m. opponens pollicis, which is innervated by the n. medianus.
   D. Only answer C is correct
   E. Only A and B are incorrect

35. **B.** MRI is the modality of choice for visualizing soft tissues such as muscles, tendons, and cartilage.
   A. A frontal x-ray would help confirm the presence or absence of a fracture, but soft tissue injuries are not visible on an x-ray.
   C. CT is excellent for visualizing bone detail but less accurate than MRI for assessing soft tissue injuries.
   D. Ultrasound is most useful for image-guided procedures and visualizing superficial tissues.

36. **E.** Injury to the long thoracic nerve inhibits the m. serratus anterior, which rotates the inferior angle of the scapula laterally, tilting the glenoid superiorly. This rotation is necessary for abduction of the arm above 90 degrees.
   A. Adducting the arm across the trunk is primarily the action of the m. pectoralis major.
   B. Touching the back of the waist requires both internal rotation and extension at the shoulder joint, which are actions of the m. latissimus dorsi in conjunction with the m. pectoralis major, m. deltoideus, and m. teres major.
   C. The m. deltoideus and m. infraspinatus are the primary external rotators of the arm.
   D. The m. deltoideus, m. pectoralis major, and m. biceps brachii are the primary flexors of the arm.

Unit VII   Lower Limb

21 Overview of the Lower Limb

The lower limb supports the weight of the entire body and therefore is designed for strength and stability. Bones, muscles, and tendons tend to be more robust and joints more stable than those found in the upper limb.

21.1 General Features

— In the anatomic position, the body is upright and supported by the lower limb. The feet are together and pointed forward.
— The regions of the lower limb **(Fig. 21.1)** include
   • the **regio glutealis,** which includes the buttocks and lateral regio coxae and overlies the **cingulum pelvicum;**

• the **thigh,** between the hip and the knee;
• the **regio genus posterior** and **regio genus anterior,** at the knee;
• the **leg,** between the knee and ankle; and
• the **foot,** which has dorsum pedis and planta pedis. The planta pedis is also called the **sole (planta)** of the foot.

— Movements of the joints of the lower limb are similar to movements of the upper limb, with some variations. They include
   • flexion—**plantar flexion** indicates flexing the foot or toes downward;
   • extension—**dorsiflexion** indicates extension of the foot, as when lifting the foot or toes upward;
   • abduction and adduction—the axis for abduction and adduction of the toes is the 2nd digit;
   • external rotation and internal rotation—movement around a longitudinal axis;
   • **inversion,** or supination of the foot—lifting the medial edge of the sole; and
   • **eversion,** or pronation of the foot lifting the lateral edge of the sole.
— As in the upper limb, muscles of the lower limb can be described as intrinsic or extrinsic:
   • Intrinsic muscles of the foot originate and insert on bones of the foot and ankle.
   • Extrinsic flexor and extensor muscles of the foot originate in the leg.
      ○ Synovial tendon sheaths surround the long flexor and extensor tendons as they cross the art. talocruralis.

21.2 Bones of the Lower Limb

Bones of the lower limb include the os coxae that articulates with the sacrum to form the pelvic girdle, the femur of the thigh, the tibia and fibula of the leg, the tarsal bones of the ankle and hindfoot, and the metatarsal bones and phalanges of the midfoot and forefoot **(Fig. 21.2).**

— The **os coxae** forms the lateral part of the cingulum pelvicum. The features of the os coxae are discussed in Section 10.2 with the bony pelvis.
— The **femur** is the long bone of the thigh **(Fig. 21.3).**
   • Proximally, its large ball-shaped **head (caput femoris)** articulates with the acetabulum of the os coxae.
   • The **collum femoris,** angled inferolaterally, connects the head with the shaft.
   • **Trochanter major** and **trochanter minor,** sites for muscle attachments, are separated by a **crista intertrochanterica** posteriorly and an **linea intertrochanterica** anteriorly.
   • The **corpus femoris** is slightly bowed anteriorly and, in the anatomic position, is angled medially.
   • **Linea aspera,** paired ridges on the posterior surface of the shaft, diverge distally as the **linea supracondylaris medialis** and **linea supracondylaris lateralis.**

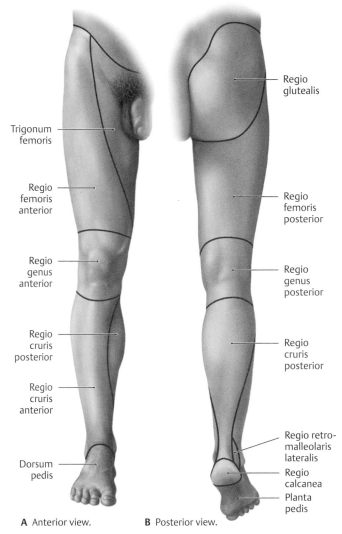

Trigonum femoris

Regio femoris anterior

Regio genus anterior

Regio cruris posterior

Regio cruris anterior

Dorsum pedis

Regio glutealis

Regio femoris posterior

Regio genus posterior

Regio cruris posterior

Regio retromalleolaris lateralis

Regio calcanea

Planta pedis

A Anterior view.   **B** Posterior view.

Fig. 21.1 Regions of the lower limb
Right limb. (From Schuenke M, Schulte E, Schumacher U. THIEME Atlas of Anatomy, Vol 1. Illustrations by Voll M and Wesker K. 3rd ed. New York: Thieme Publishers; 2020.)

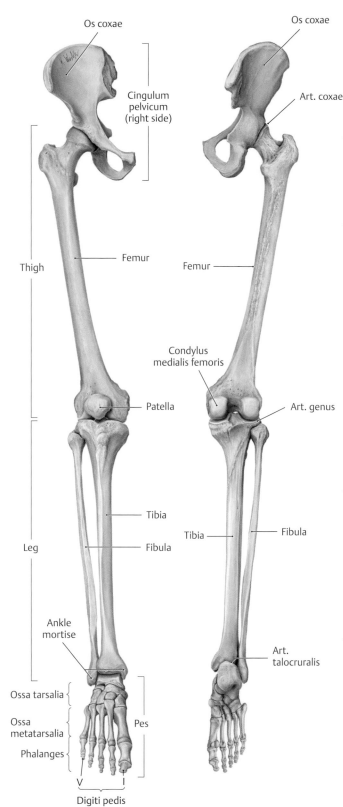

A Anterior view.   **B** Posterior view.

Fig. 21.2 Bones of the lower limb
Right limb. The skeleton of the lower limb consists of a limb girdle and an attached free limb. The free limb is divided into the thigh (femur), leg (tibia and fibula), and foot. It is connected to the pelvic girdle by the art. coxae. (From Schuenke M, Schulte E, Schumacher U. THIEME Atlas of Anatomy, Vol 1. Illustrations by Voll M and Wesker K. 3rd ed. New York: Thieme Publishers; 2020.)

- Distally, the **epicondylus medialis** and **epicondylus lateralis** are attachment sites for ligaments of the knee, and the **tuberculum adductorum** is an attachment site for muscle.
- The femur articulates with the tibia at the **condylus medialis** and **condylus lateralis,** which are separated by the **fossa intercondylaris.**
- The femur articulates with the patella anteriorly at the **facies patellaris femoris.**
— The **patella,** a large sesamoid bone, forms the kneecap (**Fig. 21.4;** see also **Fig. 22.12**).
  - It articulates with the distal femur at the art. genus.
  - Superiorly, its **base** is attached to the **tendo quadriceps femoris.**
  - Inferiorly, its **apex** is attached to the **lig. patellae.**
— The **tibia** is the large medial long bone of the leg (**Fig. 21.5**).
  - Proximally, it articulates with the femur at the **tibial plateau,** which has flat **condylus medialis** and **condylus lateralis** separated by an **eminentia intercondylaris.**
  - It articulates with the fibula proximally at the **art. tibiofibularis** and distally at the **syndesmosis tibiofibularis.**
  - A triangular **anterolateral tubercle (Gerdy's tubercle)** separates the lateral condyle from the lateral surface of the tibial shaft.
  - A **tuberositas tibiae** on the anterior surface below the tibial plateau is an attachment site for anterior thigh muscles via the patellar ligament.
  - Distally, the **malleolus medialis** forms part of the mortise of the art. talocruralis.
  - The sharp anterior border of the **shaft (corpus)** is palpable between the knee and ankle.
  - A **membrana interossea cruris** connects the corpus tibiae and corpus fibulae.
— The **fibula** is the lateral bone of the leg (see **Fig. 21.5**).
  - Proximally, the **head (caput fibulae)** articulates with the condylus lateralis of the tibia at the proximal art. tibiofibularis.
  - A narrow **neck (collum fibulae)** connects the head to the shaft.
  - A distal syndesmosis tibiofibularis binds the fibula to the distal tibia.
  - Distally, the **malleolus lateralis** forms the lateral wall of the mortise of the art. talocruralis.
— The **ossa tarsalia** consist of seven short bones of the foot (**Fig. 21.6**).
  - The **talus** is the most superior of the of the tarsal bones (ossa tarsi).
    ◦ The **body (corpus tali)** articulates with the tibia and fibula at the art. talocruralis.
    ◦ The **head (caput tali),** which articulates with the os naviculare, is the highest part of the medial arch of the foot.
    ◦ The inferior surface articulates with the calcaneus.
  - The **calcaneus** is the large tarsal bone of the heel.
    ◦ It articulates superiorly with the talus and anteriorly with the os cuboideum.
    ◦ The **sustentaculum tali,** a medial process, forms part of the arcus pedis longitudinalis (pars medialis).
  - The **os naviculare** lies anterior to the talus and forms part of the arcus pedis longitudinalis (pars medialis).
  - The **os cuboideum** lies anterior to the calcaneus on the lateral side of the foot.
  - The **os cuneiforme mediale, os cuneiforme intermedium,** and **os cuneiforme laterale** lie anterior to the os naviculare and articulate distally with the ossa metatarsi.

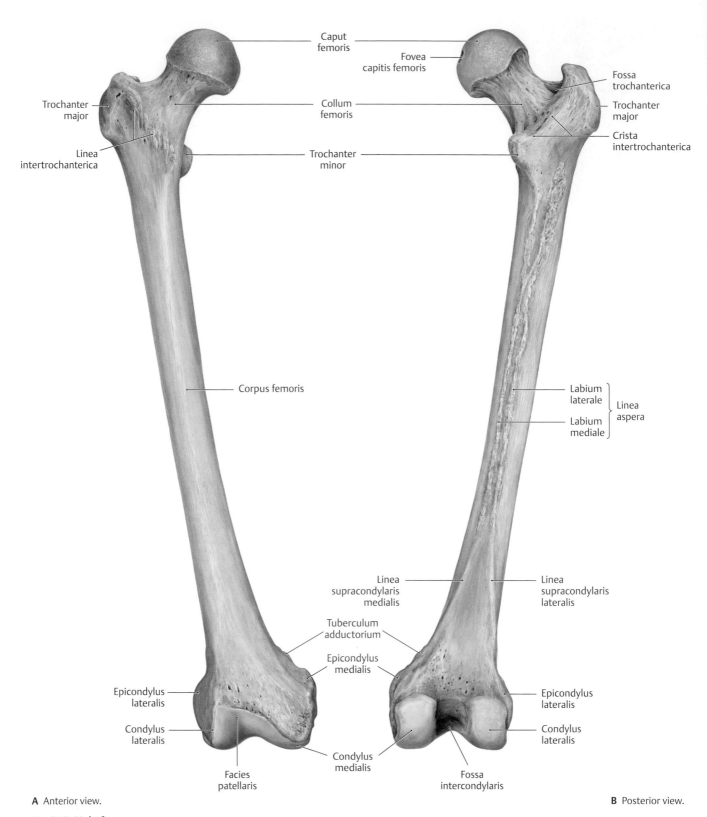

A Anterior view.

B Posterior view.

Fig. 21.3 Right femur

(From Schuenke M, Schulte E, Schumacher U. THIEME Atlas of Anatomy, Vol 1. Illustrations by Voll M and Wesker K. 3rd ed. New York: Thieme Publishers; 2020.)

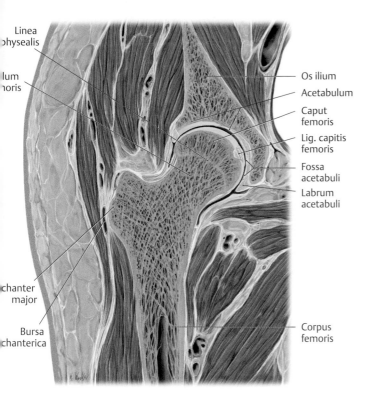

Linea
physealis

...lum
...moris

...chanter
major

Bursa
...chanterica

Os ilium

Acetabulum

Caput
femoris

Lig. capitis
femoris

Fossa
acetabuli

Labrum
acetabuli

Corpus
femoris

C Hip joint: coronal section
Right hip joint, anterior view. (From Gilroy AM et al. Atlas of Anatomy. 4th ed. 2020. Based on: Schuenke M, Schulte E, Schumacher U. THIEME Atlas of Anatomy. General Anatomy and Musculoskeletal System. Illustrations by Voll M and Wesker K. 3rd ed. New York: Thieme Medical Publishers; 2020.)

Fig. 21.3 (*continued*) **Right femur**

BOX 21.1: CLINICAL CORRELATION

FRACTURES OF THE FEMUR
Fractures of the collum femoris commonly occur following a low-energy impact in women over 60 years of age with osteoporosis. The distal fragment of bone is pulled upward by the m. quadriceps femoris, m. adductor, and mm. ischiocrurales, causing shortening and lateral (external) rotation of the limb. Femoral shaft fractures are less frequent and usually result from a major trauma.

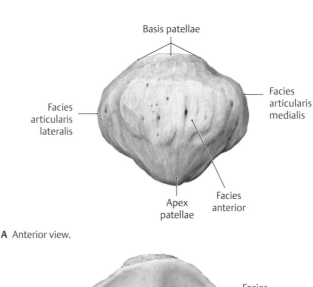

Medial femoral
neck fractures

Lateral femoral
neck fracture

Peritrochanteric
femoral fracture

Subtrochanteric
femoral fracture

(From Gilroy AM et al. Atlas of Anatomy. 4th ed. 2020. Based on: Schuenke M, Schulte E, Schumacher U. THIEME Atlas of Anatomy. General Anatomy and Musculoskeletal System. Illustrations by Voll M and Wesker K. 3rd ed. New York: Thieme Medical Publishers; 2020.)

BOX 21.2: DEVELOPMENTAL CORRELATION

BIPARTITE PATELLA
Ossification of the patella occurs at ages 3 to 6 years, usually from several ossification centers. Occasionally, one center, most commonly the upper lateral segment, fails to fuse with the larger segment, resulting in a bipartite (two-part) patella. On imaging this may appear as a patellar fracture.

(From Schuenke M, Schulte E, Schumacher U. THIEME Atlas of Anatomy, Vol 1. Illustrations by Voll M and Wesker K. 3rd ed. New York: Thieme Publishers; 2020.)

Basis patellae

Facies
articularis
lateralis

Facies
articularis
medialis

Apex
patellae

Facies
anterior

A Anterior view.

Facies
articularis

B Posterior view.

Apex patellae

Fig. 21.4 Patella
Right limb. (From Schuenke M, Schulte E, Schumacher U. THIEME Atlas of Anatomy, Vol 1. Illustrations by Voll M and Wesker K. 3rd ed. New York: Thieme Publishers; 2020.)

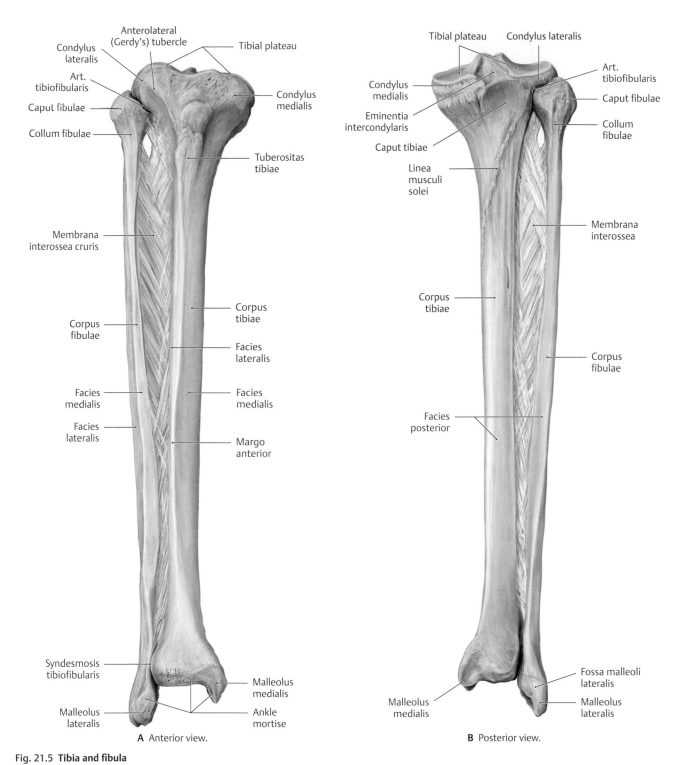

Fig. 21.5 Tibia and fibula
Right leg. (From Schuenke M, Schulte E, Schumacher U. THIEME Atlas of Anatomy, Vol 1. Illustrations by Voll M and Wesker K. 3rd ed. New York: Thieme Publishers; 2020.)

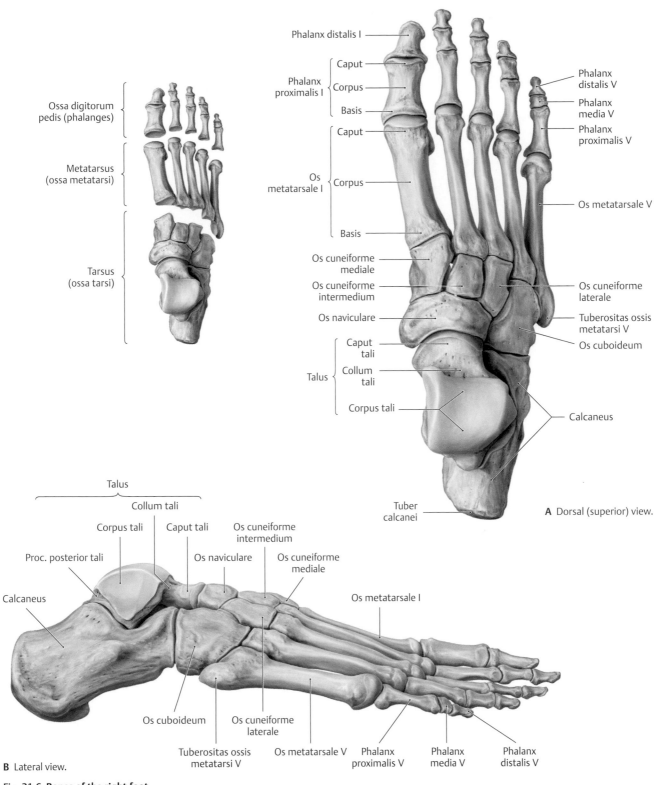

Ossa digitorum pedis (phalanges)

Metatarsus (ossa metatarsi)

Tarsus (ossa tarsi)

Phalanx distalis I

Phalanx proximalis I
- Caput
- Corpus
- Basis

Os metatarsale I
- Caput
- Corpus
- Basis

Os cuneiforme mediale

Os cuneiforme intermedium

Os naviculare

Talus
- Caput tali
- Collum tali
- Corpus tali

Phalanx distalis V

Phalanx media V

Phalanx proximalis V

Os metatarsale V

Os cuneiforme laterale

Tuberositas ossis metatarsi V

Os cuboideum

Calcaneus

Tuber calcanei

A Dorsal (superior) view.

Talus
- Corpus tali
- Collum tali
- Caput tali

Proc. posterior tali

Os cuneiforme intermedium

Os naviculare

Os cuneiforme mediale

Os metatarsale I

Calcaneus

Os cuboideum

Os cuneiforme laterale

Tuberositas ossis metatarsi V

Os metatarsale V

Phalanx proximalis V

Phalanx media V

Phalanx distalis V

B Lateral view.

Fig. 21.6 Bones of the right foot

(From Schuenke M, Schulte E, Schumacher U. THIEME Atlas of Anatomy, Vol 1. Illustrations by Voll M and Wesker K. 3rd ed. New York: Thieme Publishers; 2020.)

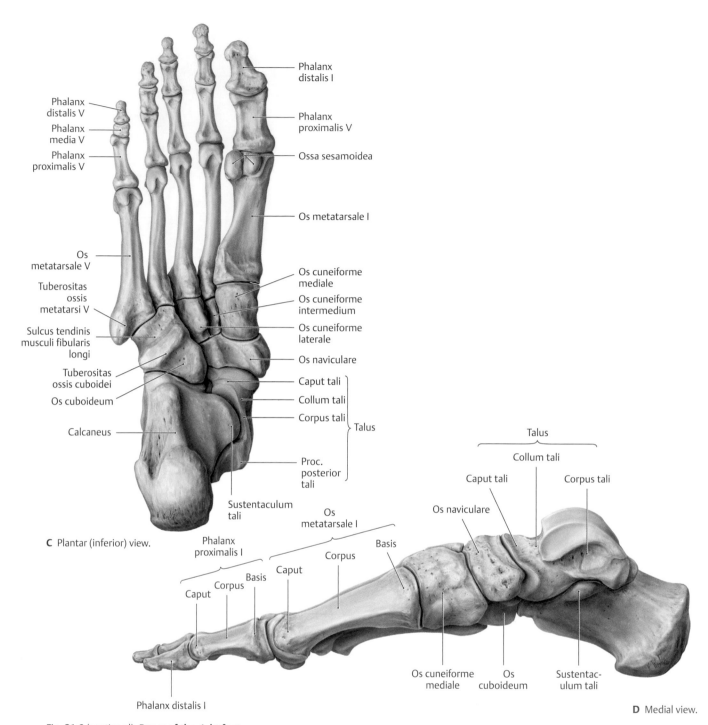

C Plantar (inferior) view.

D Medial view.

Fig. 21.6 (*continued*) **Bones of the right foot**

— The **ossa metatarsi** consist of five long bones that are designated I (medial) through V (lateral).
  - Proximally, the **basis ossis metatarsi** articulates with the ossa tarsi.
  - Distally, the **caput ossis metatarsi** articulate with the proximal phalanges.
  - The **corpus ossis metatarsi** connects the heads and bases.
  - Paired **ossa sesamoidea** are associated with the caput ossis metatarsi I.
  - A prominent tuberositas ossis metatarsi V is a site of attachment for muscles of the leg.
— The **phalanges** are small long bones of the toes.
  - The 2nd through 5th digits have a phalanx proximalis, phalanx media, and phalanx distalis.

- The 1st digit, the **hallux,** or great toe, has only a phalanx proximalis and phalanx distalis.

21.3   Fascia and Compartments of the Lower Limb

— Similar to the upper limb, the lower limb musculature is enclosed within a snug sleeve of deep fascia, which is continuous from the crista iliaca to the sole of the foot but has regional designations.
  - **Fascia lata** surrounds muscles of the thigh. Laterally, longitudinal fibers of the fascia lata form a tough band, the **tractus iliotibialis,** which extends from the crista

iliaca to the anterolateral (Gerdy's) tuberositas tibiae (see **Fig. 22.41**).

- **Fascia cruris** invests muscles of the leg, and at the ankle it forms the retinaculum extensorum and flexorum.
- Fascia on the dorsum of the foot is thin, but on the sole it forms a thickened longitudinal band, the **aponeurosis plantaris.**
- **Vaginae fibrosae digitorum pedis** are extensions of the aponeurosis plantaris onto the toes, where they enclose the flexor tendons.

— The deep fascia creates compartments that separate the limb musculature. Muscles within each compartment are usually similar in function, innervation, and blood supply. Compartments of the lower limb (see **Fig. 22.46**) include the following:

- **Anterior, medial,** and **posterior compartments** of the thigh
- **Anterior, lateral, superficial posterior,** and **deep posterior** compartments of the leg (crural compartments)
- **Medial, lateral, central,** and **interosseous compartments** on the sole of the foot
- **Dorsal compartment** on the dorsum of the foot

21.4 Neurovasculature of the Lower Limb

Arteries of the Lower Limb

Branches of the a. iliaca interna in the pelvis and the a. femoralis (a continuation of the a. iliaca externa) supply blood to the lower limb (**Fig. 21.7**).

— The branches of the a. iliaca interna that supply the lower limb include

- the **a. glutea superior and a. glutea inferior,** which exit the pelvis posteriorly through the foramen ischiadicum majus to supply the regio glutealis; and
- the **a. obturatoria,** which exits the pelvis anteriorly through the foramen obturatum to supply the medial thigh.

— The **a. femoralis** (clinically known as the a. femoralis superficialis) enters the anterior thigh deep to the lig. inguinale enclosed within a **femoral sheath** (formed by extensions of the deep fascia of the abdomen). The artery descends along the anteromedial thigh between the anterior and medial muscular compartments and ends at the **hiatus adductorius,** a gap in the tendon of the **m. adductor magnus.** Its branches include

- the **a. circumflexa ilium superficialis** and **a. epigastrica superficialis,** which supply the abdominal wall;
- the **a. pudenda externa profunda** and **superficialis,** which supply the regio inguinalis;
- the **a. descendens genus,** which contributes to the anastomosis around the knee; and
- the **a. profunda femoris,** which is the primary blood supply to the thigh.

— The a. profunda femoris, the largest branch of the a. femoralis, arises in the proximal thigh. Its branches include

- the **a. circumflexa femoris medialis,** which is the primary blood supply to the art. coxae;
- the **a. circumflexa femoris lateralis,** which supplies the art. coxae and contributes to the anastomosis around the art. genus; and

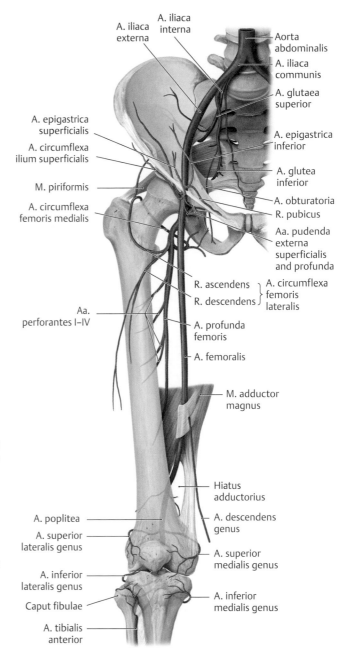

Fig. 21.7 Course and branches of the a. femoralis
(From Schuenke M, Schulte E, Schumacher U. THIEME Atlas of Anatomy, Vol 1. Illustrations by Voll M and Wesker K. 3rd ed. New York: Thieme Publishers; 2020.)

- the **aa. perforantes I–III** (or IV), which supply the anterior, medial, and posterior muscles of the thigh.

— A **cruciate anastomosis** provides a collateral blood supply to structures around the hip. Contributions to the anastomosis include

- the a. circumflexa femoris medialis and lateralis,
- the a. perforans I, and
- the a. glutea inferior.

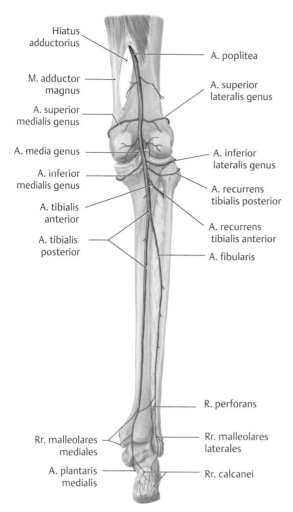

Hiatus adductorius

A. poplitea

M. adductor magnus

A. superior lateralis genus

A. superior medialis genus

A. media genus

A. inferior lateralis genus

A. inferior medialis genus

A. recurrens tibialis posterior

A. tibialis anterior

A. recurrens tibialis anterior

A. tibialis posterior

A. fibularis

R. perforans

Rr. malleolares mediales

Rr. malleolares laterales

A. plantaris medialis

Rr. calcanei

Fig. 21.8 Arteries of the knee and posterior leg
Right leg, posterior view. (From Schuenke M, Schulte E, Schumacher U. THIEME Atlas of Anatomy, Vol 1. Illustrations by Voll M and Wesker K. 3rd ed. New York: Thieme Publishers; 2020.)

BOX 21.3: CLINICAL CORRELATION

FEMORAL HEAD NECROSIS
Although the cruciate anastomosis surrounds the hip joint, only the a. circumflexa femoris medialis gives rise to branches that enter the capsule and supply the caput femoris. These end arteries are at risk during the dislocation or fracture of the collum femoris. Tearing of these vessels will result in avascular necrosis of the caput femoris.

— The **a. poplitea** is the continuation of the a. femoralis as it enters the **fossa poplitea,** a cavity posterior to the knee joint (**Fig. 21.8**).
  • Five **vv. geniculares** run medially and laterally around the knee.
  • **A. tibialis anterior** and **a. tibialis posterior,** the terminal branches of the a. poplitea, arise in the proximal part of the posterior leg compartment.
— A **genicular anastomosis (rete articulare genus)** that supplies the knee joint receives contributions from the a. media genus, a. inferior lateralis genus, a. superior lateralis genus, a. inferior medialis genus, and a. superior medialis genus;

BOX 21.4: CLINICAL CORRELATION

POPLITEAL ANEURYSM
Aneurysms of the a. poplitea are the most common peripheral arterial aneurysm. They can be distinguished by a thrill (palpable pulse) and bruits (abnormal arterial sounds) overlying the fossa poplitea. Because the artery lies deep to the n. tibialis, an aneurysm may stretch the nerve or occlude its blood supply. Pain from nerve compression is referred to the skin overlying the medial aspect of the calf, ankle, and foot. Half of all popliteal aneurysms remain asymptomatic, and ruptures are rare, but symptomatic patients present with distal leg ischemia from acute embolization or thrombosis. Fifty percent of patients with a popliteal aneurysm have an aneurysm in the contralateral artery, and 25% have an aortic aneurysm.

  • the a. descendens genus from the thigh;
  • the descending branch of the a. circumflexa femoris lateralis, and
  • the recurrent branches of a. tibialis anterior and a. tibialis posterior.
— The a. tibialis posterior descends into the deep posterior leg compartment to supply muscles in the deep and superficial posterior compartments (see **Fig. 21.8**). Its branches include
  • the **a. fibularis,** which arises in the upper leg and descends within the posterior leg compartment; and
  • the **a. plantaris medialis** and **a. plantaris lateralis,** which arise as the terminal branches posterior to the malleolus medialis (**Fig. 21.9**).
— The a. fibularis supplies muscles of the deep posterior compartment and, via small arteries that perforate the septum intermusculare, muscles of the lateral compartment. At the ankle it gives off
  • an **r. perforans** that arises at the ankle and anastomoses with the a. tibialis anterior and
  • **malleolar branches** that contribute to an anastomosis around the ankle.

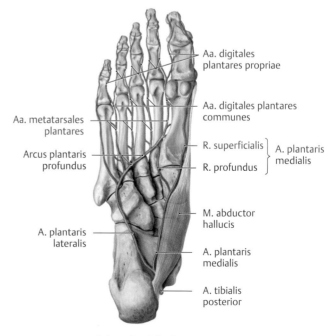

Aa. digitales plantares propriae

Aa. digitales plantares communes

Aa. metatarsales plantares

R. superficialis

Arcus plantaris profundus

R. profundus

A. plantaris medialis

M. abductor hallucis

A. plantaris lateralis

A. plantaris medialis

A. tibialis posterior

Fig. 21.9 Arteries of the sole of the foot
Right foot, plantar view. (From Schuenke M, Schulte E, Schumacher U. THIEME Atlas of Anatomy, Vol 1. Illustrations by Voll M and Wesker K. 3rd ed. New York: Thieme Publishers; 2020.)

— Arteries of the sole (**Fig. 21.9**) arise from the a. tibialis posterior and include
  • the **a. plantaris medialis,** a small branch of the a. tibialis posterior that supplies the medial part of the sole;
  • the **a. plantaris lateralis,** the largest branch of the a. tibialis posterior, which supplies the lateral side of the sole and curves medially to anastomose with the a. plantaris profunda;
  • an **arcus plantaris profundus,** which forms through the anastomosis of the a. plantaris profunda and a. plantaris lateralis; and
  • four **aa. metatarsales plantares,** which arise from the arcus plantaris profundus and their branches, the **aa. digitales plantares communes** and **aa. digitales plantares propriae,**
— The a. tibialis anterior passes through an opening in the membrana interossea cruris to supply muscles of the anterior leg compartment (**Fig. 21.10**). Its branches are
  • proximally, an **a. recurrens tibialis anterior** to the knee, and
  • distally, the **a. dorsalis pedis** as it emerges onto the back of the foot.
— Arteries of the back of the foot arise from the a. tibialis posterior and include
  • the **a. tarsalis lateralis** and **a. arcuata** which form a loop on the back of the foot;
  • the **a. plantaris profunda** which anastomoses with the a. plantaris lateralis on the sole; and
  • the **aa. metatarsales dorsales** and their branches, the **aa. digitales dorsales** which arise from the a. arcuata or the a. dorsalis pedis.

BOX 21.5: CLINICAL CORRELATION

THE DORSAL PEDAL PULSE

The a. dorsalis pedis is readily palpable on the dorsum of the foot as it runs toward the first web space lateral to the extensor hallucis tendon. Absence of the dorsal pedal pulse suggests arterial occlusion in the peripheral vasculature.

BOX 21.6: CLINICAL CORRELATION

LOWER LIMB ISCHEMIA

Ischemia of the lower extremity is almost always related to atherosclerotic disease. Intermittent claudication is a symptom of chronic ischemic disease characterized by pain while walking, which intensifies over time and disappears at rest. Chronic disease has a benign course and, in the majority of patients, is treated conservatively. Acute ischemia has an abrupt onset from an embolitic or thrombolytic origin and usually requires aggressive treatment. The six signs (P signs) of acute ischemia are pain, pallor, pulselessness, paresthesia, paralysis, and poikilothermy.

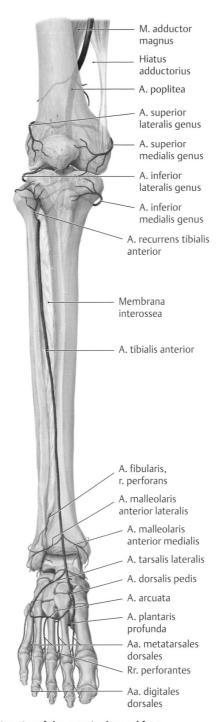

M. adductor magnus
Hiatus adductorius
A. poplitea
A. superior lateralis genus
A. superior medialis genus
A. inferior lateralis genus
A. inferior medialis genus
A. recurrens tibialis anterior
Membrana interossea
A. tibialis anterior
A. fibularis, r. perforans
A. malleolaris anterior lateralis
A. malleolaris anterior medialis
A. tarsalis lateralis
A. dorsalis pedis
A. arcuata
A. plantaris profunda
Aa. metatarsales dorsales
Rr. perforantes
Aa. digitales dorsales

Fig. 21.10 Arteries of the anterior leg and foot
Right leg, anterior view. (From Schuenke M, Schulte E, Schumacher U. THIEME Atlas of Anatomy, Vol 1. Illustrations by Voll M and Wesker K. 3rd ed. New York: Thieme Publishers; 2020.)

Veins of the Lower Limb

The lower limb has both deep and superficial venous drainages, which anastomose through vv. perforantes. Veins of both systems have numerous valves along their length.
— Veins of the deep venous system travel with the major arteries and their branches and have similar names. As in the upper limb, these deep veins usually occur as paired accompanying veins in the distal part of the limb (**Fig. 21.11**).
  • The **v. femoralis,** which drains the deep and superficial veins of the thigh and leg, passes under the lig. inguinale into the abdomen, where it becomes the v. iliaca externa.

  • **V. glutea superior** and **v. glutea inferior,** which drain the regio glutealis, pass through the foramen ischiadicum majus to empty into the v. iliaca interna of the pelvis.
— Superficial veins are located in the subcutaneous tissue and normally drain, via vv. perforantes, to the deep venous system (**Fig. 21.12**).
  • The largest superficial veins, the **v. saphena magna** and **v. saphena parva,** originate at the **arcus venosus dorsalis** on the dorsum of the foot.

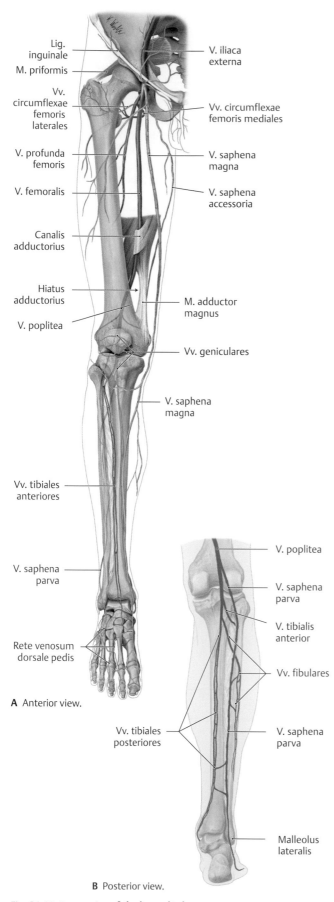

Lig. inguinale

M. priformis

Vv. circumflexae femoris laterales

V. profunda femoris

V. femoralis

Canalis adductorius

Hiatus adductorius

V. poplitea

Vv. tibiales anteriores

V. saphena parva

Rete venosum dorsale pedis

V. iliaca externa

Vv. circumflexae femoris mediales

V. saphena magna

V. saphena accessoria

M. adductor magnus

Vv. geniculares

V. saphena magna

A Anterior view.

V. poplitea

V. saphena parva

V. tibialis anterior

Vv. fibulares

Vv. tibiales posteriores

V. saphena parva

Malleolus lateralis

B Posterior view.

Fig. 21.11 Deep veins of the lower limb
Right limb. (From Schuenke M, Schulte E, Schumacher U. THIEME Atlas of Anatomy, Vol 1. Illustrations by Voll M and Wesker K. 3rd ed. New York: Thieme Publishers; 2020.)

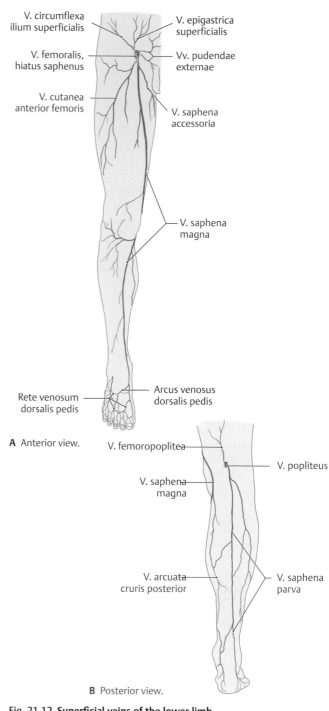

V. circumflexa ilium superficialis

V. femoralis, hiatus saphenus

V. cutanea anterior femoris

V. epigastrica superficialis

Vv. pudendae externae

V. saphena accessoria

V. saphena magna

Rete venosum dorsalis pedis

Arcus venosus dorsalis pedis

A Anterior view.

V. femoropoplitea

V. saphena magna

V. arcuata cruris posterior

V. popliteus

V. saphena parva

B Posterior view.

Fig. 21.12 Superficial veins of the lower limb
Right limb. (From Schuenke M, Schulte E, Schumacher U. THIEME Atlas of Anatomy, Vol 1. Illustrations by Voll M and Wesker K. 3rd ed. New York: Thieme Publishers; 2020.)

BOX 21.7: CLINICAL CORRELATION

DEEP VEIN THROMBOSES (DVT)
Thromboses (blood clots) in the deep veins of the leg result from stasis, the slowing or pooling of blood. This can result from prolonged inactivity (extended airplane travel, immobilization following surgery) or anatomic abnormalities such as laxity of the crural fascia. Thrombi from the legs can break off and travel to the heart and lungs, lodging in the pulmonary arterial tree as pulmonary emboli. Large clots can severely impair lung function and even cause death. Thrombophlebitis is the inflammation of a vein caused by thrombosis.

VARICOSE VEINS

Varicose disease of the vv. superficiales of the lower limb is the most common chronic venous disease, affecting 15% of the adult population. Primary varices generally result from degeneration of the wall of the vein leading to dilated, tortuous vessels and incompetent venous valves. Secondary varices can develop from chronic occlusion of the deep veins with incompetence of the perforator veins. This causes a reversal of flow through the vv. perforantes. (Normal venous drainage flows from superficial to deep systems.) As the vv. superficiales dilate with increased volume, valve leaflets separate and become incompetent.

- The v. saphena magna arises from the medial side of the arcus venosus and passes superiorly, anterior to the malleolus medialis and posteromedial to the knee. It drains into the v. femoralis at the **hiatus saphenus,** an opening in the fascia lata in the upper thigh.
- The v. saphena parva arises from the lateral side of the arcus venosus, passes posterior to the malleolus lateralis, and ascends the posterior leg. It drains into the **v. poplitea** behind the knee.
— The flow of blood from lower parts of the body must counter the downward force of gravity. In the lower limbs, venous return is assisted by

- the presence of valves in the veins,
- the pulsing of accompanying arteries, and
- the contraction of surrounding muscles.

Lymphatics of the Lower Limb

Lymph from the lower limb drains superiorly from the foot following the vv. profundae and vv. superficiales. Upward flow is facilitated by the contraction of surrounding muscles (**Fig. 21.13**).
— Lymph from deep tissues of the
  - regio glutealis drains along the gluteal vessels to nll. iliaci interni.
  - thigh drains to nll. inguinales profundi.
— Lymph from superficial tissues of the regio glutealis and thigh drains to nll. inguinales superficiales.
— Lymph from the dorsum and sole of the lateral foot and lateral leg drains along the v. saphena parva to the **nll. poplitei profundi** at the knee. These drain directly to nll. inguinales profundi.
— Lymph from the dorsum and sole of the medial foot and the medial leg drains along the v. saphena magna to nll. inguinales superficiales.
— Lymph from the thigh drains first to nll. inguinales superficiales, which in turn drain to nll. inguinales profundi.
— Nll. inguinales profundi drain sequentially to nll. iliaci externi, nll. iliaci communes, and nll. lumbales.

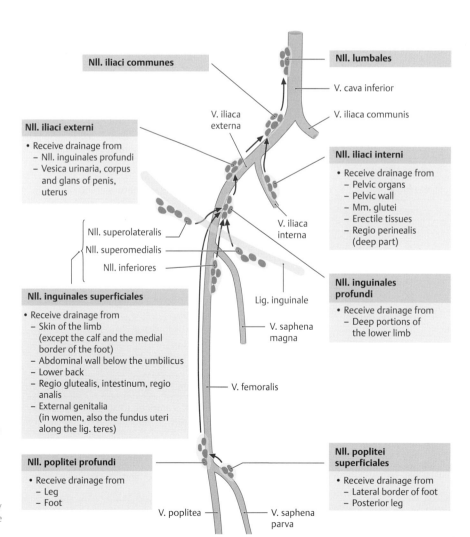

Fig. 21.13 Lymph nodes and drainage of the lower limbs
Right limb, anterior view. *Arrows*: direction of lymphatic drainage; *yellow shading*: superficial nodes; *green shading*: deep nodes.
(From Schuenke M, Schulte E, Schumacher U. THIEME Atlas of Anatomy, Vol 1. Illustrations by Voll M and Wesker K. 3rd ed. New York: Thieme Publishers; 2020.)

Nll. iliaci communes

Nll. lumbales

V. cava inferior

V. iliaca externa

V. iliaca communis

Nll. iliaci externi

- Receive drainage from
  - Nll. inguinales profundi
  - Vesica urinaria, corpus and glans of penis, uterus

Nll. iliaci interni

- Receive drainage from
  - Pelvic organs
  - Pelvic wall
  - Mm. glutei
  - Erectile tissues
  - Regio perinealis (deep part)

Nll. superolateralis

Nll. superomedialis

Nll. inferiores

V. iliaca interna

Nll. inguinales profundi

- Receive drainage from
  - Deep portions of the lower limb

Nll. inguinales superficiales

- Receive drainage from
  - Skin of the limb (except the calf and the medial border of the foot)
  - Abdominal wall below the umbilicus
  - Lower back
  - Regio glutealis, intestinum, regio analis
  - External genitalia (in women, also the fundus uteri along the lig. teres)

Lig. inguinale

V. saphena magna

V. femoralis

Nll. poplitei profundi

- Receive drainage from
  - Leg
  - Foot

Nll. poplitei superficiales

- Receive drainage from
  - Lateral border of foot
  - Posterior leg

V. poplitea

V. saphena parva

Nerves of the Lower Limb: Plexus Lumbosacralis

The plexus lumbalis and sacralis, often combined as the **plexus lumbosacralis,** innervate the lower limb (**Table 21.1; Figs. 21.14, 21.15, 21.16, 21.17**).

Nerves of the plexus lumbalis enter the limb anteriorly to supply muscles of the anterior and medial thigh.

— The **n. iliohypogastricus** (L1), **r. genitalis of n. genitofemoralis** (L1–L2), and **n. ilioinguinalis** (L1) are primarily nerves of the anterior abdominal wall and regio inguinalis. They also innervate small areas of skin over the upper lateral, anterior, and medial thigh, respectively.

— The **n. cutaneus femoris lateralis** (L2–L3), a sensory nerve that enters the lateral thigh anteromedial to the spina iliaca anterior superior, innervates skin of the lateral thigh.

— The **n. femoralis** enters the anterior thigh through the spatium retroinguinale (deep to the lig. inguinale), lateral to the a. femoralis.
  • It innervates muscles of the anterior compartment.
  • The **n. saphenus** is a sensory nerve that descends inferiorly to innervate the skin of the medial leg and foot.

BOX 21.9: CLINICAL CORRELATION

FEMORAL NERVE INJURY

Injuries of the n. femoralis can result in the following:
— Weakened flexion of the hip
— Loss of knee extension
— Loss of sensation on the anterior and medial thigh and medial side of the leg and foot
— Instability of the knee

Table 21.1 Nerves of the Lower Limb

Nerve	Level	Area of Innervation
Plexus lumbalis		
N. iliohypogastricus	L1	Skin over upper regio femoris lateralis and regio inguinalis
N. ilioinguinalis	L1	Skin over upper regio femoris anterior
N. genitofemoralis	L1, L2	Skin over upper regio femoris
N. cutaneus femoralis lateralis	L2, L3	Skin of regio femoris lateralis
N. femoralis	L2–L4	M. iliopsoas, m. pectineus, m. sartorius, m. quadriceps femoris
—N. cutaneus anterior		Skin of regio femoris anterior and medialis
—N. saphenus		Skin of regio cruris medialis and foot
N. obturatorius	L2–L4	M. obturatorius externus, m. adductor longus, m. adductor brevis, m. adductor magnus, m. gracilis, m. pectineus; skin of regio femoris medialis
Plexus sacralis		
N. gluteus superior	L4–S1	M. gluteus medius, m. gluteus minimus, m. tensor fascia latae
N. gluteus inferior	L5–S2	M. gluteus maximus
Direct branches	L5–S2	M. piriformis, m. obturator internus, mm. gemelli, m. quadratus femoris
N. cutaneus femoris posterior	S1–S3	Skin of regio femoris posterior and regio glutealis inferior
N. tibialis	L4–S3	M. biceps femoris (caput longum), m. semimembranosus, m. semitendinosus, m. adductor magnus (medial part), m. gastrocnemius, m. soleus, m. popliteus, m. tibialis posterior, m. flexor digitorum longus, m. flexor hallucis longus
—N. plantaris medialis		M. abductor hallucis, m. flexor digitorum brevis, m. flexor hallucis brevis (caput mediale), m. lumbricalis I, skin of medial sole, digiti I–III, and half of digitus IV
—N. plantaris lateralis		M. quadratus plantae, m. flexor hallucis brevis (caput laterale), m. abductor digiti minimi, m. flexor digiti minimi brevis, mm. interossei, mm. lumbricales II–IV, m. adductor hallucis, skin of lateral sole, digitus V, and half of digitus IV
N. fibularis communis	L4–S2	M. biceps femoris (caput breve)
—N. fibularis superficialis		M. fibularis longus and brevis; skin of dorsum pedis
—N. fibularis profundus		M. tibialis anterior, m. extensor hallucis longus and brevis, m. extensor digitorum longus and brevis, m. fibularis tertius; skin of web space between digitus I and II
N. pudendus	S2–S4	M. sphincter ani externus, m. transversus perinei profundus, m. transversus perinei superficialis, rr. cutanei to scrotum and labia, sensory to penis and clitoris (see Section 10.6)
N. suralis (n. tibialis and n. fibularis communis contributions)	S1	Skin of posterior and lateral leg and lateral foot

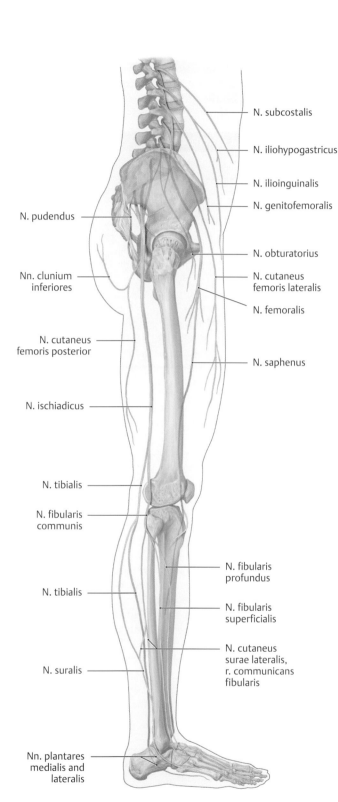

Fig. 21.14 Plexus lumbosacralis
Right side, lateral view. (From Schuenke M, Schulte E, Schumacher U.
THIEME Atlas of Anatomy, Vol 1. Illustrations by Voll M and Wesker K. 3rd
ed. New York: Thieme Publishers; 2020.)

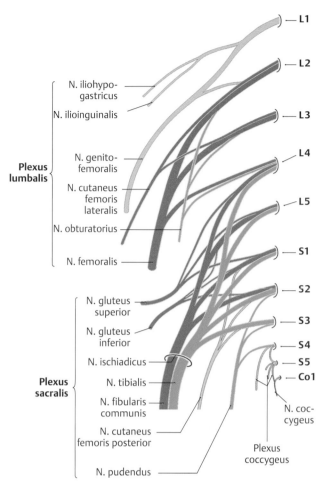

Fig. 21.15 Structure of the plexus lumbosacralis
Right side, anterior view. (From Gilroy AM et al. Atlas of Anatomy. 4th ed.
2020. Based on: Schuenke M, Schulte E, Schumacher U. THIEME Atlas of
Anatomy. General Anatomy and Musculoskeletal System. Illustrations by
Voll M and Wesker K. 3rd ed. New York: Thieme Medical Publishers; 2020.)

— The **n. obturatorius** (L2–L4) enters the medial thigh through
the foramen obturatum and innervates muscles of the medial
compartment.

BOX 21.10: CLINICAL CORRELATION

OBTURATOR NERVE INJURY
Injury to the n. obturatorius is most commonly associated with
pelvic surgery or pelvic fractures and results in the following:
— Weakened adduction of the hip (e.g., inability to move the leg
from the gas pedal to the brake)
— Weakened external rotation of the hip
— Loss of sensation over a palm-size area on the medial side of
the thigh
— Instability of the pelvis; lateral swing of the limb with
locomotion

The plexus sacralis supplies muscles of the regio glutealis, posterior thigh, and all muscular compartments of the leg and foot. Its
branches enter the lower limb through the foramen ischiadicum
majus in the regio glutealis.

BOX 21.11: CLINICAL CORRELATION

SUPERIOR GLUTEAL NERVE INJURY

When one foot is lifted off the floor, as happens during the gait cycle, abduction of the hip by the contralateral m. gluteus medius and m. gluteus minimus muscles (the supported side) stabilizes the pelvis in the horizontal position. With injury to the n. gluteus superior, the loss or weakness of abduction on that side allows the pelvis on the opposite (unsupported) side to sag. This results in a characteristic Duchenne's limp in which the weight of the trunk is shifted toward the nerve-damaged side to maintain the center of gravity.

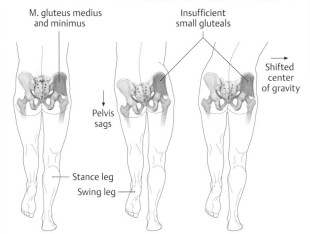

Small gluteal muscle weakness
(From Schuenke M, Schulte E, Schumacher U. THIEME Atlas of Anatomy, Vol 1. Illustrations by Voll M and Wesker K. 3rd ed. New York: Thieme Publishers; 2020.)

—   The **n. gluteus superior** (L4–S1) enters the regio glutealis above the m. piriformis and runs laterally between the deep gluteal muscles. It supplies the abductors of the art. coxae in the regio glutealis.

—   The **n. gluteus inferior** (L5–S2) enters the regio glutealis inferior to the m. piriformis and innervates the large m. gluteus maximus.

—   The **n. cutaneus femoris posterior** (L1–S3) is sensory to the thigh and posterior perineum. Its **nn. clunium inferiores** supply the inferior gluteal region.

—   The **n. ischiadicus** is made up of the **n. tibialis** (L4–S3) and **n. fibularis communis** (L4–S2), which are bound together in a common sheath along their course in the posterior thigh. The two nerves diverge at the apex of the fossa poplitea.

BOX 21.12: CLINICAL CORRELATION

SCIATIC NERVE INJURY

The n. ischiadicus can be injured by compression by the m. piriformis, misplaced intramuscular injections in the regio glutealis, pelvic fractures, or surgical procedures such as hip replacements. An injury in the regio glutealis would affect muscles of the posterior thigh and all muscular compartments of the leg, the combined effects of damage to the n. tibialis and n. fibularis communis.

—   The n. tibialis, the larger branch of the n. ischiadicus, separates from the n. fibularis communis and continues

inferiorly through the fossa poplitea into the deep posterior leg compartment.
•   It innervates all of the muscles of the posterior thigh (except the caput breve of the m. biceps femoris) and the posterior leg.
•   At the ankle, it passes posterior to the malleolus medialis, where it terminates as the **n. plantaris medialis** and **n. plantaris lateralis.**

BOX 21.13: CLINICAL CORRELATION

TIBIAL NERVE INJURY

Tibial nerve injury is unusual because the nerve is well protected in the thigh and posterior leg. Injury in the regio glutealis results in the following:
—   Impaired extension of the hip
—   Loss of flexion of the knee
In the fossa poplitea, it can be affected by aneurysms of the a. poplitea and knee trauma. These can cause the following:
—   Loss of plantar flexion at the ankle
—   Loss of plantar flexion, abduction, and adduction of the digits
—   Weakened inversion of the foot
—   Loss of sensation on the posterolateral leg to the malleolus lateralis, the sole and lateral side of the foot
—   A shuffling gait with clawing of the toes

—   The n. plantaris medialis, comparable to the n. medianus of the hand with small motor and large sensory components, is the largest branch of the n. tibialis.
•   It innervates plantar muscles on the medial side of the foot.
•   A superficial branch supplies a large area of skin on the medial side of the foot and the medial three and a half digits. It terminates as three **nn. digitales plantares.**
—   The n. plantaris lateralis, the smaller branch of the n. tibialis, is comparable to the n. ulnaris of the hand.
•   It innervates the lateral plantar muscles and most deep muscles of the foot.
•   It innervates skin on the lateral sole and lateral one and a half digits and terminates as two **nn. digitales plantares.**
—   The n. fibularis communis separates from the n. tibialis and, hugging the border of the m. biceps femoris, passes laterally around the caput fibulae where it enters the lateral leg compartment.
•   In the thigh, it innervates the caput breve of the m. biceps femoris.
•   In the lateral leg compartment, it splits into its terminal branches, the **n. fibularis superificialis** and **n. fibularis profundus.**

BOX 21.14: CLINICAL CORRELATION

COMMON FIBULAR NERVE INJURY

The n. fibularis communis is the most vulnerable of the peripheral nerves due to its exposed location around the collum fibulae. Injuries result in the following:
—   Loss of eversion of the foot
—   Loss of dorsiflexion at the ankle and digits
—   Weakened inversion of the foot
—   Loss of sensation over the lateral leg and dorsum of the foot
—   Footdrop compensated by a high-stepping gait; instability on uneven surfaces

- The n. fibularis superficialis innervates the muscles in the lateral leg compartment. At the midleg, its sensory component pierces the fascia cruralis and runs onto the dorsum of the foot.
- From its division from the n. fibularis superficialis, the n.
- fibularis profundus circles anteriorly to enter the anterior leg compartment. It descends along the membrana interossea, innervating all muscles of the compartment. It emerges onto the foot with the a. dorsalis pedis to innervate the skin on adjacent surfaces of the 1st and 2nd digits.

BOX 21.15: CLINICAL CORRELATION

SUPERFICIAL AND DEEP FIBULAR NERVE INJURY

Injury to the n. fibularis superficialis only affects eversion of the foot and sensation over the lateral leg and most of the dorsum of the foot. Injury to the n. fibularis profundus has greater functional consequences, including the loss of all dorsiflexion. This results in footdrop and the compensating high-stepping gait.

- The **n. suralis** (S1), formed by communicating branches of the n. tibialis and n. fibularis communis on the surface of the posterior leg, runs posterior to the malleolus lateralis at the ankle to innervate the skin of the lateral foot.

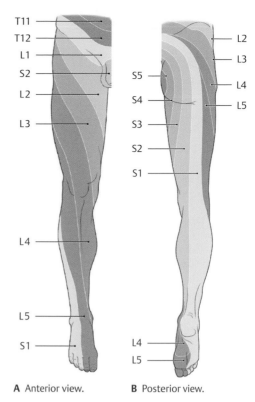

A Anterior view.   **B** Posterior view.

Fig. 21.17 Dermatomes of the lower limb
Right limb. (From Schuenke M, Schulte E, Schumacher U. THIEME Atlas of Anatomy, Vol 1. Illustrations by Voll M and Wesker K. 3rd ed. New York: Thieme Publishers; 2020.)

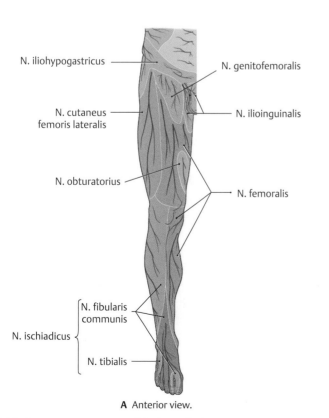

A Anterior view.

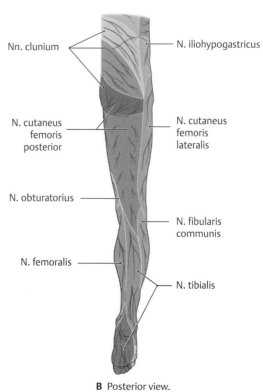

B Posterior view.

Fig. 21.16 Cutaneous innervation of the lower limb
Right limb. (From Schuenke M, Schulte E, Schumacher U. THIEME Atlas of Anatomy, Vol 1. Illustrations by Voll M and Wesker K. 3rd ed. New York: Thieme Publishers; 2020.)

22 Functional Anatomy of the Lower Limb

The strong muscles and joints of the lower limb are adapted for bipedal locomotion and, in conjunction with the muscles of the trunk, maintain the body's center of gravity.

Schematics of lower limb muscles accompany the muscle tables (origin, attachment, innervation, and action) in the appropriate chapter sections. To see the muscles in situ, view the gallery of topographic images in Section 22.9 at the end of the chapter.

22.1 The Pelvic Girdle

The ossa coxae and the os sacrum form the pelvic girdle (cingulum pelvicum, bony pelvis), which is related anatomically and functionally to the pelvis and the lower limb (**Fig. 22.1**). (See Section 14.2 for a discussion of the pelvic girdle.)

— Articulations at the art. sacroiliaca and symphysis pubica, supported by strong ligg. sacroiliacum, sacrotuberale, and sacrospinale, create a stable framework that
  • supports and encloses the viscera pelvis,
  • transfers the weight of the trunk to the lower limb, and
  • forms part of the art. coxae and provides attachment sites for lower limb muscles.

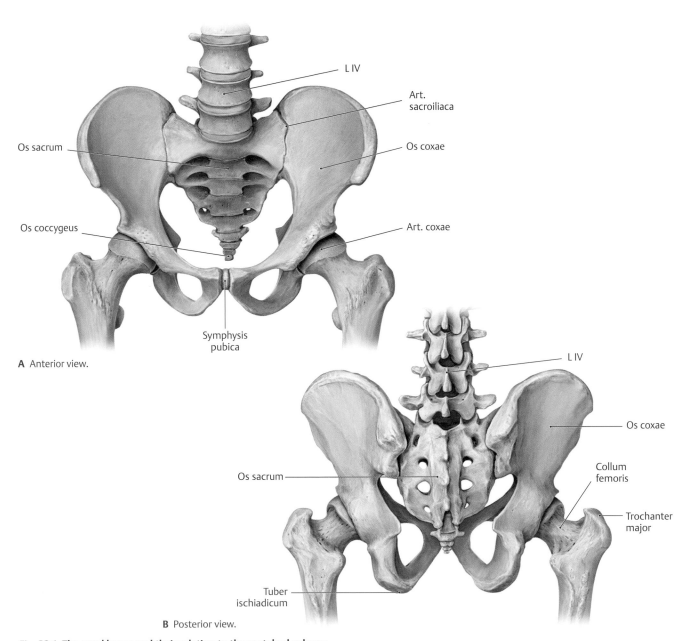

A Anterior view.

B Posterior view.

Fig. 22.1 The coxal bones and their relation to the vertebral column
(From Gilroy AM et al. Atlas of Anatomy. 4th ed. 2020. Based on: Schuenke M, Schulte E, Schumacher U. THIEME Atlas of Anatomy. General Anatomy and Musculoskeletal System. Illustrations by Voll M and Wesker K. 3rd ed. New York: Thieme Medical Publishers; 2020.)

22.2 The Gluteal Region (Regio Glutealis)

The gluteal region (regio glutealis) includes the buttock, which overlies the posterior part of the pelvic girdle, and the lateral hip region, which covers the art. coxae and extends as far anteriorly as the spina iliaca anterior superior.

— The muscular compartment of the regio glutealis contains
- muscles that laterally rotate, abduct, adduct, extend, and flex the art. coxae (**Table 22.1**);
- the n. gluteus superior, n. gluteus inferior, and n. ischiadicus; and
- the a. glutea superior and v. glutea superior and a. glutea inferior and v. glutea inferior.

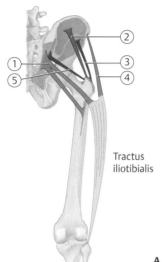

Tractus iliotibialis

A Vertically oriented gluteal muscles, right side, posterior view.

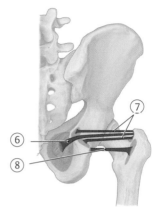

B Horizontally oriented gluteal muscles, right side, posterior view.

(From Schuenke M, Schulte E, Schumacher U. THIEME Atlas of Anatomy, Vol 1. Illustrations by Voll M and Wesker K. 3rd ed. New York: Thieme Publishers; 2020.)

Table 22.1 Gluteal Muscles

Muscle	Origin	Insertion	Innervation	Action
① M. gluteus maximus	Os sacrum (dorsal surface, lateral part), os ilium (gluteal surface, pars posterior), fascia thoracolumbalis, lig. sacrotuberale	• Upper fibers: tractus iliotibialis • Lower fibers: tuberositas glutea	N. gluteus inferior (L5–S2)	• Entire muscle: extends and externally rotates the hip in sagittal and coronal planes • Upper fibers: abduction • Lower fibers: adduction
② M. gluteus medius	Os ilium (gluteal surface below the crista iliaca between the lineae gluteae anterior and posterior)	Trochanter major of the femur (lateral surface)	N. gluteus superior (L4–S1)	• Entire muscle: abducts the hip, stabilizes the pelvis in the coronal plane
③ M. gluteus minimuss	Os ilium (gluteal surface below the origin of the m. gluteus medius)	Trochanter major of the femur (anterolateral surface)		• Anterior part: flexion and internal rotation • Posterior part: extension and external rotation
④ M. tensor fasciae latae	Spina iliaca anterior superior	Tractus iliotibialis		• Tenses the fascia lata • Art. coxae: abduction, flexion, and internal rotation
⑤ M. piriformis	Facies pelvica of os sacrum	Apex of the trochanter major of the femur	Direct branches from the plexus sacralis (S1–S2)	• External rotation, abduction, and extension of the art. coxae • Stabilizes the art. coxae
⑥ M. obturatorius internus	Inner surface of the membrana obturatoria and its bony boundaries	Medial surface of the trochanter major	Direct branches from the plexus sacralis (L5–S1)	External rotation, adduction, and extension of the art. coxae (also active in abduction, depending on the joint's position)
⑦ Mm. gemelli	• M. gemellus superior: spina ischiadica • M. gemellus inferior: tuber ischiadicum	Jointly with m. obturatorius internus tendo (medial surface, trochanter major)		
⑧ M. quadratus femoris	Lateral border of the tuber ischiadicum	Crista intertrochanterica of the femur		External rotation and adduction of the art. coxae

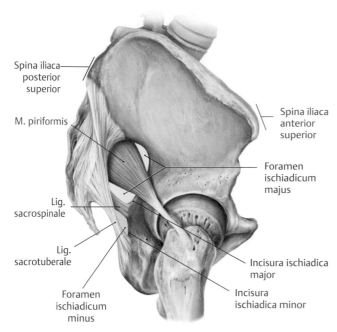

Spina iliaca posterior superior

M. piriformis

Lig. sacrospinale

Lig. sacrotuberale

Foramen ischiadicum minus

Spina iliaca anterior superior

Foramen ischiadicum majus

Incisura ischiadica major

Incisura ischiadica minor

Fig. 22.2 Foramina ischiadica
Right gluteal region. (From Schuenke M, Schulte E, Schumacher U. THIEME Atlas of Anatomy, Vol 1. Illustrations by Voll M and Wesker K. 3rd ed. New York: Thieme Publishers; 2020.)

BOX 22.1: CLINICAL CORRELATION

PIRIFORMIS SYNDROME
The n. ischiadicus normally passes into the regio glutealis inferior to the m. piriformis. Tightening or shortening of the muscle can compress and irritate the n. ischiadicus, causing pain and paresthesia (tingling and numbness) in the buttocks and posterior thigh. In some cases the n. ischiadicus, or its common fibular component, is compressed as it passes through the muscle rather than inferior to it. Piriformis syndrome should be distinguished from sciatica in which the pain and paresthesia result from compression of lumbar nerve roots by a herniated discus intervertebralis.

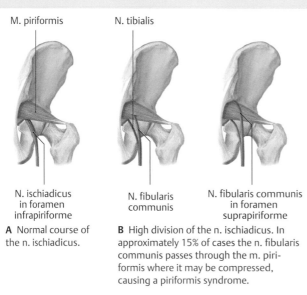

M. piriformis

N. tibialis

N. ischiadicus in foramen infrapiriforme

N. fibularis communis

N. fibularis communis in foramen suprapiriforme

A Normal course of the n. ischiadicus.

B High division of the n. ischiadicus. In approximately 15% of cases the n. fibularis communis passes through the m. piriformis where it may be compressed, causing a piriformis syndrome.

Variable course of the n. ischiadicus in the regio glutealis
(From Rauber A, Kopsch F. Anatomie des Menschen. Bd. 1-4. Stuttgart: Thieme Publishers; Bd. 1. 2nd ed. 1997; Bde. 2 u. 3 1987: Bd. 4 1988)

— Posteriorly, structures pass between the pelvis and the regio glutealis through the foramen ischiadicum majus (**Fig. 22.2**). These structures include
  - the m. piriformis,
  - the a. glutea superior and v. glutea superior and a. glutea inferior and v. glutea inferior,
  - the n. gluteus superior and n. gluteus inferior,
  - the n. ischiadicus,
  - the n. pudendus and a. pudenda interna and v. pudenda interna, and
  - the n. cutaneus femoris posterior.
— The foramen ischiadicum minus, a passageway between the regio glutealis and perineum, transmits
  - the a. pudenda interna and v. pudenda interna,
  - the n. pudendus, and
  - the tendon of the m. obturatorius internus.

22.3　The Hip and Thigh

The Hip Joint (Art. Coxae)

The **hip joint (art. coxae)** is a highly mobile, yet stable, ball-and-socket joint between the proximal femur and the acetabulum of the os coxae (**Figs. 22.3** and **22.4**). Muscles crossing the joint, particularly in the regio glutealis, provide additional stability as well as mobility.
— More than half of the large caput femoris is seated in the bony acetabulum of the os coxae, which is oriented slightly anteriorly and inferiorly.
— The axis through the neck of the femur is laterally rotated with respect to the condylar axis of the distal femur; thus, when the caput femoris is centered in the art. coxae, the distal femur and art. genus are directed slightly inward (**Figs. 22.5** and **22.6**).
— A strong capsula fibrosa surrounds the art. coxae (**Fig. 22.7**).
  - **Lig. iliofemorale**, **lig. pubofemorale**, and **lig. ischiofemorale** are extracapsular ligaments that strengthen the capsule. The lig. iliofemorale is the strongest and most supportive of these. The ligaments are arranged in a spiral around the joint. When the hip is extended, the spiral tightens, pushing the femoral head more firmly into the acetabulum and further stabilizing the joint. In hip flexion, the spiral unwinds, allowing a greater degree of joint mobility as well as vulnerability (**Fig. 22.8**).
— A fibrocartilaginous **labrum acetabuli** attached to the limbus acetabuli deepens the joint (**Fig. 22.9**).
— A weak **lig. capitis femoris** attaches to the acetabulum within the joint space but provides little support.
— Inferiorly, a **lig. transversum acetabuli** completes the circle of the C-shaped labrum acetabuli.
— Muscles of the regio glutealis and thigh move the art. coxae (**Table 22.2**).

BOX 22.2: CLINICAL CORRELATION

CONGENITAL HIP DISLOCATION
Congenital hip dislocation (also known as hip dysplasia) is a common problem that occurs when the caput femoris is not properly seated in the acetabulum. Hip abduction is impaired, and since the caput femoris sits higher than normal, the affected limb is shorter than the contralateral limb. In routine neonatal screenings, a dislocated hip will "click" when it is adducted and pushed posteriorly.

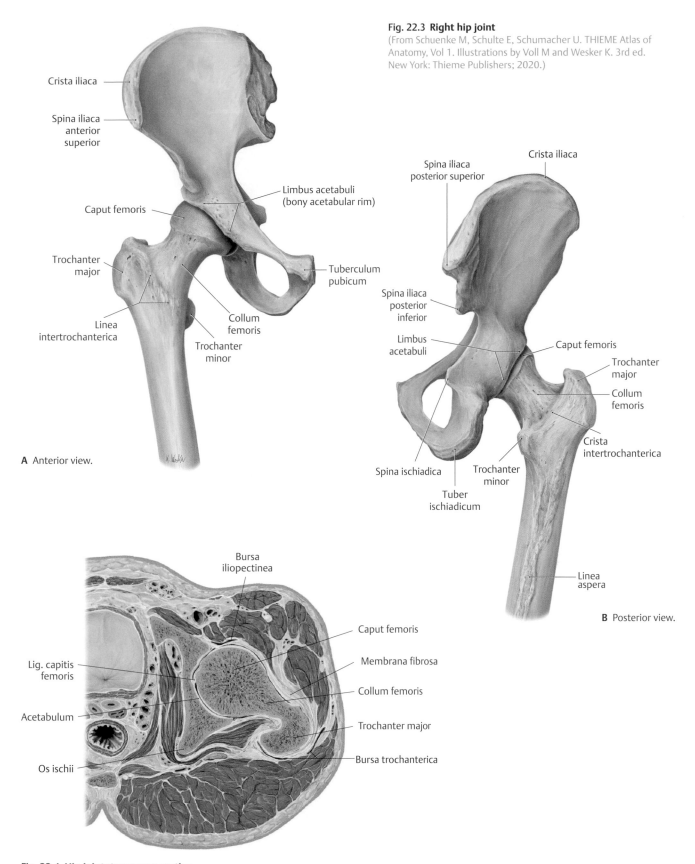

Fig. 22.3 Right hip joint
(From Schuenke M, Schulte E, Schumacher U. THIEME Atlas of Anatomy, Vol 1. Illustrations by Voll M and Wesker K. 3rd ed. New York: Thieme Publishers; 2020.)

A Anterior view.

B Posterior view.

Fig. 22.4 Hip joint: transverse section
Right hip joint, superior view. (From Schuenke M, Schulte E, Schumacher U. THIEME Atlas of Anatomy, Vol 1. Illustrations by Voll M and Wesker K. 3rd ed. New York: Thieme Publishers; 2020.)

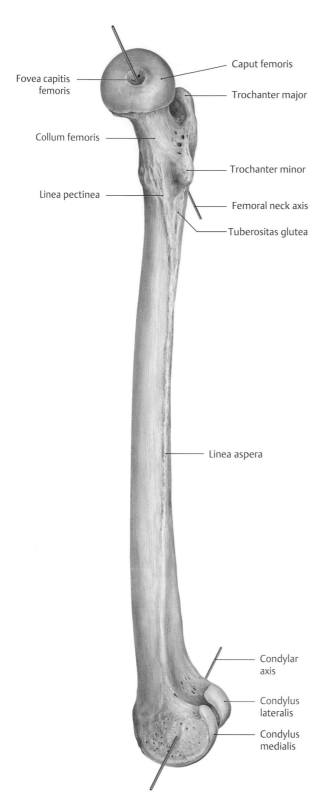

Fig. 22.5 Proximal and distal axes of rotation of the femur
Right femur. (From Schuenke M, Schulte E, Schumacher U. THIEME Atlas of Anatomy, Vol 1. Illustrations by Voll M and Wesker K. 3rd ed. New York: Thieme Publishers; 2020.)

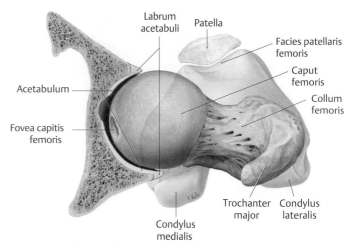

A Hip joint with caput femoris centered in the acetabulum.

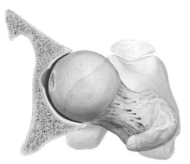

B Hip joint in external rotation.

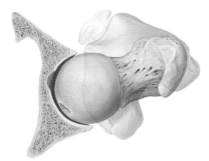

C Hip joint in internal rotation.

Fig. 22.6 Orientation of the hip joint relative to the knee joint
(From Schuenke M, Schulte E, Schumacher U. THIEME Atlas of Anatomy, Vol 1. Illustrations by Voll M and Wesker K. 3rd ed. New York: Thieme Publishers; 2020.)

BOX 22.3: CLINICAL CORRELATION

ACQUIRED HIP DISLOCATION
Acquired hip dislocation usually occurs as a result of trauma that causes the caput femoris to be displaced out of the acetabulum; anterior dislocations are rare, but posterior dislocations are common. Typically, in a head-on motor vehicle accident, the knees strike the dashboard, forcing the caput femoris posteriorly through the joint capsule and onto the lateral surface of the os ilium. The affected limb appears shortened, adducted, and internally rotated. The n. ischiadicus is particularly vulnerable to injury in these cases.

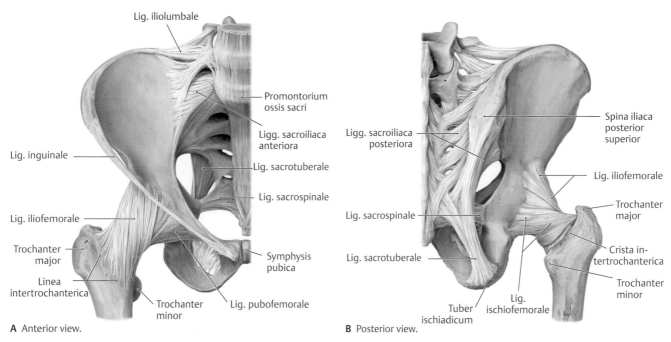

A Anterior view.

B Posterior view.

Fig. 22.7 Ligaments of the hip joint and pelvic girdle
(From Schuenke M, Schulte E, Schumacher U. THIEME Atlas of Anatomy, Vol 1. Illustrations by Voll M and Wesker K. 3rd ed. New York: Thieme Publishers; 2020.)

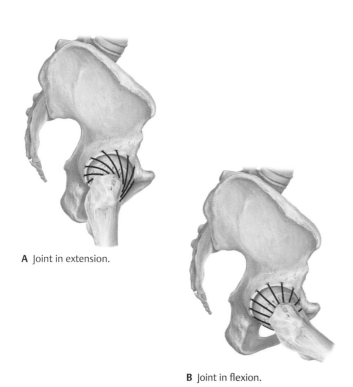

A Joint in extension.

B Joint in flexion.

Fig. 22.8 Hip ligaments as a function of joint position
Right hip, lateral view. (From Schuenke M, Schulte E, Schumacher U. THIEME Atlas of Anatomy, Vol 1. Illustrations by Voll M and Wesker K. 3rd ed. New York: Thieme Publishers; 2020.)

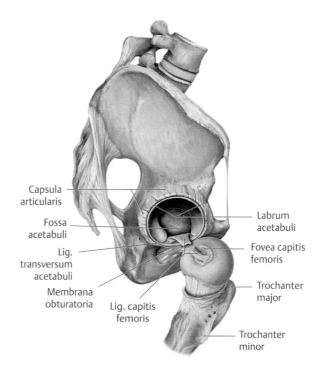

Fig. 22.9 Joint capsule of the hip joint
Lateral view. The capsule has been divided and the caput femoris dislocated to expose the cut lig. capitis femoris. (From Schuenke M, Schulte E, Schumacher U. THIEME Atlas of Anatomy, Vol 1. Illustrations by Voll M and Wesker K. 3rd ed. New York: Thieme Publishers; 2020.)

Table 22.2 Movements of the Hip Joint

Action	Primary Muscles
Flexion	M. iliopsoas
	M. tensor fascia latae
	M. sartorius
	M. rectus femoris
Extension	M. gluteus maximus
	M. adductor magnus
	M. biceps femoris, caput longus
	M. semimembranosus
	M. semitendinosus
Abduction	M. gluteus medius
	M. gluteus minimus
	M. tensor fascia latae
Adduction	M. gluteus maximus
	M. pectineus
	M. adductor longus
	M. adductor brevis
	M. adductor magnus
Internal rotation	M. gracilis
	M. gluteus medius
	M. gluteus minimus
	M. tensor fascia latae
External rotation	M. gluteus maximus
	M. pectineus
	M. sartorius
	M. quadratus femoris
	M. piriformis
	M. obturatorius externus
	M. obturatorius internus

A Flexion.

B Extension.

C Abduction.

D Adduction.   **E** Internal rotation.   **F** External rotation.

(From Schuenke M, Schulte E, Schumacher U. THIEME Atlas of Anatomy, Vol 1. Illustrations by Voll M and Wesker K. 3rd ed. New York: Thieme Publishers; 2020.)

Muscles of the Thigh

The powerful muscles of the thigh move the art. coxae and art. genus and are separated into three compartments (see **Fig. 22.45A**).
— The anterior compartment contains
  • muscles that primarily flex the art. coxae and extend the art. genus (**Tables 22.3** and **22.4**);
  • the n. femoralis; and
  • branches of the a. femoralis, the a. profunda femoris, and their accompanying veins.
— The medial compartment contains
  • muscles that primarily adduct, flex, and extend the art. coxae (**Table 22.5**);
  • the n. obturatorius and n. femoralis; and
  • the a. obturatoria and v. obturatoria and a. profunda femoris and v. profunda femoris.
— The posterior compartment contains
  • muscles that extend the art. coxae and flex the art. genus (**Table 22.6**),
  • the n. ischiadicus, and
  • branches of the a. profunda femoris and v. profunda femoris.

— Three muscles of the thigh, the **m. sartorius, m. gracilis**, and **m. semitendinosus**, cross the knee medially and join to form the **pes anserinus**, a common tendon that overlies the **bursa anserina** inferomedial to the art. genus (see **Fig. 22.37**).

BOX 22.4: CLINICAL CORRELATION

HAMSTRING STRAINS

Hamstring strains are tears of the hamstring (posterior thigh) muscles at their proximal attachment to the pelvic girdle. This is a common injury in individuals who participate in sports that involve sprinting with sudden starts and stops. Forced high kicks, especially with an extended knee, may avulse the muscle tendons from their origin at the tuber ischiadicum. Symptoms include sudden, sharp pain in the back of the thigh during physical activity, a popping or tearing feeling in the muscle, swelling, muscle weakness, and an inability to bear weight on the affected leg.

Table 22.3 Musculus Iliopsoas

Muscle		Origin	Insertion	Innervation	Action
③ M. iliopsoas*	① M. psoas major	*Superficial:* T XII–L IV and associated disci intervertebrales (lateral surfaces) *Deep:* vertebrae L I–L V (procc. stales)	Femur (trochanter minor)	Plexus lumbalis L1, L2 (L3)	Art. coxae: flexion and external rotation Lumbar spine: *unilateral* contraction (with the femur fixed) flexes the trunk laterally to the same side; *bilateral* contraction raises the trunk from the supine position
	② M. iliacus	Fossa iliaca		N. femoralis (L2, L3)	

*The m. psoas minor, present in approximately 50% of the population, is often found on the superficial surface of the m. psoas major. It is not a muscle of the lower limb. It originates, inserts, and exerts its action on the abdominal wall.

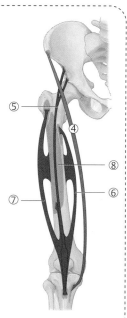

M. iliopsoas, anterior view.
(From Gilroy AM et al. Atlas of Anatomy. 4th ed. 2020. Based on: Schuenke M, Schulte E, Schumacher U. THIEME Atlas of Anatomy. General Anatomy and Musculoskeletal System. Illustrations by Voll M and Wesker K. 3rd ed. New York: Thieme Medical Publishers; 2020.)

Table 22.4 Thigh Muscles, Anterior Compartment

Muscle		Origin	Insertion	Innervation	Action
④ M. sartorius		Spina iliaca anterior superior	Medial to the tuberositas tibiae (together with m. gracilis and m. semitendinosus)	N. femoralis (L2–L3)	Art. coxae: flexion, abduction, and external rotation Art. genus: flexion and internal rotation
M. quadriceps femoris*	⑤ M. rectus femoris	Spina iliaca anterior inferior, acetabular roof of art. coxae	Tuberositas tibiae (via lig. patellae)	N. femoralis (L2–L4)	Art. coxae: flexion Art. genus: extension
	⑥ M. vastus medialis	Labium mediale lineae asperae, linea intertrochanterica (distal part)	Tuberositas tibiae via lig. patellae; patella and tuberositas tibiae via respective retinacula patellae mediale and laterale		Art. genus: extension
	⑦ M. vastus lateralis	Labium laterale lineae asperae, trochanter major (lateral surface)	Tuberositas tibiae (via lig. patellae)		
	⑧ M. vastus intermedius	Corpus femoris	Recessus suprapatellaris of capsula articularis of art. genus		
	M. articularis genus (distal fibers of m. vastus intermedius)	Anterior side of corpus femoris at level of the bursa suprapatellaris			Art. genus: extension; retracts the bursa suprapatellaris to prevent entrapment of capsule

Thigh muscles, anterior compartment, right side.
(From Schuenke M, Schulte E, Schumacher U. THIEME Atlas of Anatomy, Vol 1. Illustrations by Voll M and Wesker K. 3rd ed. New York: Thieme Publishers; 2020.)

*The entire muscle inserts on the tuberositas tibiae via the lig. patellae.

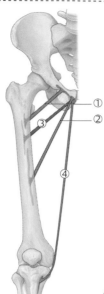
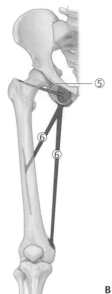
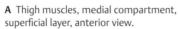

A Thigh muscles, medial compartment, superficial layer, anterior view.

B Thigh muscles, medial compartment, deep layer, anterior view.

(From Gilroy AM et al. Atlas of Anatomy. 4th ed. 2020. Based on: Schuenke M, Schulte E, Schumacher U. THIEME Atlas of Anatomy. General Anatomy and Musculoskeletal System. Illustrations by Voll M and Wesker K. 3rd ed. New York: Thieme Medical Publishers; 2020.)

Table 22.5 Thigh Muscles, Medial Compartment: Superficial and Deep Layers

Muscle	Origin	Insertion	Innervation	Action
Superficial layer				
① M. pectineus	Pecten ossis pubis	Femur (linea pectinea and the proximal linea aspera)	N. femoralis, n. obturatorius (L2, L3)	Art. coxae: adduction, external rotation, and slight flexion Stabilizes the pelvis in the coronal and sagittal planes
② M. adductor longus	Ramus superior ossis pubis and anterior side of the symphysis pubica	Femur (linea aspera, labium mediale in the middle third of the femur)	N. obturatorius (L2–L4)	Art. coxae: adduction and flexion (up to 70 degrees); extension (past 80 degrees of flexion) Stabilizes the pelvis in the coronal and sagittal planes
③ M. adductor brevis	Ramus inferior ossis pubis		N. obturatorius (L2, L3)	
④ M. gracilis	Ramus inferior ossis pubis below the symphysis pubica	Tibia (medial border of the tuberositas tibiae, along with the tendons of m. sartorius and m. semitendinosus)		Art. coxae: adduction and flexion Art. genus: flexion and internal rotation
Deep layer				
⑤ M. obturatorius externus	Outer surface of the membrana obturatoria and its bony boundaries	Fossa trochanterica of the femur	N. obturatorius (L3, L4)	Art. coxae: adduction and external rotation Stabilizes the pelvis in the sagittal plane
⑥ M. adductor magnus	Ramus inferior ossis pubis, ramus ossis ischii, and tuber ischiadicum	Deep part ("fleshy insertion"): labium mediale of the linea spine	N. obturatorius (L2–L4)	Art. coxae: adduction, extension, and slight flexion (the tendinous insertion is also active in internal rotation) Stabilizes the pelvis in the coronal and sagittal planes
		Superficial part ("tendinous insertion"): tuberculum adductorium of the femur	Tibial n. (L4)	

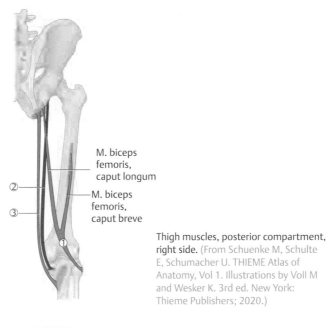

M. biceps femoris, caput longum

M. biceps femoris, caput breve

Thigh muscles, posterior compartment, right side. (From Schuenke M, Schulte E, Schumacher U. THIEME Atlas of Anatomy, Vol 1. Illustrations by Voll M and Wesker K. 3rd ed. New York: Thieme Publishers; 2020.)

Table 22.6 Thigh Muscles, Posterior Compartment

Muscle	Origin	Insertion	Innervation	Action
① M. biceps femoris	Caput longum: tuber ischiadicum, lig. sacrotuberale (common head with m. semitendinosus)	Caput fibulae	N. tibialis (L5–S2)	Art. coxae (caput longum): extends the hip, stabilizes the pelvis in the sagittal plane Art. genus: flexion and external rotation
	Caput breve: labium laterale of linea aspera in the middle third of the femur		N. fibularis communis (L5–S2)	Art. genus: flexion and external rotation
② M. semimebranosus	Tuber ischiadicum	Condylus medialis of tibia, lig. popliteum obliquum, fascia poplitea	N. tibialis (L5–S2)	Art. coxae: extends the hip, stabilizes the pelvis in the sagittal plane Art. genus: flexion and internal rotation
③ M. semitendinosus	Tuber ischiadicum and lig. sacrotuberale (common head with caput longum of m. biceps femoris)	Medial to the tuberositas tibiae in the pes anserinus (along with the tendons of m. gracilis and m. sartorius)		

Spaces of the Thigh

The n. femoralis, a. femoralis, and v. femoralis descend through narrow passages in the thigh that are created by the lig. inguinale and anterior and medial thigh muscles.

— Anteriorly, structures pass from the abdomen into the thigh through the **spatium retroinguinale**, deep to the lig. inguinale. The spatium retroinguinale is divided into a lateral muscular compartment and a medial vascular compartment (**Fig. 22.10**).

- The muscular compartment contains the n. femoralis and m. iliopsoas.
- The vascular compartment contains the femoral vessels enclosed within the **femoral sheath (vagina femoris).**
- The femoral sheath, formed by extensions of the fascia transversalis and pars psoatica fasciae iliopsoaticae, surrounds the femoral vessels as they pass under the lig. inguinale. Inferiorly, the sheath merges with the outer layer of the vessel walls (adventitia). Septa divide the sheath into compartments:

  ○ Lateral and central compartments contain the a. femoralis and v. femoralis, respectively.
  ○ A medial compartment within the sheath, the **canalis femoralis**, contains loose connective tissue, fat, and often a deep nl. inguinalis. The **anulus femoralis** defines the superior opening of the canal.

— The **trigonum femoris** is an area of the anterior thigh (**Fig. 22.11**).

- It contains the a. femoralis and v. femoralis and their branches and the terminal branches of the femoral nerve.
- Its boundaries are
  ○ superiorly, the lig. inguinale;
  ○ medially, the m. adductor longus;
  ○ laterally, the m. sartorius;
  ○ the floor, formed by the m. iliopsoas and m. pectineus; and
  ○ the apex, formed by the inferior junction of the medial and lateral borders.

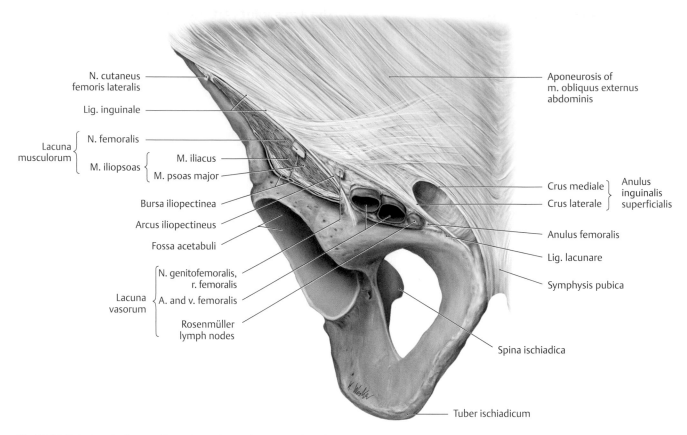

Fig. 22.10 Retroinguinal space: Muscular and vascular compartments
Right inguinal region, anterior view. (From Schuenke M, Schulte E, Schumacher U. THIEME Atlas of Anatomy, Vol 1. Illustrations by Voll M and Wesker K. 3rd ed. New York: Thieme Publishers; 2020.)

BOX 22.5: CLINICAL CORRELATION

FEMORAL HERNIAS
Femoral hernias (usually of the intestinum tenue) are always acquired and are more common in women. They pass inferior to the lig. inguinale, through the anulus femoralis and canalis femoralis, and appear in the trigonum femoris inferior and lateral to the tuberculum pubicum. They should be distinguished from inguinal hernias, which occur superior and lateral to the tuberculum pubicum (above the lig. inguinale).

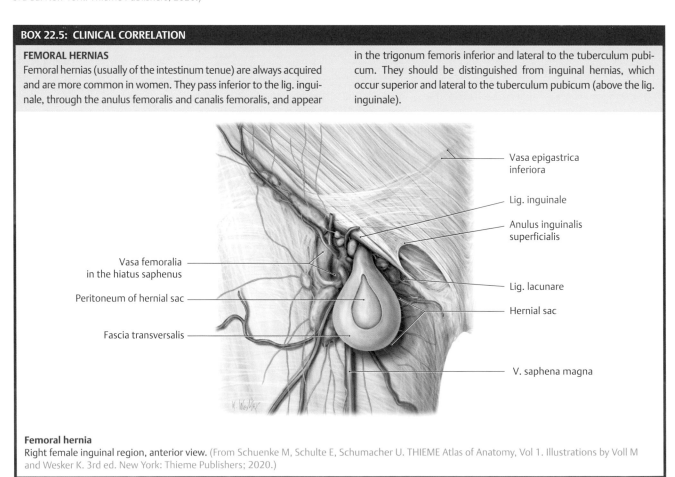

Femoral hernia
Right female inguinal region, anterior view. (From Schuenke M, Schulte E, Schumacher U. THIEME Atlas of Anatomy, Vol 1. Illustrations by Voll M and Wesker K. 3rd ed. New York: Thieme Publishers; 2020.)

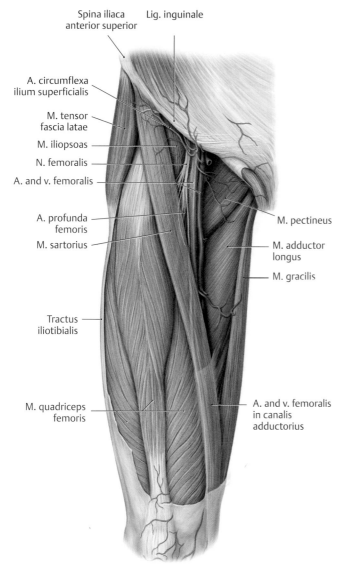

Spina iliaca anterior superior — Lig. inguinale

A. circumflexa ilium superficialis

M. tensor fascia latae

M. iliopsoas

N. femoralis

A. and v. femoralis

A. profunda femoris

M. sartorius

Tractus iliotibialis

M. quadriceps femoris

M. pectineus

M. adductor longus

M. gracilis

A. and v. femoralis in canalis adductorius

Fig. 22.11 Anterior thigh
Right thigh, anterior view. *Revealed:* Femoral triangle. *Removed:* Skin, subcutaneous tissue, and fascia lata. *Partially transparent:* Sartorius. (From Schuenke M, Schulte E, Schumacher U. THIEME Atlas of Anatomy, Vol 1. Illustrations by Voll M and Wesker K. 3rd ed. New York: Thieme Publishers; 2020.)

— The **canalis adductorius** is an intermuscular passage between the anterior and medial thigh muscles.
  • It contains the femoral vessels and the n. saphenus of the n. femoralis.
  • The canal begins at the inferior apex of the trigonum femoralis and ends at the **hiatus adductorius**, an opening in the tendon of the m. adductor magnus.

22.4 The Knee and Popliteal Region

The popliteal region connects the thigh and leg. It contains the art. genus and the fossa poplitea and its contents.

The Knee Joint (Art. Genus)

The knee joint (art. genus) is a modified hinge joint that includes the medial and lateral articulations between the condyles of the femur and tibia, and the articulation between the femur and patella (**Fig. 22.12**). Flexion and extension are the primary movements at the art. genus, but some rotation and sliding also occur.

— The patella articulates with the facies patellaris of the femur between the condylus lateralis and medialis and protects the art. genus anteriorly. The patella is embedded in the tendon of the m. quadriceps femoris, increasing the leverage of the muscle by holding the tendon away from the joint.

— Although the facies articularis of the femur and tibia are extensive, there is little congruity between the bones, and stability depends chiefly on
  • ligaments that connect the tibia and femur; and
  • muscles that surround the joint, most importantly the m. quadriceps femoris (**Figs. 22.13** and **22.14**).

— The capsula fibrosa of the art. genus is thin and incomplete and derives additional support from **retinacula patellae** (capsular ligaments that attach anteriorly to the m. quadriceps tendo), the patella, and **ligg. extracapsularia** around the joint (**Fig. 22.13**).

— Extracapsular (external) ligaments support the capsula fibrosa (**Figs. 22.15, 22.16, 22.22**).
  • The **lig. patellae**, the distal part of the m. quadriceps tendo that supports the art. genus anteriorly, extends from the patella to the tuberositas tibiae.
  • The two **ligg. collateralia** limit rotation and prevent medial and lateral dislocation of the art. genus. They are tightest in extension and slacken during flexion.
    ○ The **lig. (fibulare) collaterale laterale** is cordlike and remains unattached to the joint capsule. It extends from the epicondylus lateralis of the femur to the caput fibulae.
    ○ The **lig. (tibiale) collaterale mediale** is flat and ribbonlike and is attached to the joint capsule and meniscus medialis. It extends from the epicondylus medialis of the femur to the condylus medialis and anteromedial aspect of the tibia.

BOX 22.6: CLINICAL CORRELATION

PATELLAR TENDON REFLEX
The patellar tendon reflex is initiated by tapping the patellar tendon to elicit contraction of the m. quadriceps femoris (extension of the knee). It tests the integrity of the L2–L4 spinal cord segments carried by the n. femoralis.

  • The **lig. popliteum obliquum** is an expansion of the m. semimembranosus tendo, which supports the capsula articularis posteriorly and laterally.
  • The **lig. popliteum arcuatum** extends from the caput fibulae to the posterior art. genus and reinforces the capsula articularis posteriorly and laterally.

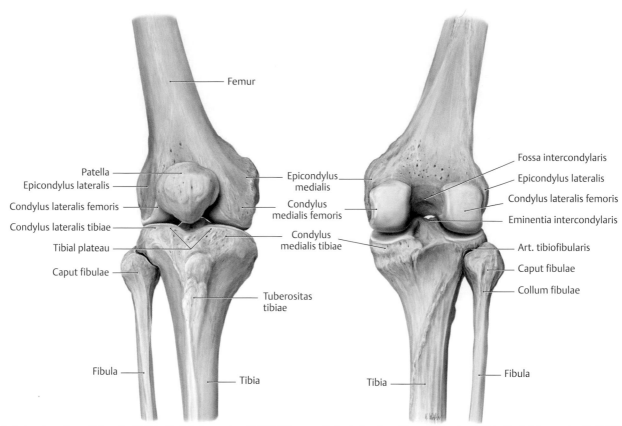

A Anterior view. (From Schuenke M, Schulte E, Schumacher U. THIEME Atlas of Anatomy, Vol 1. Illustrations by Voll M and Wesker K. 3rd ed. New York: Thieme Publishers; 2020.)

B Posterior view. (From Schuenke M, Schulte E, Schumacher U. THIEME Atlas of Anatomy, Vol 1. Illustrations by Voll M and Wesker K. 3rd ed. New York: Thieme Publishers; 2020.)

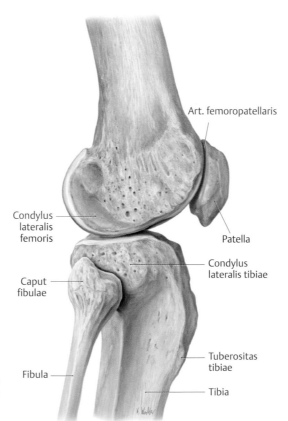

C Lateral view. (From Gilroy AM et al. Atlas of Anatomy. 4th ed. 2020. Based on: Schuenke M, Schulte E, Schumacher U. THIEME Atlas of Anatomy. General Anatomy and Musculoskeletal System. Illustrations by Voll M and Wesker K. 3rd ed. New York: Thieme Medical Publishers; 2020.)

Fig. 22.12 Right knee joint

Fig. 22.13 Ligaments of the knee joint
Right knee, anterior view. (From Schuenke M, Schulte E, Schumacher U. THIEME Atlas of Anatomy, Vol 1. Illustrations by Voll M and Wesker K. 3rd ed. New York: Thieme Publishers; 2020.)

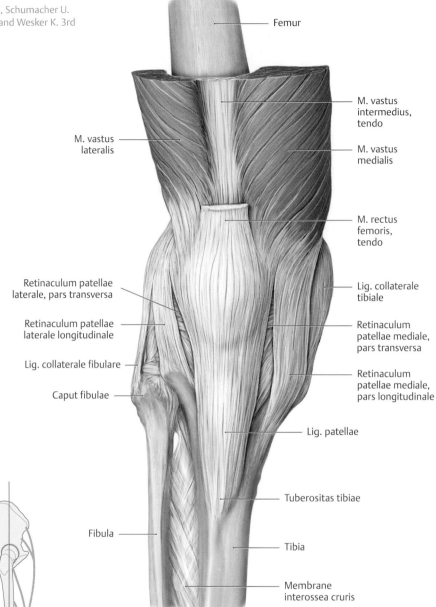

- Femur
- M. vastus intermedius, tendo
- M. vastus medialis
- M. rectus femoris, tendo
- Lig. collaterale tibiale
- Retinaculum patellae mediale, pars transversa
- Retinaculum patellae mediale, pars longitudinale
- Lig. patellae
- Tuberositas tibiae
- Tibia
- Membrane interossea cruris
- M. vastus lateralis
- Retinaculum patellae laterale, pars transversa
- Retinaculum patellae laterale longitudinale
- Lig. collaterale fibulare
- Caput fibulae
- Fibula

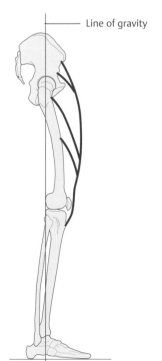

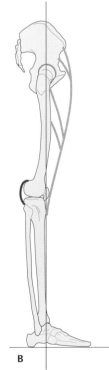

- Line of gravity

A

B

Fig. 22.14 Deficient stabilization of the knee joint due to weakness or paralysis of m. quadriceps femoris
Right lower limb, lateral view. (From Schuenke M, Schulte E, Schumacher U. THIEME Atlas of Anatomy, Vol 1. Illustrations by Voll M and Wesker K. 3rd ed. New York: Thieme Publishers; 2020.)

A When the m. quadriceps femoris is intact and the knee is in slight flexion, the line of gravity falls *behind* the transverse axis of the knee motion. As the only extensor muscle of the art. genus, the m. quadriceps femoris keeps the body from tipping backward and ensures stability.

B With the weakness or paralysis of the m. quadriceps femoris, the art. genus can no longer be actively extended. In order to stand upright, the patient must hyperextend the knee so that the line of gravity, and thus the whole-body center of gravity, is shifted forward, in front of the knee, to utilize gravity as the extending force. The joint is stabilized in this situation by the posterior capsule and ligaments of the knee.

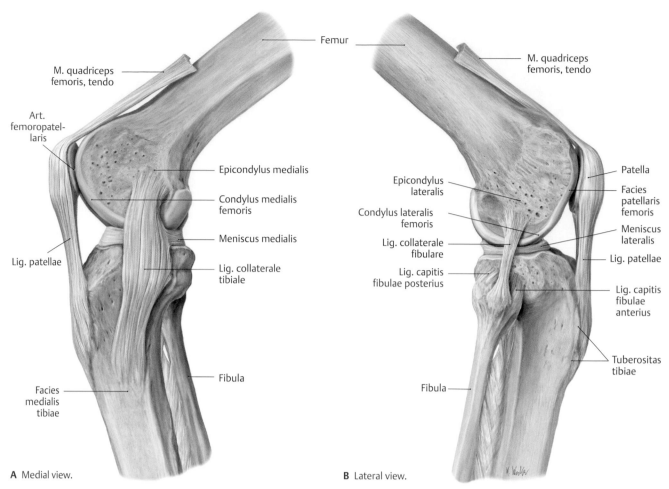

A Medial view.   **B** Lateral view.

Fig. 22.15 Ligg. collateralia and lig. patellae of the knee joint
Right art. genus. Each art. genus has ligg. collateralia mediale and tibiale. The lig. collaterale tibiale is attached to both the capsule and the meniscus medialis, whereas the lig. collaterale fibulare has no direct contact with either the capsule or the meniscus lateralis. Both ligg. collateralia are taut when the knee is in extension and stabilize the joint in the coronal plane. (From Schuenke M, Schulte E, Schumacher U. THIEME Atlas of Anatomy, Vol 1. Illustrations by Voll M and Wesker K. 3rd ed. New York: Thieme Publishers; 2020.)

— Intra-articular ligaments provide stability during movements of the joint (**Figs. 22.16** and **22.17A**).
  • Two **ligg. cruciata** are located within the joint capsule but lie external to the synovial layer. They provide stability in all positions, in addition to limiting rotation and preventing anterior and posterior dislocation of the joint.
    ◦ The **lig. cruciatum anterius** arises from the anterior intercondylar part of the tibia and extends posterolaterally to the medial aspect of the condylus lateralis of the femur.
    ◦ The **lig. cruciatum posterius** arises from the posterior intercondylar part of the tibia and extends anteromedially to the lateral aspect of the condylus medialis of the femur.
  • A **lig. transversum** connects the menisci to each other along their anterior edges.

  • A **lig. meniscofemorale posterius** joins the meniscus lateralis to the lig. cruciatum posterius and condylus medialis of the femur.
— **Menisci,** crescent-shaped fibrocartilaginous pads, deepen the articular surfaces of the tibial plateau. Wedge-shaped in cross section, they are tallest at the outer rim, where they are attached to the capsula articularis and the intercondylar ridge (**Figs. 22.17B, 22.18, 22.19**).
  • The **meniscus medialis** is C-shaped and relatively immobile due to its additional attachment to the lig. collaterale tibiale.
  • The **meniscus lateralis** is nearly circular and more mobile during flexion and extension of the joint than its medial counterpart.

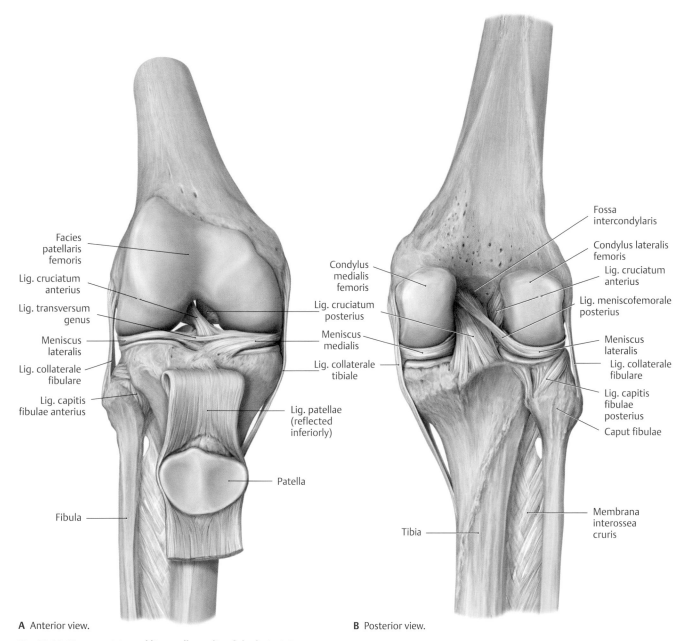

Facies
patellaris
femoris

Lig. cruciatum
anterius

Lig. transversum
genus

Meniscus
lateralis

Lig. collaterale
fibulare

Lig. capitis
fibulae anterius

Fibula

Condylus
medialis
femoris

Lig. cruciatum
posterius

Meniscus
medialis

Lig. collaterale
tibiale

Lig. patellae
(reflected
inferiorly)

Patella

Fossa
intercondylaris

Condylus lateralis
femoris

Lig. cruciatum
anterius

Lig. meniscofemorale
posterius

Meniscus
lateralis

Lig. collaterale
fibulare

Lig. capitis
fibulae
posterius

Caput fibulae

Membrana
interossea
cruris

Tibia

A Anterior view.

B Posterior view.

Fig. 22.16 Ligg. cruciata and ligg. collateralia of the knee joint
Right knee. The ligg. cruciata keep the articular surfaces of the femur and tibia in contact, while stabilizing the art. genus primarily in the sagittal plane.
Portions of the ligg. cruciata are taut in every joint position. (From Schuenke M, Schulte E, Schumacher U. THIEME Atlas of Anatomy, Vol 1. Illustrations by Voll M and Wesker K. 3rd ed. New York: Thieme Publishers; 2020.)

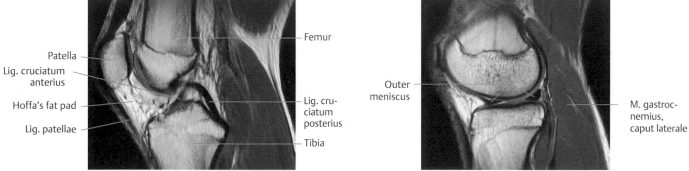

Patella

Lig. cruciatum
anterius

Hoffa's fat pad

Lig. patellae

Femur

Lig. cru-
ciatum
posterius

Tibia

Outer
meniscus

M. gastroc-
nemius,
caput laterale

A Sagittal section through the ligg. cruciata. (From Vahlensieck M, Reiser M. MRT des Bewegungsapparates. 4. Aufl. Stuttgart: Thieme Publishers; 2014.)

B Sagittal section through the meniscus lateralis. (From Vahlensieck M, Reiser M. MRT des Bewegungsapparates. 4. Aufl. Stuttgart: Thieme Publishers; 2014.)

Fig. 22.17 MRI of the knee joint

BOX 22.7: CLINICAL CORRELATION

LIGAMENTOUS INJURIES OF THE KNEE

Most knee injuries occur during physical activity and involve rupture or strain of the knee ligaments. A forceful blow to the lateral side of the knee can strain the lig. collaterale tibiale and, because of their intimate relationship, tear the meniscus medialis as well. A similar injury can result from excessive lateral rotation of the knee and is often accompanied by rupture of the lig. cruciatum anterius. The Lachman test is used to demonstrate instability of the art. genus resulting from rupture of the ligg. cruciata. Excessive anterior translation of the free-hanging tibia from under the stabilized femur is a positive anterior drawer sign, indicating anterior cruciate rupture. Posterior displacement of the tibia is a positive posterior drawer sign, indicating rupture of the lig. cruciatum posterius.

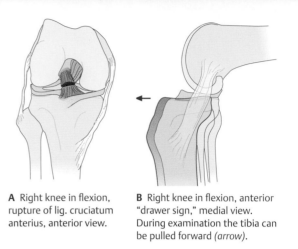

A Right knee in flexion, rupture of lig. cruciatum anterius, anterior view.

B Right knee in flexion, anterior "drawer sign," medial view. During examination the tibia can be pulled forward *(arrow)*.

Rupture of the ligamentum cruciatum anterius
(From Schuenke M, Schulte E, Schumacher U. THIEME Atlas of Anatomy, Vol 1. Illustrations by Voll M and Wesker K. 3rd ed. New York: Thieme Publishers; 2020.)

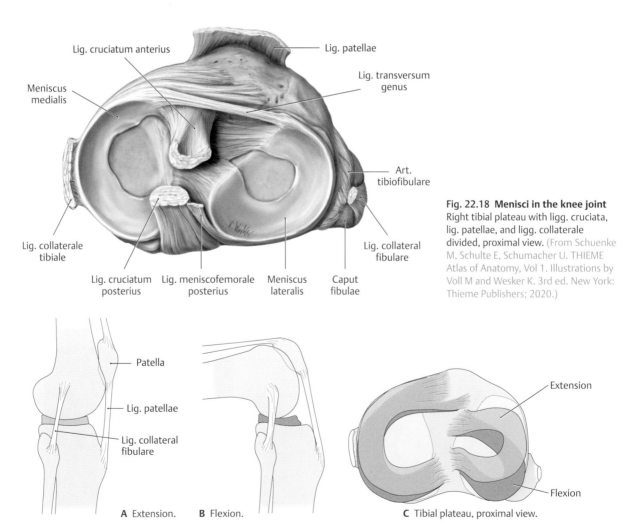

Fig. 22.18 Menisci in the knee joint
Right tibial plateau with ligg. cruciata, lig. patellae, and ligg. collaterale divided, proximal view. (From Schuenke M, Schulte E, Schumacher U. THIEME Atlas of Anatomy, Vol 1. Illustrations by Voll M and Wesker K. 3rd ed. New York: Thieme Publishers; 2020.)

A Extension.   **B** Flexion.   **C** Tibial plateau, proximal view.

Fig. 22.19 Movements of the menisci
The meniscus medialis, which is anchored more securely than the meniscus lateralis, undergoes less displacement during knee flexion. As a result, it is more susceptible to injury. (From Schuenke M, Schulte E, Schumacher U. THIEME Atlas of Anatomy, Vol 1. Illustrations by Voll M and Wesker K. 3rd ed. New York: Thieme Publishers; 2020.)

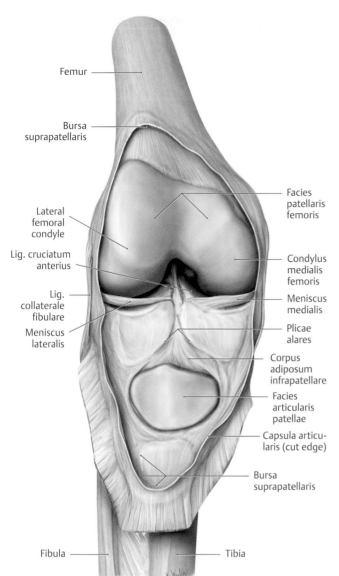

Femur
Bursa suprapatellaris
Lateral femoral condyle
Lig. cruciatum anterius
Lig. collaterale fibulare
Meniscus lateralis
Fibula
Facies patellaris femoris
Condylus medialis femoris
Meniscus medialis
Plicae alares
Corpus adiposum infrapatellare
Facies articularis patellae
Capsula articularis (cut edge)
Bursa suprapatellaris
Tibia

Fig. 22.20 Opened joint capsule of the knee
Right knee, anterior view, with patella reflected downward. (From Schuenke M, Schulte E, Schumacher U. THIEME Atlas of Anatomy, Vol 1. Illustrations by Voll M and Wesker K. 3rd ed. New York: Thieme Publishers; 2020.)

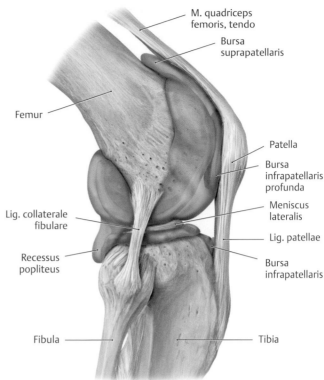

M. quadriceps femoris, tendo
Bursa suprapatellaris
Femur
Lig. collaterale fibulare
Recessus popliteus
Fibula
Patella
Bursa infrapatellaris profunda
Meniscus lateralis
Lig. patellae
Bursa infrapatellaris
Tibia

Fig. 22.21 Joint cavity of the knee
Right knee, lateral view. The cavitas articularis was demonstrated by injecting liquid plastic into the art. genus and later removing the capsule. (From Schuenke M, Schulte E, Schumacher U. THIEME Atlas of Anatomy, Vol 1. Illustrations by Voll M and Wesker K. 3rd ed. New York: Thieme Publishers; 2020.)

— An extensive synovial layer lines the internal surface of the capsula articularis. Its posterior aspect extends into the intercondylar space of the joint cavity and reflects around the ligg. intracapsularia, dividing most of the joint space into medial and lateral parts (**Figs. 22.20** and **22.21**).
— Muscles of the thigh and leg move the art. genus (**Table 22.7**).

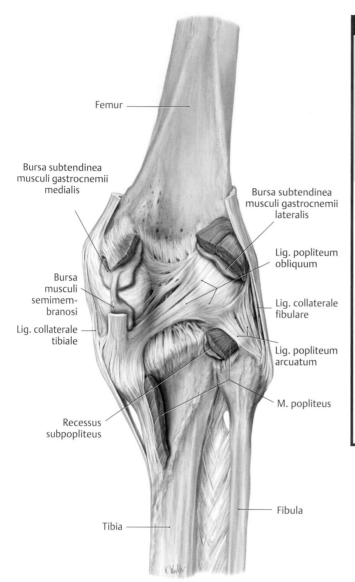

Fig. 22.22 **Capsule, ligaments, and periarticular bursae of the knee joint**
Right knee, posterior view. (From Schuenke M, Schulte E, Schumacher U. THIEME Atlas of Anatomy, Vol 1. Illustrations by Voll M and Wesker K. 3rd ed. New York: Thieme Publishers; 2020.)

— In addition to the support provided by ligg. extracapsularia, the capsule is strengthened by tendinous attachments of muscles that cross the joint (m. semitendinosus, m. semi-membranosus, m. biceps femoris, m. gastrocnemius, and

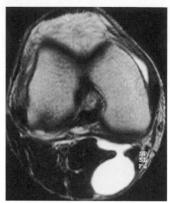
m. quadriceps femoris). Bursae associated with these muscular attachments are numerous and include

- the **bursa suprapatellaris** (pouch), which lies deep to the m. quadriceps femoris tendon and communicates with the cavity of the art. genus;
- the **bursa prepatellaris**, which is subcutaneous over the patella;
- the **bursa infrapatellaris superficialis**, which is subcutaneous over the lig. patellae;
- the **bursa infrapatellaris profundus**, which lies deep to the lig. patellae; and
- the **bursa anserina**, which lies between the pes anserinus and lig. collaterale tibiale.

— Additional bursae around the knee communicate with the joint cavity. They include the **recessus subpopliteus,** the **bursa musculi semimembranosi,** and the **bursa subtendinea musculi gastrocnemii medialis** (**Fig. 22.22**).

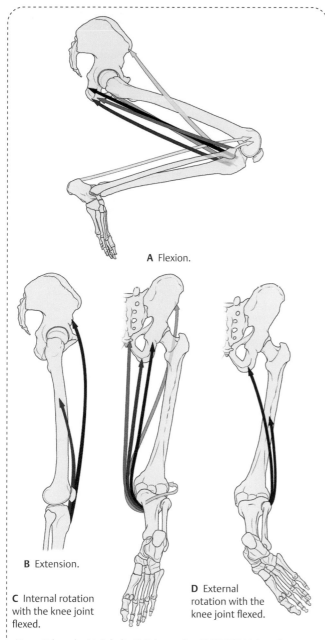

A Flexion.

B Extension.

C Internal rotation with the knee joint flexed.

D External rotation with the knee joint flexed.

(From Schuenke M, Schulte E, Schumacher U. THIEME Atlas of Anatomy, Vol 1. Illustrations by Voll M and Wesker K. 3rd ed. New York: Thieme Publishers; 2020.)

Table 22.7 Movements of the Knee Joint

Action	Primary Muscles
Flexion	M. biceps femoris—caput breve and caput longum M. semimembranosus M. semitendinosus M. sartorius M. gracilis M. gastrocnemius M. popliteus
Extension	M. quadriceps femoris
Internal rotation	M. semimembranosus M. semitendinosus M. sartorius M. gracilis M. popliteus (of nonbearing leg)
External rotation	M. biceps femoris

BOX 22.9: CLINICAL CORRELATION

GENU VARUM AND GENU VALGUM

Although the femur lies diagonally within the thigh, the tibia is nearly vertical in the leg. This creates a Q angle at the knee between the long axes of the two bones. The angle varies with developmental stage and sex, but it can also be altered by disease. Normally, the head of the femur sits over the center of the art. genus, distributing weight evenly on the tibial plateau. In genu varum (bowleg), the Q angle is smaller than normal because the femur is more vertical. This increases the weight on the medial side of the knee, putting additional stress on the meniscus medialis and lig. collaterale mediale (tibiale). When a person is standing upright with feet and ankles together, the knees are wide apart. In genu valgum (knock knee), the Q angle is larger because the femur is more diagonal. Greater weight is put on the lateral side of the knee, stressing the meniscus lateralis and lig. collaterale laterale (fibulare). In the upright position, the knees touch, but the ankles do not.

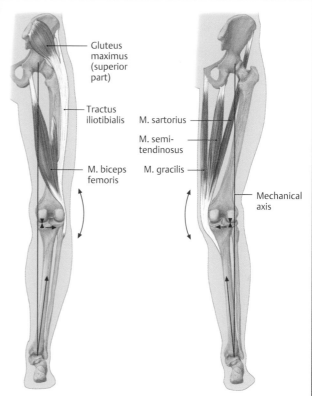

A Axis in genu varum, posterior view.

B Axis in genu valgum, posterior view.

(From Schuenke M, Schulte E, Schumacher U. THIEME Atlas of Anatomy, Vol 1. Illustrations by Voll M and Wesker K. 3rd ed. New York: Thieme Publishers; 2020.)

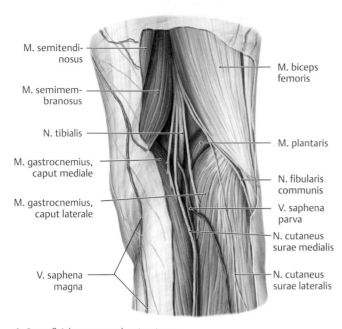

A Superficial neurovascular structures.

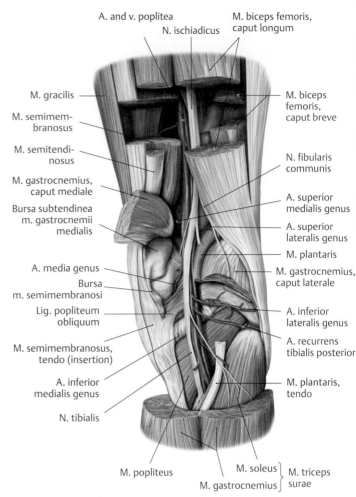

B Deep neurovascular structures.

Fig. 22.23 Popliteal fossa
Right leg, posterior view. (From Schuenke M, Schulte E, Schumacher U. THIEME Atlas of Anatomy, Vol 1. Illustrations by Voll M and Wesker K. 3rd ed. New York: Thieme Publishers; 2020.)

The Fossa Poplitea

The **fossa poplitea** is a diamond-shaped space posterior to the art. genus (**Fig. 22.22**).
— Its muscular boundaries are
  • superomedially, the m. semimembranosus;
  • superolaterally, the m. biceps femoris; and
  • inferiorly, the caput mediale and caput laterale of the m. gastrocnemius.
— The contents of the fossa, which are embedded within popliteal fat, include

  • the a. poplitea and v. poplitea and their rr. geniculares,
  • nll. poplitei, and
  • n. tibialis and n. fibularis communis.
— At the superior apex of the fossa poplitea, the n. ischiadicus splits into its two terminal branches.
  • The n. tibialis descends into the posterior leg compartment with the a. poplitea and v. poplitea.
  • The n. fibularis communis courses laterally along the edge of the m. biceps femoris to enter the lateral leg compartment.

22.5 The Leg

The leg extends from the knee to the ankle; it contains the tibia and fibula and the muscles of the leg (crural) compartments.

Tibiofibular Joints

The tibia and fibula are joined proximally at the knee and distally at the ankle. Unlike the extensive movement at the artt. radioulnares in the forearm, only slight movement occurs at each tibiofibular joint (art. tibiofibularis), and no muscles are directly associated with them.

— The **art. tibiofibularis proximalis** is a plane-type synovial joint between the caput fibulae and an articular facet of the condylus lateralis tibiae. **Lig. capitis fibulae anterius** and **posterius** secure the joint (see **Fig. 22.16**).

— The **art. tibiofibularis distalis**, a compound fibrous joint, creates a mortise formed by the malleolus medialis and malleolus lateralis that cups the talus and stabilizes the art. talocruralis. Ligaments of the art. tibiofibularis (**Fig. 22.24**) include

- a deep **lig. tibiofibulare interossea**, the primary support of the joint, which is continuous with the membrana interossea, of the leg, and
- the external **lig. tibiofibulare anterius** and **lig. tibiofibulare posterius**.

— A membrana interossea unites the corpus tibiae and corpus fibulae and provides stability to the art. tibiofibularis distalis and art. talocruralis.

Muscles of the Leg

Muscles of the leg, which move the knee, ankle, and foot, are divided into four crural compartments (see **Fig. 22.45B**).

— The anterior compartment contains
- muscles that dorsiflex the foot and toes and invert the foot (**Table 22.8**),
- the n. fibularis profundus, and
- the a. tibialis anterior and v. tibialis anterior

— The lateral compartment contains
- muscles that evert and plantar flex the foot (**Table 22.9**),
- the n. fibularis superficialis, and
- the muscular branches of the a. fibularis and v. fibularis from the posterior compartment.

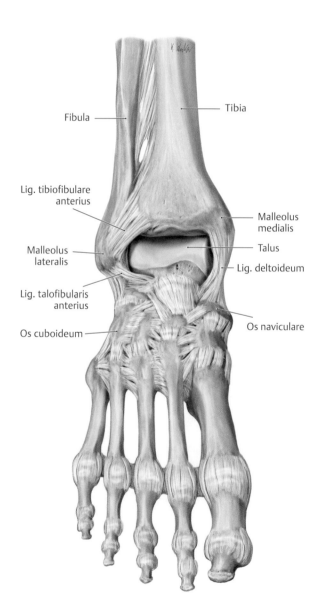

A Anterior view with art. talocruralis in plantar flexion.

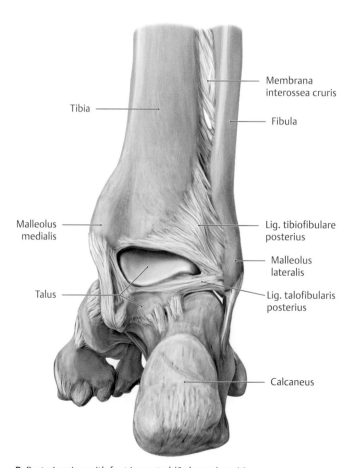

B Posterior view with foot in neutral (0-degree) position.

Fig. 22.24 Ligaments of the ankle and foot
Right foot. (From Schuenke M, Schulte E, Schumacher U. THIEME Atlas of Anatomy, Vol 1. Illustrations by Voll M and Wesker K. 3rd ed. New York: Thieme Publishers; 2020.)

BOX 22.10: CLINICAL CORRELATION

SHIN SPLINTS

Shin splints result from chronic trauma of the m. tibialis anterior, usually incurred by overuse of the muscle during athletic activities. In what is considered a mild form of anterior compartment syndrome, small tears of the periosteum cause pain and swelling over the distal two thirds of the tibial shaft.

BOX 22.11: CLINICAL CORRELATION

RUPTURE OF THE CALCANEAL TENDON

Rupture of the calcaneal tendon tends to occur following sudden forced plantar flexion of the foot, unexpected dorsiflexion of the foot, or violent dorsiflexion of a plantar-flexed foot in people unaccustomed to exercise or who exercise intermittently. The rupture disables the m. gastrocnemius, m. soleus, and m. plantaris, rendering the patient unable to plantar flex the foot.

— The superficial posterior compartment contains
  • muscles that plantar flex the foot, two of which, the m. gastrocnemius and m. soleus, form the m. triceps surae and share a common tendon of insertion, the **tendo calcaneus** (**Table 22.10**);
  • the n. tibialis; and
  • the muscular branches of the a. tibialis posterior and v. tibialis posterior from the deep posterior compartment.
— The deep posterior compartment contains
  • muscles that plantar flex the foot and toes and invert the foot (**Table 22.11**) (only one muscle, the m. popliteus, crosses the knee and laterally rotates the femur),

  • the n. tibialis, and
  • the a. tibialis posterior and a. fibularis and v. fibularis.
— Retinacula, thickened bands of the crural fascia, bind the tendons of the long extensor and flexor muscles as they cross the ankle (**Fig. 22.25**).
  • **Retinaculum musculorum extensorium superius** and **retinaculum musculorum extensorium inferius** bind muscles of the anterior compartment.
  • Medially, a **retinaculum musculorum flexorum** binds muscles of the deep posterior compartment.
  • **Retinaculum musculorum fibularium superius and retinaculum musculorum fibularium inferius** bind muscles of the lateral compartment.

Table 22.8 Leg Muscles, Compartimentum Cruris Anterius

Muscle	Origin	Insertion	Innervation	Action
① M. tibialis anterior	Tibia (upper two thirds of the facies lateralis), membrana interossea cruris, and fascia cruris superficialis (highest part)	Os cuneiforme mediale (medial and plantar surface), os metatarsi I (medial base)	N. fibularis profundus (L4, L5)	Art. talocruralis: dorsiflexion Art. subtalaris: inversion (supinatio)
② M. extensor hallucis longus	Fibula (middle third of the facies medialis), membrana interossea	Hallux (at the dorsal aponeurosis at the basis of its phalanx distalis)		Art. talocruralis: dorsiflexion Art. subtalaris: active in both eversion and inversion (pronation/supination), depending on the initial position of the foot Extends the artt. metatarsophalangeae and interphalangea of the hallux
③ M. extensor digitorum longus	Fibula (caput and facies medialis), tibia (condylus lateralis), and membrana interossea	2nd to 5th toes (at the dorsal aponeuroses at the bases of the phalanges distales)		Art. talocruralis: dorsiflexion Art. subtalaris: eversion (pronation) Extends the artt. metacarpophalangeae and interphalangeae of the 2nd to 5th digiti
④ M. fibularis tertius	Distal fibula (margo anterior)	Basis ossis metatarsi V (base)		Art. talocruralis: dorsiflexion Art. subtalaris: eversion (pronation)

Leg muscles, anterior compartment
Right leg, anterior view. (From Schuenke M, Schulte E, Schumacher U. THIEME Atlas of Anatomy, Vol 1. Illustrations by Voll M and Wesker K. 3rd ed. New York: Thieme Publishers; 2020.)

BOX 22.12: CLINICAL CORRELATION

COMPARTMENT SYNDROME

Compartment syndrome is a condition that may follow burns, hemorrhage, complex fractures, or crush injuries. Swelling, infection, or bleeding into the compartment can increase intracompartmental pressure and, when high enough, compress the small vascular structures that supply the compartment contents. Nerves are particularly vulnerable to ischemia, and permanent loss of motor and sensory functions distal to the compartment can result. Symptoms include severe pain that is out of proportion to the injury, paresthesia (tingling and numbness), pallor of the skin, paralysis of muscles affected, and loss of distal pulses in the affected limb. Treatment is prompt surgery to decompress the compartment by making long cuts through the fascia (fasciotomy).

— The **tarsal tunnel** is a passageway on the medial side of the ankle formed by the retinaculum musculorum flexorum and its attachments to the malleolus medialis and calcaneus. It transmits
- muscle tendons of the deep posterior compartment,
- a. tibialis posterior and v. tibialis posterior and their rr. plantares mediales and laterales, and
- the n. tibialis and its r. plantaris medialis and r. plantaris lateralis.

BOX 22.13: CLINICAL CORRELATION

TARSAL TUNNEL SYNDROME

Tarsal tunnel syndrome, similar to carpal tunnel syndrome of the hand, results from swelling of the vaginae synoviales of the long flexor tendons within the tarsal tunnel. Compression of the n. tibialis can result in burning pain, numbness, and tingling that radiates to the heel.

Table 22.9 Leg Muscles, Compartimentum Cruris Laterale

Muscle	Origin	Insertion	Innervation	Action
① M. fibularis longus	Fibula (caput and proximal two thirds of the facies lateralis, arising partly from the septa intermuscularia cruris)	Os cuneiforme mediale (plantar side), os metatarsi I (base)	N. fibularis superficialis (L5, S1)	Art. talocruralis: plantar flexion Art. subtalaris: eversion (pronation) Supports the arcus transversus of the foot
② M. fibularis brevis	Fibula (distal half of the facies lateralis), septa intermuscularia cruris	Os metatarsi V (tuberositas at the basis, with an occasional division to the dorsal aponeurosis of the 5th toe)		Art. talocruralis: plantar flexion Art. subtalaris: eversion (pronation)

Leg muscles, lateral compartment
Right leg and foot, anterior view.
(From Schuenke M, Schulte E, Schumacher U. THIEME Atlas of Anatomy, Vol 1. Illustrations by Voll M and Wesker K. 3rd ed. New York: Thieme Publishers; 2020.)

Table 22.10 Leg Muscles, Compartimentum Cruris Posterius: Superficial Flexors

Muscle		Origin	Insertion	Innervation	Action	
M. triceps surae	① M. gastrocnemius	Femur (caput mediale: superior posterior part of the condylus medialis femoris. caput laterale: lateral surface of condylus lateralis femoris)	Tuber calcanei via the tendo calcaneus (Achilles')	N. tibialis (S1, S2)	Art. talocruralis: plantar flexion when knee is extended (m. gastrocnemius) Art. genus: flexion (m. gastrocnemius) Art. talocruralis: plantar flexion (m. soleus)	
	② M . soleus	Fibula (caput and collum, facies posterior), tibia (linea musculi solei via an arcus tendineus)				
③ M. plantaris		Femur (epicondylus lateralis, proximal to caput laterale musculi gastrocnemii)	Tuber calcanei M. plantaris		Negligible; may act with m. gastrocnemius in plantar flexion	

Superficial flexors, posterior compartment of leg
Right leg with foot in plantar flexion, posterior view. (From Gilroy AM et al. Atlas of Anatomy. 4th ed. 2020. Based on: Schuenke M, Schulte E, Schumacher U. THIEME Atlas of Anatomy. General Anatomy and Musculoskeletal System. Illustrations by Voll M and Wesker K. 3rd ed. New York: Thieme Medical Publishers; 2020.)a

Table 22.11 Leg Muscles, Compartimentum Cruris Posterius: Deep Flexors

Muscle	Origin	Insertion	Innervation	Action	
① M. tibialis posterior	Membrana interossea cruris, adjacent borders of tibia and fibula	Tuberositas ossis navicularis; ossea cuneiformia (mediale, intermedium, and laterale); bases ossium metatarsalium II–V	N. tibialis (L4, L5)	Art. talocruralis: plantar flexion Art. subtalaris: inversion (supination) Supports the arcus longitudinalis and arcus transversus	
② M. flexor digitorum longus	Tibia (middle third of facies posterior)	Basis phalangis distalis II–V	N. tibialis (L5–S2)	Art. talocruralis: plantar flexion Art. subtalaris: inversion (supination) Artt. metatarsophalangeae and interphalangeae of the 2nd to 5th toes: plantar flexion	
③ M. flexor hallucis longus	Fibula (distal two thirds of facies posterior), adjacent membrana interossea	Basis phalangis distalis I		Art. talocruralis: plantar flexion Art. subtalaris: inversion (supination) Artt. metatarsophalangea and interphalangea of the hallux: plantar flexion Supports the medial arcus longitudinalis	
④ M. popliteus	Condylus lateralis femoris, posterior horn of the meniscus lateralis	Facies posterior corporis tibiae (above the origin at the m. soleus)	N. tibialis (L4–S1)	Art. genus: flexes and unlocks the knee by externally rotating the femur on the fixed tibia 5 degrees	

Deep flexors, posterior compartment of leg
Right leg with foot in plantar flexion, posterior view.
(From Schuenke M, Schulte E, Schumacher U. THIEME Atlas of Anatomy, Vol 1. Illustrations by Voll M and Wesker K. 3rd ed. New York: Thieme Publishers; 2020.)

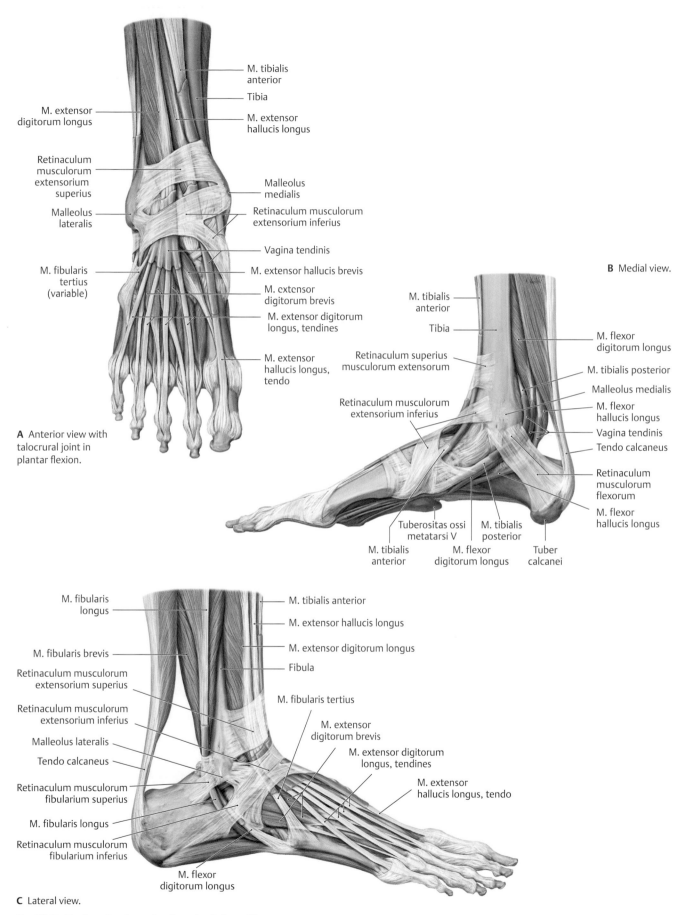

A Anterior view with talocrural joint in plantar flexion.

B Medial view.

C Lateral view.

Fig. 22.25 Tendon sheaths and retinacula of the ankle
Right foot. The retinacula musculorum extensorum superius and inferius retain the long extensor tendons, the retinacula musculorum fibularium hold the fibular muscle tendons in place, and the retinaculum musculorum flexorum retains the long flexor tendons through the canalis tarsi. (From Schuenke M, Schulte E, Schumacher U. THIEME Atlas of Anatomy, Vol 1. Illustrations by Voll M and Wesker K. 3rd ed. New York: Thieme Publishers; 2020.)

22.6 The Ankle (Talocrural) Joint

The weight of the body is transferred along the tibia of the leg, through the talus at the art. talocruralis, and onto the heel and ball of the foot. Strong bony and ligamentous supports stabilize the ankle and facilitate this transfer of weight.

The **ankle joint (art. talocruralis)** includes articulations between the distal tibia and fibula and the talus (**Figs. 22.26, 22.27, 22.28, 22.29**).

— At the art. talocruralis, the ankle mortise, which is formed by the art. tibiofibularis distalis, hugs the corpus tali. Ligg. tibiofibulares that stabilize the ankle mortise also contribute to the stability of the art. talocruralis.

— The art. talocruralis is tighter and more stable with the foot in dorsiflexion, when the wider anterior part of the trochlea (of the talus) is wedged within the ankle mortise. Accordingly, the joint is looser and less stable in plantar flexion.

— Strong ligg. collateralia articulationis talocruralis connect the tibia and fibula to the ossa tarsi and support the art. talocruralis (**Fig. 22.30**).

- The medial **lig. deltoideum** of the ankle extends from the malleolus medialis of the tibia to the talus, calcaneus, and os naviculare. Its components are
  - the **pars tibiotalaris anterior**,
  - the **pars tibiotalaris posterior**,
  - the **pars tibiocalcanea**, and
  - the **pars tibionavicularis**.
- The **lig. collaterale laterale** extends from the malleolus lateralis of the fibula to the talus and calcaneus. Its parts are
  - the **lig. talofibulare anterius**,
  - the **lig. talofibulare posterius**, and
  - the **lig. calcaneofibulare**.
- Movement at the art. talocruralis, provided by muscles of the leg, is limited primarily to dorsiflexion (extension) and plantar flexion (**Table 22.12**).

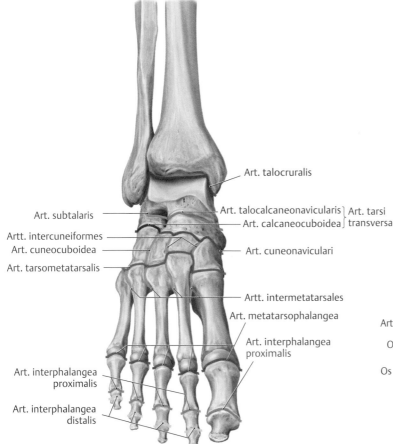

Fig. 22.26 Joints of the foot
Right foot with art. talocruralis in plantar flexion, anterior view. (From Gilroy AM et al. Atlas of Anatomy. 4th ed. 2020. Based on: Schuenke M, Schulte E, Schumacher U. THIEME Atlas of Anatomy. General Anatomy and Musculoskeletal System. Illustrations by Voll M and Wesker K. 3rd ed. New York: Thieme Medical Publishers; 2020.)

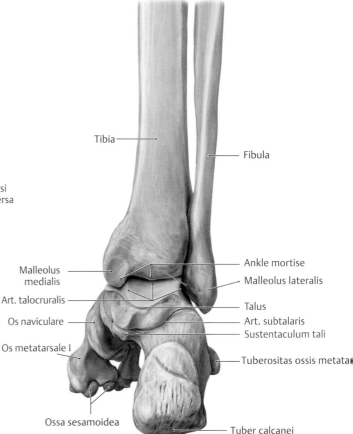

Fig. 22.27 Art. talocruralis and art. subtalaris
Right foot with foot in neutral (0-degree) position, posterior view. (From Schuenke M, Schulte E, Schumacher U. THIEME Atlas of Anatomy, Vol 1. Illustrations by Voll M and Wesker K. 3rd ed. New York: Thieme Publishers; 2020.)

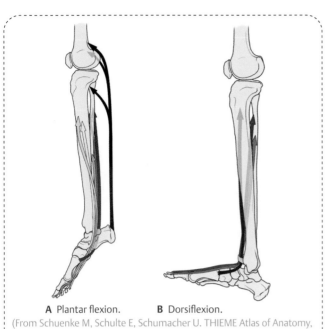

A Plantar flexion.   **B** Dorsiflexion.

(From Schuenke M, Schulte E, Schumacher U. THIEME Atlas of Anatomy, Vol 1. Illustrations by Voll M and Wesker K. 3rd ed. New York: Thieme Publishers; 2020.)

Table 22.12 Movements of the Ankle Joint

Action	Primary Muscles
Plantar flexion	M. gastrocnemius
	M. soleus
	M. tibialis posterior
	M. flexor digitorum longus
	M. flexor hallucis longus
Dorsiflexion	M. tibialis anterior
	M. extensor hallucis longus
	M. extensor digitorum longus
	M. fibularis tertius

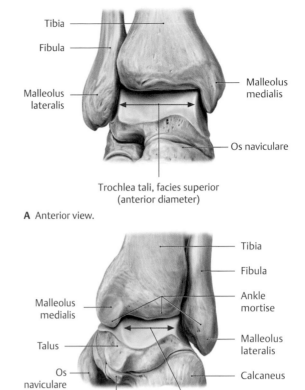

A Anterior view.

B Posterior view.

Fig. 22.28 Talocrural joint

Right foot. The art. talocruralis is tighter and more stable with the foot in dorsiflexion, when the wider, anterior part of the trochlea (of the talus) is wedged within the ankle mortise. Accordingly, the joint is looser and less stable in plantar flexion. (From Gilroy AM et al. Atlas of Anatomy. 4th ed. 2020. Based on: Schuenke M, Schulte E, Schumacher U. THIEME Atlas of Anatomy. General Anatomy and Musculoskeletal System. Illustrations by Voll M and Wesker K. 3rd ed. New York: Thieme Medical Publishers; 2020.)

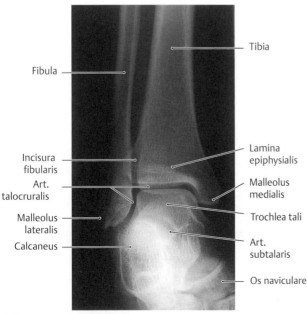

A Anteroposterior view.

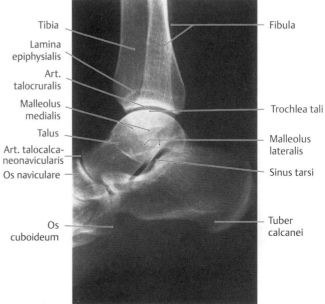

B Left lateral view.

Fig. 22.29 Radiograph of the ankle

(From Moeller TB, Reif E. Pocket Atlas of Sectional Anatomy: The Musculoskeletal System. New York: Thieme Publishers; 2009.)

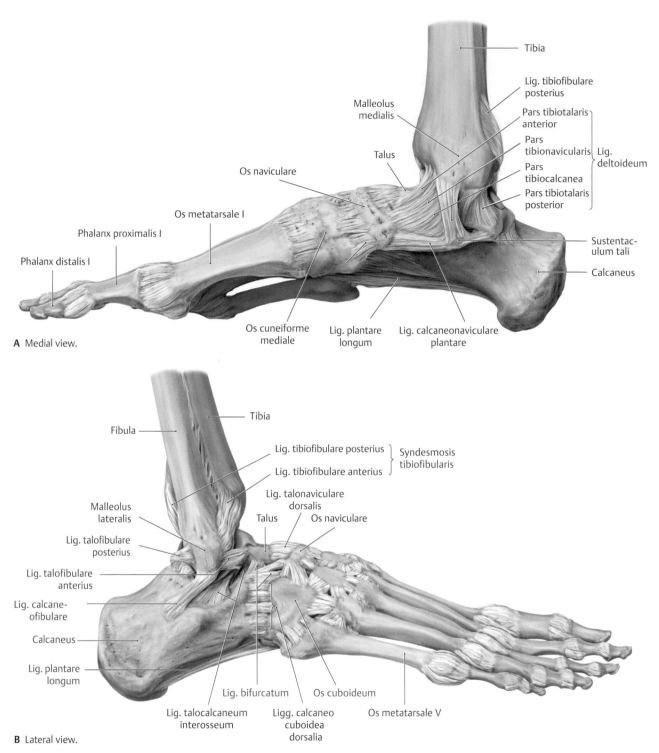

A Medial view.

B Lateral view.

Fig. 22.30 Ligaments of the ankle and foot
Right foot. (From Schuenke M, Schulte E, Schumacher U. THIEME Atlas of Anatomy, Vol 1. Illustrations by Voll M and Wesker K. 3rd ed. New York: Thieme Publishers; 2020.)

BOX 22.14: CLINICAL CORRELATION

ANKLE SPRAINS

Ankle sprains (torn ligaments) are caused most often by forced inversion of the foot (e.g., walking on uneven ground). Damage to the ligg. collateralia articulationis talocruralis is correlated with the severity of the injury and proceeds from anterior to posterior: the lig. talofibulare anterius is the most easily injured, followed by the lig. calcaneofibulare and the least frequently injured, the lig. talofibulare posterius. Fracture of the malleolus lateralis can also accompany inversion injuries.

22.7 The Foot

The numerous joints of the foot create a flexible unit that effectively absorbs shock, distributes the weight of vertical loads, and participates in locomotion.

Joints of the Foot and Toes

Movements at the joints of the foot, particularly the artt. intertarsales (art. subtalaris and art. tarsi transversa), artt. metatarsophalangeae, and artt. interphalangeae pedis, contribute to smooth locomotion and maintenance of balance (see **Fig. 22.26**).

— The **art. subtalaris** is an articulation between the inferior surface of the talus and underlying calcaneus (**Figs. 22.31** and **22.32;** see also **Fig. 22.29B**).
  • It is a compound joint that has anterior and posterior compartments.
    ○ The anterior compartment contains the talocalcaneal component of the talocalcaneonavicular articulation.
    ○ The posterior compartment contains the posterior art. talocalcanea posterius.

• A strong **lig. talocalcaneum interosseum** joins the bones and separates the anterior and posterior parts of the joint.
• This joint is the main articulation that allows inversion and eversion of the foot.

— The **art. tarsi transversa** is a compound joint that combines the talonavicular and calcaneocuboid articulations.
  • Movement at this joint rotates the front of the foot relative to the heel, augmenting the inversion and eversion at the subtalar joint.
  • This joint is a common site for surgical amputation of the foot.

— The **artt. tarsometatarsales and artt. intermetatarsales** are small and relatively immobile.

— **Artt. metatarsophalangeae** are condyloid synovial joints between the heads of the metatarsals and base of the phalanges.
  • Flexion, extension, and some abduction and adduction occur at this joint.

— **Artt. interphalangeae pedis** are hinge–type synovial joints that primarily allow flexion and extension of the toes.
  • Digits 2 through 4 have **proximal interphalangeal (PIP)** and **distal interphalangeal (DIP) joints.**
  • The great toe has only a single artt. interphalangeae pedis.

— Muscles of the leg and foot move the joints of the foot (**Tables 22.13** and **22.14**).

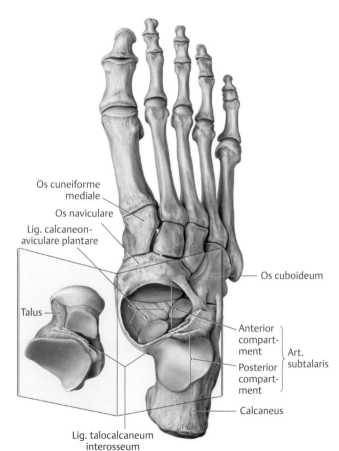

Os cuneiforme mediale
Os naviculare
Lig. calcaneon-aviculare plantare
Os cuboideum
Talus
Anterior compartment
Posterior compartment
Art. subtalaris
Calcaneus
Lig. talocalcaneum interosseum

Fig. 22.31 Articulatio subtalaris and ligaments
Right foot with opened art. subtalaris, dorsal view. The art. subtalaris consists of two distinct articulations separated by the interosseous lig. talocalcaneus interosseum: the posterior compartment (art. talocalcaneus) and the anterior compartment (art. talocalcaneonavicularis). (From Schuenke M, Schulte E, Schumacher U. THIEME Atlas of Anatomy, Vol 1. Illustrations by Voll M and Wesker K. 3rd ed. New York: Thieme Publishers; 2020.)

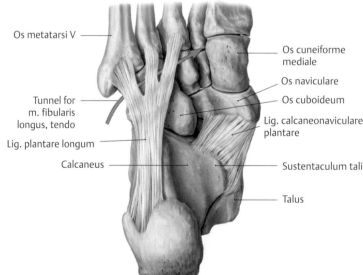

Os metatarsi V
Tunnel for m. fibularis longus, tendo
Lig. plantare longum
Calcaneus
Os cuneiforme mediale
Os naviculare
Os cuboideum
Lig. calcaneonaviculare plantare
Sustentaculum tali
Talus

Fig. 22.32 Ligaments of the plantar surface
Plantar view. The lig. calcaneonaviculare plantare completes the bony socket of the art. talocalcaneus. The long plantar ligament converts the tuberosity of the os cuboideum into a tunnel for the tibialis longus tendon (*arrow*). (From Gilroy AM et al. Atlas of Anatomy. 4th ed. 2020. Based on: Schuenke M, Schulte E, Schumacher U. THIEME Atlas of Anatomy. General Anatomy and Musculoskeletal System. Illustrations by Voll M and Wesker K. 3rd ed. New York: Thieme Medical Publishers; 2020.)

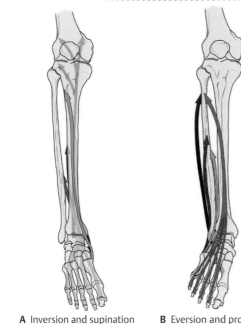

A Inversion and supination (lifting the medial border of the foot).   **B** Eversion and pronation (lifting the lateral border of the foot).

(From Schuenke M, Schulte E, Schumacher U. THIEME Atlas of Anatomy, Vol 1. Illustrations by Voll M and Wesker K. 3rd ed. New York: Thieme Publishers; 2020.)

Table 22.13 Movements of the Subtalor and Transverse Tarsal Joints

Action	Primary Muscles
Inversion and supination	M. tibialis anterior
	M. tibialis posterior
	M. flexor hallucis longus
	M. flexor digitorum longus
Eversion and pronation	M. fibularis longus
	M. fibularis brevis
	M. fibularis tertius

Table 22.14 Movements of the Metatarsophalangeal (MTP) and Interphalangeal (IP) Joints

Action	Primary Muscles
Flexion (MTP and IP joints)	M. flexor hallucis longus
	M. flexor hallucis brevis
	M. flexor digitorum longus
	M. flexor digitorum brevis
	Mm. lumbricales pedis
	Mm. interossei dorsales and palmares pedis
Extension (MTP and IP joints)	M. extensor hallucis longus
	M. extensor hallucis brevis
	M. extensor digitorum longus
	M. extensor digitorum brevis
Abduction (MTP joints)	M. abductor hallucis
	M. abductor digiti minimi
	Mm. interossei dorsales pedis
Adduction (MTP joints)	M. adductor hallucis
	Mm. interossei plantares

- The arcus lateralis is flatter than the arcus medialis and is formed by the calcaneus, os cuboideum, and lateral ossa metatarsi.
— The arcus transversus, formed by the os cuboideum, ossa cuneiformes, and bases of the ossa metatarsi, crosses the midfoot (**Fig. 22.34**).
— The arches are supported by active and passive stabilizers (**Fig. 22.35**).
  - The primary active stabilizers of the arches are muscles of the leg and foot:
    ◦ The m. tibialis posterior and m. fibularis longus of the leg
    ◦ The short flexors, abductors, and adductors of the foot
  - The primary passive stabilizers of the arches are ligaments of the foot:
    ◦ The aponeurosis plantaris
    ◦ The **lig. calcaneonaviculare plantare** (spring ligament)
    ◦ The **lig. plantare longum**

Arches of the Foot

The ossa tarsi and ossa metatarsi form flexible arcus pedis longitudinalis and transversus on the sole of the foot.
— The arches function as a unit to
  • distribute weight onto the heel and ball of the foot,
  • act as shock absorbers during locomotion, and
  • enhance the flexibility of the foot when planted on uneven surfaces.
— The arcus longitudinalis has medial and lateral parts (**Fig. 22.33**).
  • The arcus medialis is the highest part of the arcus longitudinalis, formed by the talus, os naviculare, three ossa cuneiformes, and medial ossa metatarsi. The head of the talus is the keystone of the arch.

BOX 22.15: CLINICAL CORRELATION

PES PLANUS

Pes planus, or flatfoot, is a condition in which both the active and the passive stabilizers of the medial arcus longitudinalis are lax or absent. Because the head of the talus is not supported, it can displace inferomedially, and the forefoot everts and abducts, putting increased stress on the lig. calcaneonaviculare plantare. Pes planus commonly occurs in older individuals who stand for long periods. Flatfoot is normal in children younger than 3 years, but this resolves with maturity.

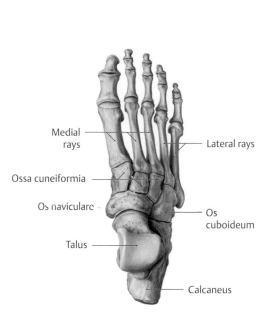

Fig. 22.33 Plantar vault
Right foot, dorsal view. The forces of the foot are distributed between two lateral and three medial rays. The arrangement of these rays creates a longitudinal and transverse arch in the sole of the foot, helping the foot absorb vertical loads. (From Schuenke M, Schulte E, Schumacher U. THIEME Atlas of Anatomy, Vol 1. Illustrations by Voll M and Wesker K. 3rd ed. New York: Thieme Publishers; 2020.)

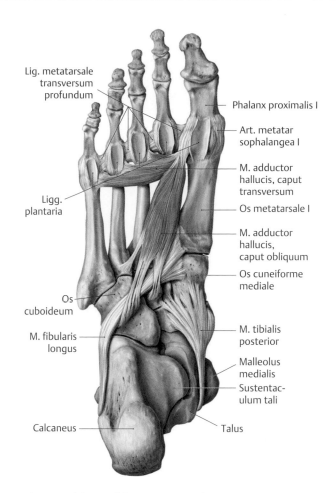

Fig. 22.34 Stabilizers of the transverse arch
Right foot, plantar view. The arcus pedis transversus is supported by both active and passive stabilizing structures (muscles and ligaments, respectively). *Note:* The arch of the forefoot has only passive stabilizers, whereas the arcus ossis metatarsi and arcus ossis tarsi have only active stabilizers. (From Schuenke M, Schulte E, Schumacher U. THIEME Atlas of Anatomy, Vol 1. Illustrations by Voll M and Wesker K. 3rd ed. New York: Thieme Publishers; 2020.)

A Passive stabilizers of the longitudinal arch. The main passive stabilizers of the longitudinal arch are the plantar aponeurosis (strongest component), the lig. plantare longum (see **Fig. 22.32**), and the lig. calcaneocuboideum plantare (weakest component).

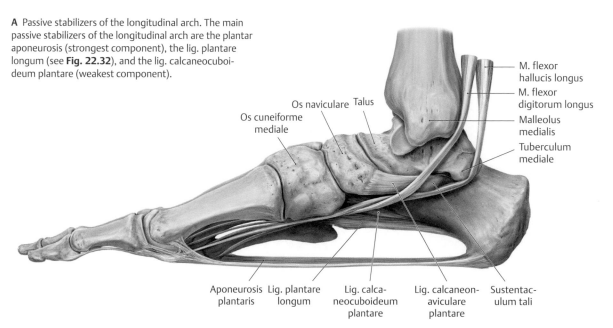

Fig. 22.35 Stabilizers of the longitudinal arch
Right foot, medial view. (From Schuenke M, Schulte E, Schumacher U. THIEME Atlas of Anatomy, Vol 1. Illustrations by Voll M and Wesker K. 3rd ed. New York: Thieme Publishers; 2020.)

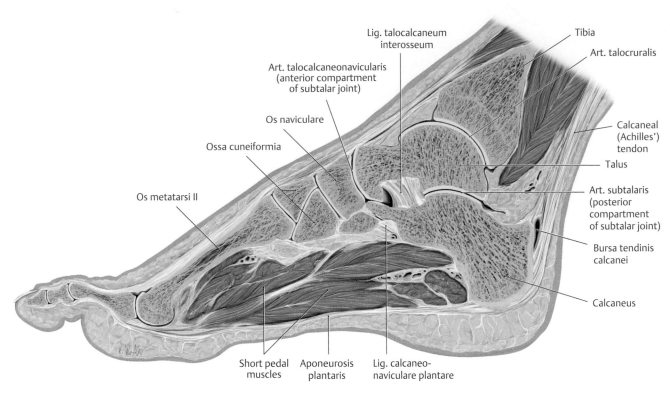

Lig. talocalcaneum interosseum

Art. talocalcaneonavicularis (anterior compartment of subtalar joint)

Os naviculare

Ossa cuneiformia

Os metatarsi II

Tibia

Art. talocruralis

Calcaneal (Achilles') tendon

Talus

Art. subtalaris (posterior compartment of subtalar joint)

Bursa tendinis calcanei

Calcaneus

Short pedal muscles

Aponeurosis plantaris

Lig. calcaneo-naviculare plantare

B Active stabilizers of the longitudinal arch. The main active stabilizers are the short muscles of the foot: m. abductor hallucis, m. flexor hallucis brevis, m. flexor digitorum brevis, m. quadratus plantae, and m. abductor digiti minimi.

Fig. 22.35 (*continued*) **Stabilizers of the longitudinal arch**

Dorsum of the Foot

— Surface anatomy on the dorsum of the foot reveals
  • skin that is thin and loose,
  • a superficial arcus venosus dorsalis pedis that is the origin of the v. saphena magna and v. saphena parva, and

  • tendons of extensor muscles of the anterior leg compartment.
— A **dorsal muscular compartment** of the foot contains two intrinsic muscles, the **m. extensor digitorum brevis** and the **m. extensor hallucis brevis,** which extend the toes (**Table 22.15**).

Table 22.15 Intrinsic Muscles of the Dorsum of the Foot

Muscle	Origin	Insertion	Innervation	Action
① M. extensor digitorum brevis	Calcaneus (facies dorsalis)	Digiti pedis II–IV (at dorsal aponeuroses and bases phalangum medianum)	N. fibularis profundus (L5, S1)	Extension of the artt. metatarsophalangeae and proximal artt. interphalangeae of the digiti pedis II–IV
② M. extensor hallucis brevis		Hallux (at dorsal aponeurosis and phalanx proximalis)		Extension of the art. metatarsophalangea of the hallux

Intrinsic muscles of the dorsum of the foot, right foot, dorsal view. (From Gilroy AM et al. Atlas of Anatomy. 4th ed. 2020. Based on: Schuenke M, Schulte E, Schumacher U. THIEME Atlas of Anatomy. General Anatomy and Musculoskeletal System. Illustrations by Voll M and Wesker K. 3rd ed. New York: Thieme Medical Publishers; 2020.)

Sole of the Foot

— Surface anatomy on the sole of the foot reveals
  • tough, thickened skin, particularly on the heel, lateral side, and ball of the foot;
  • skin that is firmly attached to the underlying plantar aponeurosis; and
  • subcutaneous tissue divided by fibrous septa into fat-filled areas that act as shock absorbers, especially in the heel.
— The tough, longitudinal aponeurosis plantaris (see **Fig. 22.42**)
  • attaches tightly to the skin of the sole,
  • originates at the calcaneus and is continuous distally with the fibrous digital sheaths that contain the flexor tendons of the toes,

• protects the sole of the foot from injury, and
• acts as a tie rod that supports the arches of the foot.
— The musculature of the sole is usually described as having four layers (**Tables 22.16** and **22.17**). However, as in the palm of the hand, the deep fascia separates the muscles of the sole into four fascial compartments:
  • The **medial compartment,** which contains the abductor and flexors of the 1st digit (hallux)
  • The **central compartment,** which contains the short and long flexors of the 2nd through 4th digits, the m. adductor hallucis, the mm. lumbricales, and the m. quadratus plantae
  • The **lateral compartment,** which contains the abductor and flexor of the 5th digit
  • The **interosseous compartment,** which contains the mm. interossei

Table 22.16 Intrinsic Muscles of the Sole of the Foot: Superficial Layer

Muscle	Origin	Insertion	Innervation	Action
① M. abductor hallucis	Tuber calcanei (proc. medialis); retinaculum musculorum flexorum pedis, aponeurosis plantaris	Hallux (basis phalangis proximalis via the medial os sesamoideum)	N. plantaris medialis (S1, S2)	1st art. metatarsophalangea: flexion and abduction of the hallux. Supports the arcus pedis longitudinalis
② M. flexor digitorum brevis	Tuber calcanei (proc. medialis), aponeurosis plantaris	Digiti pedis II–V (sides of phalanges mediae)		Flexes the artt. metatarsophalangea and interphalangea (proximalis) of the digiti pedis II–V. Supports the arcus pedis longitudinalis
③ M. abductor digiti minimi		Digitus pedis V (basis phalangis proximalis), os metatarsi V (at tuberositas)	N. plantaris lateralis (S1–S3)	Flexes the art. metatarsophalangea of the digitus pedis V. Abducts the digitus V. Supports the arcus pedis longitudinalis

Superficial intrinsic muscles of the sole of the foot, right foot, first layer, plantar view. (From Gilroy AM et al. Atlas of Anatomy. 4th ed. 2020. Based on: Schuenke M, Schulte E, Schumacher U. THIEME Atlas of Anatomy. General Anatomy and Musculoskeletal System. Illustrations by Voll M and Wesker K. 3rd ed. New York: Thieme Medical Publishers; 2020.)

BOX 22.16: CLINICAL CORRELATION

PLANTAR FASCIITIS
Inflammation of the aponeurosis plantaris is a common and painful affliction of runners that is characterized by tenderness on the sole, particularly on the calcaneus. Pain is usually greatest following rest and may dissipate with activity.

BOX 22.17: CLINICAL CORRELATION

THE PLANTAR REFLEX
The plantar reflex tests the integrity of the radices of nn. spinales L4–S2. It is performed by firmly stroking the lateral aspect of the sole from the heel and across the foot to the base of the big toe. In the normal individual, this elicits flexion of the toes. Extension of the big toe with flaring of the 2nd through 5th digits is called the Babinski sign, an abnormal response in adults, indicating brain damage. Because of the immaturity of their central nervous system, the Babinski sign is a normal response in young children (under 4 years).

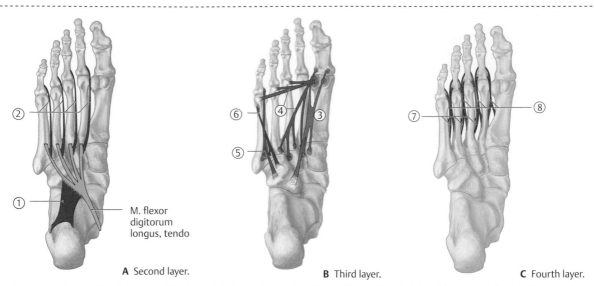

A Second layer.   **B** Third layer.   **C** Fourth layer.

Deep intrinsic muscles of the sole of the foot, right foot, plantar view. (From Gilroy AM et al. Atlas of Anatomy. 4th ed. 2020. Based on: Schuenke M, Schulte E, Schumacher U. THIEME Atlas of Anatomy. General Anatomy and Musculoskeletal System. Illustrations by Voll M and Wesker K. 3rd ed. New York: Thieme Medical Publishers; 2020.)

Table 22.17 Intrinsic Muscles of the Sole of the Foot: Deep Layer

Muscle	Origin	Insertion	Innervation	Action
① M. quadratus plantae	Tuber calcanei (medial and plantar borders on plantar side)	M. flexor digitorum longus tendon (lateral border)	N. plantaris lateralis (S1–S3)	Redirects and augments the pull of m. flexor digitorum longus
② Mm. lumbri- cales (four muscles)	M. flexor digitorum longus tendons (medial borders)	Digiti pedis II–V (at dorsal aponeuroses)	M. lumbricalis I: n. plantaris medialis (S2, S3)	Flexes the artt. metatarsophalangeae of digiti pedis II–V Extension of artt. interphalangeae of digiti pedis II–V Adducts digiti pedis II–V toward the hallux
			Mm. lumbricales II–IV: n. plantaris lateralis (S2, S3)	
③ M. flexor hallucis brevis	Os cuboideum, os cuneiforme laterale, and lig. calcaneocuboideum plantare	Hallux (at basis phalangis proximalis via medial and lateral ossa sesamoidea)	Caput mediale: n. plantaris medialis (S1, S2)	Flexes the first art. metatarsophalangea Supports the arcus pedis longitudinalis
			Caput laterale: n. plantaris lateralis (S1, S2)	
④ M. adductor hallucis	Caput obliquum: Ossa metatarsi II–IV (at bases) os cuboideum and os cuneiforme laterale	Phalanx proximalis I (at base, by a common tendon via the lateral os sesamoideum)	R. profundus nervi plantaris lateralis (S2, S3)	Flexes the first art. metatarsophalangea Adducts hallux Caput transversum: supports arcus pedis transversus distalis Caput obliquum: supports arcus pedis longitudinalis
	Caput transversum: Artt. metatarsophalangeae of digiti III–V, lig. metatarsale transversum profundum			
⑤ M. flexor digiti minimi brevis	Basis ossis metatarsi V, lig. plantare longum	Basis phalangis proximalis V	R. superficialis nervi plantaris lateralis (S2, S3)	Flexes the art. metatarsophalangea of the little toe
⑥ M. opponens digiti minimi*	Lig. plantare longum; m. fibularis longus (at plantar tendon sheath)	Os metatarsi V		Pulls os metatarsi V in plantar and medial direction
⑦ Mm. interossei plantares (three muscles)	Ossa metatarsi III–V (medial border)	Digiti pedis III–V (medial basis phalangis proximalis)	N. plantaris lateralis (S2, S3)	Flexes the artt. metatarsophalangeae of digiti pedis III–V Extension of artt. interphalangeae of digiti pedis III–V Adducts digiti III–V toward digitus II
⑧ Mm. interossei dorsales (four muscles)	Ossa metatarsi I–V (by two heads on opposing sides)	M. interosseus dorsalis I: Phalanx proximalis II (medial base)		Flexes the artt. metatarsophalangeae of digiti pedis II–IV Extension of artt. interphalangeae of digiti pedis II–IV Abducts digiti pedis III–IV from digitus II
		Mm. interossei dorsales II–IV: Phalanges proximales II–IV (lateral basis), digiti pedis II–IV (at dorsal aponeuroses)		

*May be absent.

22.8 The Gait Cycle

Gait is a complex activity that requires the coordinated action of muscles of the hip, thigh, and leg. **Table 22.18** provides a summary of muscle action during the gait cycle.

— Gait is described in two phases: in normal walking, the stance phase makes up ~ 60%, and the swing phase makes up ~ 40%.
— One cycle of gait consists of the action of one leg through each of the two phases.

Table 22.18 Muscle Action Sequence During the Gait Cycle

Activity	Active Muscle Groups
Stance phase	
This phase begins with the heel strike.	Hip extensors Dorsiflexors
The foot begins to accept the weight of the body, and the pelvis is stabilized.	Hip adductors Knee extensors Plantar flexors
At midstance, the pelvis, knee, and ankle are stabilized.	Hip abductors Knee extensors Plantar flexors
This phase ends with the push off that includes "heel lift" and "toe off." Pelvis is stabilized.	Hip abductors Plantar flexors
Throughout the stance phase, the arches of the foot are preserved.	Long tendons of the foot Intrinsic muscles of the foot
Swing phase	
This phase begins with forward acceleration of the thigh.	Hip flexors
The foot needs to clear the ground as it swings forward.	Dorsiflexors
The thigh decelerates in preparation for landing.	Hip extensors
As the foot prepares for heel strike, the knee extends and positions the foot.	Knee extensor Dorsiflexors

22.9   Topographic Anatomy of Lower Limb Musculature

Thigh, Hip, and Gluteal Region

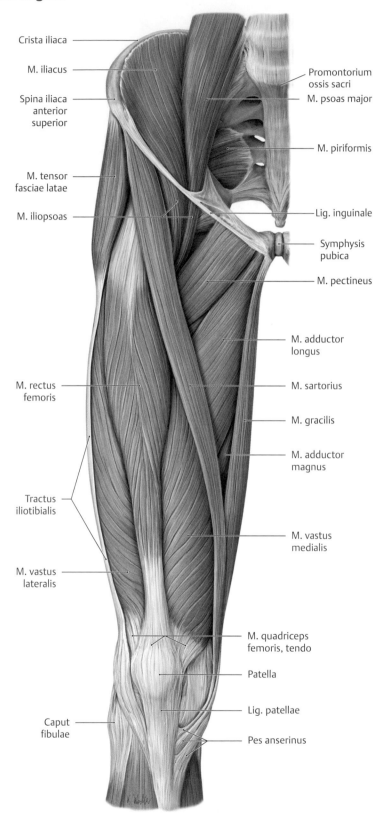

Crista iliaca

M. iliacus

Spina iliaca anterior superior

M. tensor fasciae latae

M. iliopsoas

Promontorium ossis sacri

M. psoas major

M. piriformis

Lig. inguinale

Symphysis pubica

M. pectineus

M. adductor longus

M. rectus femoris

M. sartorius

M. gracilis

M. adductor magnus

Tractus iliotibialis

M. vastus medialis

M. vastus lateralis

M. quadriceps femoris, tendo

Patella

Lig. patellae

Caput fibulae

Pes anserinus

Fig. 22.36 Muscles of the hip and thigh
Right limb, anterior view. Muscle origins are shown in *red*, insertions in *gray*.
Removed: Fascia lata of the thigh (to the lateral tractus iliotibialis). (From Schuenke M, Schulte E, Schumacher U. THIEME Atlas of Anatomy, Vol 1. Illustrations by Voll M and Wesker K. 3rd ed. New York: Thieme Publishers; 2020.)

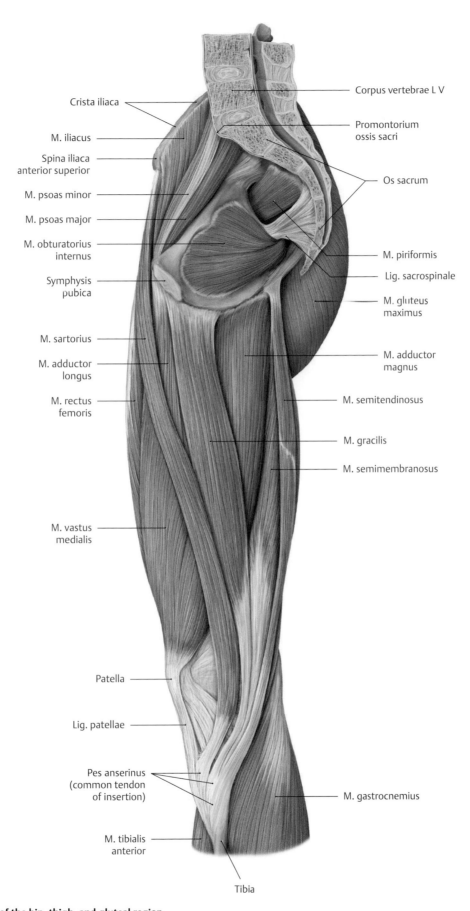

Crista iliaca

M. iliacus

Spina iliaca
anterior superior

M. psoas minor

M. psoas major

M. obturatorius
internus

Symphysis
pubica

M. sartorius

M. adductor
longus

M. rectus
femoris

M. vastus
medialis

Patella

Lig. patellae

Pes anserinus
(common tendon
of insertion)

M. tibialis
anterior

Tibia

Corpus vertebrae L V

Promontorium
ossis sacri

Os sacrum

M. piriformis

Lig. sacrospinale

M. gluteus
maximus

M. adductor
magnus

M. semitendinosus

M. gracilis

M. semimembranosus

M. gastrocnemius

Fig. 22.37 Muscles of the hip, thigh, and gluteal region
Midsagittal section, medial view. (From Gilroy AM et al. Atlas of Anatomy. 4th ed. 2020. Based on: Schuenke M, Schulte E, Schumacher U. THIEME Atlas of Anatomy. General Anatomy and Musculoskeletal System. Illustrations by Voll M and Wesker K. 3rd ed. New York: Thieme Medical Publishers; 2020.)

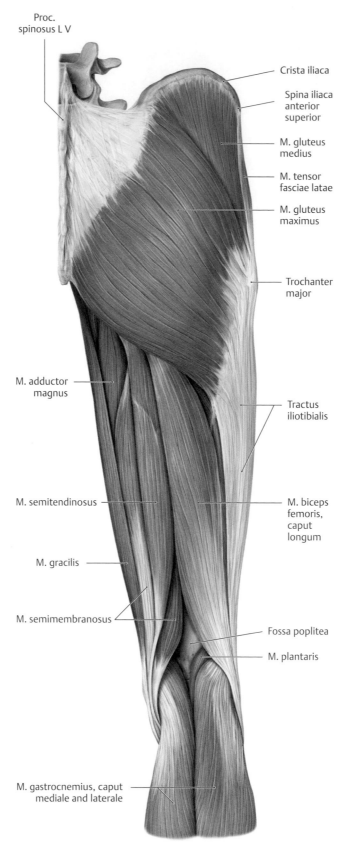

Fig. 22.38 Muscles of the hip, thigh, and gluteal region
Right limb, posterior view.
Removed: Fascia lata (to tractus iliotibialis). (From Schuenke M, Schulte E, Schumacher U. THIEME Atlas of Anatomy, Vol 1. Illustrations by Voll M and Wesker K. 3rd ed. New York: Thieme Publishers; 2020.)

The Leg

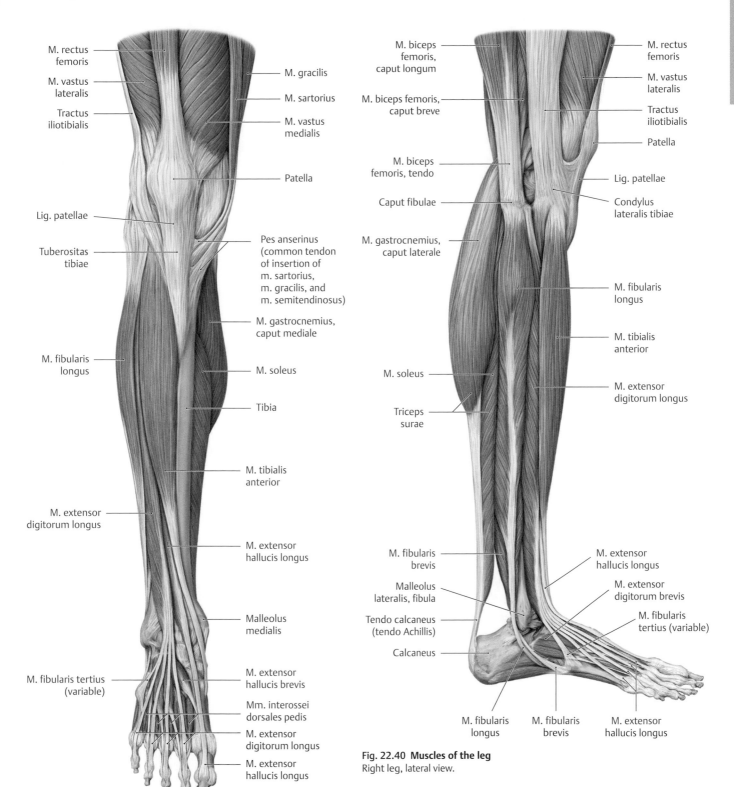

Fig. 22.39 Muscles of the leg
Right leg, anterior view. (From Schuenke M, Schulte E, Schumacher U. THIEME Atlas of Anatomy, Vol 1. Illustrations by Voll M and Wesker K. 3rd ed. New York: Thieme Publishers; 2020.)

Fig. 22.40 Muscles of the leg
Right leg, lateral view.

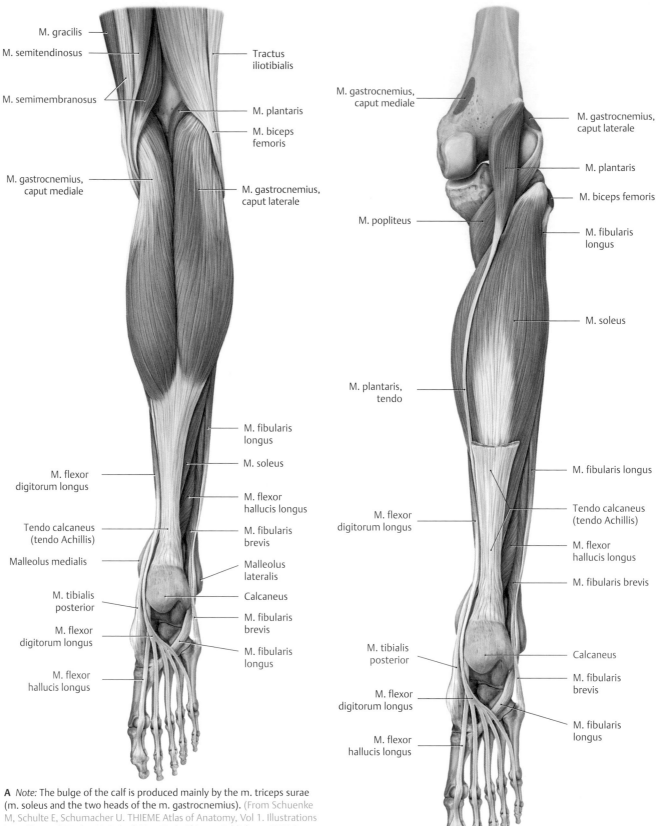

A *Note:* The bulge of the calf is produced mainly by the m. triceps surae (m. soleus and the two heads of the m. gastrocnemius). (From Schuenke M, Schulte E, Schumacher U. THIEME Atlas of Anatomy, Vol 1. Illustrations by Voll M and Wesker K. 3rd ed. New York: Thieme Publishers; 2020.)

Fig. 22.41 Muscles of the leg
Right leg, posterior view.

B *Removed:* M. gastrocnemius (both heads). (From Gilroy AM, MacPherson BR, Wikenheiser JC. Atlas of Anatomy. Illustrations by Voll M and Wesker K. 4th ed. New York: Thieme Publishers; 2020.)

The Foot

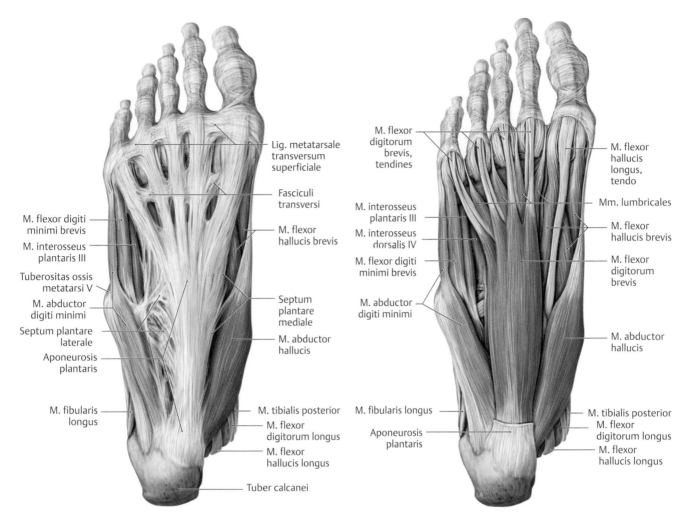

Fig. 22.42 Aponeurosis plantaris
Right foot, plantar view. The aponeurosis plantaris is a tough aponeurotic sheet, thickest at the center, that blends with the dorsal fascia (not shown) at the borders of the foot. (From Schuenke M, Schulte E, Schumacher U. THIEME Atlas of Anatomy, Vol 1. Illustrations by Voll M and Wesker K. 3rd ed. New York: Thieme Publishers; 2020.)

Fig. 22.43 Intrinsic muscles of the sole of the foot
Right foot, plantar view.
Superficial (first) layer. *Removed:* Aponeurosis plantaris, including the lig. metacarpale transversum superficiale. (From Schuenke M, Schulte E, Schumacher U. THIEME Atlas of Anatomy, Vol 1. Illustrations by Voll M and Wesker K. 3rd ed. New York: Thieme Publishers; 2020.)

Compartments of the Thigh and Leg

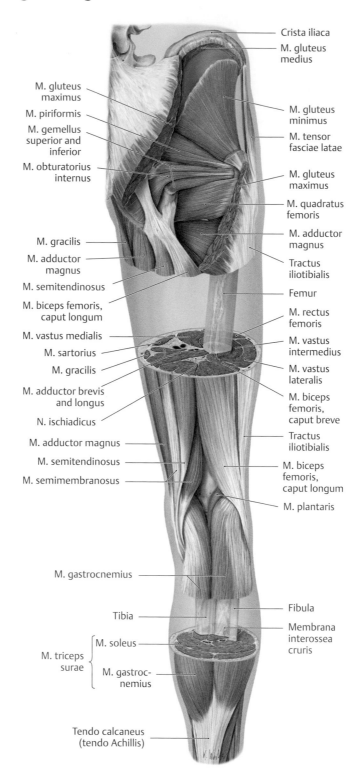

Fig. 22.44 Windowed dissection
Right limb, posterior view. (From Schuenke M, Schulte E, Schumacher U. THIEME Atlas of Anatomy, Vol 1. Illustrations by Voll M and Wesker K. 3rd ed. New York: Thieme Publishers; 2020.)

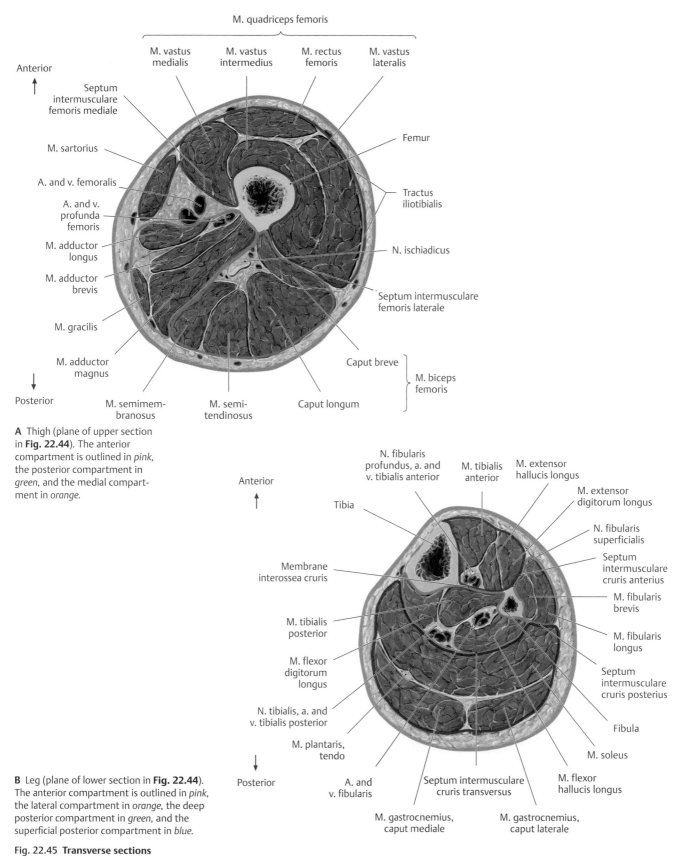

A Thigh (plane of upper section in **Fig. 22.44**). The anterior compartment is outlined in *pink*, the posterior compartment in *green*, and the medial compartment in *orange*.

B Leg (plane of lower section in **Fig. 22.44**). The anterior compartment is outlined in *pink*, the lateral compartment in *orange*, the deep posterior compartment in *green*, and the superficial posterior compartment in *blue*.

Fig. 22.45 Transverse sections
Right limb, proximal (superior) view. (From Schuenke M, Schulte E, Schumacher U. THIEME Atlas of Anatomy, Vol 1. Illustrations by Voll M and Wesker K. 3rd ed. New York: Thieme Publishers; 2020.)

23 Clinical Imaging Basics of the Lower Limb

As in the upper extremity, radiographs are always the first imaging choice in evaluation of bones and joints in the setting of trauma or pain, and magnetic resonance imaging (MRI) is the primary method for evaluating the soft tissue components of the joints. In infants, ultrasound is used to diagnose developmental hip dysplasia and to assess for abnormal joint fluid (**Table 23.1**).

The principles and practices used in evaluating images of bones, joints, and soft tissues in the lower limb are similar to those used in the upper limb, except lower limb radiographs are often obtained with the patient standing or in a weight-bearing position. This distinction is important especially in the evaluation of weight-bearing joints (hips, knees, and ankles) because the joint is evaluated under the stress of everyday use (**Figs. 23.1** and **23.2**). MRIs cannot be taken with the patient in a weight-bearing position; nonetheless, they provide excellent detail of the internal soft tissue structures of the joint (**Fig. 23.3**).

Table 23.1 Suitability of Imaging Modalities for the Lower Limb

Modality	Clinical Uses
Radiographs (x-rays)	First-line imaging evaluation tool for the extremities; used primarily to evaluate for fractures, bone lesions, and alignment of joints
CT (computed tomography)	Reserved as a troubleshooting tool to evaluate for subtle nondisplaced fractures
MRI (magnetic resonance imaging)	One of the most important imaging modalities for the evaluation of joints, specifically the non-osseous components of the joint, e.g., cartilage, ligaments, tendons, and muscles
Ultrasound	In children, due to their small size, it plays a larger role in diagnosis of hip disorders (developmental dysplasia, toxic synovitis, or joint effusion) and in evaluation of cartilaginous growth plates. Ultrasound has a limited role in evaluation of superficial soft tissue abnormalities and for guidance of interventional procedures involving the joints.

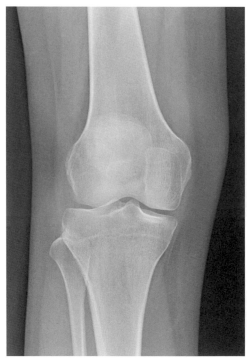 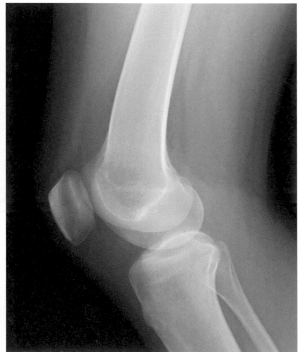

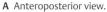

A Anteroposterior view.   **B** Lateral view.

Fig. 23.1 Radiograph of the right knee
Knee radiographs are usually performed with the patient upright in order to assess the knee joint in a weight-bearing stance. The articular surfaces of the bones should be smooth and the medial and lateral joint compartments should be equally spaced. There should be no bone fragments in the joint spaces. The cortical edge of each bone should be traced around the entire bone and should be smooth. Note how the patella overlaps the femur in the frontal projection (A) and is difficult to see clearly. The lateral view (B) affords a non-overlapping view of the patella. (Courtesy of Joseph Makris, MD, Baystate Medical Center.)

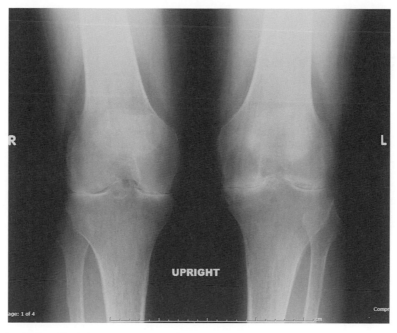

Fig. 23.2 Standing frontal radiographs of both knees in a 60-year-old man with chronic knee pain
Note the "bone on bone" appearance of the joint due to marked joint space narrowing. Compare this with the normal joint space appearance in
Fig. 23.1. Although we don't see articular cartilage itself on an x-ray, we do see the space it creates between the bones, or, in this case, we see the
results of chronic degenerative cartilage loss. (From Garcia G, ed. RadCases: Musculoskeletal Radiology 2nd ed. New York: Thieme Publishers; 2017.)

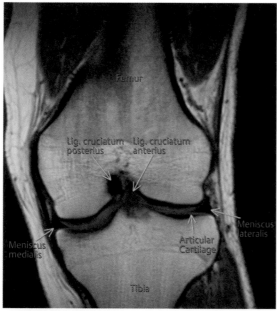

A Coronal section.

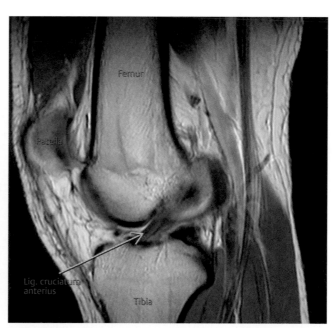

B Midsagittal section.

Fig. 23.3 MRI of the knee
In this sequence fat is bright (*white*), cortical bone is *black*, most normal ligaments and tendons are dark gray or black, and muscle is *dark gray*. The
normal lig. cruciatum anterius has a unique striated appearance due to its linear bands of fibers. Note that the bone marrow is white because of its high
fat content. (Courtesy of Joseph Makris, MD, Baystate Medical Center)

Unit VII   Review Questions: Lower Limb

1. A young girl has recovered well from the severe injuries she sustained in a motor vehicle accident 9 months ago, but because of some lingering nerve problems, she still has difficulty walking. She is balanced during the midstance phase but has difficulty bringing her limb forward to initiate movement. What nerve seems to be affected?
    A. N. gluteus superior
    B. N. gluteus inferior
    C. N. femoralis
    D. N. obturatorius
    E. N. tibialis

2. A young woman searching for driftwood walked several miles on the soft sandy beach of a Caribbean island. While walking on this uneven surface, the balance between inversion and eversion at her art. subtalaris was maintained by the opposing actions of the m. fibularis longus and the
    A. m. fibularis brevis
    B. m. fibularis tertius
    C. m. soleus
    D. m. tibialis anterior
    E. m. extensor digitorum longus

3. Structures at the knee that are *not* attached to the capsula articularis include the
    A. meniscus medialis
    B. lig. collaterale tibiale
    C. lig. collaterale fibulare
    D. retinacula patellae
    E. All of the above (A–D) are attached to the capsula articularis.

4. A woman in her early 40s discovered a small lump at the top of her thigh that was later diagnosed as a femoral hernia. Where would this hernia be located?
    A. Spatium retroinguinale
    B. Canalis femoralis
    C. Femoral sheath
    D. Anulus femoralis
    E. All of the above

5. An elderly woman shopping with her daughter fell in the mall parking lot. After examining the woman, the paramedics who responded to the call noted that the limb was pulled upward, and the hip was rotated laterally. They confided to the daughter that it appeared that the woman had fractured her collum femoris. Which of the following muscles would be responsible for the lateral (external) rotation?
    A. M. gluteus medius
    B. M. tensor of the fascia lata
    C. M. pectineus
    D. M. vastus lateralis
    E. All of the above

6. The strongest and most supportive ligament of the art. coxae is the
    A. lig. transversum acetabuli
    B. lig. capitis femoris
    C. lig. pubofemorale
    D. lig. ischiofemorale
    E. lig. iliofemorale

7. A young man running on the beach severely lacerated his foot when he accidentally stepped into a pit with broken glass left by late-night partygoers. Surgery was required to remove the glass fragments and treat the lacerations. You opt to use regional anesthesia, injecting anesthetic near each of the nerves that cross the ankle. Where would you anesthetize the n. suralis?
    A. Anterior to the malleolus medialis
    B. Posterior to the malleolus medialis
    C. Posterior to the malleolus lateralis
    D. Anterior to the malleolus lateralis
    E. First web space

8. Sensation along the lateral side of the first toe is transmitted by branches of the
    A. n. saphenus
    B. n. plantaris medialis
    C. n. fibularis profundus
    D. n. fibularis superficialis
    E. n. plantaris lateralis

9. Superficial veins of the lower limb
    A. lie deep to the fascia lata
    B. include the v. saphena magna that terminates at the v. poplitea
    C. include the v. saphena parva whose course runs anterior to the malleolus lateralis
    D. drain to deep veins via vv. perforantes
    E. originate from the arcus venosus plantaris

10. The a. dorsalis pedis is a continuation of the
    A. a. tibialis posterior
    B. a. fibularis
    C. a. tibialis anterior
    D. a. poplitea
    E. a. inferior medialis genus

11. The arcus plantaris profundus is an anastomosis between the a. dorsalis pedis and which structure on the sole of the foot?
    A. A. fibularis
    B. A. plantaris lateralis
    C. Aa. metatarsales plantares
    D. Aa. digitales plantares
    E. A. arcuata

12. An obese woman suffers from peripheral edema (swelling of the legs) and large varicose veins in her leg. Which of the following might be coexisting symptoms related to her condition?
    A. Incompetent valves in the v. saphena magna
    B. Reversed flow in the vv. perforantes
    C. Deep vein thrombosis
    D. Thrombophlebitis
    E. All of the above

13. "Footdrop" occurs when the plantar flexor muscles are unopposed. This condition may be caused by damage to which of the following nerves?
  A. N. fibularis superficialis
  B. N. fibularis profundus
  C. N. suralis
  D. N. tibialis
  E. N. plantaris medialis

14. As she was riding her bike home from her job as a camp counselor, Kristin was sideswiped by a large pickup trunk. She suffered multiple bruises, a fractured tibia, and a fractured pelvis. Several months later she still had an area of numbness on the medial side of her thigh and walked with a lateral swing to her gait. Which muscle was affected by her injury?
  A. M. gluteus medius
  B. M. gluteus maximus
  C. M. semimembranosus
  D. M. adductor longus
  E. M. rectus femoris

15. In the anatomy laboratory you have just dissected the regio glutealis of your cadaver. You are surprised to discover that in your cadaver the lateral component of the n. ischiadicus passes *through* the m. piriformis instead of *inferior* to it. Being a dedicated student, you investigate this further and find this anomaly can cause a piriformis syndrome in which the nerve is compressed by contraction of the muscle. What symptom might this particular patient have experienced?
  A. Paresthesia (tingling) on the sole of the foot
  B. Loss of knee flexion
  C. Loss of knee extension
  D. Foot drop
  E. Sagging of the unsupported hip when walking

16. The m. adductor magnus
  A. extends and adducts the art. coxae
  B. is innervated by the n. femoralis and n. obturatorius
  C. inserts on the linea aspera of the femur and tuberculum adductorium of the tibia
  D. forms the anterior wall of the canalis adductorius
  E. originates from the r. superior ossis pubis

17. Which muscle(s) of the lower limb is/are capable of producing flexion at one joint and extension at a second joint?
  A. M. semimembranosus
  B. M. rectus femoris
  C. Mm. lumbricales of the foot
  D. Caput longum of m. biceps femoris
  E. All of the above

18. During a street fight between two local gangs, one boy received a violent blow to the anterior knee that knocked him to the ground. In the emergency department, the physical exam of his knee revealed a positive posterior drawer sign. What structure appears to be injured?
  A. Lig. cruciatum anterius
  B. Lig. cruciatum posterius
  C. Lig. patellae
  D. Lig. collaterale tibiale
  E. Lig. collaterale fibulare

19. A single woman looking for adventure signed up for a walking tour of the Scottish highlands. She was unprepared for the effort that it required but kept up with the more experienced walkers. After a few days she began to experience extreme tenderness in her anterior leg deep to the ridge of the tibia. The tour guide had seen this in previous clients and suggested that her pain was due to shin splints. Her pain originated from overuse of the
  A. m. extensor digitorum longus
  B. m. extensor digitorum brevis
  C. m. extensor hallucis longus
  D. m. fibularis tertius
  E. m. tibialis anterior

20. Which fibrous structure on the sole of the foot originates at the calcaneus and continues distally as digital fibrous sheaths?
  A. Aponeurosis plantaris
  B. Lig. calcaneonaviculare plantare
  C. Lig. plantare longum
  D. Lig. plantare breve
  E. Lig. deltoideum

21. A man was on a hunting trip with friends when he was accidentally shot in the midthigh. He bled profusely from his a. femoralis until his friends applied constant pressure over the wound and drove him to a local emergency clinic. Although examination of the wound site in surgery revealed a badly torn a. femoralis, the man continued to have distal pulses in his leg. What vessel arises proximal to the injury site and can provide collateral blood supply to the distal limb?
  A. A. circumflexa femoris medialis
  B. A. circumflexa femoris lateralis
  C. A. obturatoria
  D. A. descendens genus
  E. A. poplitea

22. An elderly woman slipped on a patch of ice in her driveway when she went to pick up the morning newspaper. Her neighbor witnessed the accident and called an ambulance. In the emergency department, X-rays revealed that she had fractured the collum femoris. Her physician explained to her that avascular necrosis was a common complication of this injury in elderly women and convinced her to agree to a hip replacement. What vessel contributes most significantly to the blood supply of the art. coxae?
  A. A. obturatoria
  B. A. glutea superior
  C. A. glutea inferior
  D. A. circumflexa femoris medialis
  E. A. circumflexa femoris lateralis

23. Which of the following spaces contain the n. femoralis?
  A. Femoral sheath
  B. Hiatus adductorius
  C. Fossa poplitea
  D. Canalis femoralis
  E. Spatium retroinguinale

24. The n. gluteus inferior innervates the
  A. m. gluteus maximus
  B. m. gluteus medius
  C. m. gluteus minimus
  D. m. piriformis
  E. All of the above

25. Which of the following muscles insert on the tractus iliotibialis?
   A. M. gluteus maximus
   B. M. gluteus medius
   C. M. gluteus minimus
   D. M. quadratus femoris
   E. None of the above

26. Your 13-year-old son who studies martial arts is particularly flexible and is praised for his high kicks. After several weeks of training in preparation for an upcoming tournament, he complains of tenderness in his lower buttocks during practice and even when he sits on the hard stadium benches. As his pediatrician, how do you explain his problem?
   A. Inflammation of the tuberositas ischii
   B. Rupture of the m. obturatorius internus tendon from its insertion
   C. Compression of the n. ischiadicus in the regio glutealis
   D. Irritation of the n. tibialis in the thigh
   E. Irritation of the n. gluteus inferior

27. Which of the following muscles are involved in knee flexion?
   A. M. flexor hallucis longus
   B. M. soleus
   C. M. tibialis posterior
   D. M. biceps femoris
   E. M. rectus femoris

28. The lateral border of the trigonum femoris is formed by the
   A. M. tensor fasciae latae
   B. N. femoralis
   C. M. sartorius
   D. M. adductor longus
   E. M. rectus femoris

29. An 18-year-old marathon runner finished fourth in the Detroit marathon but limped away from the finish line. He had been suffering from excruciating pain on the sole of his foot and immediately sought advice from the medical volunteers. Following a thorough exam, the EMTs explained that the muscle tendons running through his tarsal tunnel had swollen and were compressing the nerve that accompanies them. What bones form the wall of this tunnel?
   A. Os naviculare and talus
   B. Os cuboideum and calcaneus
   C. Talus and calcaneus
   D. Malleolus medialis of the tibia and calcaneus
   E. Talus and base of the 1st metatarsal

30. An experienced 24-year-old backpacker has spent the last 4 months hiking the entire Appalachian trail. Although he has sturdy hiking boots, he often changes to the lightweight sneakers he brought as a backup. For the last few miles of the trek, he has been experiencing shooting pain along the side of his foot at the apex of his arcus medialis. What structure is probably the cause of the pain?
   A. Lig. calcaneonaviculare plantare
   B. Lig. deltoideum
   C. Lig. talofibulare posterius
   D. Retinaculum musculorum extensorum superius pedis
   E. Tendon of m. fibularis longus

31. After retirement your uncle quickly grew bored with home activities and began working at a local hardware store. He was a social person and enjoyed remaining active in the community but the long hours of standing on his feet was difficult. At his recent physical exam, he complained of foot pain and his physician explained that he was suffering from pes planus, or flatfoot. Which of the following are characteristics of this condition?
   A. Increased laxity of the active stabilizers of the medial longitudinal arch
   B. Increased laxity of the passive stabilizers of the medial longitudinal arch
   C. Eversion of the forefoot puts additional stress on the lig. calcaneonaviculare plantare
   D. Inferomedial displacement of the talus
   E. All of the above

32. Crests, prominences, and depressions on bones are important for the attachment sites they provide for muscles or the passageways used by nerves and vessels. Which of the following are correctly paired with the bone to which they belong?
   A. Malleolus medialis: tibia
   B. Linea aspera: fibula
   C. Eminentia intercondylaris: femur
   D. Sustentaculum tali: talus
   E. Tuberculum adductorium: tibia

33. A 19-year-old soccer player felt a sudden pain in his knee when, with his right foot planted, he pivoted to the left to avoid an opposing player. Later at the emergency clinic, he learned that he would be out for the remainder of the season because he had ruptured his lig. cruciatum anterius and one of the menisci. The orthopedist informed him that this was a fairly common type of knee injury. Which of the menisci is most likely injured and why?
   A. The meniscus lateralis because it's tightly adherent to the fibrous capsule and lig. collaterale laterale
   B. The meniscus lateralis because it's more mobile during flexion of the knee
   C. The meniscus medialis because it's relatively immobile and attached to the lig. collaterale tibiale
   D. The meniscus medialis because it's more mobile during flexion and extension of the knee

34. Following an explosion at the local fertilizer factory, you volunteered to triage patients at the local hospital. A young female victim was brought in with minor burns on her lower torso and a broken leg that appeared to be the cause of her intense pain. After a quick exam of the limb that revealed paresthesia and absence of a dorsal pedal pulse, you recognize that she was suffering from a compartment syndrome of her deep posterior compartment and called in the trauma surgeon. Without swift intervention, what would likely be the functional outcome of this case?
   A. Weakening of the medial arch of the foot
   B. Loss of dorsiflexion during the swing phase of gait
   C. Weakened eversion of the foot
   D. Loss of sensation on the dorsum of the foot
   E. All of the above

35. Malia has been experiencing constant nagging pain in her left knee ever since she landed the high jump in her track meet a week ago. An initial x-ray series did not reveal any obvious fractures or dislocations, but since the pain persists, her physician is concerned about the possibility of a meniscal tear. What further imaging studies would be useful?

    A. CT
    B. MRI
    C. Ultrasound
    D. Additional radiographic (x-ray) views

Answers and Explanations

1. **C.** Forward movement at the beginning of the swing phase depends on the action of her hip flexors, particularly the m. rectus femoris, which is innervated by the n. femoralis (Sections 22.2, 22.3, and 22.8).
    A. The n. gluteus superior innervates the abductors of the hip. Damage to this nerve would cause a sagging of the hip on the contralateral side just before the midstance.
    B. The n. gluteus inferior innervates the m. gluteus maximus. Injury to this nerve would affect the deceleration of the swing phase.
    D. Injury to the n. obturatorius, which innervates the adductors of the hip, would cause an outward swing of the limb but would not inhibit acceleration of the thigh.
    E. The n. tibialis innervates the hamstring muscles of the posterior thigh, which are responsible for the deceleration at the end of the swing phase.

2. **D.** The m. tibialis anterior and m. tibialis posterior are the strong inverters of the foot that counter the action of the m. fibularis longus and m. fibularis brevis (Section 22.7).
    A. The m. fibularis brevis, in the lateral crural compartment, inserts on the base of the os metatarsale V, which allows it to evert the foot.
    B. The m. fibularis tertius, a muscle of the anterior crural compartment, inserts on the base of the os metatarsale V and everts the foot.
    C. The m. soleus, in the posterior crural compartment, plantar flexes the foot.
    E. The m. extensor digitorum, in the anterior crural compartment, everts the foot.

3. **C.** The lig. collaterale fibulare is an extracapsular ligament that extends from the epicondylus lateralis of the femur to the caput fibulae and remains separate from the capsula articularis of the knee (Section 22.4).
    A. The meniscus medialis and meniscus lateralis attach along their outer rims to the capsula articularis.
    B. The lig. collaterale tibiale is a capsular ligament that extends from the epicondylus medialis of the femur to the condylus medialis tibiae and superior part of the medial tibia. It attaches to the capsula articularis and to the meniscus medialis.
    D. The retinacula patellae are fibrous expansions of the tendons of the m. quadriceps femoris. They form the capsula articularis on either side of the patella.
    E. Only the lig. collaterale fibulare (C) is correct.

4. **E.** A vascular compartment of the spatium retroinguinale contains the femoral sheath and the canalis femoralis. The anulus femoralis defines the upper edge of the canalis femoralis. A femoral hernia protrudes into the canalis femoralis (Section 22.3).
    A. The spatium retroinguinale contains the canalis femoralis, the site of the femoral hernia. B through D are also correct (E).
    B. The canalis femoralis is a space within the femoral sheath that normally contains loose connective tissue, fat, and often a nl. inguinalis profundus. A, C, and D are also correct (E).
    C. The femoral sheath contains the femoral vessels and the canalis femoralis. A, B, and D are also correct (E).
    D. The anulus femoralis defines the superior opening of the canalis femoralis. A, B, and C are also correct (E).

5. **C.** The m. pectineus in the medial thigh compartment adducts and laterally rotates the hip (Section 22.3).
    A. The m. gluteus medius is an abductor of the hip.
    B. The m. tensor fasciae latae abducts, flexes, and internally rotates the hip.
    D. The m. vastus lateralis extends the knee and has no influence over the art. coxae.
    E. A, B, and D are incorrect.

6. **E.** The lig. iliofemorale attaches proximally to the spina iliaca anterior inferior and rim of the acetabulum and distally to the linea intertrochanterica of the femur. It supports the art. coxae during standing (Section 22.3).
    A. The lig. transversum completes the rim of the C-shaped acetabulum inferiorly.
    B. The lig. capitis femoris attaches to the acetabulum within the joint but provides little support. A small artery runs within the ligament to the caput femoris.
    C. The lig. pubofemorale runs laterally from the inferior aspect of the acetabular rim to merge with the lig. iliofemorale. It assists the lig. iliofemorale and limits abduction of the joint.
    D. The lig. ischiofemorale is the weakest of the three ligaments of the capsule. It arises from the ischial part of the acetabular rim and spirals anteriorly to insert on the collum femoris.

7. **C.** The n. suralis innervates the lateral side of the foot and runs posterior to the malleolus lateralis (Section 21.4).
    A. The n. saphenus runs anterior to the malleolus medialis.
    B. The n. tibialis courses through the tarsal tunnel posterior to the malleolus medialis.
    D. The n. fibularis superficialis runs onto the dorsum of the foot anterior to the malleolus lateralis.
    E. The n. fibularis profundus accompanies the a. dorsalis pedis onto the dorsum of the foot. It innervates the skin of the first web space.

8. **C.** The n. fibularis profundus, a branch of the n. fibularis communis, supplies cutaneous innervation to the first web space, including the skin adjacent to the first and second digits. It also supplies motor innervation to the muscles of the anterior compartment of the leg (Section 21.4).
    A. The n. saphenus transmits sensation from the medial side of the foot.

B. The r. plantaris medialis of the n. tibialis supplies cutaneous innervation to a large area of skin on the medial side of the foot and the medial three and a half digits.

D. The n. fibularis superficialis supplies cutaneous innervation to the dorsum of the foot.

E. The r. plantaris lateralis supplies cutaneous innervation to the lateral foot and the lateral one and a half digits.

9. **D.** Similar to superficial veins of the upper limb, superficial veins of the lower limb drain to deep veins via vv. perforantes (Section 15.4).

A. Superficial veins lie in the subcutaneous tissue, superficial to the deep fascia (fascia lata).

B. The v. saphena magna pierces the fascia lata at the hiatus saphenus in the proximal thigh and terminates in the v. femoralis.

C. The v. saphena parva runs posterior to the lateral malleolus and superiorly to the fossa poplitea.

E. The large superficial veins, the v. saphena magna and v. saphena parva, originate from the arcus venosus on the dorsum of the foot.

10. **C.** The a. tibialis anterior descends within the anterior crural compartment and emerges onto the dorsum of the foot as the a. dorsalis pedis (Section 21.4).

A. The a. tibialis posterior descends within posterior crural compartment and branches into the a. plantaris medialis and a. plantaris lateralis that supply the sole of the foot.

B. The a. fibularis arises in the lateral part of the posterior leg and anastomoses with the a. tibialis anterior to supply the ankle.

D. The a. poplitea lies posterior to the knee. It gives rise to the aa. geniculares and a. tibialis.

E. The a. media genus inferior is a branch of the a. poplitea and supplies blood to the patella and insertions of the m. sartorius, m. gracilis, and m. semitendinosus.

11. **B.** The a. plantaris lateralis, similar to the a. ulnaris in the hand, is the largest branch of the a. tibialis posterior. It supplies the lateral side of the foot and forms the arcus plantaris profundus with the a. dorsalis pedis (Section 21.4).

A. The a. fibularis supplies muscles in the posterior and lateral compartments of the leg and forms an anastomosis with the a. tibialis anterior at the ankle, but it has no branches on the sole of the foot.

C. The aa. metatarsales plantares arise from the arcus plantaris profundus.

D. aa. digitales propriae arise from the aa. metatarsales plantares, which are branches of the arcus plantaris profundus.

E. The a. arcuata, a branch of the a. dorsalis pedis, forms a loop on the dorsum of the foot and supplies the aa. metatarsales dorsales II, III, and IV.

12. **E.** Varicose, or dilated, veins can occur in conjunction with deep vein thromboses. When the deep veins are obstructed, the normal superficial-to-deep flow in the vv. perforantes reverses. With the increased volume, the superficial veins dilate, and their valves become incompetent. Thrombophlebitis, or venous inflammation, often occurs with thrombus formation (Section 21.4).

A. When valvulae venosa are incompetent, upward flow is impeded, and blood pools in the veins. The resulting dilated veins are known as varicose veins. B through D are also correct (E).

B. Superficial veins normally drain into the deep venous system through the vv. perforantes. If the deep veins are obstructed by thrombus, blood flows outward through the perforating veins into the superficial system, dilating the superficial veins. A, C, and D are also correct (E).

C. When thrombus obstructs the deep veins of the leg, blood flows outward into the superficial veins, causing them to dilate. A, B, and D are also correct (E).

D. Inflammation of veins can occur with thrombus formation. A through C are also correct (E).

13. **B.** Footdrop is caused by an injury to the n. fibularis profundus (or communis) causing paralysis of the dorsiflexor muscles in the foot, leaving the plantar flexor muscles unopposed (Section 21.4).

A. Injury to the superficial fibular nerve results in an inability to evert the foot and therefore an overall loss of balance and loss of sensation on the dorsum of the foot.

C. Injury to the n. suralis causes loss of sensation over the skin on the lateral side of the foot.

D. Injury to the n. tibialis causes paralysis of all of the muscles of the posterior thigh (except the caput breve of m. biceps femoris) and posterior leg.

E. Injury to the n. plantaris medialis causes paralysis of the muscles on the medial side of the foot and loss of sensation over a large area of skin on the medial side of the foot and the medial three and a half digits.

14. **D.** A lateral swinging gait is caused by unopposed hip abduction, which occurs when the adductors are paralyzed. The n. obturatorius innervates the adductor muscles of the thigh and can be injured by pelvic fractures. The area of numbness on the medial thigh also suggests an injury to the n. obturatorius (Section 21.4).

A. The m. gluteus medius is an abductor of the hip. Injury to this muscle results in a gluteal, or waddling, gait.

B. The injury to the n. gluteus inferior, which innervates the gluteus maximus, impairs extension of the hip but does not cause any sensory loss.

C. Injury to the m. semimembranosus or its nerve, the n. tibialis, impairs hip extension, knee flexion, and sensation on the sole of the foot.

E. Injury to the n. femoralis, which innervates the m. rectus femoris, weakens flexion of the hip and extension of the knee. There is a sensory loss from the anterior thigh and the medial side of the leg and foot.

15. **D.** The n. fibularis communis is the lateral component of the n. ischiadicus. Compression will affect the dorsiflexors of the anterior leg compartment (through the n. fibularis profundus), resulting in footdrop (Sections 21.4 and 22.2).

A. Paresthesia on the sole of the foot would be a consequence of compression of the n. tibialis.

B. The n. tibialis, the medial component of the n. ischiadicus, innervates the hamstring muscles, which flex the knee. This action would remain intact.

C. The knee extensors on the anterior thigh extend the knee and would not be affected by this anomaly.

E. Sagging of the unsupported hip is characteristic of an injury to the n. gluteus superior.

16. **A.** The m. adductor magnus is the largest adductor of the hip but also works with the m. gluteus maximus to provide powerful extension of the art. coxae (Section 22.3).

B. The m. adductor magnus has a dual innervation, the n. obturatorius and n. tibialis.

C. The m. adductor magnus inserts entirely on the femur; the tuberculum adductorium is a feature on the distal femur.

D. The canalis adductorius passes between the anterior and medial thigh compartments. The m. vastus medialis forms the anterior wall, and the adductor muscles form the posterior wall.

E. The m. adductor magnus originates on the r. ischiopubicus, which includes the r. pubicus inferior and r. ischii.

17. **E.** M. semimembranosus (A) produces flexion at the art. genus and extension at the art. coxae. M. rectus femoris (B) produces flexion at the art. coxae and extension at the art. genus. The mm. lumbricales of the foot (C) produce flexion of the artt. metacarpophalangeae of the 2nd to 5th toes and extension of the artt. interphalangeae of the 2nd to 5th toes. The caput longum of the m. biceps femoris (D) produces extension of the art. coxae and flexion of the art. genus (Sections 22.3 and 22.7).

    A. Semimembranosus produces flexion at the art. genus and extension at the art. coxae. B through D are also correct (E).

    B. M. rectus femoris produces flexion at the art. coxae and extension at the art. genus. A, C, and D are also correct (E).

    C. The mm. lumbricales of the foot produce flexion of the artt. metacarpophalangeae of the 2nd to 5th toes and extension of the artt. interphalangeae of the 2nd to 5th toes. A, B, and D are also correct (E).

    D. The caput longum of the m. biceps femoris produces extension of the hip joint and flexion of the art. genus. A through C are also correct (E).

18. **B.** The posterior displacement of the tibia is a positive posterior drawer sign that indicates an injury to the lig. cruciatum posterius (Section 22.4).

    A. Injury to the lig. cruciatum anterius is recognized by the positive anterior drawer sign in which the tibia can be pulled anteriorly from under the femur.

    C. A positive drawer sign suggests anterior or posterior displacement of the tibia relative to the femur. Rupture of the lig. patellae destabilizes the art. genus but does not disrupt the alignment of the tibia and femur.

    D. Although the lig. collaterale tibiale may be damaged by a forceful blow, it is not diagnosed by a posterior drawer sign.

    E. The lig. collaterale fibulare is unlikely to be damaged by a blow to the anterior knee and is not diagnosed by either anterior or posterior drawer signs.

19. **E.** Shin splints are a result of inflammation of the m. tibialis anterior and small tears of the periosteum where the muscle attaches to the bone (Section 22.5).

    A. The m. extensor digitorum originates from the caput fibulae, condylus lateralis of the tibia, and membrana interossea.

    B. The m. extensor digitorum brevis is an intrinsic muscle of the foot. It arises from the calcaneus.

    C. The m. extensor hallucis longus arises from the middle of the corpus fibulae and the membrana interossea.

D. M. fibularis tertius is a lateral muscle within the anterior compartment that arises from the distal fibula.

20. **A.** The aponeurosis plantaris is a thick fibrous band on the sole that is continuous with the fascia profunda cruris (Section 22.7).

    B. The lig. calcaneonaviculare plantare, or spring ligament, supports the head of the talus and maintains the medial side of the arcus longitudinalis.

    C. The lig. plantare longum supports the lateral side of the arcus longitudinalis and extends from the calcaneus to the bases of the ossa metatarsi I, II, and III.

    D. The lig. calcaneocuboideum plantare, supports the arcus lateralis pedis.

    E. The lig. deltoideum is a four-part ligament that supports the medial side of the art. talocruralis.

21. **B.** The a. circumflexa femoris lateralis arises from the a. profunda femoris in the proximal thigh. It supplies structures around the hip as well as a descending branch that anastomoses with the aa. geniculares at the knee. Reverse flow in these branches could supply the a. poplitea and its branches in the leg (Section 21.4).

    A. The a. circumflexa femoris medialis arises from the a. profunda femoris and supplies the art. coxae. It does not anastomose with the a. poplitea or other branches of the knee and leg.

    C. The a. obturatoria supplies the medial compartment of the thigh and does not anastomose with vessels of the leg.

    D. The a. descendens genus is a branch of the a. femoralis, but it arises distal to the site of injury and therefore cannot provide collateral circulation.

    E. The a. poplitea anastomoses with the proximal a. femoralis only through the a. circumflexa femoris lateralis.

22. **D.** Although the a. circumflexa femoris mediales and laterales and a. glutea inferior anastomose around the hip, branches that supply the art. coxae arise primarily from the a. circumflexa femoris medialis (Section 21.4).

    A. The a. obturatoria supplies the medial thigh muscles and a small artery to the caput femoris. It is not a significant blood supply to the joint.

    B. The a. glutea superior supplies muscles of the regio glutealis but does not supply the art. coxae.

    C. The a. glutea inferior contributes to an anastomosis around the hip and primarily supplies muscles of the regio glutealis.

    E. The a. circumflexa femoris lateralis anastomoses with the a. circumflexa femoris medialis around the collum femoris, but it contributes less to the art. coxae and more to the muscles of the lateral thigh.

23. **E.** The n. femoralis enters the anterior thigh through the muscular compartment of the spatium retroinguinale. It branches immediately to innervate the muscles of the anterior thigh (Section 21.4).

    A. The femoral sheath encloses only the a. femoralis and v. femoralis.

    B. The a. femoralis and v. femoralis pass through the hiatus adductorius into the fossa poplitea.

    C. The fossa poplitea contains the n. tibialis and n. fibularis communis.

    D. The canalis femoralis lies medially within the femoral sheath and contains only loose connective tissue, fat, and lymph nodes.

24. **A.** The n. gluteus inferior innervates only the m. gluteus maximus (Section 21.4).
     B. The n. gluteus superior innervates the m. gluteus medius and m. gluteus minimus and m. tensor fasciae latae.
     C. The n. gluteus superior innervates the m. gluteus medius and m. gluteus minimus and m. tensor fasciae latae.
     D. The m. piriformis is innervated by the S1 and S2 branches of the plexus sacralis.
     E. B, C, and D are incorrect

25. **A.** The upper fibers of the m. gluteus maximus insert onto the tractus iliotibialis (Section 22.2).
     B. M. gluteus medius inserts onto the lateral surface of the trochanter major of the femur.
     C. M. gluteus minimus inserts onto the anterolateral surface of the trochanter major of the femur.
     D. M. quadratus femoris inserts onto the intertrochanteric crest of the femur.
     E. Not applicable.

26. **A.** The hamstring muscles originate at the tuberositas ischii and insert on the tibia and fibula. Repetitive stretching of these muscles over two joints (the flexed hip and extended knee) can irritate the site of origin (Section 22.3).
     B. Pain from a tear at the insertion site of the m. obturatorius internus tendon would be focused over the trochanter major of the femur.
     C. The n. ischiadicus emerges from behind the m. piriformis and can be compressed at this location. However, pain would reflect the sensory areas of the n. tibialis and n. fibularis communis, which include the anterolateral and posterior leg and the dorsum and sole of the foot.
     D. Irritation of the n. tibialis would manifest as pain in the sole of the foot.
     E. The n. gluteus inferior does not have a sensory component. Injury to the nerve would affect the m. gluteus maximus muscle and manifest as weakened extension and lateral rotation.

27. **D.** The m. biceps femoris is one of the hamstring muscles (m. biceps femoris, m. semitendinosus, m. semimembranosus), which are the primary flexors of the knee (Section 22.3).
     A. The m. flexor hallucis longus flexes the 1st digit and plantar flexes the foot.
     B. The m. soleus does not cross the art. genus and only plantar flexes the foot at the ankle.
     C. The m. tibialis posterior plantar flexes and inverts the foot.
     E. The m. rectus femoris extends the leg at the knee.

28. **C.** The borders of the trigonum femoris are the m. sartorius, m. adductor longus, and lig. inguinale (Section 22.3).
     A. The m. tensor fasciae latae is the lateral boundary of the anterior thigh. The trigonum femoris lies between the anterior and medial thigh compartments.
     B. The n. femoralis is one of the contents (lateral) of the trigonum femoris but not a boundary.
     D. The m. adductor longus is the medial border of the trigonum femoris.
     E. The m. rectus femoris is lateral to the trigonum femoris and lies inside the anterior compartment of the thigh.

29. **D.** The tarsal tunnel is formed by the retinaculum musculorum flexorum pedis and its attachments to the calcaneus and malleolus medialis of the tibia (Section 22.5).
     A. The os naviculare and talus lie distal to the tarsal tunnel, and neither provide attachment for the retinaculum musculorum flexorum pedis, which forms the roof of the tunnel.
     B. The os cuboideum lies on the lateral side of the foot; the tarsal tunnel lies on the medial side of the ankle.
     C. The talus is not part of the tarsal tunnel.
     E. Neither the talus nor os metatarsale I is part of the tarsal tunnel.

30. **A.** The lig. calcaneonaviculare plantare supports the head of the talus, which forms the apex of the arcus longitudinalis medialis (Section 22.7).
     B. The lig. deltoideum is the collateral ligament on the medial side of the ankle. It is not associated with the arcus medialis.
     C. The lig. talofibularis posterius is part of the lateral ligament of the ankle and is not associated with the arcus medialis.
     D. The retinaculum musculorum extensorum superius pedis restrains the tendons on the dorsum of the foot (dorsiflexors).
     E. The tendon of the m. fibularis longus supports the arcus transversus on the lateral side of the sole of the foot.

31. **E.**
     A, B. Pes planus is a condition that occurs most commonly in older adults who stand for long periods. It's characterized by laxity in both active and passive stabilizers of the medial arch.
     C. As the forefoot everts and abducts, additional pressure is put on the lig. calcaneonaviculare plantare.
     D. The lack of support for the head of the talus causes it to displace inferiorly and medially.

32. **A.** The malleolus medialis of the distal tibia forms part of the talocrural joint (Section 21.2 and 22.6).
     B. The linea aspera are paired ridges on the posterior surface of the femur that serve as attachments sites for thigh muscles.
     C. The eminentia intercondylaris, part of the tibial plateau, separates the condylus medialis and condylus lateralis.
     D. The sustentaculum tali is a part of the calcaneus, which forms part of the medial arch of the foot.
     E. The tuberculum adductorium is an attachment site for the m. adductor magnus on the distal femur.

33. **C.** The meniscus medialis is relatively immobile during flexion and extension because of its attachment to the lig. collaterale tibiale. This makes it more vulnerable to injury and is frequently injured in conjunction with the lig. cruciatum anterius and lig. collaterale tibiale (Section 22.4).
     A. The meniscus lateralis is attached to the capsula articularis but not to the lig. collaterale.
     B. The meniscus lateralis is more mobile during movements of the art. genus and therefore less vulnerable to injury.
     D. The meniscus medialis is relatively immobile during movements at the knee.

34. **A.** The n. tibialis, which passes through the deep posterior compartment, innervates many of the active stabilizers of the medial longitudinal arch including the m. tibialis posterior and intrinsic muscles of the foot (Section 22.5 and 22.7).

B. Dorsiflexion is a function of muscles of the anterior compartment, which would remain intact in this patient.

C. Eversion of the foot is a function primarily of muscles of the lateral compartment.

D. Sensation on the dorsum of the foot is mediated by the branches of the n. fibularis (peroneus) superficialis, which travel in the anterior and lateral compartments.

35. **B.** The soft tissue contrast of MRI makes it the most effective imaging modality for assessing non-osseous structures, such as ligaments, tendons and cartilaginous structures like menisci (Chapter 23).

A. CT would be most useful for evaluating subtle fractures but MRI is the modality of choice for assessing the integrity of cartilaginous structures.

C. Ultrasound is useful for evaluating superficial soft tissue abnormalities but is limited by the depth of structures and doesn't provide the soft tissue contrast of MRIs.

D. Cartilaginous structures are not visible on x-rays.

Unit VIII   Head and Neck

24 Overview of the Head and Neck

The head and neck region contains the brain, cranial meninges, cranial nerves, and sensory organs, as well as components of the respiratory, gastrointestinal, and endocrine systems. The skull encloses the brain (encephalon), provides the bony framework for soft tissues of the head, and contains the cavitas nasi and cavitas oralis and bony orbitae. The head and neck communicate with the thorax through the apertura thoracis superior and with the upper limb through the canalis cervicoaxillaris.

24.1 Bones of the Head: The Skull

The skull (cranium) is made up of two parts: the large **neurocranium** and the smaller **viscerocranium (Fig. 24.1** and **Table 24.1)**.
— The neurocranium, which makes up the largest part of the skull, houses and protects the brain.

— The viscerocranium includes the lower jaw and the thin-walled bones of the facial skeleton.

The Neurocranium

The neurocranium is formed by eight bones: the os frontale, os occipitale, os sphenoidale, and os ethmoidale, and paired ossa parietales and ossa temporales.
— The **os frontale (Figs. 24.2** and **24.3)** forms the forehead, the roof, and the superior rim of the orbita (eye socket), and the floor of the fossa cranii anterior.
— The paired **ossa parietales** (see **Figs. 24.2, 24.5, 24.6)** are flat bones that form the superolateral parts of the calvaria. Their internal surface has grooves for the a. meningea and the sinus sagittalis superior.

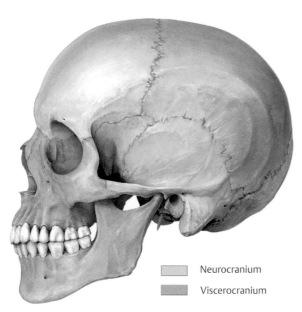

Fig. 24.1 Bones of the neurocranium and viscerocranium
Left lateral view. (From Schuenke M, Schulte E, Schumacher U. THIEME Atlas of Anatomy, Vol 3. Illustrations by Voll M and Wesker K. 3rd ed. New York: Thieme Publishers; 2020.)

Neurocranium
Viscerocranium

Table 24.1 Bones of the Neurocranium and Viscerocranium

Neurocranium	Viscerocranium
• Os frontale	• Os nasale
• Os sphenoidale (excluding the proc. pterygoideus)	• Os lacrimale
• Os temporale (partes petrosa and squamosa)	• Os ethmoidale (excluding the lamina cribrosa)
• Os parietale	• Os sphenoidale (proc. pterygoideus)
• Os occipitale	• Maxilla
• Os ethmoidale (lamina cribrosa)	• Os zygomaticum
• Auditory ossicles	• Os temporale (proc. styloideus ossis temporalis)
	• Mandibula
	• Vomer
	• Concha nasi inferior
	• Os palatinum
	• Os hyoideum

Most of the os ethmoidale is in the viscerocranium; most of the os sphenoidale is in the neurocranium. The os temporale is divided between the two (see **Fig. 24.1**).

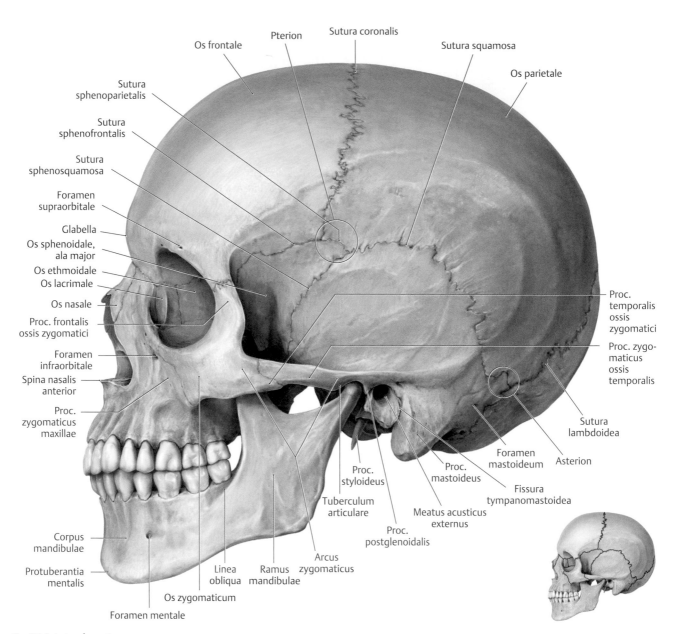

Fig. 24.2 Lateral cranium
Left lateral view. (From Schuenke M, Schulte E, Schumacher U. THIEME Atlas of Anatomy, Vol 3. Illustrations by Voll M and Wesker K. 3rd ed. New York: Thieme Publishers; 2020.)

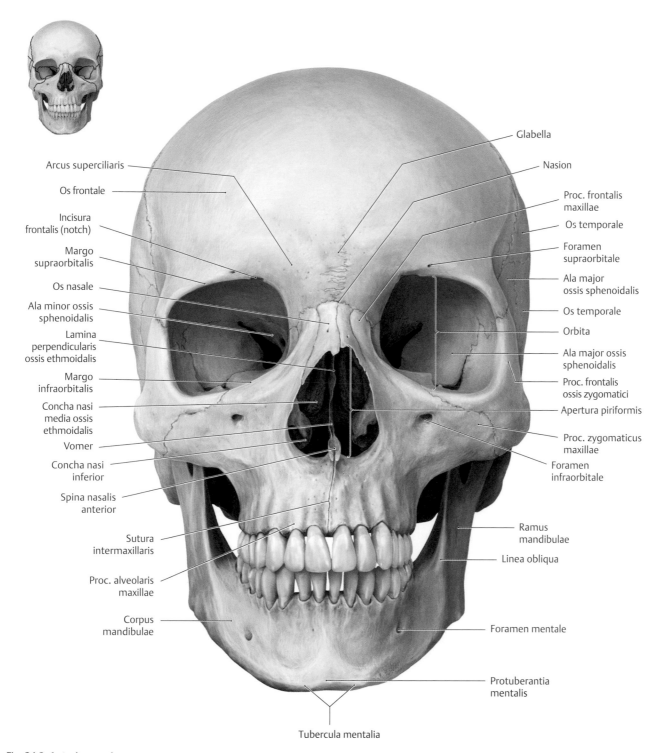

Glabella

Nasion

Arcus superciliaris

Os frontale

Proc. frontalis maxillae

Os temporale

Incisura frontalis (notch)

Foramen supraorbitale

Margo supraorbitalis

Ala major ossis sphenoidalis

Os nasale

Os temporale

Ala minor ossis sphenoidalis

Orbita

Lamina perpendicularis ossis ethmoidalis

Ala major ossis sphenoidalis

Margo infraorbitalis

Proc. frontalis ossis zygomatici

Concha nasi media ossis ethmoidalis

Apertura piriformis

Vomer

Proc. zygomaticus maxillae

Concha nasi inferior

Foramen infraorbitale

Spina nasalis anterior

Ramus mandibulae

Sutura intermaxillaris

Linea obliqua

Proc. alveolaris maxillae

Corpus mandibulae

Foramen mentale

Protuberantia mentalis

Tubercula mentalia

Fig. 24.3 Anterior cranium
Anterior view. (From Schuenke M, Schulte E, Schumacher U. THIEME Atlas of Anatomy, Vol 3. Illustrations by Voll M and Wesker K. 3rd ed. New York: Thieme Publishers; 2020.)

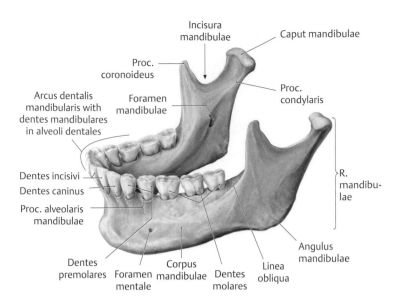

Incisura mandibulae

Caput mandibulae

Proc. coronoideus

Proc. condylaris

Arcus dentalis mandibularis with dentes mandibulares in alveoli dentales

Foramen mandibulae

Dentes incisivi

Dentes caninus

Proc. alveolaris mandibulae

R. mandibu-lae

Dentes premolares

Foramen mentale

Corpus mandibulae

Dentes molares

Linea obliqua

Angulus mandibulae

Fig. 24.4 Mandibula
Oblique, left lateral view. (From Schuenke M, Schulte E, Schumacher U. THIEME Atlas of Anatomy, Vol 3. Illustrations by Voll M and Wesker K. 3rd ed. New York: Thieme Publishers; 2020.)

BOX 24.1: CLINICAL CORRELATION

FRACTURES OF THE FACE
The framelike construction of the facial skeleton leads to characteristic patterns for fracture lines (classified as Le Fort I, II, and III fractures).

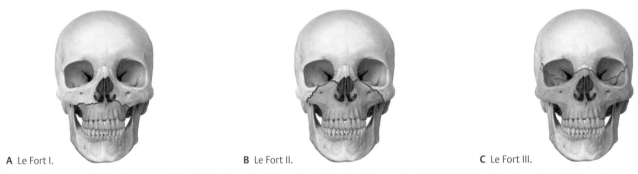

A Le Fort I.   **B** Le Fort II.   **C** Le Fort III.

(From Gilroy AM et al. Atlas of Anatomy. 4th ed. 2020. Based on: Schuenke M, Schulte E, Schumacher U. THIEME Atlas of Anatomy. Head, Neck, and Neuroanatomy. Illustrations by Voll M and Wesker K. 3rd ed. New York: Thieme Medical Publishers; 2020.)

— The **os occipitale (Figs. 24.6, 24.7, 24.8)** forms the fossa cranii posterior of the skull base.
  • A small anterior portion is called the **clivus**.
  • Foramina (openings) include the large **foramen magnum** and the **canales condylares**. The **foramina jugulares**, is formed partly by the os occipitale and partly by the pars petrosa of the os temporale.
  • Inferiorly, **condyli occipitales** articulate with vertebra C I.
  • The internal surface has grooves for the sinus sigmoideus and sinus transversus.
  • The external surface is marked with the **linea nuchalis superior** and **linea nuchalis inferior** and the **protuberantia occipitalis externa**.
— The paired **ossa temporales (Figs. 24.2, 24.7, 24.8, 24.9, 24.10)** form part of the fossa cranii media and fossa cranii posterior.
  • An outer **pars squamosa** forms the lateral skull, an inner **pars petrosa** encloses the auris media and interna, (neurocranium), and a **pars tympanica** encloses the external auditory canal (meatus acusticus externus) and membrana tympanica.
  • Processes include a **proc. mastoideus** composed of a mesh of **cellulae mastoideae**, the posterior part of the **arcus zygomaticus**, and a long, pointed **proc. styloideus**.

• Foramina (openings) include **meatus acusticus internus**, **meatus acusticus externus**, **canalis caroticus**, and **foramen stylomastoideum**.
• A **fossa mandibularis** and **tuberculum articulare** articulate with the mandibula.
— The **os sphenoidale (Figs. 24.11 and 24.12)** forms the posterior part of the orbita and the floor and the lateral wall of the fossa cranii media between the os frontale and os temporale.
  • It has two **alae majores** that form parts of the fossa cranii media and lateral walls of the skull.
  • Two **alae minores** form the posterior part of the fossa cranii anterior and end in **procc. clinoidei anteriores**.
  • The **corpus sphenoidalis** encloses the **sinus sphenoidalis**.
  • A midline saddle-shaped formation, the **sella turcica**, contains the **fossa hypophysiales** and is limited anteriorly by the **tuberculum sellae** and posteriorly by the **dorsum sellae** and its **processus clinoideus posterior**.
  • Paired **procc. pterygoidei**, each with a **lamina medialis** and **lamina lateralis**, project inferiorly (viscerocranium).
  • Paired openings include the **canalis opticus**, **fissura orbitalis superior**, **foramen rotundum**, **foramen ovale**, and **foramen spinosum**.

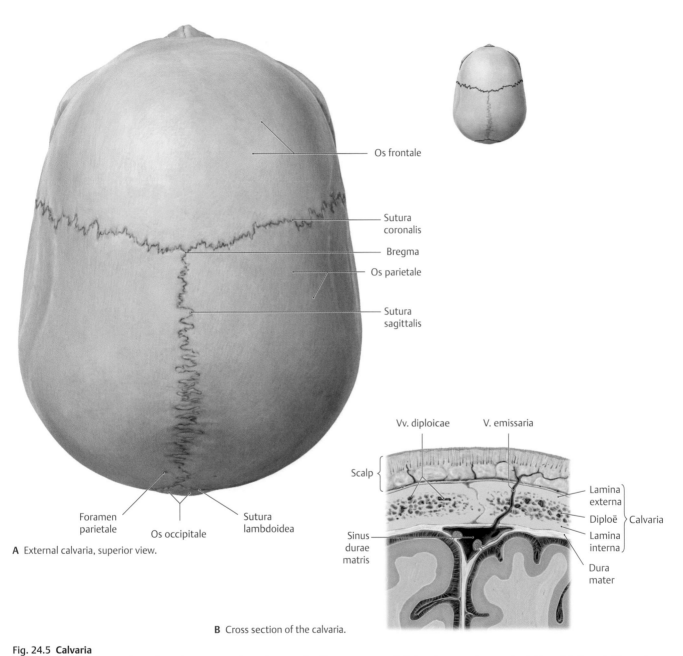

A External calvaria, superior view.

B Cross section of the calvaria.

Fig. 24.5 Calvaria

The bones of the calvaria—the os frontale, os occipitale, and ossa parietalia—are composed of three layers: a dense outer table, a thin inner table, and a middle diploë layer. (From Schuenke M, Schulte E, Schumacher U. THIEME Atlas of Anatomy, Vol 3. Illustrations by Voll M and Wesker K. 3rd ed. New York: Thieme Publishers; 2020.)

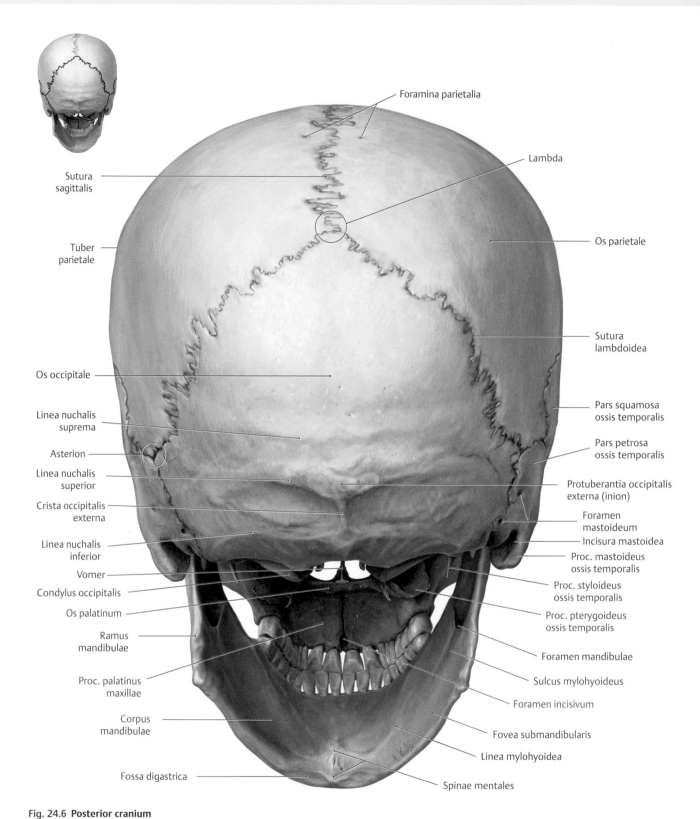

Foramina parietalia

Lambda

Sutura sagittalis

Tuber parietale

Os parietale

Os occipitale

Sutura lambdoidea

Linea nuchalis suprema

Pars squamosa ossis temporalis

Asterion

Pars petrosa ossis temporalis

Linea nuchalis superior

Protuberantia occipitalis externa (inion)

Crista occipitalis externa

Foramen mastoideum

Linea nuchalis inferior

Incisura mastoidea

Vomer

Proc. mastoideus ossis temporalis

Condylus occipitalis

Proc. styloideus ossis temporalis

Os palatinum

Proc. pterygoideus ossis temporalis

Ramus mandibulae

Foramen mandibulae

Proc. palatinus maxillae

Sulcus mylohyoideus

Corpus mandibulae

Foramen incisivum

Fovea submandibularis

Linea mylohyoidea

Fossa digastrica

Spinae mentales

Fig. 24.6 Posterior cranium
Posterior view. (From Schuenke M, Schulte E, Schumacher U. THIEME Atlas of Anatomy, Vol 3. Illustrations by Voll M and Wesker K. 3rd ed. New York: Thieme Publishers; 2020.)

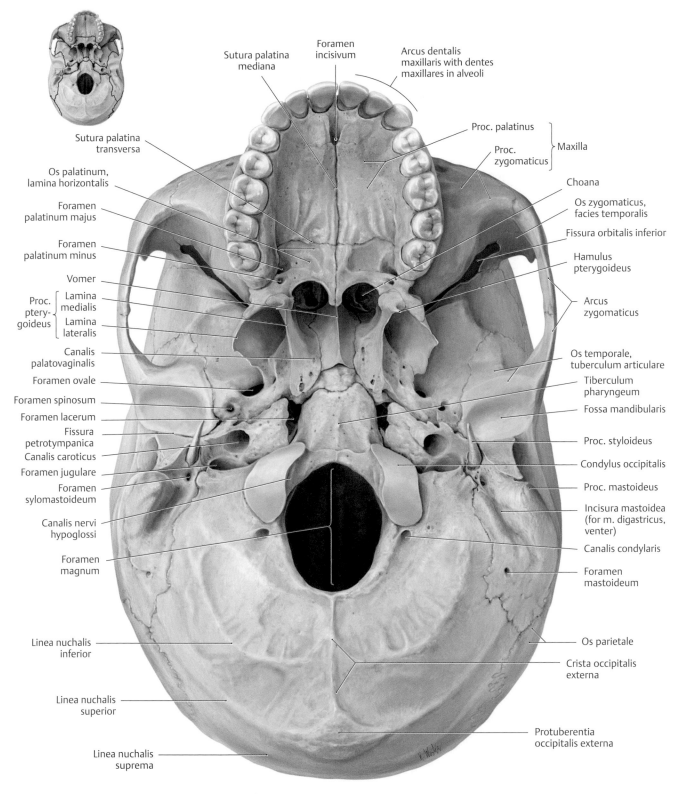

Sutura palatina mediana

Foramen incisivum

Arcus dentalis maxillaris with dentes maxillares in alveoli

Sutura palatina transversa

Proc. palatinus

Proc. zygomaticus

Maxilla

Os palatinum, lamina horizontalis

Choana

Foramen palatinum majus

Os zygomaticus, facies temporalis

Foramen palatinum minus

Fissura orbitalis inferior

Vomer

Hamulus pterygoideus

Proc. pterygoideus

Lamina medialis

Lamina lateralis

Arcus zygomaticus

Canalis palatovaginalis

Os temporale, tuberculum articulare

Foramen ovale

Tiberculum pharyngeum

Foramen spinosum

Fossa mandibularis

Foramen lacerum

Fissura petrotympanica

Proc. styloideus

Canalis caroticus

Condylus occipitalis

Foramen jugulare

Proc. mastoideus

Foramen sylomastoideum

Incisura mastoidea (for m. digastricus, venter)

Canalis nervi hypoglossi

Canalis condylaris

Foramen magnum

Foramen mastoideum

Linea nuchalis inferior

Os parietale

Crista occipitalis externa

Linea nuchalis superior

Protuberentia occipitalis externa

Linea nuchalis suprema

Fig. 24.7 Basis cranii: exterior
Inferior view. (From Schuenke M, Schulte E, Schumacher U. THIEME Atlas of Anatomy, Vol 3. Illustrations by Voll M and Wesker K. 3rd ed. New York: Thieme Publishers; 2020.)

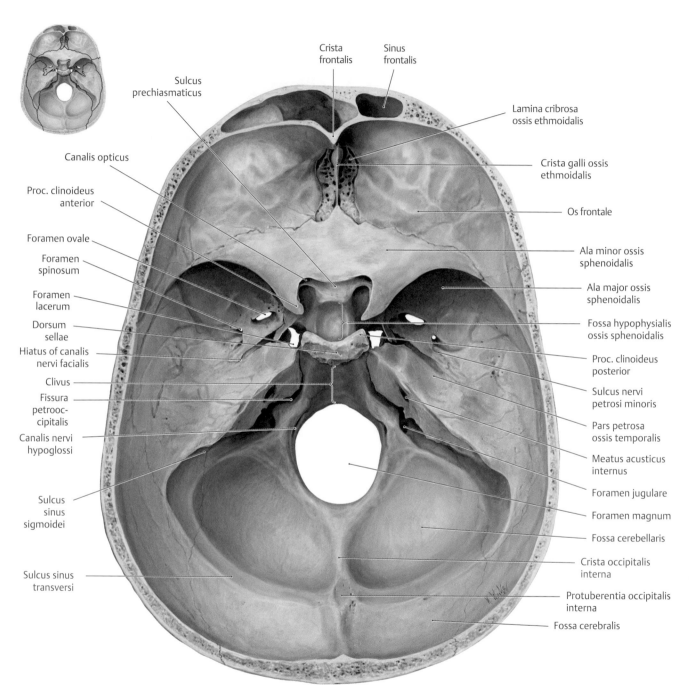

Crista
frontalis

Sinus
frontalis

Sulcus
prechiasmaticus

Lamina cribrosa
ossis ethmoidalis

Canalis opticus

Crista galli ossis
ethmoidalis

Proc. clinoideus
anterior

Os frontale

Foramen ovale

Ala minor ossis
sphenoidalis

Foramen
spinosum

Ala major ossis
sphenoidalis

Foramen
lacerum

Fossa hypophysialis
ossis sphenoidalis

Dorsum
sellae

Proc. clinoideus
posterior

Hiatus of canalis
nervi facialis

Sulcus nervi
petrosi minoris

Clivus

Fissura
petrooc-
cipitalis

Pars petrosa
ossis temporalis

Canalis nervi
hypoglossi

Meatus acusticus
internus

Foramen jugulare

Sulcus
sinus
sigmoidei

Foramen magnum

Fossa cerebellaris

Crista occipitalis
interna

Sulcus sinus
transversi

Protuberentia occipitalis
interna

Fossa cerebralis

Fig. 24.8 Basis cranii: Interior
Superior view. (From Schuenke M, Schulte E, Schumacher U. THIEME Atlas of Anatomy, Vol 3. Illustrations by Voll M and Wesker K. 3rd ed. New York: Thieme Publishers; 2020.)

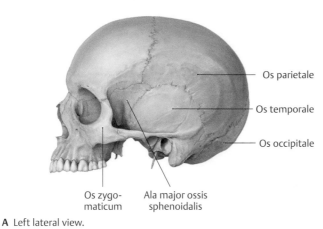

A Left lateral view.

- Os parietale
- Os temporale
- Os occipitale
- Os zygomaticum
- Ala major ossis sphenoidalis

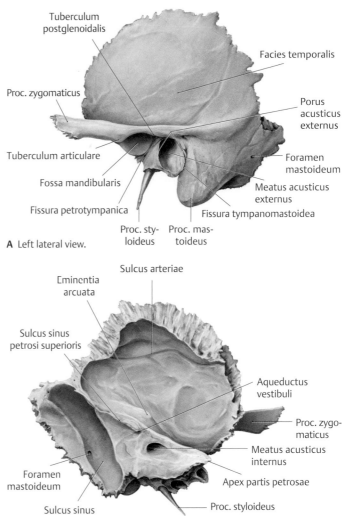

A Left lateral view.

- Tuberculum postglenoidalis
- Facies temporalis
- Proc. zygomaticus
- Porus acusticus externus
- Tuberculum articulare
- Foramen mastoideum
- Fossa mandibularis
- Meatus acusticus externus
- Fissura petrotympanica
- Fissura tympanomastoidea
- Proc. styloideus
- Proc. mastoideus

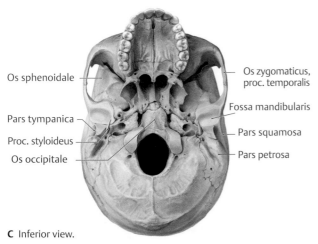

B Superior view.

- Os sphenoidale
- Pars squamosa
- Pars petrosa
- Os parietale
- Os occipitale

B Medial view.

- Sulcus arteriae
- Eminentia arcuata
- Sulcus sinus petrosi superioris
- Aqueductus vestibuli
- Proc. zygomaticus
- Meatus acusticus internus
- Foramen mastoideum
- Apex partis petrosae
- Proc. styloideus
- Sulcus sinus sigmoidei

C Inferior view.

- Os sphenoidale
- Os zygomaticus, proc. temporalis
- Fossa mandibularis
- Pars tympanica
- Pars squamosa
- Proc. styloideus
- Pars petrosa
- Os occipitale

Fig. 24.9 Os temporale in situ
Pars squamosa (*light green*), pars petrosa (*pale green*), pars tympanica (*dark green*). (From Schuenke M, Schulte E, Schumacher U. THIEME Atlas of Anatomy, Vol 3. Illustrations by Voll M and Wesker K. 3rd ed. New York: Thieme Publishers; 2020.)

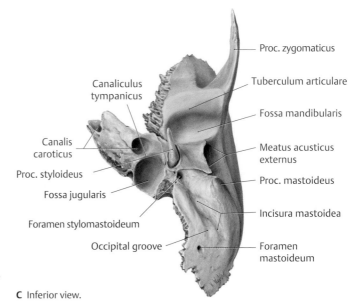

C Inferior view.

- Proc. zygomaticus
- Tuberculum articulare
- Fossa mandibularis
- Canaliculus tympanicus
- Meatus acusticus externus
- Canalis caroticus
- Proc. styloideus
- Proc. mastoideus
- Fossa jugularis
- Incisura mastoidea
- Foramen stylomastoideum
- Occipital groove
- Foramen mastoideum

Fig. 24.10 Os temporale
(From Schuenke M, Schulte E, Schumacher U. THIEME Atlas of Anatomy, Vol 3. Illustrations by Voll M and Wesker K. 3rd ed. New York: Thieme Publishers; 2020.)

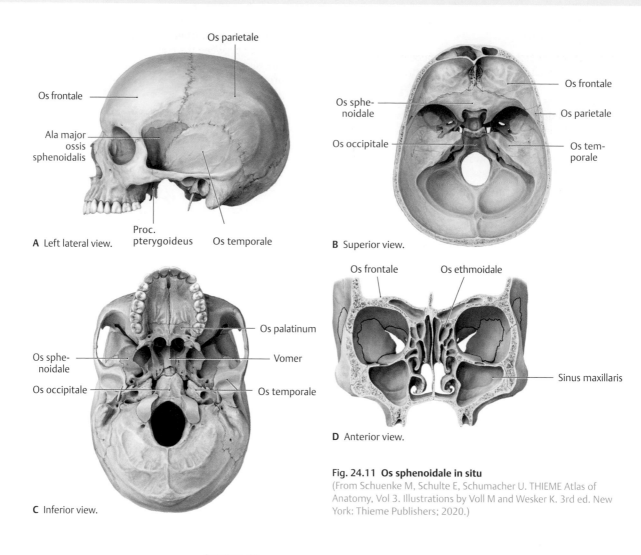

A Left lateral view.

B Superior view.

C Inferior view.

D Anterior view.

Fig. 24.11 Os sphenoidale in situ
(From Schuenke M, Schulte E, Schumacher U. THIEME Atlas of Anatomy, Vol 3. Illustrations by Voll M and Wesker K. 3rd ed. New York: Thieme Publishers; 2020.)

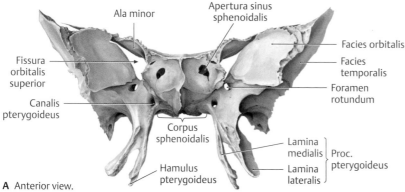

A Anterior view.

Fig. 24.12 Os sphenoidale
(From Schuenke M, Schulte E, Schumacher U. THIEME Atlas of Anatomy, Vol 3. Illustrations by Voll M and Wesker K. 3rd ed. New York: Thieme Publishers; 2020.)

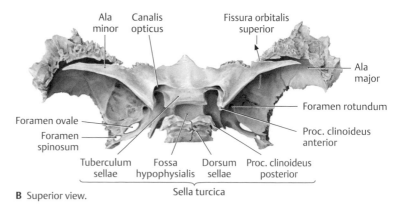

B Superior view.

The Viscerocranium

The **viscerocraniun**, or facial skeleton, is composed of 15 bones: the os ethmoideum, mandibula, and vomer, and the paired concha nasi inferior, maxilla, os nasale, os lacrimale, os zygomaticum, and os palatinum (see **Figs. 24.2, 24.3, 24.15**).

— The **os ethmoidale** (**Figs. 24.13** and **24.14**) forms part of the fossa cranii anterior, the medial walls of the orbitae, and parts of the septum nasi and lateral nasal walls.
  - The **lamina cribrosa** (neurocranium) sits in the fossa cranii anterior above the cavitas nasi.
  - The **lamina perpendicularis** forms part of the septum nasi.
  - Ethmoid processes include the **crista galli** superiorly and **concha nasi superior and concha nasi media** inferiorly on the lateral wall of the cavitas nasi.
  - Numerous thin-walled **cellulae ethmoidales** form the **ethmoid sinuses**.
— Paired **maxillary bones** (maxilla) (**Figs. 24.2, 24.3, 24.15**) form the upper jaw, floors of the orbitae, and parts of the nose and palate.
  - The **arcus dentalis maxillaris** contains **alveoli dentales** (sockets) for the upper teeth.
  - The **proc. palatinus** form the anterior part of the palate, and **proc. frontalis** form part of the external nose.
  - An **foramen infraorbitale** opens onto the face.
  - A large **sinus maxillaris** within the maxilla sits below each orbita.
— The **mandibula** (**Figs. 24.2** and **24.4**) forms the lower jaw.
  - A horizontal **corpus mandibulae** connects posteriorly with a vertical **ramus mandibulae** on each side.

- An **angulus mandibulae** forms on each side at the junction between the body and the ramus.
- The superior end of each ramus has an anterior **proc. coronoideus** that is separated from the posterior **proc. condylaris** by a **incisura mandibulae**.
- The **caput** of the proc. condylaris articulates with the fossa mandibularis of the os temporale.
- Foramina include a **foramen mentale** externally and a **foramen mandibulae** internally.
- The **arcus dentalis mandibularis** contains alveoli that house the lower teeth.

— Paired **ossa nasales** (**Fig. 24.3**) form the bridge of the nose.
— Paired **ossa lacrimales** (**Fig. 24.2**) form the anterior medial walls of the orbitae and contain **fossae sacci lacrimalis**.
— Paired **ossa zygomatica** (**Fig. 24.2**) form the bony prominences of the cheeks, anterior parts of the arcus zygomaticus, and lateral walls of the orbitae.
— Paired **ossa palatina** (**Fig. 24.7**) have vertical parts that form the posterior lateral walls of the cavitas nasi and **laminae horizontales** that form the posterior parts of the palatum.
— The **vomer** (**Fig. 24.15**) forms the inferior and posterior part of septum nasi.
— Paired **conchae nasales inferiores** (**Fig. 24.15**) form the lowest scroll-like processes on the lateral walls of the cavitas nasi.

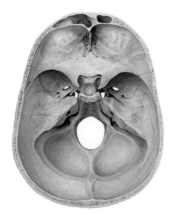

A Superior view.

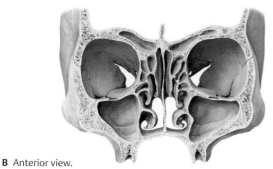

B Anterior view.

Fig. 24.13 Os ethmoidale in situ
(From Schuenke M, Schulte E, Schumacher U. THIEME Atlas of Anatomy, Vol 3. Illustrations by Voll M and Wesker K. 3rd ed. New York: Thieme Publishers; 2020.)

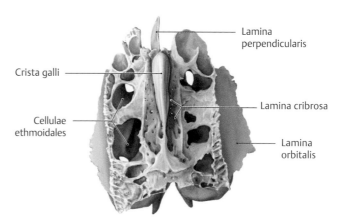

A Superior view.

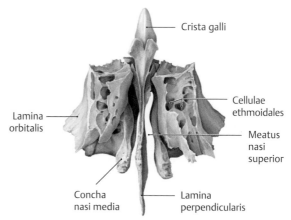

B Anterior view.

Fig. 24.14 Os ethmoidale
(From Schuenke M, Schulte E, Schumacher U. THIEME Atlas of Anatomy, Vol 3. Illustrations by Voll M and Wesker K. 3rd ed. New York: Thieme Publishers; 2020.)

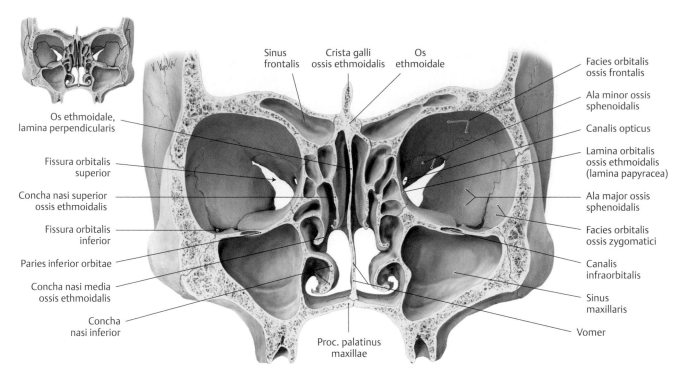

Fig. 24.15 Bones of the orbita and cavitas nasi
Coronal section, anterior view. (From Schuenke M, Schulte E, Schumacher U. THIEME Atlas of Anatomy, Vol 3. Illustrations by Voll M and Wesker K. 3rd ed. New York: Thieme Publishers; 2020.)

Sutures of the Skull

— During development, the bones of the calvaria grow outward from their center toward adjacent bones; the bones eventually fuse to form fibrous joints called **sutures (suturae cranii)**.
— Although there are many smaller sutures, the major sutures of the calvaria (see **Figs. 24.2, 24.3, 24.5, 24.6**) are
  • the **sutura sagittalis** between the ossa parietales,
  • the **sutura coronalis** between the os frontale and os parietale,
  • the **sutura lambdoidea** between the os occipitale and os parietale, and
  • the **sutura squamosa** between the os parietale and os temporale.
— At birth, growth of the ossa cranii and formation of the sutures are incomplete. Large fibrous areas, known as **fonticuli cranii**, remain between the bones and allow for continued growth of the brain. The largest of these, the **fonticulus anterior** at the junction of the os frontale and os parietale, closes between 18 and 24 months of age (**Fig. 24.16**).

BOX 24.2: DEVELOPMENTAL CORRELATION

CRANIOSYNOSTOSIS
Premature closure of the cranial sutures, a condition known as craniosynostosis, results in a variety of skull malformations, the shape of which depends on the suture involved. *Plagiocephaly*, the most common deformity, indicates premature closure of the sutura coronalis and sutura lambdoidea on one side and creates an asymmetrical appearance. *Scaphocephaly* is characterized by a long, narrow cranium produced by early closure of the sagittal suture. If untreated, craniosynostosis may lead to increased intracranial pressure, seizures, and delayed development of the skull and brain. Surgery is typically the recommended treatment to reduce the intracranial pressure and correct the deformities of the face and skull bones.

— Junctions of the sutures and other prominent points of the skull are useful for measuring growth of the skull and brain; determining race, gender, and age; and locating deep cranial structures (**Table 24.2**).

BOX 24.3: CLINICAL CORRELATION

SKULL FRACTURES AT THE PTERION
The thin bones that make up the pterion overlie the anterior branches of the middle meningeal artery, a branch of the a. maxillaris that runs deep to the bone in the spatium epidurale. Because of this relationship, skull fractures at the pterion can lead to a life-threatening epidural hemorrhage (see **Box 26.3**).

Table 24.2 Landmarks of the Cranium

Landmark	Location of Point or Area
Nasion	Junction of sutura frontonasalis and sutura internasalis
Glabella	Most anterior prominence of os frontale above the nasum
Bregma	Junction of sutura coronalis and sutura sagittalis
Pterion	Area encompassing junction of os frontale, os parietale, os sphenoidale, and os temporale along the sutura sphenoparietalis
Vertex	Most superior point of the skull along the sutura sagittalis
Lambda	Junction of sutura lambdoidea and sutura sagittalis
Asterion	Junction of suturae joining os occipitale, os temporale, and os parietale

(see **Figs. 24.2, 24.3, 24.5, 24.6**)

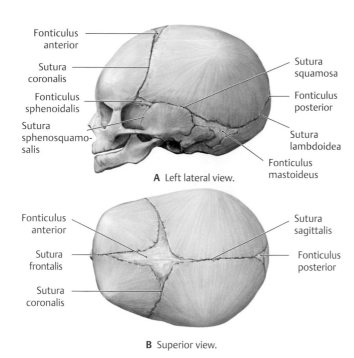

A Left lateral view.

B Superior view.

Fig. 24.16 The neonatal skull
(From Schuenke M, Schulte E, Schumacher U. THIEME Atlas of Anatomy, Vol 3. Illustrations by Voll M and Wesker K. 3rd ed. New York: Thieme Publishers; 2020.)

Fossae Cranii

— The floor of the cavitas crani is divided into three fossae, or spaces (**Fig. 24.17**; see also **Fig. 24.8**).
  • The **fossa cranii anterior**, formed by the os frontale and os ethmoidale, and ala minor ossis sphenoidalis, contains the lobus frontalis of the brain and the bulbi olfactorii (see Section 26.2 for a description of the brain).
  • The **fossa cranii media**, formed by the ala major and ala minor ossis sphenoidalis and pars squamosa and pars petrosa ossis temporalis, contains the lobi temporales, the chiasma opticum, and the glandula pituitaria. The fossa hypophysialis separates the right and left halves of the fossa cranii media.
  • The **fossa cranii posterior**, formed primarily by the os occipitale and pars petrosa ossis temporalis, contains the pons, medulla oblongata, and cerebellum of the brain. The medulla oblongata exits the skull through the foramen magnum located on the floor of the fossa, and grooves on

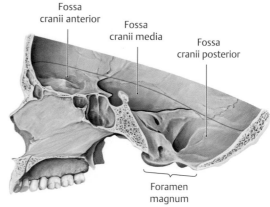

A Midsagittal section, left lateral view.

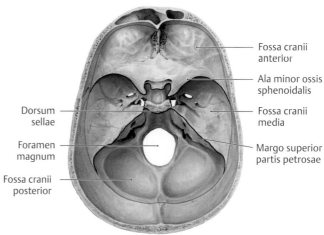

B Superior view of opened skull.

Fig. 24.17 Fossae cranii
The interior of the skull base consists of three successive fossae that become progressively deeper in the frontal-to-occipital direction.
(From Schuenke M, Schulte E, Schumacher U. THIEME Atlas of Anatomy, Vol 3. Illustrations by Voll M and Wesker K. 3rd ed. New York: Thieme Publishers; 2020.)

the posterior and lateral walls accommodate the sinus transversus and sinus sigmoideus.
— Foramina within the anterior, middle, and posterior fossae allow blood vessels and nerves to pass through the skull (**Fig. 24.18**). (See Sections 24.3, 24.4 and 26.3 for aa. capitis, vv. capitis, and nn. craniales, respectively.)

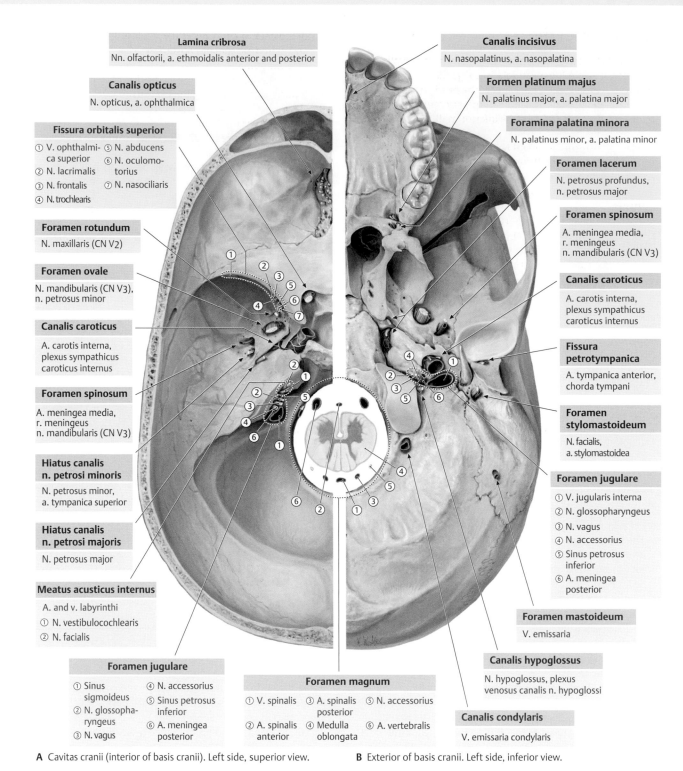

Lamina cribrosa
Nn. olfactorii, a. ethmoidalis anterior and posterior

Canalis opticus
N. opticus, a. ophthalmica

Fissura orbitalis superior
① V. ophthalmi-   ⑤ N. abducens
  ca superior   ⑥ N. oculomo-
② N. lacrimalis   torius
③ N. frontalis   ⑦ N. nasociliaris
④ N. trochlearis

Foramen rotundum
N. maxillaris (CN V2)

Foramen ovale
N. mandibularis (CN V3),
n. petrosus minor

Canalis caroticus
A. carotis interna,
plexus sympathicus
caroticus internus

Foramen spinosum
A. meningea media,
r. meningeus
n. mandibularis (CN V3)

**Hiatus canalis
n. petrosi minoris**
N. petrosus minor,
a. tympanica superior

**Hiatus canalis
n. petrosi majoris**
N. petrosus major

Meatus acusticus internus
A. and v. labyrinthi
① N. vestibulocochlearis
② N. facialis

Foramen jugulare
① Sinus   ④ N. accessorius
  sigmoideus   ⑤ Sinus petrosus
② N. glossopha-   inferior
  ryngeus   ⑥ A. meningea
③ N. vagus   posterior

Foramen magnum
① V. spinalis   ③ A. spinalis   ⑤ N. accessorius
                      posterior
② A. spinalis   ④ Medulla   ⑥ A. vertebralis
  anterior   oblongata

Canalis incisivus
N. nasopalatinus, a. nasopalatina

Formen platinum majus
N. palatinus major, a. palatina major

Foramina palatina minora
N. palatinus minor, a. palatina minor

Foramen lacerum
N. petrosus profundus,
n. petrosus major

Foramen spinosum
A. meningea media,
r. meningeus
n. mandibularis (CN V3)

Canalis caroticus
A. carotis interna,
plexus sympathicus
caroticus internus

**Fissura
petrotympanica**
A. tympanica anterior,
chorda tympani

**Foramen
stylomastoideum**
N. facialis,
a. stylomastoidea

Foramen jugulare
① V. jugularis interna
② N. glossopharyngeus
③ N. vagus
④ N. accessorius
⑤ Sinus petrosus
  inferior
⑥ A. meningea
  posterior

Foramen mastoideum
V. emissaria

Canalis hypoglossus
N. hypoglossus, plexus
venosus canalis n. hypoglossi

Canalis condylaris
V. emissaria condylaris

A Cavitas cranii (interior of basis cranii). Left side, superior view.   **B** Exterior of basis cranii. Left side, inferior view.

Fig. 24.18 Neurovascular structures entering or exiting the cavitas cranii
(From Schuenke M, Schulte E, Schumacher U. THIEME Atlas of Anatomy, Vol 3. Illustrations by Voll M and Wesker K. 3rd ed. New York: Thieme Publishers; 2020.)

24.2 Bones of the Neck

Most bones of the neck are parts of the columna vertebralis, thoracic skeleton, or cingulum pectorale (see **Fig. 1.5A**).

— The seven cervical vertebrae support the head on the columna vertebralis and provide attachment for neck muscles.
— The manubrium sterni forms the inferior midline boundary of the anterior neck.
— The claviculae form the lateral boundaries of the neck.
— The **os hyoideum**, a small U-shaped bone, lies anterior to the vertebra C III in the neck (**Fig. 24.19**).
   • It has a **corpus ossis hyoidei** and **cornu minus** and **cornu majus**.
   • The os hyoideum does not articulate directly with any other bones of the skeleton, but muscles and ligaments attach it to the mandibula, procc. styloidei ossis temporalis, larynx, claviculae, sternum, and scapulae.

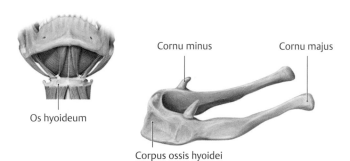

Cornu minus   Cornu majus

Os hyoideum

Corpus ossis hyoidei

Fig. 24.19 Os hyoideum
The os hyoideum is suspended in the neck by muscles between the floor of the mouth and the larynx. (From Schuenke M, Schulte E, Schumacher U. THIEME Atlas of Anatomy, Vol 3. Illustrations by Voll M and Wesker K. 3rd ed. New York: Thieme Publishers; 2020.)

24.3 Arteries of the Head and Neck

Arteries of the head and neck are branches of **a. subclavia dextra** and **a. subclavia sinistra** and **a. carotis communis** (see **Fig. 5.6**).

— The truncus brachiocephalicus arises from the arcus aortae and divides behind the art. sternoclavicularis dextra to form the a. subclavia dextra and a. carotis communis dextra.
— The a. subclavia sinistra and a. carotis communis sinistra are direct branches of the arcus aortae in the mediastinum superior of the thorax.

The Arteriae Subclavia

The aa. subclaviae enter the neck through the apertura thoracis superior and pass laterally between the m. scalenus anterior and m. scalenus medius. Two branches, the a. vertebralis and the truncus thyrocervicalis, arise medial to the m. scalenus anterior on each side and supply structures in the head and neck (**Fig. 24.20**). Other branches supply structures at the base of the neck and thoracic outlet.

— The **a. vertebralis** passes posteriorly in the neck to ascend through the foramen transversarium vertebrae cervicales C I–C VI and enters the foramen magnum at the basis cranii.

   • In the neck, it contributes the single a. spinalis anterior and paired aa. spinales posteriores that supply the upper medulla spinalis.
   • In the skull, it gives off the **a. inferior posterior cerebelli**.
   • It terminates by joining the contralateral a. vertebralis to form a single **a. basilaris**, which supplies the posterior circulation of the brain.

— The **truncus thyrocervicalis** is a short trunk that branches into four arteries:
   • the **a. thyroidea inferior**, the largest branch, which turns medially to supply the larynx, trachea, oesophagus, gl. thyroidea, and gl. parathyroidea;
   • the **a. suprascapularis** and **a. transversa colli**, which supply muscles of the back and regio scapularis; and
   • the **a. cervicalis ascendens**, a small branch that supplies muscles in the neck.

— The **truncus costocervicalis** arises posteriorly from the a. subclavia and branches into
   • the **a. cervicalis profunda**, which supplies muscles of the posterior neck.
   • the **a. intercostalis suprema**, which supplies the muscles of the first intercostal space.

— The a. thoracica interna arises from the inferior side of the a. subclavia. It descends into the thorax on either side of the sternum to supply muscles of the thorax and sternum (see Section 5.2).

BOX 24.4: CLINICAL CORRELATION

SUBCLAVIAN STEAL SYNDROME

"Subclavian steal" usually results from a stenosis of the left a. subclavia located proximal to the origin of the a. vertebralis. When the left arm is exercised, there may be insufficient blood flow to the arm. As a result, blood is "stolen" from the a. vertebralis circulation, causing a reversal of flow in the a. vertebralis on the *affected* side. This leads to a deficient blood flow in the a. basilaris and may deprive the brain of blood, producing a feeling of lightheadedness.

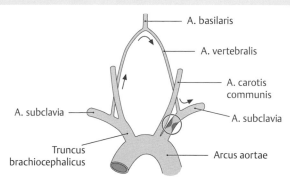

A. basilaris

A. vertebralis

A. carotis communis

A. subclavia

A. subclavia

Truncus brachiocephalicus

Arcus aortae

Subclavian steal syndrome
Red circle indicates area of stenosis; *arrows* indicate direction of blood flow. (From Schuenke M, Schulte E, Schumacher U. THIEME Atlas of Anatomy, Vol 3. Illustrations by Voll M and Wesker K. 3rd ed. New York: Thieme Publishers; 2020.)

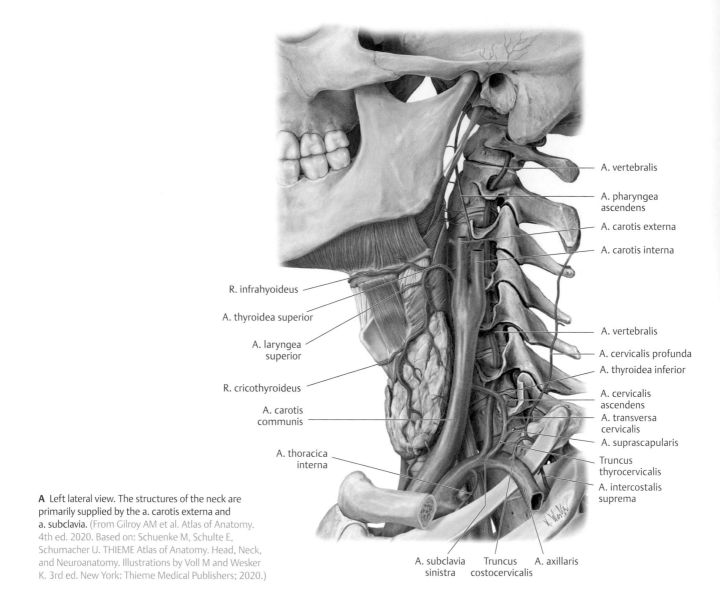

A. vertebralis

A. pharyngea ascendens

A. carotis externa

A. carotis interna

R. infrahyoideus

A. thyroidea superior

A. laryngea superior

A. vertebralis

A. cervicalis profunda

A. thyroidea inferior

R. cricothyroideus

A. cervicalis ascendens

A. carotis communis

A. transversa cervicalis

A. suprascapularis

A. thoracica interna

Truncus thyrocervicalis

A. intercostalis suprema

A. subclavia sinistra   Truncus costocervicalis   A. axillaris

A Left lateral view. The structures of the neck are primarily supplied by the a. carotis externa and a. subclavia. (From Gilroy AM et al. Atlas of Anatomy. 4th ed. 2020. Based on: Schuenke M, Schulte E, Schumacher U. THIEME Atlas of Anatomy. Head, Neck, and Neuroanatomy. Illustrations by Voll M and Wesker K. 3rd ed. New York: Thieme Medical Publishers; 2020.)

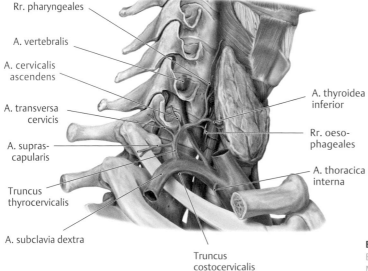

Rr. pharyngeales

A. vertebralis

A. cervicalis ascendens

A. transversa cervicis

A. thyroidea inferior

Rr. oeso-phageales

A. supras-capularis

A. thoracica interna

Truncus thyrocervicalis

A. subclavia dextra

Truncus costocervicalis

B Branches of the truncus thyrocervicalis. (From Schuenke M, Schulte E, Schumacher U. THIEME Atlas of Anatomy, Vol 3. Illustrations by Voll M and Wesker K. 3rd ed. New York: Thieme Publishers; 2020.)

Fig. 24.20 Arteries of the neck

The Carotid Artery System

The carotid artery system supplies structures of the neck, face, skull, and brain and consists of paired aa. carotis communes, aa. carotis externae, and aa. carotis internae and their branches.

— The **a. carotis communis** enters the neck from the thorax and ascends, with the v. jugularis interna and n. vagus, within a fascial sleeve, the **vagina carotica**.

- Its only branches, the **a. carotis externa** and **a. carotis interna**, arise from its bifurcation at the C IV vertebral level (**Fig. 24.21**).

— The **a. carotis externa** supplies most structures of the face and head except the brain and the orbitae. Six branches arise from the a. carotis externa in the neck before it passes behind the mandibula and finally bifurcates into two terminal branches, the **a. maxillaris** and **a. temporalis superficialis** (**Table 24.3**).

1. The **a. thyroidea superior** supplies the gl. thyroidea and, through its **a. laryngea superior**, the larynx.
2. The **a. lingualis** supplies the posterior tongue and floor of the mouth, parts of the cavitas oris, the tonsil, soft palate, epiglottis, and gl. sublingualis.

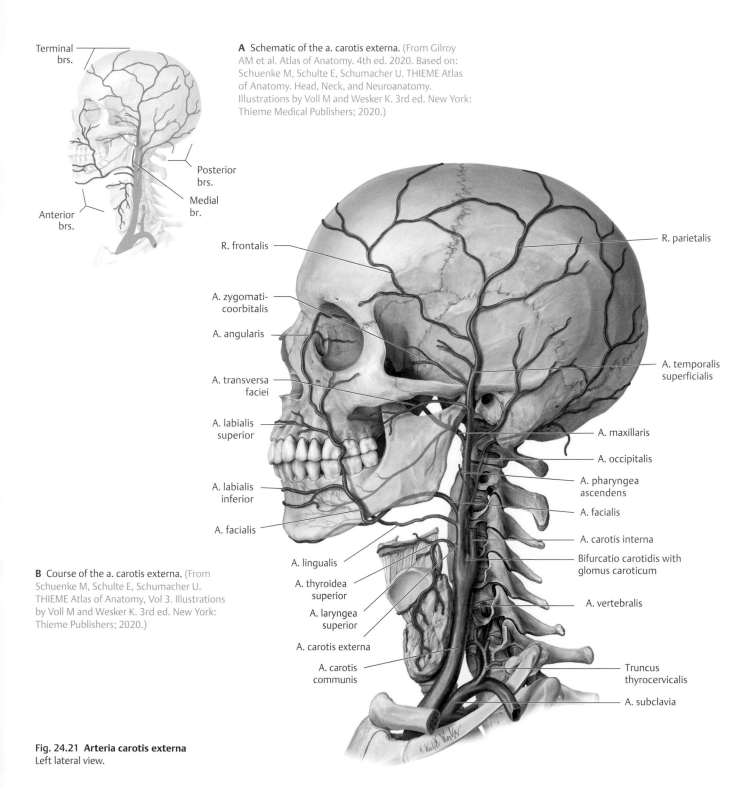

A Schematic of the a. carotis externa. (From Gilroy AM et al. Atlas of Anatomy. 4th ed. 2020. Based on: Schuenke M, Schulte E, Schumacher U. THIEME Atlas of Anatomy. Head, Neck, and Neuroanatomy. Illustrations by Voll M and Wesker K. 3rd ed. New York: Thieme Medical Publishers; 2020.)

Terminal brs.

Posterior brs.

Medial br.

Anterior brs.

R. frontalis

R. parietalis

A. zygomaticoorbitalis

A. angularis

A. temporalis superficialis

A. transversa faciei

A. labialis superior

A. maxillaris

A. occipitalis

A. labialis inferior

A. pharyngea ascendens

A. facialis

A. facialis

A. carotis interna

A. lingualis

Bifurcatio carotidis with glomus caroticum

A. thyroidea superior

A. vertebralis

A. laryngea superior

A. carotis externa

A. carotis communis

Truncus thyrocervicalis

A. subclavia

B Course of the a. carotis externa. (From Schuenke M, Schulte E, Schumacher U. THIEME Atlas of Anatomy, Vol 3. Illustrations by Voll M and Wesker K. 3rd ed. New York: Thieme Publishers; 2020.)

Fig. 24.21 Arteria carotis externa
Left lateral view.

3. The **a. facialis** ascends deep to the gl. submandibularis, which it supplies, and crosses the mandibula from below to enter the face. It passes lateral to the corners of the mouth and terminates near the medial angle of the eye as the **a. angularis**. The branches of the a. facialis include
   ◦ the **a. submentalis** and **a. tonsillaris** in the neck, and
   ◦ the **a. labialis superior** and **a. labialis inferior** and an **a. nasalis lateralis** on the face.
4. The **a. occipitalis** supplies branches to the posterior neck muscles.
5. The **a. pharyngea ascendens** sends branches to the pharynx, ear, and deep neck muscles.
6. The **a. auricularis posterior** passes posteriorly to supply the scalp behind the ear.

— The a. maxillaris arises posterior to the mandibula and passes medially through the **fossa infratemporalis** and **fossa pterygopalatina** (see Sections 27.5 and 27.6). Branches from its three parts, the **pars mandibularis**, **pars ptery-goidea**, and **pars pterygopalatina**, supply most structures of the face (**Table 24.4; Figs. 24.22** and **24.23**).

— The a. temporalis superficialis passes superiorly through the regio temporalis anterior to the ear and terminates as **the a. frontalis** and **a. parietalis** on the scalp. Its branches on the face (**Fig. 24.21**; see **Table 24.4**) include the following:

• The **a. transversa faciei**, which supplies the glandula parotidea and ductus parotideus and crosses anteriorly to supply the skin of the face

• The **a. zygomaticoorbitalis**, which supplies the lateral orbita
• The **a. temporalis media**, which supplies the regio temporalis

— The **a. carotis interna** is the continuation of the a. carotis communis (**Figs. 24.24** and **24.25**).

• It is described in four parts:
   ◦ A pars cervicalis in the neck that has no branches
   ◦ A pars petrosa that courses within the canalis caroticus of the os temporale
   ◦ A pars cavernosa that passes through the **sinus cavernosus** (a sinus venosus lateral to the sella turcica; see **Figs. 26.6** and **26.7**)
   ◦ A pars cerebralis that emerges into the fossa cranii media posterior to the orbita

• Two receptors are located within the a. carotis interna near its origin.
   ◦ The **sinus caroticus**, a baroreceptor that responds to changes in arterial pressure, is noticeable as a small dilation near the origin of the a. carotis interna.
   ◦ The **glomus caroticum**, a small mass of tissue located near the sinus caroticus, is a chemoreceptor that monitors blood oxygen levels. Stimulation of the glomus caroticum initiates an increase in heart rate, respiration rate, and blood pressure.

Table 24.3 Anterior, Medial, and Posterior Branches of the Arteria Carotis Externa

Branch	Artery	Divisions and Distributions
Anterior brs.	A. thyroidea superior	Rr. glandulares (to gl. thyroidea); a. laryngea superior; r. sternocleidomastoideus
	A. lingualis	Rr. dorsales linguae (to basis linguae, arcus palatoglossus, tonsilla palatina, palatum molle and epiglottis), a. sublingualis (to gl. sublingualis, lingua, oral floor, cavitas oris); r. sublingualis to gl. sublingualis; a. profunda linguae
	A. facialis	A. palatina ascendens (to pharyngeal wall, palatum molle, tuba auditiva); r. tonsillaris (to tonsillae palatinae); a. submentalis (to oral floor, gl. submandibularis); aa. labiales; a. angularis (to radix nasi)
Medial br.	A. pharyngea ascendens	Rr. pharyngeales; a. tympanica inferior (to mucosa of auris interna); a. meningea posterior
Posterior brs.	A. occipitalis	Rr. occipitales; r. descendens (to posterior neck muscles)
	A. auricularis posterior	A. stylomastoidea (to n. facialis in canalis nervi facialis); a. tympanica posterior; r. auricularis; r. occipitalis; r. parotideus

Note: For terminal brs., see **Table 24.4**.

Table 24.4 Terminal Branches of the Arteria Carotis Externa

Artery		Divisions and Distribution
A. temporalis superficialis		A. transversa faciei (to soft tissues below the arcus zygomaticus); r. frontalis; r. parietalis; a. zygomaticoorbitalis (to paries lateralis orbitae)
A. maxillaris	Pars mandibularis	A. alveolaris inferior (to mandibula, dentes, gingiva); a. meningea media; a. auricularis profunda (to art. temporomandibularis, porus acusticus externus); a. tympanica anterior
	Pars pterygoideus	A. masseterica; aa. temporales profundae; rr. pterygoidei; a. buccalis
	Pars pterygopalatina	A. alveolaris superior posterior (to dentes molares maxillares, sinus maxillaris, gingiva); a. infraorbitalis (to alveoli dentales maxillae)
	A. palatina descendens	A. palatina major (to palatum durum)
		Aa. palatinae minores (to palatum molle, tonsilla palatina, pharyngeal wall)
	A. sphenopalatina	Aa. nasales posteriores laterales (to lateral wall of cavitas nasi, conchae)
		Rr. septales posteriores (to septum nasi)

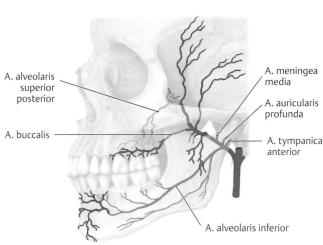

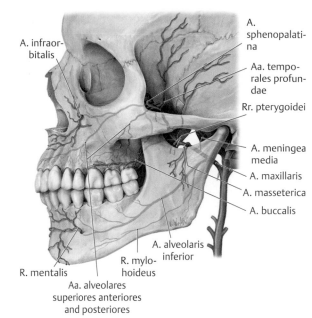

A Divisions of a. maxillaris: pars mandibularis (*blue*), pars pterygoidea (*green*), pars pterygopalatina (*yellow*). (From Gilroy AM et al. Atlas of Anatomy. 4th ed. 2020. Based on: Schuenke M, Schulte E, Schumacher U. THIEME Atlas of Anatomy. Head, Neck, and Neuroanatomy. Illustrations by Voll M and Wesker K. 3rd ed. New York: Thieme Medical Publishers; 2020.)

B Course of a. maxillaris. (From Schuenke M, Schulte E, Schumacher U. THIEME Atlas of Anatomy, Vol 3. Illustrations by Voll M and Wesker K. 3rd ed. New York: Thieme Publishers; 2020.)

Fig. 24.22 Rami profundi of arteria maxillaris
Left lateral view.

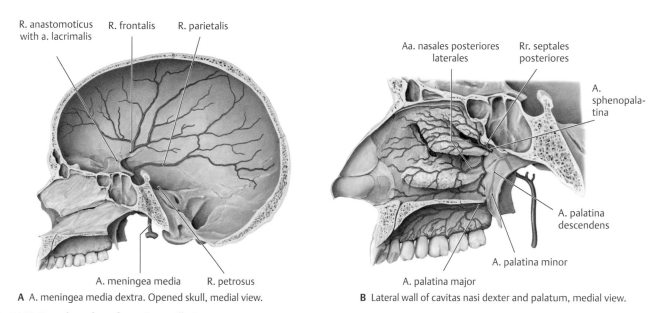

A A. meningea media dextra. Opened skull, medial view.

B Lateral wall of cavitas nasi dexter and palatum, medial view.

Fig. 24.23 Deep branches of arteria maxillaris
(From Schuenke M, Schulte E, Schumacher U. THIEME Atlas of Anatomy, Vol 3. Illustrations by Voll M and Wesker K. 3rd ed. New York: Thieme Publishers; 2020.)

- The **a. ophthalmica**, which arises within the skull as the first major branch of the a. carotis interna, passes through the canalis opticus to supply the orbital contents, including the retina of the eye through its **a. centralis retinae**.
  - Branches of the a. ophthalmica, the **a. supraorbitalis** and **a. supratrochlearis** to the anterior scalp and **aa. ethmoidales** to the cavitas nasi, anastomose with branches of the a. carotis externa **(Box 24.5)**.
- The **a. cerebri anterior** and **a. cerebri media** arise from the a. carotis interna to supply the anterior circulation of the brain (see Section 26.2).

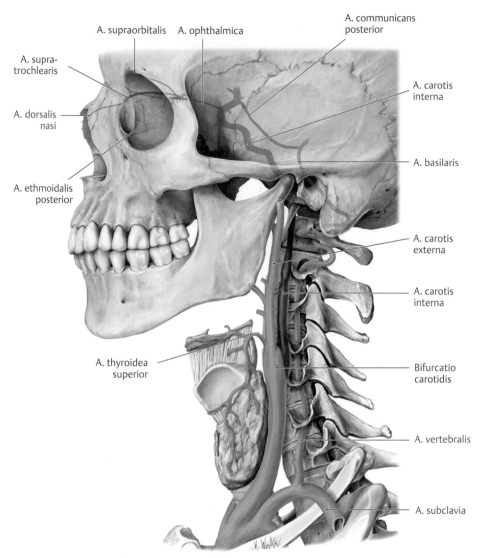

A. supra-
trochlearis

A. supraorbitalis

A. ophthalmica

A. communicans
posterior

A. dorsalis
nasi

A. carotis
interna

A. ethmoidalis
posterior

A. basilaris

A. carotis
externa

A. carotis
interna

A. thyroidea
superior

Bifurcatio
carotidis

A. vertebralis

A. subclavia

Fig. 24.24 Arteria carotis interna
Left lateral view. (From Gilroy AM et al.
Atlas of Anatomy. 4th ed. 2020. Based on:
Schuenke M, Schulte E, Schumacher U.
THIEME Atlas of Anatomy. Head, Neck,
and Neuroanatomy. Illustrations by Voll M
and Wesker K. 3rd ed. New York: Thieme
Medical Publishers; 2020.)

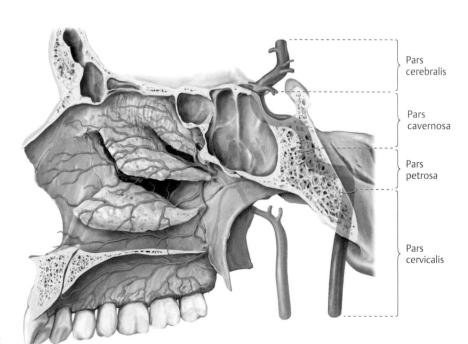

Pars
cerebralis

Pars
cavernosa

Pars
petrosa

Pars
cervicalis

**Fig. 24.25 Course of the arteria carotis
interna in the cranium**
Right side, medial view. (From Schuenke M,
Schulte E, Schumacher U. THIEME Atlas of
Anatomy, Vol 3. Illustrations by Voll M and
Wesker K. 3rd ed. New York: Thieme Publishers;
2020.)

BOX 24.5: CLINICAL CORRELATION

ANASTOMOSES BETWEEN ARTERIA CAROTIS EXTERNA AND ARTERIA CAROTIS INTERNA

The a. carotis externa artery supplies superficial and deep regions of the face, the cavitas nasi and cavitas oris, and the neck, while the a. carotis interna supplies the brain and the orbita. There are areas of overlap and important anastomoses between these circulations that can become clinically significant, such as the collateralization of blood supply to the brain, the transmission of infections from the face to the cerebral circulation, and accurate ligation of the source of a nosebleed. Primary areas of anastomoses include branches of the a. facialis and a. ophthalmica in the orbita and the a. sphenopalatina and a. ethmoidale on the septum nasi.

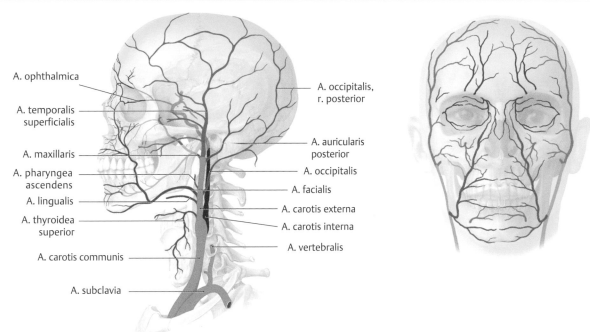

A. ophthalmica
A. temporalis superficialis
A. maxillaris
A. pharyngea ascendens
A. lingualis
A. thyroidea superior
A. carotis communis
A. subclavia

A. occipitalis, r. posterior
A. auricularis posterior
A. occipitalis
A. facialis
A. carotis externa
A. carotis interna
A. vertebralis

A Left lateral view.

B Anterior view.

Anastomoses between branches of the arteria carotis externa and arteria carotis interna
Branches of the a. carotis externa are grouped by color: anterior = red; medial = blue; posterior = green; terminal = brown. Branches of the a. carotis externa (e.g. the a. facialis, red) communicate with terminal branches of the a. carotis interna (e.g. the a. ophthalmica, purple). (From Schuenke M, Schulte E, Schumacher U. THIEME Atlas of Anatomy, Vol 3. Illustrations by Voll M and Wesker K. 3rd ed. New York: Thieme Publishers; 2020.)

24.4 Veins of the Head and Neck

— Superficial and deep veins of the head and neck drain almost exclusively to the v. jugularis externa and interna, although some also communicate with the plexus venosus vertebralis of the columna vertebralis (**Figs. 24.26** and **24.27**).
— Superficial veins generally follow the course of the arteries, but the veins are usually more numerous, more variable, and more interconnected than the arteries.
— The most prominent superficial veins on each side of the head include
  • the **v. supratrochlearis** and **v. supraorbitalis**, which drain to the v. angularis;
  • the **v. angularis**, which joins with the v. profunda faciei and continues inferiorly as the v. facialis;
  • the **plexus venosus pterygoideus**, which drains areas supplied by the a. maxillaris, including the orbita, cavitas nasi, and cavitas oris (it drains to the v. maxillaris and v. profunda faciei);
  • the **v. profunda faciei**, which arises from the plexus venosus pterygoideus and drains to the v. facialis;
  • the **v. facialis**, which drains to the **v. jugularis interna**;
  • the **v. temporalis superficialis** and **v. maxillaris**, which join to form the v. retromandibularis;

  • the **v. retromandibularis,** which joins the **v. auricularis posterior** to form the **v. jugularis externa**; and
  • the **v. occipitalis**, which drains to the v. jugularis externa.
— v. jugularis externa dextra and sinistra form posterior to the angulus mandibularis by the union of the vv. auriculares posteriores and the posterior division of the vv. retromandibulares.
  • They cross the m. sternocleidomastoideus in the neck and drain into the v. subclavia.
  • They drain the scalp and side of the face.
  • Their tributaries include the v. retromandibularis, v. auricularis posterior, v. occipitalis, v. transversa cervicalis, v. suprascapularis, and v. jugularis anterior.
— A **v. jugularis interna** dextra and sinistra forms at the foramen jugulare at the skull base and descends within the vagina carotica with the a. carotis communis and n. vagus.
  • It joins the v. subclavia in the root of the neck to form the v. brachiocephalica. The junction of the v. jugularis interna and v. subclavia is called the **jugulosubclavian junction,** or **venous angle.** The ductus thoracicus and ductus lymphaticus dexter terminate at this junction, respectively.
  • It drains the brain, the anterior face and scalp, and the viscera and deep muscles of the neck.

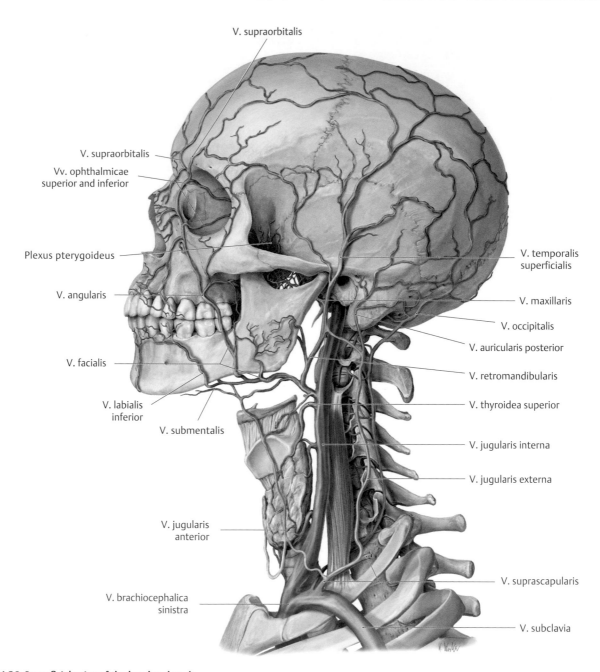

Fig. 24.26 Superficial veins of the head and neck
Left lateral view. (From Gilroy AM et al. Atlas of Anatomy. 4th ed. 2020. Based on: Schuenke M, Schulte E, Schumacher U. THIEME Atlas of Anatomy. Head, Neck, and Neuroanatomy. Illustrations by Voll M and Wesker K. 3rd ed. New York: Thieme Medical Publishers; 2020.)

- Its tributaries include the sinus durae matris, v. facialis, v. lingualis, vv. pharyngei, and v. thyroidea superior and media.
- A small **v. jugularis anterior** originates from superficial veins on each side near the os hyoideum.
  - It descends to the base of the neck and terminates in the v. jugularis externa or v. subclavia.

- A **arcus venosus jugularis** may connect the v. jugularis anterior dextra and sinistra at the basis colli, above the sternum.
- Deep veins of the orbita and brain drain to **sinus durae matris**, venous channels formed within the dura mater that have no arterial counterpart (see Section 18.1). Sinus durae matris drain eventually to the v. jugularis interna.

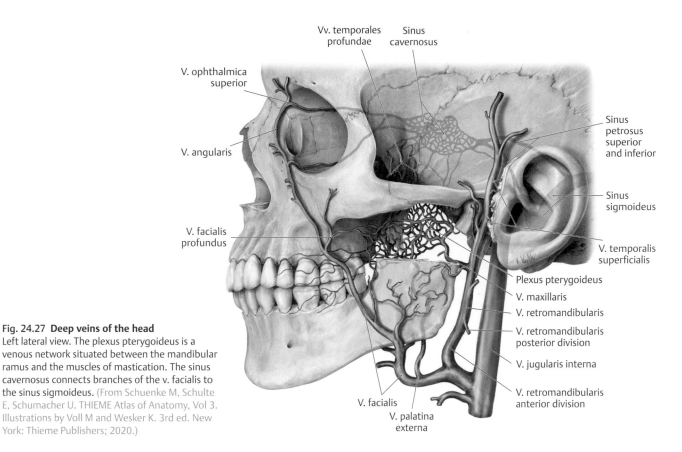

Fig. 24.27 Deep veins of the head
Left lateral view. The plexus pterygoideus is a venous network situated between the mandibular ramus and the muscles of mastication. The sinus cavernosus connects branches of the v. facialis to the sinus sigmoideus. (From Schuenke M, Schulte E, Schumacher U. THIEME Atlas of Anatomy, Vol 3. Illustrations by Voll M and Wesker K. 3rd ed. New York: Thieme Publishers; 2020.)

BOX 24.6: CLINICAL CORRELATION

VENOUS ANASTOMOSES AS PORTALS OF INFECTION
The extensive anastomoses between superficial veins of the face, and the deep veins of the head (e.g., pterygoid plexus) and dural sinuses (e.g., sinus cavernosus) is clinically very important. Veins in the triangular danger zone of the face are, in general, valveless.

Thus, bacterial infections from the face are easily disseminated into the cavitas cranii. An infection on the lip, for example, may travel via the v. facialis to the sinus cavernosus, resulting in a sinus cavernosus thrombosis (infection leading to clot formation that may occlude the sinus) or even meningitis.

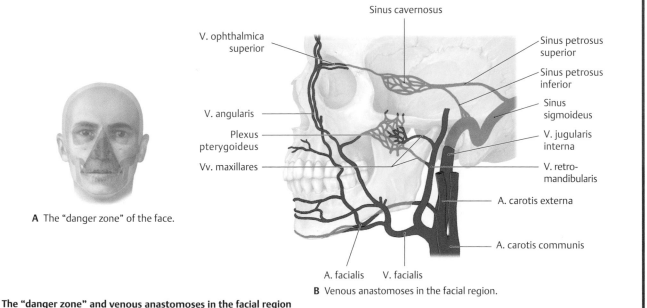

A The "danger zone" of the face.

B Venous anastomoses in the facial region.

The "danger zone" and venous anastomoses in the facial region
(From Schuenke M, Schulte E, Schumacher U. THIEME Atlas of Anatomy, Vol 3. Illustrations by Voll M and Wesker K. 3rd ed. New York: Thieme Publishers; 2020.)

24.5   Lymphatic Drainage of the Head and Neck

— Nll. superficiales of the head and neck extend along the v. jugularis externa.
  • They receive lymph from local areas and drain to the nll. cervici profundi.
  • Superficial node groups include nll. occipitales, nll. retroauriculares, nll. mastoidei, nll. parotidei, nll. cervicales anteriores, and nll. cervicales laterales (**Fig. 24.28; Table 24.5**).

Table 24.5 Nll. Cervicales Superficiales

Nll.	Drainage Region
Nll. retroauriculares	Regio occipitalis
Nll. occipitales	
Nll. mastoidei	
Nll. parotidei superficiales	Regio parotideo auricularis
Nll. parotidei profundi	
Nll. cervicales anteriores superficiales	Regio sternocleidomastoidea
Nll. cervicales laterales superficiales	

— Lymph from structures in the head and neck ultimately drains into **nll. cervicales profundi** that lie along the v. jugularis interna deep to the m. sternocleidomastoideus (**Fig. 24.29; Table 24.6**). There are two groups of nll. cervicales profundi:
  • **Nll. cervicales profundi superiores**, known as the jugulodigastric group, lie near the v. facialis and v. jugularis interna and venter posterior of m. digastricus. Nll. submandibulares and nll. submentales also drain to this group. Nll. cervicales laterales profundi superiores drain either to the nll. cervicales profundi inferiores or directly to the trunci lymphatici jugulares.
  • **Nll. cervicales profundi inferiores** are usually associated with the lower v. jugularis interna, but some nodes also reside in the area around the v. subclavia and plexus brachialis. Nll. cervicales profundi inferiores drain directly to the trunci lymphatici jugulares.
— Lymphatic vessels from the nll. cervicales profundi join to form **trunci lymphatici jugulares**.
  • On the right, these trunks drain directly or indirectly (via the ductus lymphaticus dexter) into the right jugulosubclavian junction (right venous angle).
  • On the left, these trunks join the ductus thoracicus, which drains into the left jugulosubclavian junction (left venous angle).

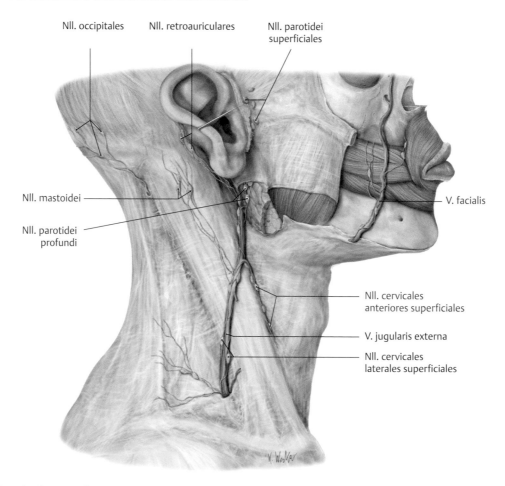

Fig. 24.28 Nodi lymphoidei cervicales superficiales
Right lateral view. (From Schuenke M, Schulte E, Schumacher U. THIEME Atlas of Anatomy, Vol 3. Illustrations by Voll M and Wesker K. 3rd ed. New York: Thieme Publishers; 2020.)

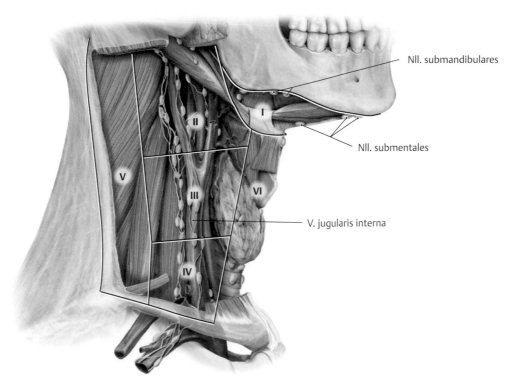

Fig. 24.29 Nodi lymphoidei cervicales profundi
Right lateral view. (From Schuenke M, Schulte E, Schumacher U. THIEME Atlas of Anatomy, Vol 3. Illustrations by Voll M and Wesker K. 3rd ed. New York: Thieme Publishers; 2020.)

Table 24.6 Nll. Cervicales Profundi

Level	Nll.		Drainage Region
I	Nll. submentales		Face
	Nll. submandibulares		
II	Nll. jugulares laterales	Upper lateral group	Nuchal region, laryngo-tracheo-thyroidal region
III		Middle lateral group	
IV		Lower lateral group	
V	Nll. trigoni cervicalis posterior		Nuchal region
VI	Nll. cervicales anteriores		Laryngo-tracheo-thyroidal region

24.6 Nerves of the Head and Neck

Innervation of head and neck structures is a complex combination of somatic and autonomic nerves arising from the cervical spinal cord, nn. craniales, and the truncus sympathicus. A brief overview is provided here. For more detailed discussions see Section 26.3 (nn. craniales), Section 26.4 (autonomic innervation), and Section 25.4 (nerves of the neck).

— Somatic nerves of the head and neck include the following:
  • Nn. spinales C1 through C4, which innervate structures in the head and neck
    ◦ The **plexus nervosus cervicalis** is derived from rami anteriores of nn. spinales C1–C4.
    ◦ The **n. suboccipitalis**, **n. occipitalis major**, and **n. occipitalis tertius** are derived from posterior rami of cervical nervi spinales.
  • Nn. spinales C5 through T1, whose rami anteriores form the plexus brachialis that innervates the upper limb (see Section 18.4)
  • Nn. craniales (CN I to CN XII), which arise from the brain.

— Autonomic nerves of the head and neck include
  • parasympathetic nerves, which arise in association with four of the nn. craniales (CN III, VII, XI, and X), and
  • sympathetic nerves, which arise from the truncus sympathicus cervicalis.

25 The Neck

The neck extends from the base of the skull to the clavicula and manubrium sterni. It contains vital neurovascular structures that supply the head, the thorax, and the upper limb. The neck also contains musculoskeletal elements that support and move the head and viscera of the gastrointestinal, respiratory, and endocrine systems.

25.1 Regions of the Neck

The regions of the neck, defined by muscular and skeletal boundaries, are largely descriptive rather than functional, but they are useful for understanding the topographic relationships in the neck, which often play a significant role in medical practice **(Table 25.1; Figs. 25.1)**. Refer to Section 25.8 for detailed anatomic relations of these regions.

— The **trigonum cervicale anterius** (anterior triangle) extends from the midline of the neck to the anterior margin of the m. sternocleidomastoideus.
  • The region is further divided into **trigonum submandibulare**, **trigonum submentale**, **trigonum musculare**, and **trigonum caroticum**.
  • The anterior region contains most of the cervical viscera, which includes the lower pharynx, esophagus, larynx, trachea, gl. thyroidea, and gll. parathyroideae.
— The **regio sternocleidomastoidea** is a narrow area defined by the anterior margin and posterior margin of the m. sternocleidomastoideus.
  • Inferiorly, the caput sternale and caput claviculare of the muscle define the small **fossa supraclavicularis minor**.
  • This region contains parts of the major vascular structures of the neck.
— The **regio cervicalis lateralis** (trigonum cervicale posterius) extends from the posterior margin of m. sternocleidomastoideusto the anterior margin of m. trapezius.
  • The venter posterior of m. omohyoideus divides this region into the **trigonum omoclaviculare** and **trigonum occipitale**.
  • The m. scaleneim, and plexus cervicalis and plexus brachialis are located in this region.
— The **regio cervicalis posterior** extends from the anterior margin of m. trapezius to the posterior midline of the neck.
  • It contains the m. trapezius and m. suboccipitalis, the a. vertebralis, and rami posteriores of the plexus cervicalis.
— The **root of neck,** a transition area for structures passing between the thorax and neck, is enclosed by the apertura thoracica superior, which is formed by the manubrium, costae I and their cartilagines costales, and vertebra T I.
  • It contains the trachea, oesophagus, a. carotis communis and a. subclavia, vv. brachiocephalicae, n. vagus and n. phrenicus, the truncus sympathicus, the ductus thoracicus, and the apex pulmonis.

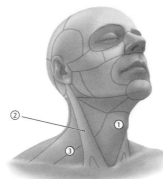
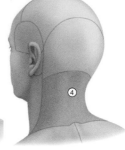

A Right anterior oblique view. (From Schuenke M, Schulte E, Schumacher U. THIEME Atlas of Anatomy, Vol 3. Illustrations by Voll M and Wesker K. 3rd ed. New York: Thieme Publishers; 2020.)

B Left posterior oblique view. (From Schuenke M, Schulte E, Schumacher U. THIEME Atlas of Anatomy, Vol 3. Illustrations by Voll M and Wesker K. 3rd ed. New York: Thieme Publishers; 2020.)

Table 25.1 Regions of the Neck

Region	Divisions	Contents
① Trigonum cervicale anterius	Trigonum submandibulare (digastric)	Gl. submandibularis and nll. submandibulares, n. hypoglossus (CN XII), a. and v. facialis
	Trigonum submentale	Nll. submentales
	Trigonum musculare	M. sternothyroideus and m. sternohyoideus, gl. thyroidea and gll. parathyroideae
	Trigonum caroticum	Bifurcatio carotidis, glomus caroticum, n. hypoglossus (CN XII) and n. vagus (CN X)
② Regio sternocleidomastoidea*		M. sternocleidomastoideus, a. carotis communis, v. jugularis interna, n. vagus (CN X), nll. jugulares laterales
③ Regio cervicalis lateralis (trigonum cervicale posterius)	Trigonum omoclaviculare	A. subclavia, a. subscapularis, nll. supraclaviculares
	Trigonum occipitale	N. accessorius (CN XI), trunci of plexus brachialis, a. transversa cervicis, plexus cervicalis (rr. dorsales)
④ Regio cervicalis posterior		Nuchal muscles, a. vertebralis, plexus cervicalis

* The regio sternocleidomastoidea also contains the fossa supraclavicularis minor.

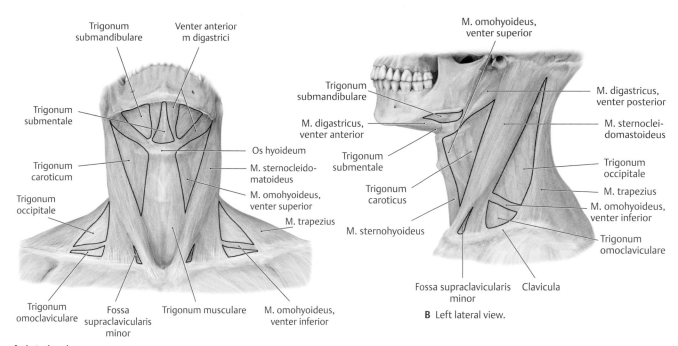

A Anterior view.

Fig. 25.1 Cervical regions
(From Gilroy AM et al. Atlas of Anatomy. 4th ed. 2020. Based on: Schuenke M, Schulte E, Schumacher U. THIEME Atlas of Anatomy. Head, Neck, and Neuroanatomy. Illustrations by Voll M and Wesker K. 3rd ed. New York: Thieme Medical Publishers; 2020.)

25.2 Deep Fascia of the Neck

The **fascia cervicalis** is divided into four layers that surround and compartmentalize the structures of the neck (**Fig. 25.2; Table 25.2**).

— The **lamina superficialis of fascia cervicalis**, a thin layer that lies deep to the skin, surrounds the entire neck but splits to enclose the m. sternocleidomastoideus and m. trapezius and contains cutaneous nerves, superficial vessels, and superficial lymphatics of the neck.
— The **lamina pretrachealis** in the anterior neck has a muscular lamina (layer) that encloses the mm. infrahyoidei and a visceral lamina that encloses the viscera of the anterior neck.

— The **prevertebral fascia** surrounds the columna vertebralis and the deep neck muscles and is continuous with the **nuchal fascia** posteriorly.
— The **vagina carotica**, a condensation of the fascia pretrachealis, fascia prevertebralis, and fascia superficialis, forms a narrow cylindrical tube that encloses the neurovascular bundle of the neck: the v. jugularis interna, a. carotis communis, and n. vagus.
— The **spatium retropharyngeum**, a potential space between the lamina visceralis of fascia pretrachealis and the fascia prevertebralis, extends from the basis cranii superiorly to the mediastinum superior inferiorly.

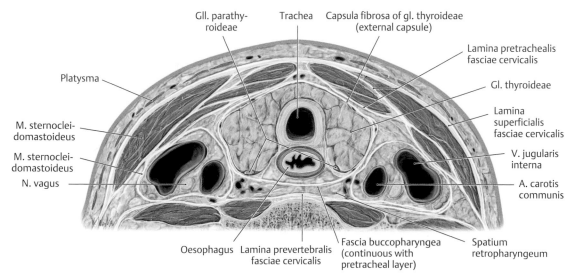

Fig. 25.2 Fascial layers in the anterior neck
Transverse section of the neck at the level of C6, superior view. (From Schuenke M, Schulte E, Schumacher U. THIEME Atlas of Anatomy, Vol 3. Illustrations by Voll M and Wesker K. 3rd ed. New York: Thieme Publishers; 2020.)

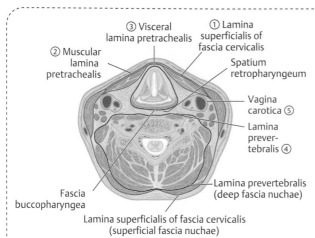

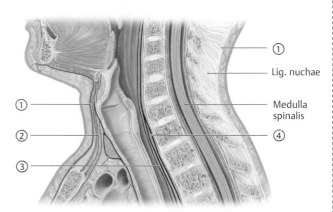

A Transverse section at level of C5 vertebra. (From Gilroy AM et al. Atlas of Anatomy. 4th ed. 2020. Based on: Schuenke M, Schulte E, Schumacher U. THIEME Atlas of Anatomy. Head, Neck, and Neuroanatomy. Illustrations by Voll M and Wesker K. 3rd ed. New York: Thieme Medical Publishers; 2020.)

B Midsagittal section, left lateral view. (From Gilroy AM et al. Atlas of Anatomy. 4th ed. 2020. Based on: Schuenke M, Schulte E, Schumacher U. THIEME Atlas of Anatomy. Head, Neck, and Neuroanatomy. Illustrations by Voll M and Wesker K. 3rd ed. New York: Thieme Medical Publishers; 2020.)

Table 25.2 Fascia cervicalis
The fascia cervicalis is divided into four laminae that enclose the structures of the neck.

Layer	Type of Fascia	Description
● ① Lamina superficialis	Muscular	Envelopes entire neck; splits to enclose m. sternocleidomastoideus and m. trapezius
Lamina pretrachealis	● ② Muscular	Encloses mm. infrahyoidei
	● ③ Visceral	Surrounds gl. thyroidea, larynx, trachea, pharynx, and oesophagus
● ④ Lamina prevertebralis	Muscular	Surrounds cervical columna vertebralis and associated muscles
● ⑤ Vagina carotica	Neurovascular	Encloses a. carotis communis, v. jugularis interna, and n. vagus

25.3   Muscles of the Neck

— Three muscles form the most superficial muscular layer of the neck (**Fig. 25.3; Table 25.3**):
  • The **platysma,** enclosed within the superficial fascia of the neck, is a muscle of facial expression, and therefore a subcutaneous muscle, that extends onto the anterolateral surfaces of the neck.
  • The **m. sternocleidomastoideus**, enclosed within the investing layer of the fascia cervicalis, is a visible landmark that divides the neck into regio cervicalis anterior and regio cervicalis lateralis.
  • The **m. trapezius**, also within the investing fascial layer, is a muscle of the cingulum pectorale that extends onto the neck and forms the posterior margin of the regio cervicalis lateralis.
— Muscles attached to the os hyoideum lie between the superficial and deep neck muscles.
  • **Mm. suprahyoidei**, the **m. digastricus**, **m. stylohyoideus**, **m. mylohyoideus**, and **m. hyoglossus**, form the floor of the mouth and elevate the os hyoideum and larynx during swallowing and phonation (see **Table 27.9**).

  • **Mm. infrahyoidei** in the neck, **m. omohyoideus**, **m. sternohyoideus**, **m. sternothyroideus**, and **m. thyrohyoideus**, depress the os hyoideum and larynx during swallowing and phonation (**Fig. 25.4; Table 25.4**).
— The deep muscles of the neck lie deep to the fascia prevertebralis and include the mm. prevertebrales and mm. scalenei (**Fig. 25.5; Table 25.5**).

BOX 25.1: CLINICAL CORRELATION

CONGENITAL TORTICOLLIS
Congenital torticollis (wryneck) is a condition in which one of the mm. sternocleidomastoidei (SCM) is abnormally short, causing the head to tilt to one side with the chin pointing upward to the opposite side. This shortening is thought to be the result of trauma at birth (tears or stretching of the SCM muscle) causing bleeding and swelling within the muscle and subsequent scar tissue formation.

Fig. 25.3 Superficial musculature of the neck

Left lateral view. (From Schuenke M, Schulte E, Schumacher U. THIEME Atlas of Anatomy, Vol 3. Illustrations by Voll M and Wesker K. 3rd ed. New York: Thieme Publishers; 2020.)

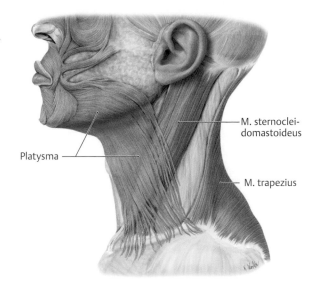

M. sternocleidomastoideus

Platysma

M. trapezius

Table 25.3 Superficial Muscles of the Neck

Muscle		Origin	Insertion	Innervation	Action
Platysma		Skin over lower neck and upper lateral thorax	Mandibula (inferior border), skin over lower face and angle of mouth	R. cervicalis of n. facialis (CN VII)	Depresses and wrinkles skin of lower face and mouth, tenses skin of neck, aids forced depression of mandibula
M. sternocleido-mastoideus	Caput sternale	Manubrium sterni	Os temporale (proc. mastoideus), os occipitale (linea nuchalis superior)	*Motor:* N. accessorius (CN XI) *Pain and proprioception:* Plexus cervicalis (C2, C3, [C4])	*Unilateral:* Tilts head to same side, rotates head to opposite side *Bilateral:* Extends head, aids in respiration when head is fixed
	Caput claviculare	Clavicula (medial one third)			
M. trapezius	Pars descendens	Os occipitale, procc. spinosi of C I–C VII	Clavicula (lateral one third)		Draws scapula obliquely upward, rotates cavitas glenoidalis superiorly

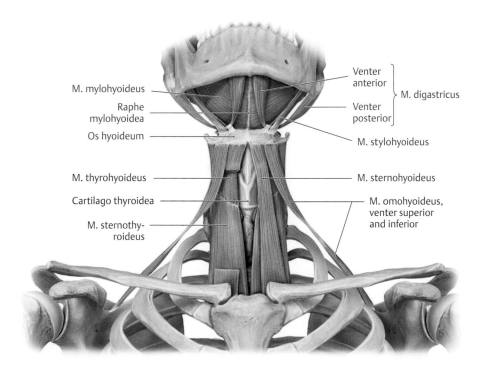

M. mylohyoideus

Raphe mylohyoidea

Os hyoideum

M. thyrohyoideus

Cartilago thyroidea

M. sternothy-roideus

Venter anterior

Venter posterior

M. digastricus

M. stylohyoideus

M. sternohyoideus

M. omohyoideus, venter superior and inferior

Fig. 25.4 Musculi suprahyoidei and musculi infrahyoidei

Anterior view. The m. sternohyoideus has been cut on the right side. See **Table 27.9** for the mm. suprahyoidei. (From Schuenke M, Schulte E, Schumacher U. THIEME Atlas of Anatomy, Vol 3. Illustrations by Voll M and Wesker K. 3rd ed. New York: Thieme Publishers; 2020.)

Table 25.4 Musculi Infrahyoidei

Muscle	Origin	Insertion	Innervation	Action
M. omohyoideus	Scapula (margo superior)	Os hyoideum (corpus) (body)	Ansa cervicalis of plexus cervicalis (C1–C3)	Depresses (fixes) os hyoideum, draws larynx and os hyoideum down for phonation and terminal phases of swallowing*
M. sternohyoideus	Manubriaum sterni and art. sternoclavicularis (posterior surface)			
M. sternothyroideus	Manubrium sterni (posterior surface)	Cartilago thyroidea (linea obliqua)	Ansa cervicalis (C1–C3)	
M. thyrohyoideus	Cartilago thyroidea (linea obliqua)	Os hyoideum (corpus)	C1 via n. hypoglossus (CN XII)	Depresses and fixes os hyoideum, raises the larynx during swallowing

*The m. omohyoideus also tenses the fascia cervicalis (with an intermediate tendon).

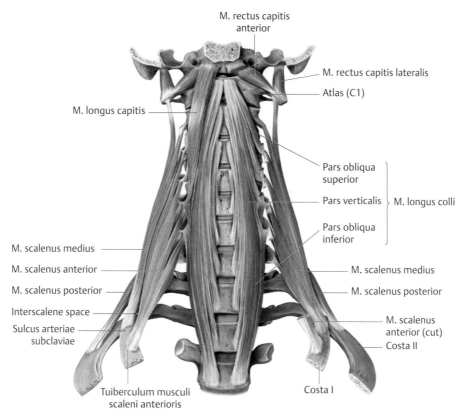

Fig. 25.5 Deep muscles of the neck
Prevertebral and mm. scaleni, anterior view. *Removed from left side:* M. longus capitis and m. scalenus anterior. (From Schuenke M, Schulte E, Schumacher U. THIEME Atlas of Anatomy, Vol 3. Illustrations by Voll M and Wesker K. 3rd ed. New York: Thieme Publishers; 2020.)

Table 25.5 Deep Muscles of the Neck

Muscles		Origin	Insertion	Innervation	Action
Prevertebral muscles					
M. longus capitis		C III–C VI (tubercula anteriora of procc. transversi)	Pars basilaris ossis occipitalis	Rr. anteriores of C1–C3	Flexion of head at artt. atlantooccipitales
M. longus colli	Pars recta (intermediate part)	C V–T III (anterior surfaces of corpora vertebrarum)	C II–C IV (anterior surfaces)	Rr. anteriores of C2–C6	*Unilateral:* Tilts and rotates cervical spine to opposite side
	Pars obliqua superior	C III–C V (tubercula anteriora of procc. transversi)	Tuberculum anterius atlantis		*Bilateral:* Forward flexion of cervical spine
	Pars obliqua inferior	T I–T III (anterior surfaces of corpora vertebrarum)	C V–C VI (tubercula anteriora of procc. transversi)		

Table 25.5 (*continued*) **Deep Muscles of the Neck**

Muscles	Origin	Insertion	Innervation	Action
M. rectus capitis anterior	Massa lateralis atlantis	Pars basilaris ossis occipitalis	Rr. anteriores of C1 and C2	*Unilateral:* Lateral flexion of the head at the art. atlantooccipitalis
M. rectus capitis lateralis	Proc. transversus atlantis	Pars basilaris ossis occipitalis, lateral to condyli occipitales		*Bilateral:* Flexion of the head at the art. atlantooccipitalis
Scalene muscles				
M. scalenus anterior	C III–C VI (tubercula anteriora of procc. transversi)	Costa I (tuberculum musculi scaleni anterioris)	Rr. anteriores of C4–C6	*With ribs mobile:* Elevates upper costae (during forced inspiration)
M. scalenus medius	C I–C II (procc. transversi), C III–C VII (tubercula posteriora of procc. transversi)	Costa I (posterior to sulcus arteriae subclaviae)	Rr. anteriores of C3–C8	*With ribs fixed:* Flexes cervical spine to same side (unilateral), flexes neck (bilateral)
M. scalenus posterior	C V–C VII (tubercula posteriora of procc. transversi)	Costa II (outer surface)	Rr. anteriores of C6–C8	

25.4 Nerves of the Neck

Nerves of the neck include cervical and thoracic spinal nerves, nerves from the truncus sympathicus cervicis, and nn. craniales.

Nn. Cervicales

The C1–C4 nn. spinales supply the regions of the neck (**Table 25.6**).

— Rami posteriores of C1–C4 cervical spinal nerves form the **plexus cervicalis,** which has sensory and motor components.
  • The sensory nerves of the plexus, the **n. occipitalis minor** (C2), **n. auricularis magnus** (C2–C3), **n. transversus cervicalis** (C2–C3), and **nn. supraclaviculares** (C3–C4), innervate the skin of the anterior and lateral neck and lateral scalp. They emerge from behind the midpoint of the posterior margin of the m. sternocleidomastoideus, a location known as the **nerve point of the neck** (or Erb's point) (**Fig. 25.6**).
  • The **ansa cervicalis** (C1–C3), the motor part of the plexus, which has a superior and inferior root, innervates all of the mm. infrahyoidei except the m. thyrohyoideus and usually lies anterior to the v. jugularis interna (**Fig. 25.7**).
— The n. phrenicus, which arises from rami anteriores of C3–C5 nn. spinales, descends on the surface of the m. scalenus anterior and enters the thorax, where it supplies the diaphragma with sensory and motor innervation. It also transmits sensation from the mediastinal and diaphragmatic pleura and fibrous and parietal pericardium.

— Posterior rami of cervical spinal nerves C1 through C3 form three nerves that provide motor and cutaneous innervation to the posterior neck and scalp: the **n. suboccipitalis** (C1), **n. occipitalis major** (C2), and **n. occipitalis tertius** (C3) (**Fig. 25.8**).

Plexus Brachialis

The plexus brachialis, which innervates the upper limb, forms from the rami anteriores of C5–T1. It emerges through the **spatium interscalenum** (the space between the m. scalenus anterior and m. scalenus medius) in the lateral region of the neck before continuing into the axilla (see Section 18.4). Normally four branches arise from the supraclavicular part of the plexus to supply muscles of the shoulder and pectoral girdle as it traverses the neck: the n. dorsalis scapulae, n. suprascapularis, n. to the subclavius, and n. thoracicis longus.

The Cervical Sympathetic Trunk

The cervical sympathetic trunk, a continuation of the thoracic sympathetic trunk, extends into the neck to the level of vertebra C I, where it lies anterolateral to the columna vertebralis and posterior to the vagina carotis (see **Figs. 25.18** and **25.20**).

— The cervical sympathetic trunk receives no rr. communicantes albi from cervical spinal nerves. The preganglionic fibers that synapse in the ganglia cervicales originate in thoracic spinal nerves and ascend in the truncus sympathicus to the regio cervicalis.

Table 25.6 Branches of the Nervi Spinales in the Neck

Rami Posteriores

	Nerve	Sensory Function	Motor Function
C1	N. suboccipitalis	No C1 dermatome	Innervate intrinsic nuchal muscles
C2	N. occipitalis major	Innervate C2 dermatome	
C3	N. occipitalis tertius	Innervate C3 dermatome	

Rami Anteriores

	Sensory Branches	Sensory Function	Motor Branches	Motor Function
C1	–	–	Form ansa cervicalis (motor part of plexus cervicalis)	Innervate mm. infrahyoidei (except m. thyrohyoideus)
C2	N. occipitalis minor	Form sensory part of plexus cervicalis, innervate anterior and lateral neck		
C2, C3	N. auricularis major			
	N. transversus colli			
C3, C4	Nn. supraclavicularis		Contribute to n. phrenicus*	Innervate diaphragma and pericardium*

* The radices anteriores of C3–C5 combine to form the n. phrenicus.

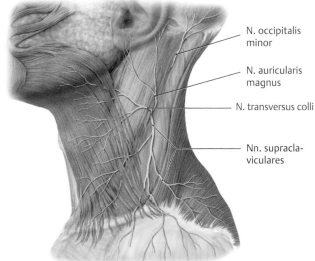

(From Gilroy AM et al. Atlas of Anatomy. 4th ed. 2020. Based on: Schuenke M, Schulte E, Schumacher U. THIEME Atlas of Anatomy. Head, Neck, and Neuroanatomy. Illustrations by Voll M and Wesker K. 3rd ed. New York: Thieme Medical Publishers; 2020.)

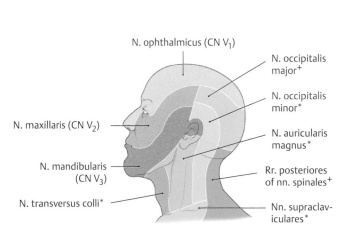

A Cutaneous nerve territories. N. trigeminus, CN V₃ (*orange*), rr. posteriores (+), rr. anteriores (*).

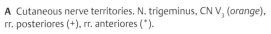

B Sensory branches of the plexus cervicalis.

Fig. 25.6 Sensory innervation of the anterolateral neck
Left lateral view. (From Gilroy AM et al. Atlas of Anatomy. 4th ed. 2020. Based on: Schuenke M, Schulte E, Schumacher U. THIEME Atlas of Anatomy. Head, Neck, and Neuroanatomy. Illustrations by Voll M and Wesker K. 3rd ed. New York: Thieme Medical Publishers; 2020.)

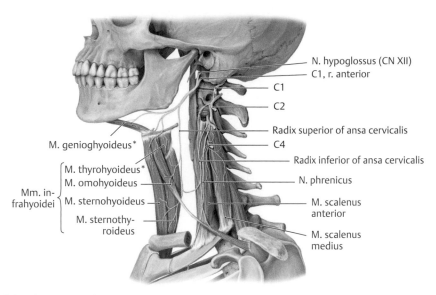

Fig. 25.7 Motor nerves of the plexus cervicalis
Left lateral view. *Innervated by the r. anterior of C1 (distributed by the n. hypoglossus). (From Schuenke M, Schulte E, Schumacher U. THIEME Atlas of Anatomy, Vol 3. Illustrations by Voll M and Wesker K. 3rd ed. New York: Thieme Publishers; 2020.)

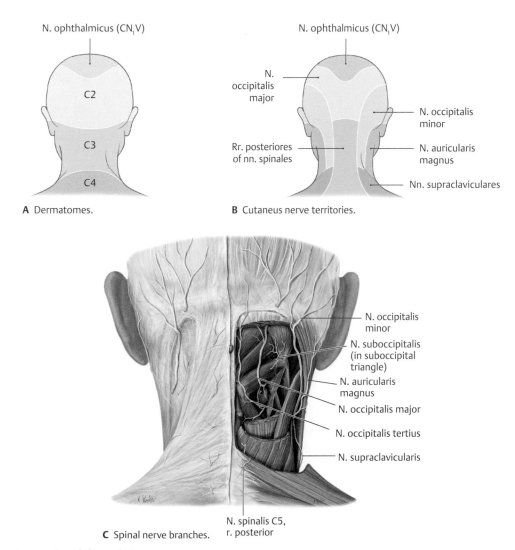

Fig. 25.8 Sensory innervation of the nuchal region
Posterior view. (From Gilroy AM et al. Atlas of Anatomy. 4th ed. 2020. Based on: Schuenke M, Schulte E, Schumacher U. THIEME Atlas of Anatomy. Head, Neck, and Neuroanatomy. Illustrations by Voll M and Wesker K. 3rd ed. New York: Thieme Medical Publishers; 2020.)

- Postganglionic fibers from the ganglia cervicales are distributed along three routes:
  - Via rami communicantes grisei to join cervical spinal nerves
  - Via nn. cardiaci cervicales (cardiopulmonary) to the plexus cardiacus in the thorax
  - Via sympathetic nerve plexuses surrounding vessels (plexus periarterialis), especially along the a. carotis externa, a. carotis interna, and a. vertebralis, to supply structures of the head and neck (see Section 26.4)
- The cervical sympathetic trunk has ganglion cervicale superius, medium, and inferioris.
  - The **ganglion cervicale superius** lies anterior to vertebra C I and posterior to the a. carotis interna. Its branches include
    - the **n. cardiacus cervicalis superior**,
    - branches to the **plexus pharyngeus**,
    - an **n. caroticus internus** that forms the **plexus caroticus internus**, and
    - an **n. caroticus externus** that forms the **plexus caroticus externus**.
    - rami communicantes grisei to rami anteriores of C1–C4 nn. spinales.
  - The **ganglion cervicale medium** lies at the level of vertebra C VI and gives off the **n. cardiacus cervicalis medius**, which joins the plexus cardiacus in the thorax, and rami communicantes grisei to rami anteriores of C5 and C6 nn. spinales.
  - The **ganglion cervicale inferioris** usually combines with the most superior ganglion thoracica (T1) to form the **ganglion stellatum**, which lies anterior to the proc. transversus of vertebra C VII. It gives off the **n. cardiacus cervicalis inferior**, which descends into the thorax, and rami communicantes grisei to rami anteriores of C7 and C8 nn. spinales.

Nervi Craniales in the Neck

Four of the nn. craniales are found in the neck.
- The n. glossopharyngeus (CN IX) sends branches to the tongue and pharynx in the head and descends into the neck to innervate the carotid body and carotid sinus (see **Fig. 26.28**). It innervates one muscle, the m. stylopharyngeus.
- The n. vagus (CN X) descends within the vagina carotica in the neck before entering the thorax. Its branches to cervical structures arise from both thoracic and cervical parts of the nerve (see **Fig. 26.30**).
  - **A n. laryngeus superior** arises from the cervical part of each vagus nerve and innervates the upper larynx through its internal and external branches.
  - The **n. laryngeus recurrens dexter** arises from the inferior cervical part of the n. vagus dexter and recurs around the a. subclavia in the neck.
  - The **n. laryngeus recurrens sinister** arises from the thoracic part of the n. vagus sinister. It recurs around the arcus aortae and ascends in the neck between the trachea and oesophagus.
  - **Nn. cardiaci cervicales** carry visceral motor (presynaptic parasympathetic) fibers and visceral sensory fibers to the plexus cardiacus.
- The n. accessorius (CN XI), which is derived from roots of the upper cervical spinal cord segments, enters the skull through the foramen magnum. After exiting the skull through the foramen jugulare, it innervates the m. sternocleiodmastoideus, then crosses the lateral region of the neck to innervate the m. trapezius (see **Fig. 26.31**).
  - The cranial root joins the n. vagus.
  - The spinal root innervates the m. sternocleidomastoideus, then crosses the lateral region of the neck to innervate the m. trapezius.
- The n. hypoglossus (CN XII), which exits the skull through the canalis nervi hypoglossi and courses anteriorly to the submandibular region, enters the cavitas oris to innervate muscles of the tongue.
  - Along its course, fibers from C1 join the n. hypoglossus briefly, eventually diverging from it to innervate the m. geniohyoideus and m. thyrohyoideus and to form the radix superior of the ansa cervicalis (see **Fig. 25.7**).

25.5 Oesophagus

The oesophagus is a muscular tube that connects the pharynx in the neck to the stomach in the abdomen (see Section 7.7).
- The pars cervicalis begins at the C VI vertebral level, which corresponds to the inferior border of the cartilago cricoidea. The cervical esophagus is posterior to the trachea, anterior to the vertebrae cervicales, and continuous with the laryngopharynx superiorly.
- At the pharyngoesophageal junction, the **m. cricopharyngeus**, the lowest part of the m. constrictor pharyngis inferior, forms the superior oesophageal sphincter.
- The aa. thyroideae inferior, branches of the a. subclavia via the trunci thyrocervicales, supply the pars cervicalis of the oesophagus. Veins of similar name accompany the arteries.
- Lymphatic vessels from the cervical esophagus drain to nll. paratracheales and nll. cervicales profundi.
- The nn. laryngei recurrentes, branches of the n. vagus (CN X), and vasomotor fibers from the cervical sympathetic trunk innervate the oesophagus in the neck.

25.6 Larynx and Trachea

The larynx, part of the upper airway, is responsible for sound production. It communicates superiorly with the pharynx and inferiorly with the trachea and lies anterior to vertebrae C III–C VI. The trachea, the upper part of the arbor tracheobronchialis, descends into the thorax, where it is continuous with the bronchi of the lungs.

Laryngeal Skeleton

Three single cartilages and two sets of paired cartilages form the laryngeal skeleton (**Fig. 25.9**). All except the epiglottis (elastic cartilage) are formed of hyaline cartilage.
- The **cartilago thyroidea**, the largest of the nine cartilages, has two **laminae** that join at the midline to form a **prominentia laryngea** (Adam's apple). The **cornu superius** of the cartilago thyroidea attaches to the os hyoideum, and the **cornu inferius** articulates with the cartilago cricoidea at the **art. cricothyroidea**.
- The **cartilago cricoidea**, the only part of the laryngeal skeleton to form a complete ring around the airway, articulates superiorly with the cartilago thyroidea and is attached inferiorly to the first tracheal ring. The anterior part of the cartilago cricoidea, the **arch**, is short, and the **lamina,** its posterior part, is tall.
- The **epiglottis,** a leaf-shaped cartilage that forms the anterior wall of the laryngeal inlet at the root of the tongue, is attached inferiorly to the cartilago thyroidea and anteriorly to the os hyoideum.

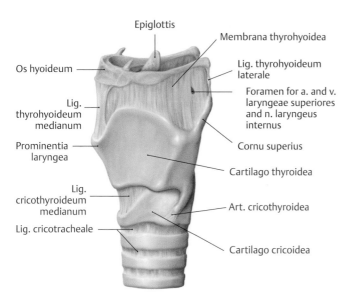

A Left anterior oblique view. (From Schuenke M, Schulte E, Schumacher U. THIEME Atlas of Anatomy, Vol 3. Illustrations by Voll M and Wesker K. 3rd ed. New York: Thieme Publishers; 2020.)

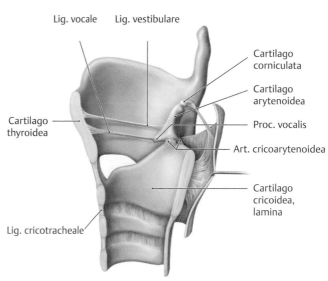

B Sagittal section viewed from the left medial aspect. *Removed:* Os hyoideum and lig. thyrohyoideum medianum. Cartilago arytenoidea alters the position of the plicae vocales during phonation. (From Schuenke M, Schulte E, Schumacher U. THIEME Atlas of Anatomy, Vol 3. Illustrations by Voll M and Wesker K. 3rd ed. New York: Thieme Publishers; 2020.)

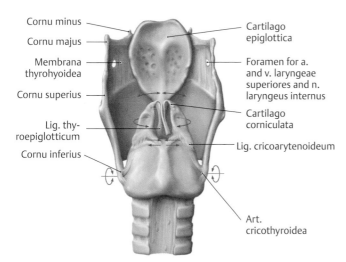

C Posterior view. *Arrows* indicate the direction of movement in the various joints. (From Schuenke M, Schulte E, Schumacher U. THIEME Atlas of Anatomy, Vol 3. Illustrations by Voll M and Wesker K. 3rd ed. New York: Thieme Publishers; 2020.)

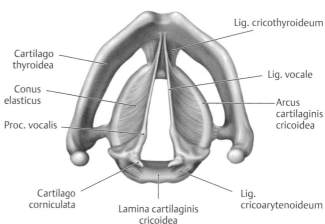

D Superior view of cartilago thyroidea, cartilago cricoidea, and cartilago corniculata. (From Schuenke M, Schulte E, Schumacher U. THIEME Atlas of Anatomy, Vol 3. Illustrations by Voll M and Wesker K. 3rd ed. New York: Thieme Publishers; 2020.)

Fig. 25.9 Structure of the larynx

- The paired pyramidal **cartilagines arytenoideae,** which articulate with the sumargo superior of lamina cricoidea, have an apex that articulates with the tiny **cartilagines corniculatae** and a **proc. vocalis** that attaches to the cartilago thyroidea through the **ligg. vocale**.
- The small, paired cartilagines corniculatae and **cartilagines cuneiformes** appear as tubercles within the **plica aryepiglottica.** Although the cartilagines corniculatae articulate with the cartilagines arytenoideae, the cartilagines cuneiformes do not articulate with the other cartilages.

Membranes and Ligaments of the Larynx

Membranes of the larynx connect the cartilagines laryngis to each other and to the os hyoideum and trachea (**Figs. 25.9, 25.10, 25.11**).

- The **membrana thyrohyoidea** attaches the cartilago thyroidea to the os hyoideum superiorly.
- The **lig. cricothyroideum** attaches the cartilago cricoidea to the first tracheal ring inferiorly.
- The **membrana quadrangularis** extends posteriorly from the lateral border of the epiglottis to the cartilago arytenoidea on each side.
  - The superior free margin of this membrane forms the **aryepiglottic ligament,** which, when covered by mucosa, is known as the **plica aryepiglottica**.
  - The inferior free margin is the **lig. vestibulare**, which, when covered by mucosa, is known as the **plica vestibularis** or false vocal cord.
- The **membrana cricothyroidea** connects the cartilago cricoidea and cartilago thyroidea and extends superiorly deep to the cartilago thyroidea as the **conus elasticus** (see **Figs. 25.9D and 25.12C**).

— The free superior border of the conus elasticus forms the **lig. vocale**, which extends from the midpoint of the cartilago thryoidea to the procc. vocales of the cartilago arytenoidea. The lig. vocale and the **m. vocalis** form the **plica vocalis** or **vocal cord.**

BOX 25.2:   CLINICAL CORRELATION

TRACHEOSTOMY AND CRICOTHYROIDOTOMY

When the upper airway is obstructed, airway access can be reestablished using two different approaches. *Tracheostomy* is a surgical procedure in which a tracheostomy tube is inserted through an incision in the proximal trachea. This procedure is generally used for long-term management of the airway. *Cricothyroidotomy* is a related procedure in which an incision is made in the cricothyroid membrane. This procedure, usually performed in emergency situations, is less technically difficult than tracheostomy and has fewer complications.

Cavitas Laryngis

The cavitas laryngis begins at the aditus laryngis and extends to the inferior margin of the cartilago cricoidea (see **Figs. 25.10** and **25.11**).

— The plicae vestibulares and plicae vocales define spaces within the cavitas laryngis.
- The **vestibulum laryngis**, or supraglottic space lies above the plicae vestibulares.
- The **rima vestibuli** is the aperture between the two plicae vestibulares.
- The **ventriculi laryngis** are recesses of the cavitas laryngis between the plicae vestibulares and plicae vocales.
- **Sacculi laryngis** are the blind ends of the ventriculi laryngis.
- The **rima glottidis** is the aperture between the two plicae vocales.
- The **cavitas infraglottica** is the pars inferior of the cavitas laryngis, which lies below the plicae vocales and extends to the inferior margin of the cartilago cricoidea.

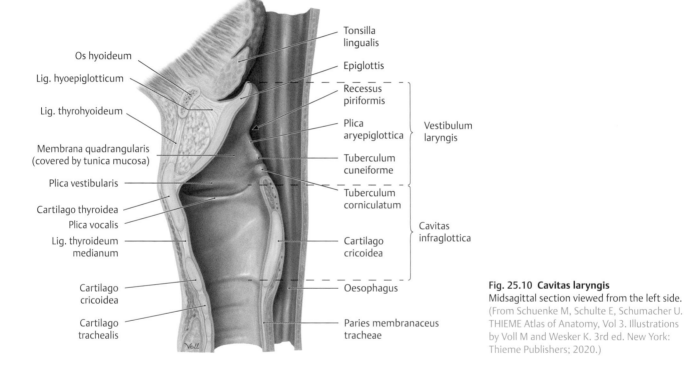

Fig. 25.10   Cavitas laryngis
Midsagittal section viewed from the left side. (From Schuenke M, Schulte E, Schumacher U. THIEME Atlas of Anatomy, Vol 3. Illustrations by Voll M and Wesker K. 3rd ed. New York: Thieme Publishers; 2020.)

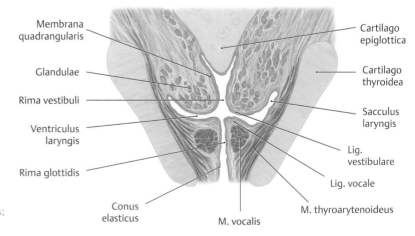

Fig. 25.11   Vestibular and vocal folds
Coronal section. (From Schuenke M, Schulte E, Schumacher U. THIEME Atlas of Anatomy, Vol 3. Illustrations by Voll M and Wesker K. 3rd ed. New York: Thieme Publishers; 2020.)

— Sound is produced as air passes through the cavitas laryngis between the plicae vocales. Variations in sound arise from changes in the position, tension, and length of these folds.
— The plicae vestibulares protect the airway but have no role in sound production.

Muscles of the Larynx

The larynx has extrinsic and intrinsic muscle groups.
— Extrinsic muscles are attached to the os hyoideum and move the larynx and os hyoideum together. These include the mm. suprahyoidei (see **Table 27.9**), which form the floor of the mouth and elevate the larynx, and the mm. suprahyoidei (see **Table 25.4**), which depress the larynx.
— Intrinsic muscles move the cartilagines laryngis, which changes the length and tension of the ligg. vocales and size of the rima glottidis (**Table 25.7; Fig. 25.12**).
— Two muscles are particularly clinically and anatomically significant:
   • The **m. cricoarytenoideus posterior** is the only muscle that abducts the plicae vocales and opens the rima glottidis.
   • The **m. cricothyroideus**, innervated by the external branch of the n. laryngeus superior, is the only intrinsic muscle that is not innervated by the n. laryngeus inferior (a continuation of the recurrent n. laryngeus recurrens).

Neurovasculature of the Larynx (Figs. 25.13, 25.15, 25.16)

— a. laryngea superior and a. laryngea inferior are branches of the a. thyroidea superior and a. thyroidea inferior, respectively. Veins of the larynx follow the arteriae laryngis and join the vv. thyroideae.

— The superior and inferior laryngeal branches of the vagus nerve (CN X) provide all of the motor and sensory innervation of the larynx.
   • The n. laryngeus superior splits into an internal sensory branch, which supplies the mucosa of the vestibule and superior surface of the plicae vocales, and r. externus, which innervates the m. cricothyroideus.
   • The **n. laryngeus inferior**, a continuation of the n. laryngeus recurrens, supplies the mucosa of the infraglottic larynx and innervates all intrinsic muscles of the larynx except the m. cricothyroideus.

BOX 25.3: CLINICAL CORRELATION

RECURRENT LARYNGEAL NERVE PARALYSIS WITH THYROIDECTOMY
The n. laryngeus recurrens in the neck are vulnerable to damage during thyroidectomy because they run immediately posterior to the gl. thyroidea. Unilateral damage results in hoarseness; bilateral damage causes respiratory distress and aphonia (inability to speak). Aspiration pneumonia may occur as a complication.

Trachea

The trachea, the extension of the airway inferior to the larynx, extends from the inferior margin of the cartilago cricoidea to the level of the dici intervertebrales T IV–T V disci intervertebrales in the thorax, where it bifurcates into the two primary bronchi of the lungs (see Section 7.7). In the cervical region (see **Fig. 25.18**)
— it lies deep to the lamina superficialis fasciae cervicalis and fascia cervicalis, and m. sternohyoid and m. sternothyroid.
— the isthmus of the gl. thyroidea crosses its 2nd to 4th tracheal cartilages. The lobes of the thyroid are lateral to it and descend to the fifth or sixth tracheal cartilage.
— the oesophagus lies posterior and separates it from the columna vertebralis.

Table 25.7 Actions of the Musculi Laryngis

Muscle	Action	Effect on Rima Glottidis
① M. cricothyroideus*	Tightens the plicae vocales	None
② M. vocalis		
③ M. thyroarytenoideus	Adducts the plicae vocales	Closes
④ M. arytenoideus transversus		
⑤ M. cricoarytenoideus posterior	Abducts the plicae vocales	Opens
⑥ M. cricoarytenoideus lateralis	Adducts the plicae vocales	Closes

*The m. cricothyroideus is innervated by the n. laryngeus externus
All other intrinsic mm. are innervated by the n. laryngeus recurrens.

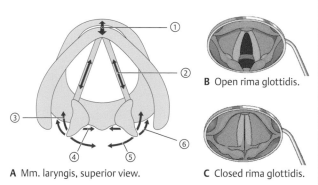

A Mm. laryngis, superior view.

B Open rima glottidis.

C Closed rima glottidis.

(From Schuenke M, Schulte E, Schumacher U. THIEME Atlas of Anatomy, Vol 3. Illustrations by Voll M and Wesker K. 3rd ed. New York: Thieme Publishers; 2020.)

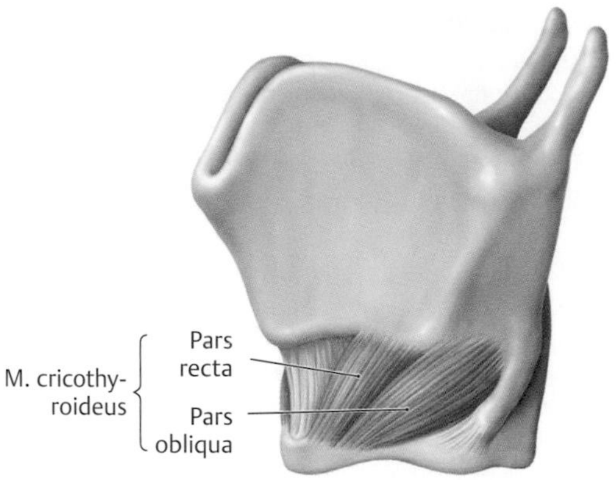

M. thyroarytenoideus,
pars thyroepiglottica

Plica
aryepiglottica

Tuberculum
cuneiforme

M. thyroary-
tenoideus

Tuberculum
corniculatum

M. cricoary-
tenoideus
lateralis

M. cricoary-
tenoideus
posterior

M. cricothy-
roideus
{ Pars
recta

Pars
obliqua }

A Extrinsic mm. laryngis, left lateral oblique view.
Removed: Epiglottis.

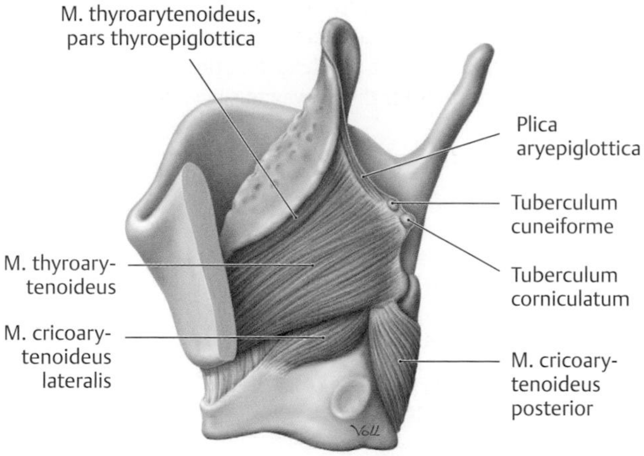

B Intrinsic mm. laryngis, left lateral view. Removed: Cartilago
thyroidea (left lamina). *Revealed:* Epiglottis and m. thyroarytenoideus.

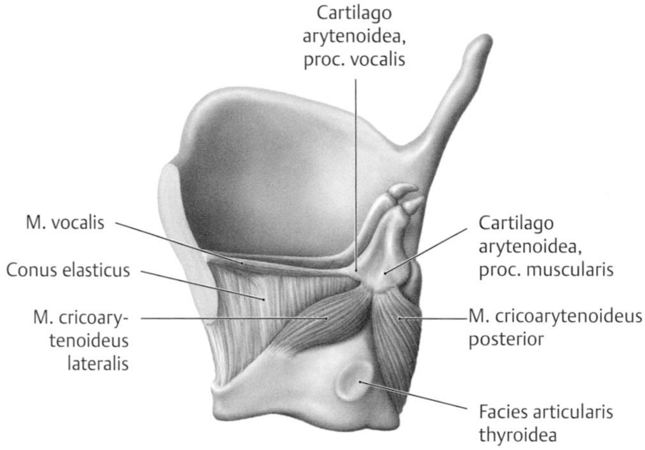

Cartilago
arytenoidea,
proc. vocalis

Epiglottis

M. vocalis

Cartilago
arytenoidea,
proc. muscularis

Plica
aryepiglottica

Conus elasticus

M. ary-
tenoideus
obliquus

Tuberculum
cuneiforme

M. cricoary-
tenoideus
lateralis

M. cricoarytenoideus
posterior

M. ary-
tenoideus
transversus

M. thyroary-
tenoideus

Facies articularis
thyroidea

M. ary-
tenoideus
obliquus

M. cricoary-
tenoideus
posterior

C Left lateral view. *Removed:* Cartilago thyroidea (left lamina) and epiglottis.

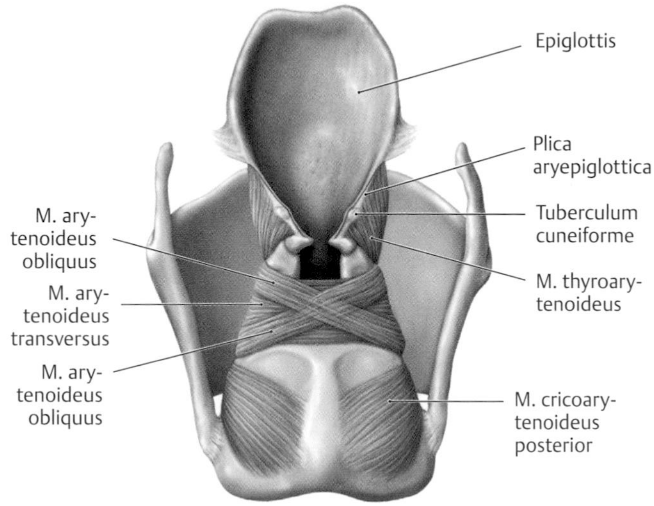

D Posterior view.

Fig. 25.12 Musculi laryngis

The mm. laryngis move the laryngeal cartilages relative to one another, affecting the tension and/or position of the plicae vocales. (From Schuenke M, Schulte E, Schumacher U. THIEME Atlas of Anatomy, Vol 3. Illustrations by Voll M and Wesker K. 3rd ed. New York: Thieme Publishers; 2020.)

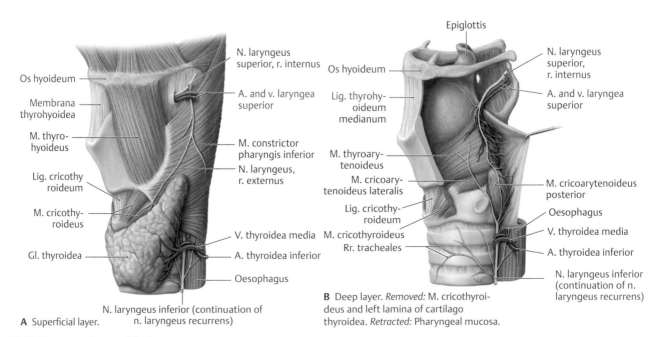

Os hyoideum

N. laryngeus
superior, r. internus

Epiglottis

N. laryngeus
superior,
r. internus

Membrana
thyrohyoidea

A. and v. laryngea
superior

Os hyoideum

Lig. thyrohy-
oideum
medianum

A. and v. laryngea
superior

M. thyro-
hyoideus

M. constrictor
pharyngis inferior

N. laryngeus,
r. externus

M. thyroary-
tenoideus

Lig. cricothy-
roideum

M. cricoary-
tenoideus lateralis

M. cricoarytenoideus
posterior

M. cricothy-
roideus

Lig. cricothy-
roideum

Oesophagus

Gl. thyroidea

V. thyroidea media

M. cricothyroideus

Rr. tracheales

V. thyroidea media

A. thyroidea inferior

A. thyroidea inferior

Oesophagus

N. laryngeus inferior (continuation of
n. laryngeus recurrens)

N. laryngeus inferior
(continuation of n.
laryngeus recurrens)

A Superficial layer.

B Deep layer. *Removed:* M. cricothyroideus and left lamina of cartilago thyroidea. *Retracted:* Pharyngeal mucosa.

Fig. 25.13 Neurovasculature of the larynx

Left lateral view. (From Schuenke M, Schulte E, Schumacher U. THIEME Atlas of Anatomy, Vol 3. Illustrations by Voll M and Wesker K. 3rd ed. New York: Thieme Publishers; 2020.)

- the aa. carotides communes ascend lateral to it.
- the nn. laryngei recurrentes ascend lateral or posterolateral to it (in the groove between the trachea and oesophagus).
- it is supplied by the a. thyroidea inferior and drained by the vv. thyroideae inferiores.
- lymph drains to nll. pretracheales and nll. paratracheales.
- it receives innervation from branches of the n. vagus and the truncus sympathicus.

25.7 Thyroid and Parathyroid Glands

The gl. thyroidea and gll. parathyroideae are endocrine glands that reside in the regio cervicalis anterior (**Fig. 25.14**).

The Thyroid Gland (Gl. Thyroidea)

The **thyroid gland (gl. thyroidea)**, the largest endocrine gland in the body, secretes **thyroid hormone**, which regulates the rate of metabolism, and **calcitonin,** which regulates the metabolism of calcium.

- The gl. thyroidea lies deep to the m. sternohyoideus and m. sternothyroideus (mm. infrahyoidei) and anterolateral to the larynx and trachea between C V and T I vertebral levels.
- The gl. thyroidea has right and left (lateral) lobes connected by a narrow **isthmus** that lies anterior to the second and third tracheal rings.
- A **lobus pyramidalis**, present in ~ 50% of the population, is a vestigium ductus thyroglossi that extends from the isthmus toward the os hyoideum.

> **BOX 25.4: DEVELOPMENTAL CORRELATION**
>
> **THYROGLOSSAL DUCT CYST**
> A thyroglossal duct cyst is a fluid-filled cavity in the midline of the neck, just inferior to the os hyoideum. It results from the proliferation of epithelium left behind from the ductus thyroglossus during the descent of the gl. thyroidea from its embryonic origin on the tongue to its postnatal position in the neck. The cyst can enlarge and press on the trachea and oesophagus, in which case it can be surgically removed.

- A capsula fibrosa encloses the gl. thyroidea. The fascia pretrachealis of the neck lies outside the capsula thyroidea (see **Fig. 25.2**).

The Parathyroid Glands (Gll. Parathyroideae)

Parathyroid glands (gll. parathyroideae), small, ovoid glandulae endocrinae that lie on the posterior surface of the gl. thyroidea, secrete **parathormone,** which regulates the metabolism of phosphorus and calcium (**Fig. 25.14B**).

- There are normally four glands, two superior and two inferior, although the number can range from two to six glands.
- The gll. parathyroideae superiores are constant in position near the inferior margin of the cartilago cricoidea. The position of the gll. parathyroideae inferiores may vary, ranging from the lower pole of the gl. thyroidea to the mediastinum superius.

Neurovasculature of the Thyroid and Parathyroid Glands

- The a. thyroidea superior, a branch of the a. carotis externa, and the a. thyroidea inferior from the truncus thyrocervicalis supply the gl. thyroidea (**Fig. 25.15**). The a. thyroidea inferior is usually the main supply to the gll. parathyroideae.
- **V. thyroidea superior** and **v. thyroidea inferior** drain into the vv. jugulares internae; **vv. thyroideae inferiores** drain into the vv. brachiocephalicae in the mediastinum (**Fig. 25.16**). Venous drainage from the gll. parathyroideae joins the thyroid veins.
- Lymphatic vessels of the gl. thyroidea may drain directly into the nll. cervicales superiores profundi and inferiores profundi or indirectly, passing first through nll. prelaryngei, nll. pretracheales, and nll. paratracheales.
- The gll. parathyroideae drain with the gl. thyroidea into the nll. cervicales inferiores profundi and nll. paratracheales.
- Cardiac and superior and inferior thyroid sympathetic plexuses arise from the superior, middle, and inferior cervical sympathetic ganglia to supply vasomotor innervation to the gll. thyroidea and parathyroidea.
- The gll. thyroidea and parathyroidea are under hormonal control and therefore lack secretomotor innervation.

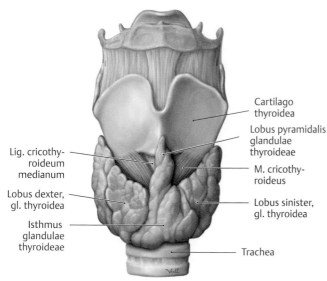

A Gl. thyroidea. Anterior view. (From Gilroy AM et al. Atlas of Anatomy. 4th ed. 2020. Based on: Schuenke M, Schulte E, Schumacher U. THIEME Atlas of Anatomy. Head, Neck, and Neuroanatomy. Illustrations by Voll M and Wesker K. 3rd ed. New York: Thieme Medical Publishers; 2020.)

Fig. 25.14 Glandulae thyroideae and glandulae parathyroideae

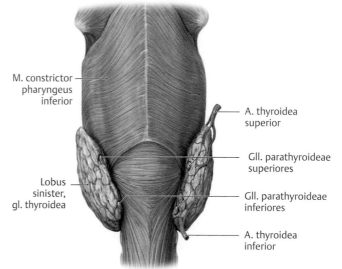

B Gll. thyroideae and gll. parathyroideae, posterior view. (From Schuenke M, Schulte E, Schumacher U. THIEME Atlas of Anatomy, Vol 3. Illustrations by Voll M and Wesker K. 3rd ed. New York: Thieme Publishers; 2020.)

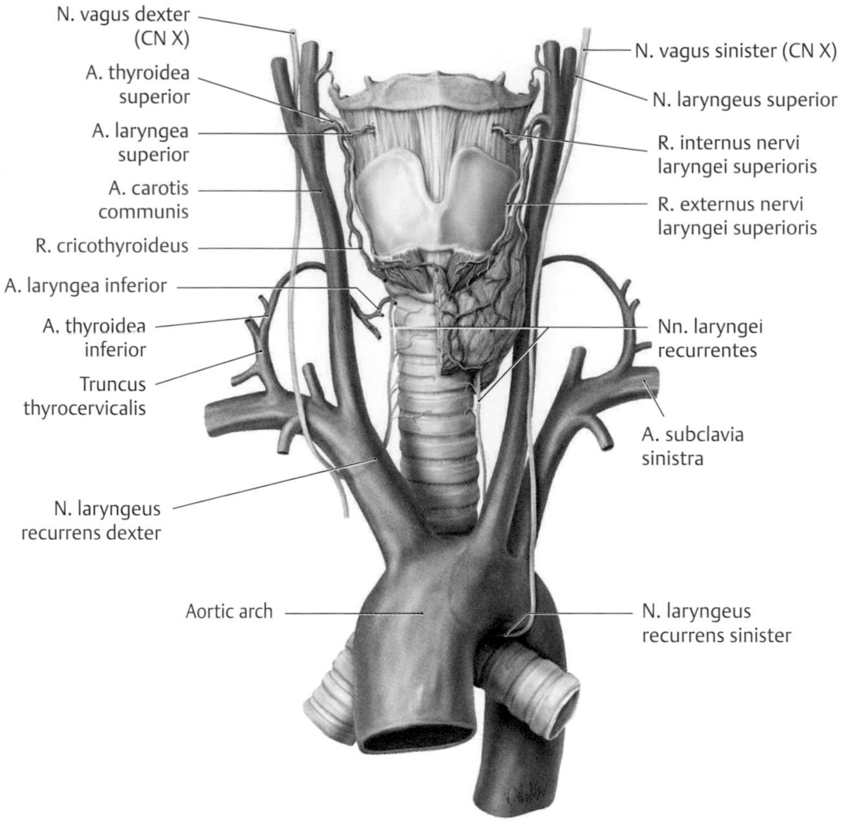

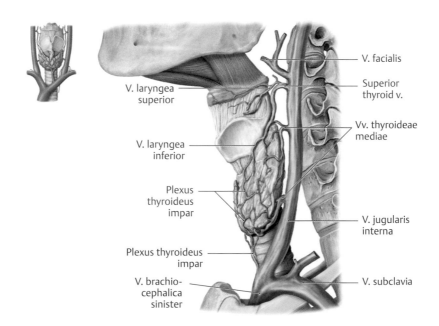

Fig. 25.15 Arteries and nerves of the larynx, thyroid, and parathyroids
Anterior view. *Removed:* Gl. thyroidea (right half). (From Gilroy AM et al. Atlas of Anatomy. 4th ed. 2020. Based on: Schuenke M, Schulte E, Schumacher U. THIEME Atlas of Anatomy. Head, Neck, and Neuroanatomy. Illustrations by Voll M and Wesker K. 3rd ed. New York: Thieme Medical Publishers; 2020.)

Fig. 25.16 Veins of the larynx, glandula thyroidea, and glandulae parathyroideae
Left lateral view. *Note:* The v. thyroidea inferior generally drains into the v. brachiocephalica sinister. (From Schuenke M, Schulte E, Schumacher U. THIEME Atlas of Anatomy, Vol 3. Illustrations by Voll M and Wesker K. 3rd ed. New York: Thieme Publishers; 2020.)

25.8 Topography of the Neck

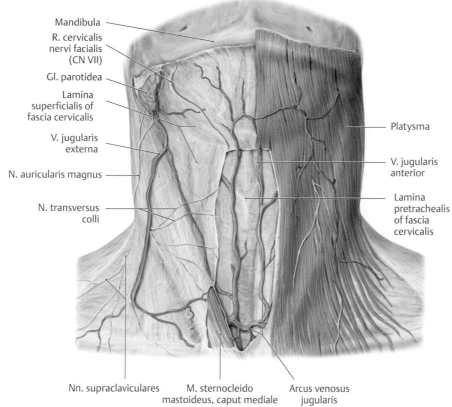

Mandibula

R. cervicalis nervi facialis (CN VII)

Gl. parotidea

Lamina superficialis of fascia cervicalis

V. jugularis externa

N. auricularis magnus

N. transversus colli

Platysma

V. jugularis anterior

Lamina pretrachealis of fascia cervicalis

Nn. supraclaviculares

M. sternocleido mastoideus, caput mediale

Arcus venosus jugularis

A Superficial dissection. (From Schuenke M, Schulte E, Schumacher U. THIEME Atlas of Anatomy, Vol 3. Illustrations by Voll M and Wesker K. 3rd ed. New York: Thieme Publishers; 2020.)

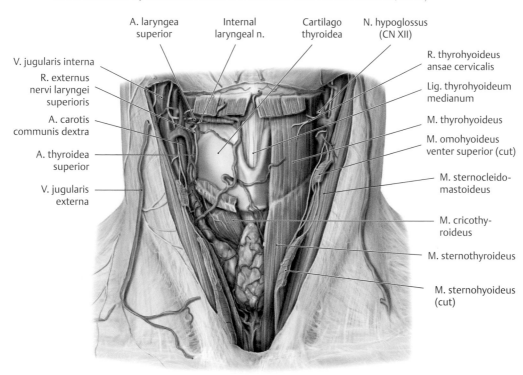

A. laryngea superior

Internal laryngeal n.

Cartilago thyroidea

N. hypoglossus (CN XII)

V. jugularis interna

R. externus nervi laryngei superioris

A. carotis communis dextra

A. thyroidea superior

V. jugularis externa

R. thyrohyoideus ansae cervicalis

Lig. thyrohyoideum medianum

M. thyrohyoideus

M. omohyoideus venter superior (cut)

M. sternocleido-mastoideus

M. cricothy-roideus

M. sternothyroideus

M. sternohyoideus (cut)

B Deep dissection. (From Gilroy AM et al. Atlas of Anatomy. 4th ed. 2020. Based on: Schuenke M, Schulte E, Schumacher U. THIEME Atlas of Anatomy. Head, Neck, and Neuroanatomy. Illustrations by Voll M and Wesker K. 3rd ed. New York: Thieme Medical Publishers; 2020.)

Fig. 25.17 Topography of the anterior cervical region (*continued on page 470*)
Anterior view.

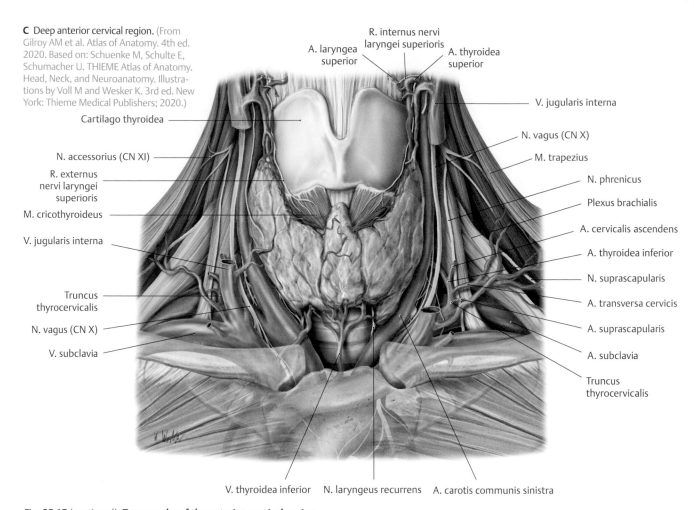

C Deep anterior cervical region. (From Gilroy AM et al. Atlas of Anatomy. 4th ed. 2020. Based on: Schuenke M, Schulte E, Schumacher U. THIEME Atlas of Anatomy. Head, Neck, and Neuroanatomy. Illustrations by Voll M and Wesker K. 3rd ed. New York: Thieme Medical Publishers; 2020.)

- A. laryngea superior
- R. internus nervi laryngei superioris
- A. thyroidea superior
- Cartilago thyroidea
- V. jugularis interna
- N. accessorius (CN XI)
- N. vagus (CN X)
- R. externus nervi laryngei superioris
- M. trapezius
- M. cricothyroideus
- N. phrenicus
- V. jugularis interna
- Plexus brachialis
- A. cervicalis ascendens
- Truncus thyrocervicalis
- A. thyroidea inferior
- N. vagus (CN X)
- N. suprascapularis
- V. subclavia
- A. transversa cervicis
- A. suprascapularis
- A. subclavia
- Truncus thyrocervicalis
- V. thyroidea inferior
- N. laryngeus recurrens
- A. carotis communis sinistra

Fig. 25.17 (*continued*) **Topography of the anterior cervical region**

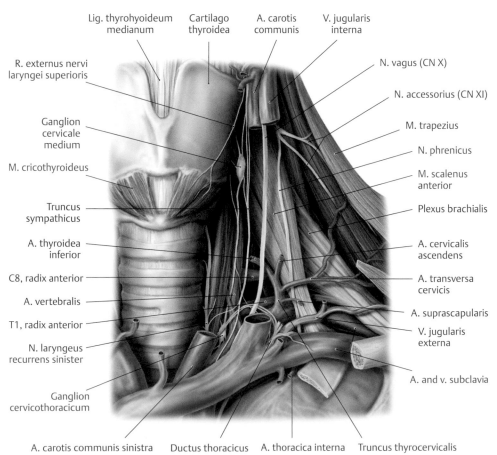

- Lig. thyrohyoideum medianum
- Cartilago thyroidea
- A. carotis communis
- V. jugularis interna
- R. externus nervi laryngei superioris
- N. vagus (CN X)
- N. accessorius (CN XI)
- Ganglion cervicale medium
- M. trapezius
- M. cricothyroideus
- N. phrenicus
- M. scalenus anterior
- Truncus sympathicus
- Plexus brachialis
- A. thyroidea inferior
- A. cervicalis ascendens
- C8, radix anterior
- A. transversa cervicis
- A. vertebralis
- A. suprascapularis
- T1, radix anterior
- V. jugularis externa
- N. laryngeus recurrens sinister
- A. and v. subclavia
- Ganglion cervicothoracicum
- A. carotis communis sinistra
- Ductus thoracicus
- A. thoracica interna
- Truncus thyrocervicalis

Fig. 25.18 Root of the neck
Anterior view, left side. The gl. thyroidea has been removed and the a. carotis communis and v. jugularis interna have been cut to reveal the deep structures in the root of the neck. (From Schuenke M, Schulte E, Schumacher U. THIEME Atlas of Anatomy, Vol 3. Illustrations by Voll M and Wesker K. 3rd ed. New York: Thieme Publishers; 2020.)

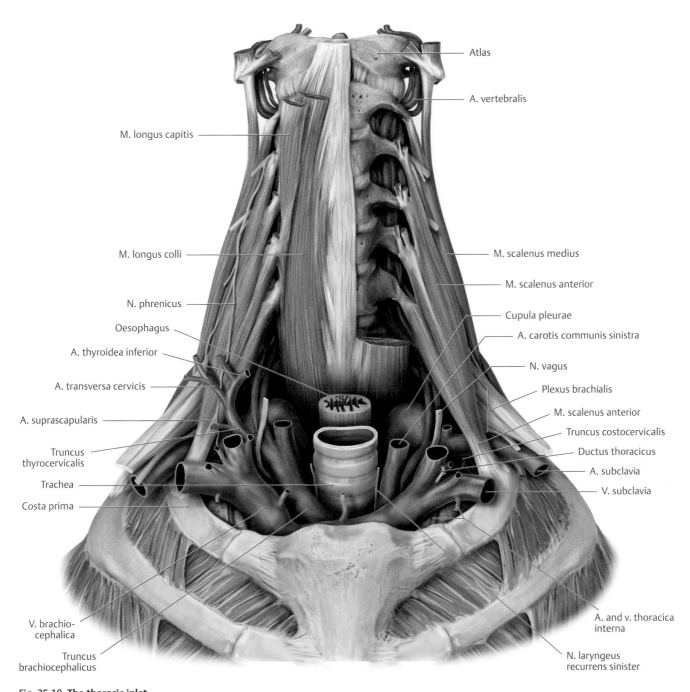

Atlas

A. vertebralis

M. longus capitis

M. longus colli

N. phrenicus

Oesophagus

A. thyroidea inferior

A. transversa cervicis

A. suprascapularis

Truncus thyrocervicalis

Trachea

Costa prima

V. brachio-cephalica

Truncus brachiocephalicus

M. scalenus medius

M. scalenus anterior

Cupula pleurae

A. carotis communis sinistra

N. vagus

Plexus brachialis

M. scalenus anterior

Truncus costocervicalis

Ductus thoracicus

A. subclavia

V. subclavia

A. and v. thoracica interna

N. laryngeus recurrens sinister

Fig. 25.19 The thoracic inlet
Anterior view. The viscera of the neck have been removed and the oesophagus, trachea, a. carotis communis, and v. jugularis interna have been dissected to show the relations of structures passing through the thoracic inlet. The prevertebral muscles on the left side have been cut to show the course of the a. vertebralis. (From Schuenke M, Schulte E, Schumacher U. THIEME Atlas of Anatomy, Vol 3. Illustrations by Voll M and Wesker K. 3rd ed. New York: Thieme Publishers; 2020.)

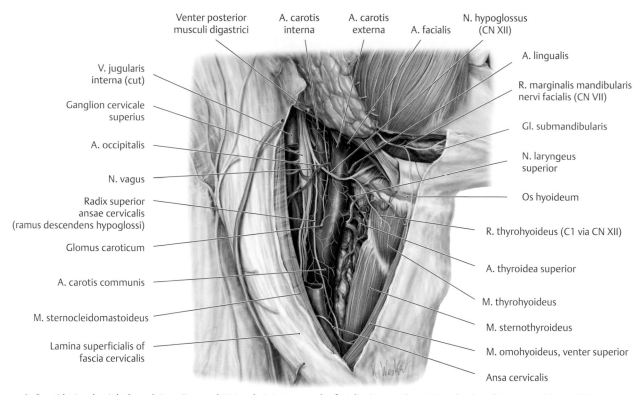

Venter posterior
musculi digastrici

A. carotis
interna

A. carotis
externa

A. facialis

N. hypoglossus
(CN XII)

A. lingualis

R. marginalis mandibularis
nervi facialis (CN VII)

Gl. submandibularis

N. laryngeus
superior

Os hyoideum

R. thyrohyoideus (C1 via CN XII)

A. thyroidea superior

M. thyrohyoideus

M. sternothyroideus

M. omohyoideus, venter superior

Ansa cervicalis

V. jugularis
interna (cut)

Ganglion cervicale
superius

A. occipitalis

N. vagus

Radix superior
ansae cervicalis
(ramus descendens hypoglossi)

Glomus caroticum

A. carotis communis

M. sternocleidomastoideus

Lamina superficialis of
fascia cervicalis

A Carotid triangle, right lateral view. *Removed:* V. jugularis interna and v. facialis. (From Gilroy AM et al. Atlas of Anatomy. 4th ed. 2020. Based on: Schuenke M, Schulte E, Schumacher U. THIEME Atlas of Anatomy. Head, Neck, and Neuroanatomy. Illustrations by Voll M and Wesker K. 3rd ed. New York: Thieme Medical Publishers; 2020.)

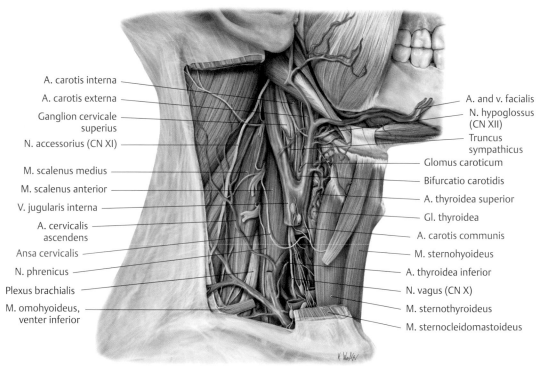

A. carotis interna

A. carotis externa

Ganglion cervicale
superius

N. accessorius (CN XI)

M. scalenus medius

M. scalenus anterior

V. jugularis interna

A. cervicalis
ascendens

Ansa cervicalis

N. phrenicus

Plexus brachialis

M. omohyoideus,
venter inferior

A. and v. facialis

N. hypoglossus
(CN XII)

Truncus
sympathicus

Glomus caroticum

Bifurcatio carotidis

A. thyroidea superior

Gl. thyroidea

A. carotis communis

M. sternohyoideus

A. thyroidea inferior

N. vagus (CN X)

M. sternothyroideus

M. sternocleidomastoideus

B The m. sternocleidomastoideus has been cut to reveal structures in the carotid triangle and root of the neck. (From Schuenke M, Schulte E, Schumacher U. THIEME Atlas of Anatomy, Vol 3. Illustrations by Voll M and Wesker K. 3rd ed. New York: Thieme Publishers; 2020.)

Fig. 25.20 Lateral cervical region
Right lateral view.

26 Meninges, Brain, and Nervi Craniales

The cranial meninges continuous with the meninges of the spinal cord (medulla spinalis), as well as the 12 nn. craniales that arise from the brain, are essential parts of the gross anatomy of the head and neck region and are discussed in detail in this unit. The study of the brain, however, is generally confined to the neuroanatomy curriculum, and only a brief overview is provided here.

26.1 The Meninges

The cranial meninges, coverings that protect the brain, consist of the external fibrous **dura mater,** the thin intermediate **arachnoidea mater,** and the delicate inner **pia mater** (Fig. 26.1).

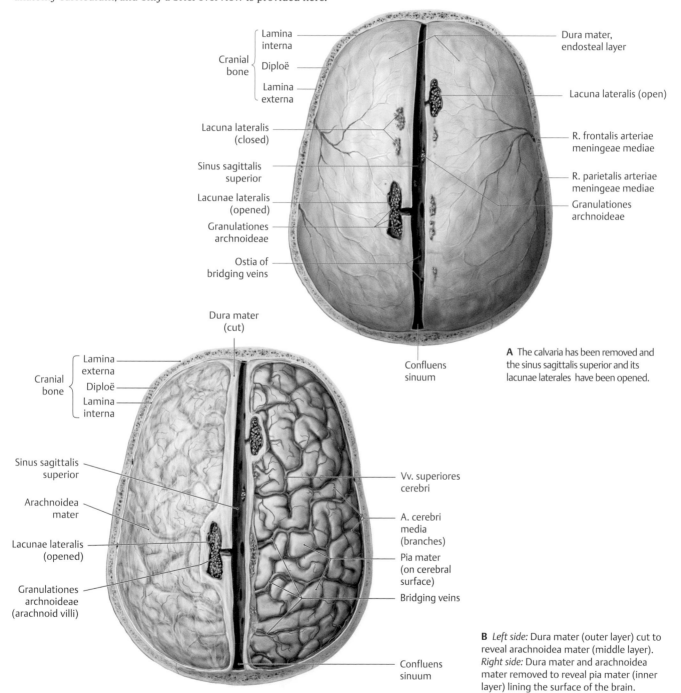

A The calvaria has been removed and the sinus sagittalis superior and its lacunae laterales have been opened.

B *Left side:* Dura mater (outer layer) cut to reveal arachnoidea mater (middle layer). *Right side:* Dura mater and arachnoidea mater removed to reveal pia mater (inner layer) lining the surface of the brain.

Fig. 26.1 Layers of the meninges
Opened cranium, superior view. Granulationes archnoideae, sites for reabsorption of cerebral spinal fluid into the venous blood, are protrusions of the arachnoid layer of the meninges into the venous sinus system. (From Schuenke M, Schulte E, Schumacher U. THIEME Atlas of Anatomy, Vol 3. Illustrations by Voll M and Wesker K. 3rd ed. New York: Thieme Publishers; 2020.)

Dura mater

— The dura mater, or dura, a tough outer membrane surrounding the brain, is composed of a **periosteal (endosteal) layer** and a **meningeal layer.** The two layers are inseparable except where they enclose the sinus durae matris that drain the brain (e.g., the sinus sagittalis superior; see **Fig. 26.4**).
  • The outer periosteal layer, formed by the periosteum of the skull, adheres tightly to the inner surface of the skull, particularly at the sutures. This layer ends at the foramen magnum and is not continuous with the dura around the medulla spinalis.
  • The inner meningeal layer, a strong membranous sheet that adheres to the inner surface of the periosteal layer, provides sheaths for the nn. craniales as they pass through the skull foramina. It is closely applied, although not attached, to the underlying **arachnoidea mater.** It continues into the canalis vertebralis as dura mater spinalis (**Fig. 26.2**).
— The a. meningea media, from the a. maxillaris, supply most of the dura, with contributions from the a. ophthalmica, a. occipitalis, and a. vertebralis. Veins accompany the arteries and drain into the plexus venosus pterygoideus.
— Branches of the n. trigeminus (n. cranialis [CN] V) transmit sensation from the dura of the fossa cranii anterior and media. Nn. spinales C1, C2, and C3 and small branches of the n. vagus (CN X) innervate the dura of the fossa cranii posterior.

Dural Partitions

Infoldings of the meningeal layer of the dura form incomplete membranous partitions that separate and support parts of the brain (**Fig. 26.3**).
— The **falx cerebri,** a vertical sickle-shaped partition separating the hemispherium cerebri dexter and hemispherium cerebri sinister, is attached anteriorly to the crista galli and the crista frontalis of os frontale and is continuous posteriorly with the tentorium cerebelli. The inferior, free edge of the falx cerebri is unattached.
— The **tentorium cerebelli,** a horizontal continuation of the falx cerebri, separates the lobi occipitales from the hemispheria cerebelli in the fossa cranii posterior.

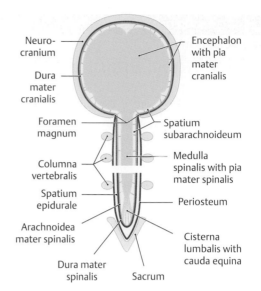

Fig. 26.2 Meninges in the cavitas cranii and canalis vertebralis
The two layers of the dura mater (periosteal and meningeal) form a single structural unit in the cavitas cranii that adheres to the inner surface of the skull. In the medulla spinalis, however, the dura is separated from the periosteum of the vertebrae by the spatium epidurale. (From Schuenke M, Schulte E, Schumacher U. THIEME Atlas of Anatomy, Vol 3. Illustrations by Voll M and Wesker K. 3rd ed. New York: Thieme Publishers; 2020.)

  • It is attached to the procc. clinoidei posteriores and pars petrosa ossis temporalis anteriorly and to the os parietale and os occipitale posterolaterally.
  • A U-shaped **incisura tentorii** separates the attachments to the petrous ridge on each side and connects the fossa cranii media and fossa cranii posterior.
— The **falx cerebelli,** a vertical partition separating the hemispheria cerebelli, is continuous superiorly with the tentorium cerebelli and is attached posteriorly to the crista occipitalis.
— The **diaphragma sellae,** a small dural fold attached to the proc. clinoideus anterior and posterior, forms a roof over the sella turcica, which encloses the hypophysis (gl. pituitaria).

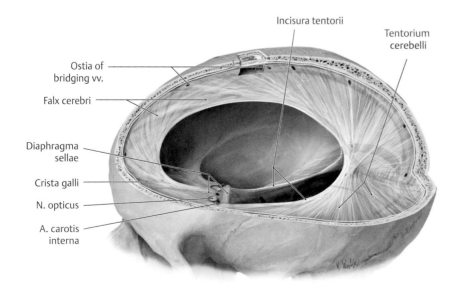

Fig. 26.3 Dural septa (folds)
Left anterior oblique view. (From Schuenke M, Schulte E, Schumacher U. THIEME Atlas of Anatomy, Vol 3. Illustrations by Voll M and Wesker K. 3rd ed. New York: Thieme Publishers; 2020.)

BOX 26.1: CLINICAL CORRELATION

TENTORIAL HERNIATION

Increased pressure within the fossa cranii media created by edema or a space-occupying lesion such as a tumor can squeeze the brain tissue and force part of the lobus temporalis to herniate through the incisura tentorii. Pressure on the adjacent truncus encephali can be fatal in this situation. The n. oculomotorius (CN III) can also be stretched or damaged, leading to fixed pupil dilation (loss of parasympathetic function) and a "down and out" gaze due to paralysis of most of the mm. externi bulbi oculi.

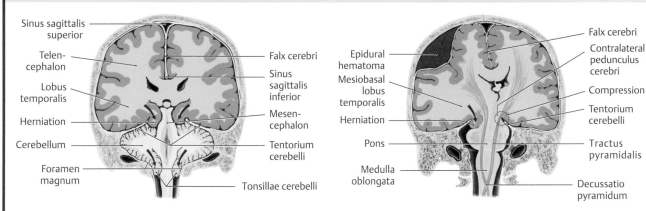

A Axial herniations are usually caused by general brain edema and can be life threatening. As the lower parts of the lobi temporales are pushed through the incisura tentorii, pressure is exerted on the truncus encephali, which contains the respiratory and circulatory centers.

B Lateral herniations are caused by a unilateral mass (e.g., tumor or intracranial hemorrhage). As one lobus temporalis herniates through the incisura tentorii, the contralateral side can be compressed against the edge of the tentorium, resulting in symptoms developing on the side opposite the injury.

Potential sites of herniation beneath the free edges of the meninges
Coronal section, anterior view. (From Schuenke M, Schulte E, Schumacher U. THIEME Atlas of Anatomy, Vol 3. Illustrations by Voll M and Wesker K. 3rd ed. New York: Thieme Publishers; 2020.)

Sinus Durae Matris

Sinus durae matris are valveless venous spaces that form as a result of the separation of the periosteal and meningeal layers of the dura. Most of the large veins of the brain, skull, orbita, and auris interna drain through the sinus dura matris and into the vv. jugulares internae in the neck (**Figs. 26.4** and **26.5; Table 26.1**).

— The **confluens sinuum** at the posterior edge of the tentorium cerebelli is a junction of the sinus sagittalis superior, sinus rectus, sinus occipitalis, and sinus transversus.
— The **sinus sagittalis superior** runs in the attached superior border of the falx cerebri and ends in the confluens sinuum.
— The **sinus sagittalis inferior** runs in the free inferior edge of the falx cerebri and ends in the sinus rectus.

— The **sinus rectus** runs in the space formed by the union of the falx cerebri and tentorium cerebelli. It receives the sinus sagittalis inferior and **v. magna cerebri** and drains into the confluens sinuum.
— The paired **sinus transversus** run along the attached posterolateral margins of the tentorium cerebelli. Posteriorly, they join at the confluens sinuum, and anteriorly they drain into the sinus sigmoideus, forming grooves in the os occipitale and os parietale along their course.
— The paired **sinus sigmoideus** run in deep grooves of the os occipitale and os temporale and drain into the vv. jugulares internae at the foramen jugulare.
— The **sinus occipitalis** runs in the free edge of the falx cerebelli and ends in the confluens sinuum.

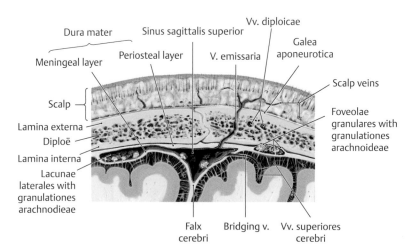

Fig. 26.4 Structure of a sinus durae matris
Sinus sagittalis superior, coronal section, anterior view. (From Schuenke M, Schulte E, Schumacher U. THIEME Atlas of Anatomy, Vol 3. Illustrations by Voll M and Wesker K. 3rd ed. New York: Thieme Publishers; 2020.)

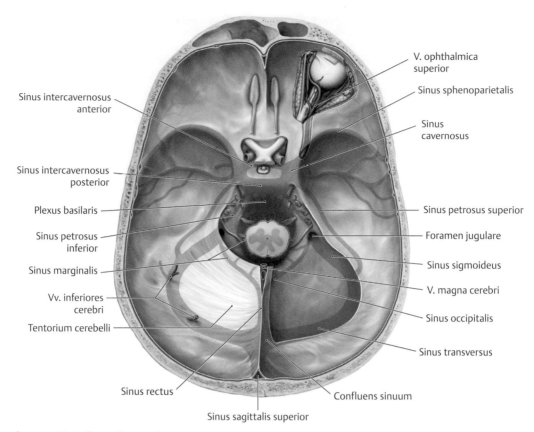

Fig. 26.5 Sinus durae matris in the cavitas cranii
Opened cavitas cranii with dural sinus system ghosted in *blue*, superior view. *Removed from the right side:* Tentorium cerebelli and roof of the orbita. (From Schuenke M, Schulte E, Schumacher U. THIEME Atlas of Anatomy, Vol 3. Illustrations by Voll M and Wesker K. 3rd ed. New York: Thieme Publishers; 2020.)

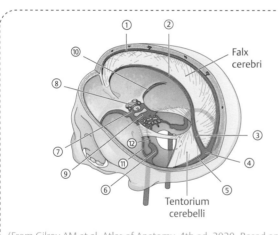

(From Gilroy AM et al. Atlas of Anatomy. 4th ed. 2020. Based on: Schuenke M, Schulte E, Schumacher U. THIEME Atlas of Anatomy. Head, Neck, and Neuroanatomy. Illustrations by Voll M and Wesker K. 3rd ed. New York: Thieme Medical Publishers; 2020.)

Table 26.1 Principal Dural Sinuses

Upper Group	Lower Group
① Sinus sagittalis superior	⑦ Sinus cavernosus
② Sinus sagittalis inferior	⑧ Sinus intercavernosus anterior
③ Sinus rectus	⑨ Sinus intercavernosus posterior
④ Confluens sinuum	⑩ Sinus sphenoparietalis
⑤ Sinus transversus	⑪ Sinus petrosus superior
⑥ Sinus sigmoideus	⑫ Sinus petrosus inferior

Note: The sinus occipitalis is also included in the upper group.

— The paired **sinus cavernosus**, located on either side of the sella turcica, have characteristics that distinguish them from other sinus durae matris (**Figs. 26.6** and **26.7**).
  • Each sinus cavernosus contains a large plexus of thin-walled veins.
  • Several important structures are associated with each sinus cavernosus:
    ○ A. carotis interna, which is surrounded by the plexus nervosus caroticus internus
    ○ N. oculomotorius (CN III)
    ○ N. trochlearis (CN IV)
    ○ N. ophthalmicus and n. maxillaris (CN V$_1$, V$_2$) of the n. trigeminus (CN V)
    ○ N. abducens (CN VI)

BOX 26.2: CLINICAL CORRELATION

CAVERNOUS SINUS THROMBOPHLEBITIS
Cavernous sinus thrombophlebitis can occur secondary to thrombophlebitis of the v. facialis. Although blood from the angle of the eye, lips, nose, and face usually drains inferiorly, it can also drain through the veins of the orbita to the sinus cavernosus. Infections from the face, particularly from the danger zone of the face (which extends from the bridge of the nose to the angles of the mouth) can spread infected thrombi to the sinus cavernosus (see **Box 24.6**). This can affect the nerves that traverse the sinus (CN III, CN IV, CN V1 and V2, and CN VI) and result in acute meningitis.

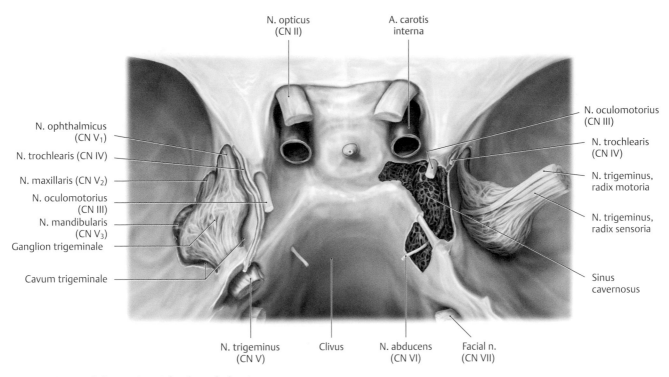

Fig. 26.6 Course of the nervi craniales through the sinus cavernosus
Cranial view.
Sella turcica with partially opened sinus cavernosus on the right side. On the right side, the lateral dural wall and roof of the sinus cavernosus is removed and the ganglion trigeminale is cut and retracted laterally. CN = cranial nerves (nn. craniales). (From Schuenke M, Schulte E, Schumacher U. THIEME Atlas of Anatomy, Vol 3. Illustrations by Voll M and Wesker K. 3rd ed. New York: Thieme Publishers; 2020.)

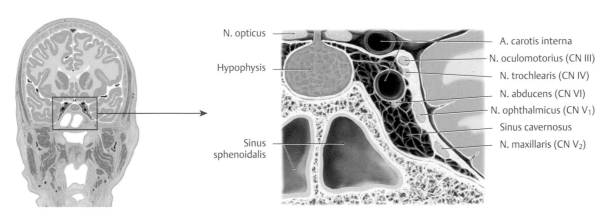

Fig. 26.7 Sinus cavernosus
Fossa cranii media, coronal section, anterior view. (From Gilroy AM et al. Atlas of Anatomy. 4th ed. 2020. Based on: Schuenke M, Schulte E, Schumacher U. THIEME Atlas of Anatomy. Head, Neck, and Neuroanatomy. Illustrations by Voll M and Wesker K. 3rd ed. New York: Thieme Medical Publishers; 2020.)

- The sinus cavernosus receive the v. ophthalmica superior and inferior, the sinus sphenoparietalis, the vv. media superficiales cerebri, and the vv. centrales retinae.
- The sinus cavernosus drain into the sinus petrosus superior and sinus petrosus inferior posteriorly and the plexus venosus pterygoideus inferiorly.
- **Sinus intercavernosus anterior** and **sinus intercavernosus posterior** (see **Fig. 26.5**) connect the sinus cavernosus dexter and sinus cavernosus sinister.

– Paired **sinus petrosus superior**, which drain the sinus cavernosus, travel within the attached margins of the tentorium cerebelli along the top of the pars petrosa of the os temporale and empty into the sinus sigmoideus.
– Paired **sinus petrosus inferior** drain the sinus cavernosus, passing through a groove between the pars petrosa of the os temporale and the pars basilaris of the os occipitale and emptying into the sinus sigmoideus at the origin of the v. jugularis interna. The sinus petrosus inferior communicate, through a **plexus basilaris**, with the plexus venosus vertebralis.

Arachnoidea Mater and Pia Mater (see Figs. 26.1, 26.4, 26.8)

— **Arachnoidea mater,** or **arachnoid**, is a thin, avascular, fibrous layer underlying the meningeal layer of the dura.
  • Liquor cerebrospinalis in the subarachnoid space presses the arachnoid against the overlying dura, but the two layers are not attached. Weblike **trabeculae arachnoideae** attach the arachnoid to the underlying **pia mater.**
  • Delicate fingers of the arachnoid layer, the **arachnoid villi,** pierce the dura to allow the reabsorption of liquor cerebrospinalis into the venous circulation and are especially numerous in the sinus sagittalis superior. They form aggregations called **granulationes arachnoideae** that protrude into the largest sinus durae matris and can push the dura ahead of them into the os parietale, forming "pits."
  • Congregations of arachnoid granulations also occur in **lacunae laterales,** lateral expansions of the sinus sagittalis superior.
— **Pia mater,** or pia, is a thin, highly vascular layer that adheres to the surface of the brain and closely follows its contours.

Meningeal Spaces (Fig. 26.8)

— The **spatium epidurale** between the cranium and dura is not a natural space because the dura adheres to the skull. Meningeal vessels that supply the skull and dura travel in this space.
— The **spatium subdurale** between the dura and arachnoid is a potential space, open only in pathologic conditions such as

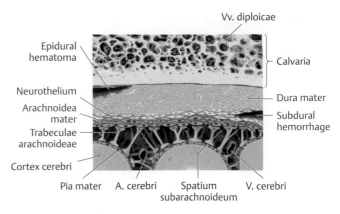

Fig. 26.8 Meningeal spaces
Meninges, coronal section, anterior view. (From Schuenke M, Schulte E, Schumacher U. THIEME Atlas of Anatomy, Vol 3. Illustrations by Voll M and Wesker K. 3rd ed. New York: Thieme Publishers; 2020.)

a subdural hematoma. Superficial cerebral veins ("bridging veins") cross this space, connecting the venous circulation of the brain with the sinus durae matris.

— The **subarachnoid space,** between the arachnoid and pia layers, contains cerebrospinal fluid, arteries, and veins.
  • **Cisternae subarachnoideae** are spaces that form where the spatium subarachnoideum enlarges around large infoldings of the brain. The largest of these include the **cisterna cerebromedullaris, cisterna pontocerebellaris, cisterna interpeduncularis, cisterna chiasmatica, cisterna quadrigeminalis,** and **cisterna ambiens** (see Section 26.2; see **Fig. 26.11**).

BOX 26.3: CLINICAL CORRELATION

EXTRACEREBRAL HEMORRHAGE
Bleeding from vessels between the bony skull and the brain (extracerebral hemorrhage) increases intracranial pressure and can damage brain tissue. Three types of cerebral hemorrhages are distinguished based on their relationship to the meningeal layers.

Epidural hemorrhages commonly originate from a torn a. meningea media following a skull fracture at the pterion and result in bleeding into the epidural space. The hemorrhagic spread is usually limited by suture lines because the dura is attached to the skull at these points. As a result, the local accumulation of blood causes compression of the brain in that area.

Subdural hematomas result from tearing of the bridging veins as they traverse the gap between the dural sinus and cere-

bral cortex. The elderly are more susceptible to this type of hemorrhage because with brain shrinkage these veins bridge a larger gap and are more vulnerable to injury from head trauma. This condition may mimic a slowly evolving stroke with a fluctuating level of consciousness and localizing neurologic signs.

Most subarachnoid hemorrhages occur due to the rupture of aneurysms associated with vessels of the circle of Willis and most frequently with vessels of the anterior cerebral circulation. These hemorrhages into the spatium subarachnoideum begin with a sudden, severe headache, neck stiffness, and drowsiness but can progress to severe consequences such as hemiplegia and coma.

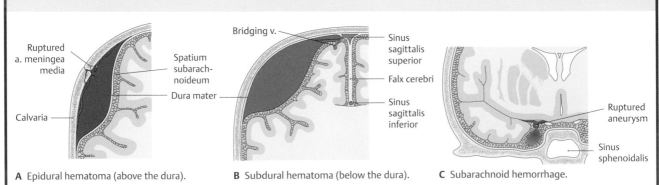

A Epidural hematoma (above the dura).   **B** Subdural hematoma (below the dura).   **C** Subarachnoid hemorrhage.

Extracerebral hemorrhages
(From Schuenke M, Schulte E, Schumacher U. THIEME Atlas of Anatomy, Vol 3. Illustrations by Voll M and Wesker K. 3rd ed. New York: Thieme Publishers; 2020.)

26.2 The Brain

The brain, enclosed within the bony skull, is the largest part of the central nervous system. It communicates with the peripheral nervous system through the medulla spinalis and nn. spinales and through the 12 pairs of nn. craniales.

Regions of the Brain

The major regions of the brain are the cerebrum, diencephalon, truncus encephali (mesencephalon, pons, medulla oblongata), and cerebellum **(Fig. 26.9)**.

— The **cerebrum** is the largest part of the brain and the center for integration within the central nervous system.
  • The falx cerebri lies in the **fissura longitudinalis cerebri** between the **right** and **hemispherium cerebri**.

• Each hemispherium cerebri is further divided into **lobus frontalis**, **lobus parietalis**, **lobus occipitalis**, and **lobus temporalis** that occupy the fossae cranii anterior and media.
• Posteriorly, the cerebrum rests on the tentorium cerebelli.
• The surface layer of the cerebrum (cortex) forms **gyri cerebri** (folds) separated by **sulci cerebri** (grooves).

— The **diencephalon** forms the central core of the brain and consists of the **thalamus, hypophysis,** and **hypothalamus.**
— The **mesencephalon** (midbrain), the most anterior part of the truncus encephali, passes through the incisura tentorii between the fossa cranii media and fossa cranii posterior.
  • It is associated with the n. oculomotorius (CN III) and n. trochlearis (CN IV).
— The **pons,** the middle part of the truncus encephali, lies in the anterior part of the fossa cranii posterior below the mesencephalon.

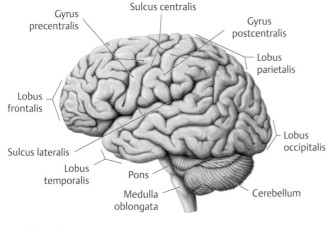

A Left lateral view.

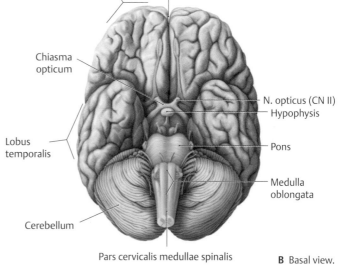

B Basal view.

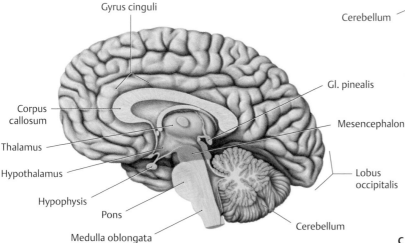

C Midsagittal section, medial view of the right hemisphere.

Fig. 26.9 Adult brain
(From Gilroy AM et al. Atlas of Anatomy. 4th ed. 2020. Based on: Schuenke M, Schulte E, Schumacher U. THIEME Atlas of Anatomy. Head, Neck, and Neuroanatomy. Illustrations by Voll M and Wesker K. 3rd ed. New York: Thieme Medical Publishers; 2020.)

- Several ascending and descending fiber tracts connect the pons to the cerebellum.
- The pons is associated with the n. trigeminus (CN V), n. abducens (CN VI), and n. facialis (CN VII).
— The **medulla oblongata,** the most posterior part of the truncus encephali, connects the brain and medulla spinalis.
  - It contains nuclei for the n. vestibulocochlearis (CN VIII), n. glossopharyngeus (CN IX), n. vagus (CN X), and n. hypoglossus (XII).
— The **cerebellum,** which occupies most of the fossa cranii posterior, lies inferior to the cerebrum and is separated from it by the tentorium cerebelli.
  - It consists of paired hemispheres and a small middle section, the vermis.

Ventricular System and Cerebrospinal Fluid

The brain and medulla spinalis are suspended in cerebrospinal fluid (liquor cerebrospinalis, CSF). The buoyant environment created by the CSF reduces the pressure of the brain on the nerves and vessels on its inferior surface.

— CSF is produced in the **plexus choroideus**, vascular networks within four ventricles (spaces) of the brain. The first two of these ventricles are large and paired; the third and fourth are smaller and lie in the midline (**Fig. 26.10**).
  - The **ventriculi laterales**, paired cavities that occupy a large portion of each hemispherium cerebri, communicate with the ventriculus tertius through the **foramina intraventriculares**.
  - The **ventriculus tertius**, a slitlike space between the two halves of the diencephalon, communicates posteriorly

with the ventriculus quartus through a narrow passage, the **aqueductus cerebri**, which passes through the mesencephalon.
  - The **ventriculus quartus**, a pyramidally shaped space that extends from the pons to the medulla oblongata, is continuous with the canalis spinalis inferiorly and with the spatium subarachnoideum through the **apertura mediana** and **apertura lateralis** in its tegmen.
— CSF circulates through the ventricles and passes into the spatium subarachnoideum and cisterna subarachnoideae through the apertura mediana and apertura lateralis ventriculus quatrus. It flows superiorly through the fissures and sulci of the cerebrum and is reabsorbed into the venous circulation through the granulationes arachnoideae that protrude into the sinus sagittalis superior (**Fig. 26.11**).

BOX 26.4: CLINICAL CORRELATION

HYDROCEPHALUS

Hydrocephalus, an excessive accumulation of cerebrospinal fluid (liquor cerebrospinalis, CSF) in the ventricles of the brain, can occur as a result of partial obstruction of the flow of CSF within the ventricular system, interference of CSF reabsorption into the venous circulation, or, in rare cases, overproduction of CSF. Excess CSF in the ventricles causes them to dilate and exert pressure on the surrounding cortex, causing the bones of the calvaria to separate, thus creating the characteristic increase in head size. Treatment involves the placement of a shunt between the ventricles and the abdomen, which allows CSF to drain to the cavitas peritonealis, where it can be easily absorbed.

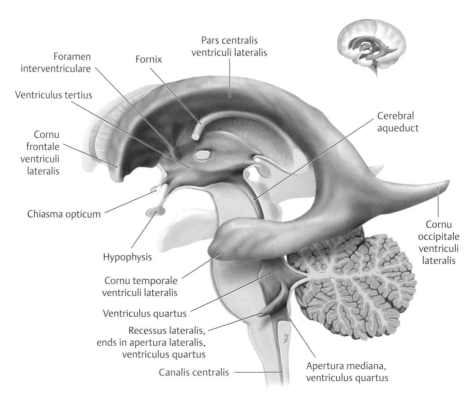

Fig. 26.10 Ventricular system in situ
Ventricular system with neighboring structures, left lateral view. (From Schuenke M, Schulte E, Schumacher U. THIEME Atlas of Anatomy, Vol 3. Illustrations by Voll M and Wesker K. 3rd ed. New York: Thieme Publishers; 2020.)

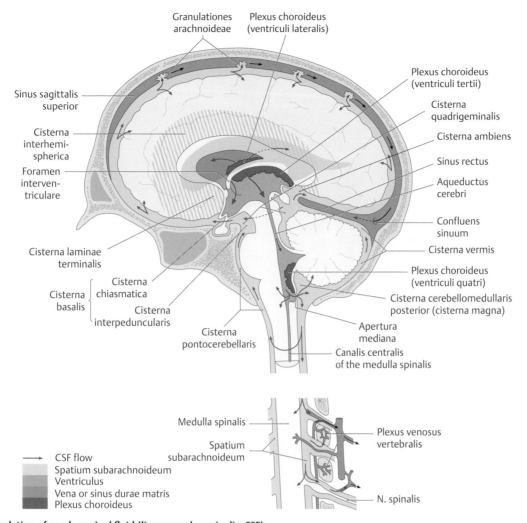

Fig. 26.11 **Circulation of cerebrospinal fluid (liquor cerebrospinalis, CSF)**
(From Schuenke M, Schulte E, Schumacher U. THIEME Atlas of Anatomy, Vol 3. Illustrations by Voll M and Wesker K. 3rd ed. New York: Thieme Publishers; 2020.)

Arteries of the Brain

As a result of its high metabolic demand, the brain receives one sixth of the cardiac output and one fifth of the oxygen consumed by the body at rest. This blood supply, derived from the a. carotis interna and a. vertebralis, is divided into **anterior** and **posterior cerebral circulations** (**Fig. 26.12**), which unite on the ventral surface of the brain to form a **cerebral arterial circle** (**circulus arteriosus cerebri**, circle of Willis).

— The internal carotid artery supplies the anterior cerebral circulation (see **Fig. 24.25**).
  • Its **pars petrosa** has a tortuous course as it enters the skull and follows the canalis caroticus horizontally and medially within the os temporale. Small branches pass into the auris media and canalis pterygoideus.
  • The **pars cavernosa** crosses over the foramen lacerum and runs anteriorly within the sinus cavernosus (**Fig. 26.13**). Small branches supply the meninges, hypophysis, and nn. craniales within the sinus cavernosus.
  • The **pars cerebralis** in the fossa cranii media gives off the a. ophthalmica (see **Fig. 28.12**) and immediately makes a U-turn to run posteriorly, where it divides into the a. cerebri anterior and a. cerebri media.
— The a. vertebralis and a. basilaris supply the posterior cerebral circulation.

• The a. vertebralis enters the skull through the foramen magnum and supplies branches to the medulla spinalis and cerebellum before merging with the opposite a. vertebralis to form a single a. basilaris.
  ○ Intracranial branches of the a. vertebralis include the a. inferior posterior cerebelli and the a. spinalis anterior and a. spinalis posterior.

BOX 26.5: CLINICAL CORRELATION

STROKE

A stroke is the manifestation of a neurologic deficiency resulting from a cerebral vascular impairment. *Ischemic strokes* are usually caused by an embolus obstructing one of the major cerebral arteries. Although the vessels of the circle of Willis can provide collateral circulation to circumvent the obstruction, anastomoses between the vessels are often incomplete or of insufficient size to provide adequate flow. *Hemorrhagic strokes* are usually due to rupture of an aneurysm, most often a saccular, or berry, aneurysm that bleeds into the spatium subarachnoideum. Symptoms occur shortly after the cerebral event and relate to the area of brain affected. They may include difficulty speaking, understanding language, or walking; vision problems; contralateral paralysis or numbness; and headache.

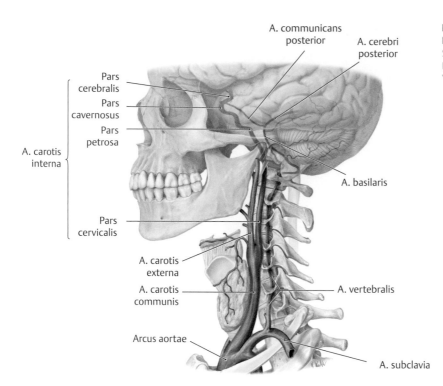

Fig. 26.12 Arteria carotis interna
Left lateral view. (From Schuenke M, Schulte E, Schumacher U. THIEME Atlas of Anatomy, Vol 3. Illustrations by Voll M and Wesker K. 3rd ed. New York: Thieme Publishers; 2020.)

- The **a. basilaris** ascends on the ventral surface of the truncus encephali, distributing branches to the truncus encephali, cerebellum, and cerebrum. It terminates as the right and left **a. cerebri posterior.**
  - Major branches of the a. basilaris are the **a. inferior anterior cerebelli** and **a. superior cerebelli**.
- The **cerebral arterial circle** (**circulus arteriosus cerebri**, circle of Willis), an important arterial anastomosis on the ventral surface of the brain, supplies the brain and connects the circulations of the a. carotis internus and a. vertebralis (**Figs. 26.14** and **26.15**).
  - A small **a. communicans anterior** connects the two aa. cerebri anteriores, linking the right and left anterior cerebral circulations.
  - A pair of **aa. communicans posteriores** connects the a. carotis interna and a. cerebri posterior on each side, completing the communication between the anterior and posterior cerebral circulations.
  - The vessels that form the circle are
    - the aa. communicans anteriores,
    - the aa. cerebri anteriores,
    - the aa. carotis internae,
    - the aa. communicans posteriores, and
    - the aa. cerebri posteriores.
- The aa. cerebri that arise from the cerebral arterial circle provide the blood supply to the hemispherium cerebri (**Table 26.2**).

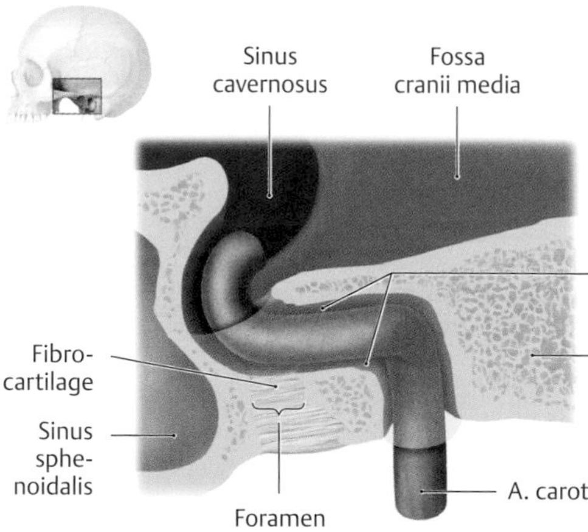

Fig. 26.13 The foramen lacerum and the arteria carotis interna in the canalis caroticus
Left lateral view. The foramen lacerum is not a true aperture, being occluded in life by a layer of fibrocartilage; it appears as an opening only in the dried skull. It is closely related to the a. carotis interna that traverses the canal. (From Schuenke M, Schulte E, Schumacher U. THIEME Atlas of Anatomy, Vol 3. Illustrations by Voll M and Wesker K. 3rd ed. New York: Thieme Publishers; 2020.)

Table 26.2 Distribution of the Arteriae Cerebri

Artery	Origin	Distribution
A. cerebri anterior	A. carotis interna	Frontal pole and medial and superior surfaces of the hemispherium cerebri
A. cerebri media	A. carotis interna	Most of the lateral surfaces of the hemispherium cerebri
A. cerebri posterior	A. basilaris	Occipital pole and inferior part of lobus temporalis

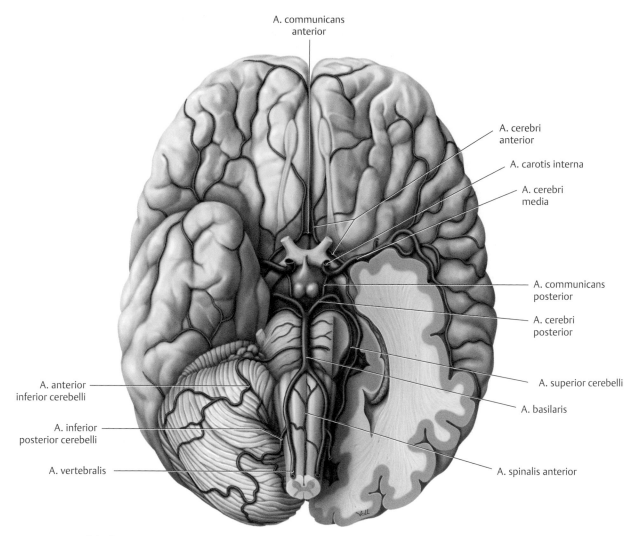

Fig. 26.14 Arteries of the brain
Inferior (basal) view. (From Schuenke M, Schulte E, Schumacher U. THIEME Atlas of Anatomy, Vol 3. Illustrations by Voll M and Wesker K. 3rd ed. New York: Thieme Publishers; 2020.)

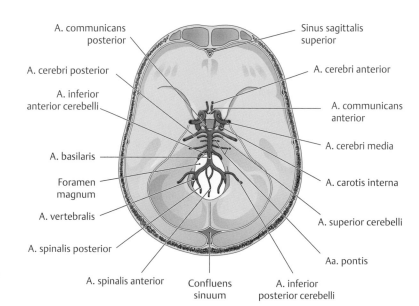

Fig. 26.15 Projection of the circle of Willis (circulus arteriosus cerebri) onto the basis cranii
Superior view. (From Schuenke M, Schulte E, Schumacher U. THIEME Atlas of Anatomy, Vol 3. Illustrations by Voll M and Wesker K. 3rd ed. New York: Thieme Publishers; 2020.)

Veins of the Brain

Veins that drain the brain are thin-walled and valveless and usually drain into a sinus durae matris (**Fig. 26.16**).
— Superficial (external) veins that drain the hemispherium cerebri include
  • the **vv. superior cerebri**, which drain the supralateral and medial aspects. These "bridging veins" traverse the spatium subdurale and drain into the sinus sagittalis superior (**Fig. 26.17**);
  • the **vv. media cerebri**, which drain the lateral hemispheres and empty into the sinus cavernosus and from there into the sinus petrosus and sinus transversus; and

• the **vv. inferiores cerebri**, which drain inferior aspects of the brain and join either the vv. superior cerebri or the **vv. basales**.
— Vv. basales drain the small vv. anteriores cerebri and vv. media profunda cerebri.
— **Vv. internae cerebri** drain the ventriculus tertius and ventriculus quatrus and deep parts of the cerebrum. These unite to form the **v. magna cerebri**.
— The v. magna cerebri receives the basilar veins and merges with the sinus sagittalis inferior to form the sinus rectus.
— **Vv. superior cerebelli** and **vv. inferiores cerebelli** drain the cerebellum into adjacent sinus durae matris or superficially into the v. magna cerebri.

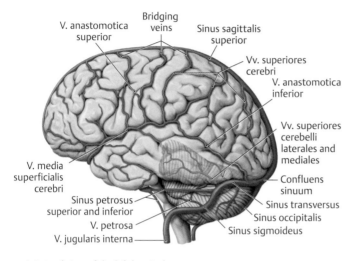

A Lateral view of the left hemisphere.

B Medial view of the right hemisphere.

Fig. 26.16 Venae cerebri
(From Schuenke M, Schulte E, Schumacher U. THIEME Atlas of Anatomy, Vol 3. Illustrations by Voll M and Wesker K. 3rd ed. New York: Thieme Publishers; 2020.)

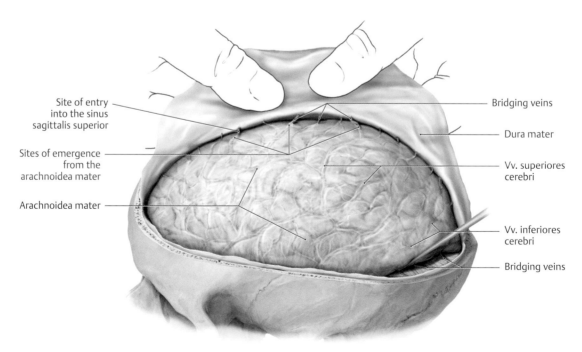

Fig. 26.17 Bridging veins
Viewed from upper left; the dura has been opened and reflected upward. Before vv. superficiales cerebri terminate in the dural sinus, they leave the spatium subarachnoideum for a short distance and course between the arachnoidea mater and meningeal layers of the dura to the sinus sagittalis superior. Injury to these segments of cerebral veins, called "bridging veins," leads to subdural hemorrhage. (From Schuenke M, Schulte E, Schumacher U. THIEME Atlas of Anatomy, Vol 3. Illustrations by Voll M and Wesker K. 3rd ed. New York: Thieme Publishers; 2020.)

26.3 Nervi Craniales

The 12 nn. craniales arise from the base of the brain **(Figs. 26.18 and 26.19; Tables 26.3** and **26.4)**. Like nn. spinales, nn. craniales can stimulate muscles or transmit sensation from a peripheral structure to the central nervous system. Some nn. craniales also carry fibers from the cranial portion of the parasympathetic nervous system. Seven types of nerve fibers are found (alone or in combination) in nn. craniales.

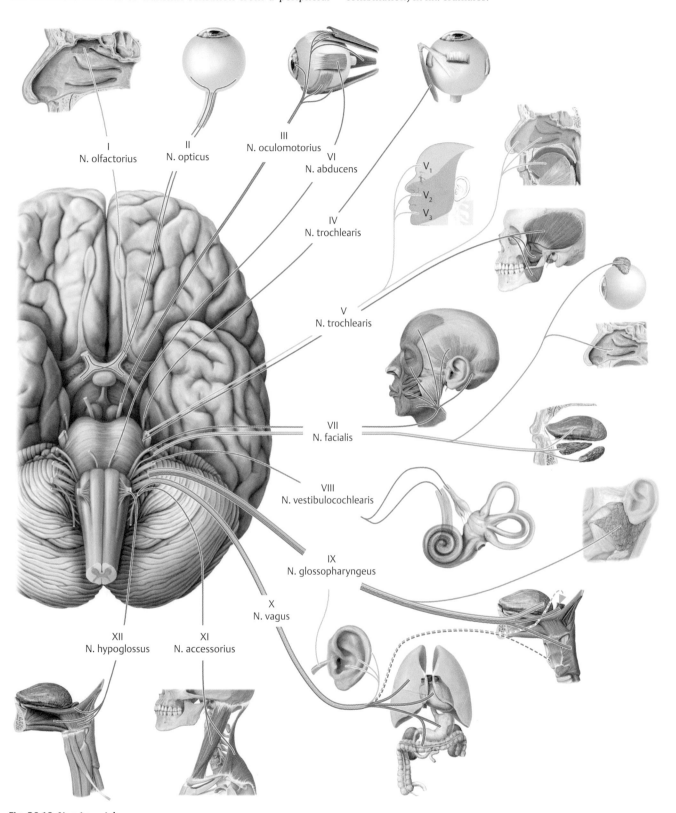

I
N. olfactorius

II
N. opticus

III
N. oculomotorius

VI
N. abducens

IV
N. trochlearis

V_1
V_2
V_3

V
N. trochlearis

VII
N. facialis

VIII
N. vestibulocochlearis

IX
N. glossopharyngeus

X
N. vagus

XII
N. hypoglossus

XI
N. accessorius

Fig. 26.18 Nervi craniales
Inferior (basal) view. The 12 pairs of nn. craniales (CN) are numbered according to their emergence from the truncus encephali. *(See **Table 26.3** for explanation of color coding.)* (From Gilroy AM et al. Atlas of Anatomy. 4th ed. 2020. Based on: Schuenke M, Schulte E, Schumacher U. THIEME Atlas of Anatomy. Head, Neck, and Neuroanatomy. Illustrations by Voll M and Wesker K. 3rd ed. New York: Thieme Medical Publishers; 2020.)

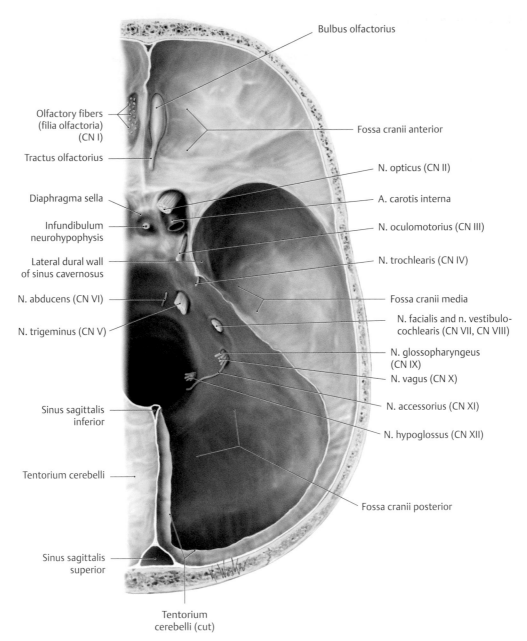

Fig. 26.19 Nervi craniales exiting the cavitas cranii
Cavitas cranii (superior view of interior skull base), right side. *Removed:* Brain and tentorium cerebelli. The ends of the nn. craniales have been cut to reveal the fissures, fossa, or dural cave where they pass through the cranial fossa. (From Schuenke M, Schulte E, Schumacher U. THIEME Atlas of Anatomy, Vol 3. Illustrations by Voll M and Wesker K. 3rd ed. New York: Thieme Publishers; 2020.)

Table 26.3 Classification of Cranial Nerve Fibers

Fiber Type	Function
General somatomotor	● Innervate voluntary muscle
General visceromotor (parasympathetic)	● Constitute the cranial component of the parasympathetic system, innervate involuntary muscles and glands
Special visceromotor (branchiomotor)	● Innervate muscles that developed from the primitive pharynx (pharyngeal arches)
General somatosensory	● Carry sensations such as touch, temperature, pain, and pressure
Special somatosensory	● Carry impulses from the eye for sight and from the ear for hearing and balance
General viscerosensory	● Transmit information from viscera such as carotid bodies, the cor, oesophagus, trachea, and gastrointestinal tract
Special viscerosensory	● Transmit information regarding smell and taste

See **Fig. 26.18** for explanation of color coding.

Table 26.4 Nervi Craniales: Function Overview

Nervi craniales		Passage Through Skull	Sensory Territory (Afferent)/Target Organ (Efferent)
CN I: N. olfactorius		Os ethmoidale (lamina cribrosa)	Smell: special viscerosensory fibers from olfactory mucosa of cavitas nasi
CN II: N. opticus		Canalis opticus	Sight: special somatosensory fibers from retina
CN III: N. oculomotorius		Fissura orbitalis superior	Somatomotor innervation: to m. levator palpebrae superioris and four mm. externi bulbi oculi (m. recti superior, m. recti medialis, and m. recti inferior, and m. obliquus inferior)
			Parasympathetic innervation: preganglionic fibers to ganglion ciliare; postganglionic fibers to mm. interni bulbi oculi (m. ciliaris and m. sphincter pupillae)
CN IV: N. trochlearis		Fissura orbitalis superior	Somatomotor innervation: to one m. externus bulbus oculus (m. obliquus superior)
CN V: N. trigeminus	CN V$_1$	Fissura orbitalis superior	General somatic sensation: from orbita, cavitas nasi, paranasal sinuses, dura of fossa cranii anterior and fossa cranii media, and face
	CN V$_2$	Foramen rotundum	General somatic sensation: from cavitas nasi, paranasal sinuses, superior nasopharynx, upper cavitas oris, dura of fossa cranii anterior and fossa cranii media, and face
	CN V$_3$	Foramen ovale	General somatic sensation: from lower cavitas oris, ear, dura of fossa cranii anterior and fossa cranii media, and face
			Branchiomotor innervation: to the eight mm. derived from the 1st pharyngeal (branchial) arch (including mm. of mastication)
CN VI: N. abducens		Fissura orbitalis superior	Somatomotor innervation: to one m. externus bulbus oculus (m. rectus lateralis)
CN VII: N. facialis		Meatus acusticus internus	General somatic sensation: from auris externa
			Taste: special viscerosensory fibers from tongue (anterior two thirds) and soft palate
			Parasympathetic innervation: preganglionic fibers to ganglion pterygopalatinum or submandibulare; postganglionic fibers to glands (e.g., gll. lacrimalis, submandibularis, sublingualis, palatina) and mucosa of cavitas nasi, palate, and paranasal sinuses
			Branchiomotor innervation: to mm. derived from the 2nd pharyngeal arch (including mm. of facial expression, stylohyoid, posterior digastric, and stapedius)
CN VIII: N. vestibulocochlearis		Meatus acusticus internus	Hearing and balance: special somatosensory fibers from cochlea (hearing) and vestibular apparatus (balance)
CN IX: N. glossopharyngeus		Foramen jugulare	General somatic sensation: from cavitas oris, pharynx, tongue (posterior third), and auris media
			Taste: special visceral sensation from tongue (posterior third)
			General visceral sensation: from carotid body and sinus
			Parasympathetic innervation: preganglionic fibers to otic ganglion; postganglionic fibers to gl. parotidea and gll. buccales and labiales
			Branchiomotor innervation: to the one m. derived from the 3rd arcus pharyngeus (m. stylopharyngeus)
CN X: N. vagus		Foramen jugulare	General somatic sensation: from ear and dura of fossa cranii posterior
			Taste: special visceral sensation from epiglottis and root of tongue
			General visceral sensation: from aortic body, laryngopharynx and larynx, respiratory tract, and thoracoabdominal viscera
			Parasympathetic innervation: preganglionic fibers to small, unnamed ganglia near target organs or embedded in smooth muscle walls; postganglionic fibers to glands, mucosa, and smooth muscle of pharynx, larynx, and thoracic and abdominal viscera
			Branchiomotor innervation: to m. pharyngeus and m. laryngeus derived from the 4th and 6th arcus pharyngei; also distributes branchiomotor fibers from CN XI
CN XI: N. accessorius		Foramen jugulare	Spinal root: somatomotor innervation: to m. trapezius and m. sternocleidomastoid
			Cranial root (now considered part of the n. vagus (CN X): branchiomotor innervation: to mm. laryngei (except m. cricothyroideus) via plexus pharyngeus and CN X
CN XII: N. hypoglossus		Canalis nervi hypoglossi	Somatomotor innervation: to all intrinsic and extrinsic lingual mm. (except m. palatoglossus)

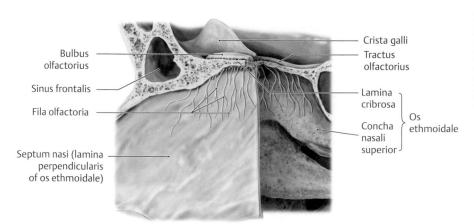

Bulbus olfactorius

Sinus frontalis

Fila olfactoria

Septum nasi (lamina perpendicularis of os ethmoidale)

Crista galli

Tractus olfactorius

Lamina cribrosa

Concha nasali superior

Os ethmoidale

Fig. 26.20 Nervus olfactorius (CN I)
Fila olfactoria, bulbus olfactorius, and tractus olfactorius. Portion of left septum nasi and lateral wall of right cavitas nasi, left lateral view. (From Schuenke M, Schulte E, Schumacher U. THIEME Atlas of Anatomy, Vol 3. Illustrations by Voll M and Wesker K. 3rd ed. New York: Thieme Publishers; 2020.)

CN I, the **n. olfactorius**, carries special sensory fibers that transmit sensation of smell from the superior aspect of the lateral and septal walls of the cavitas nasi **(Fig. 26.20)**.
— Olfactory neurons pass through the lamina cribrosa of the os ethmoidale and synapse with secondary neurons in the **bulbus olfactorius**.
  • The axons of these secondary neurons form the **tractus olfactorius**.
  • The bulbus olfactorius and tractus olfactorius are extensions of the cortex cerebri.

CN II, the **n. opticus**, is a collection of special sensory nerve fibers that originate on the **retina** of the eye and converge at the **discus opticus** at the back of the eyeball (bulbus oculi) **(Fig. 26.21;** see also Section 28.1).
— The nerve exits the orbita through the canalis opticus and joins the contralateral n. opticus to form the **chiasma opticum.**
— The chiasma opticum is a redistribution center where nerve fibers from the medial half of each n. opticus cross to the opposite side.
— Two **tractus opticus** diverge from the chiasm. Each tract contains nerve fibers from the medial half of one eye and the lateral half of the other eye.

CN III, the **n. oculomotorius**; **CN IV,** the **n. trochlearis**; and **CN VI,** the **n. abducens** innervate structures of the orbita **(Fig. 26.22;** see also Section 28.1). They pass through the sinus cavernosus before entering the orbita through the fissura orbitalis superior.
— The n. oculomotorius has somatic and visceral components.
  • General somatic motor fibers innervate four of the mm. externi bulbi oculi (m. rectus superior, m. rectus medius, m. rectus inferior, and m. obliquus inferior), which move the bulbus oculi, and the m. levator palpebrae superioris, which elevates the eyelid (palpebra).
  • General visceral motor fibers carry preganglionic parasympathetic fibers that synapse in the **ganglion ciliare** and innervate the **m. sphincter pupillae** (which constricts the pupil) and **corpus ciliare** (which changes the curvature of the lens of the eye) (see **Fig. 28.7**).
— The n. trochlearis carries general somatic motor fibers and innervates the m. obliquus superior, which depresses and medially rotates the eye.
— The n. abducens carries general somatic motor fibers and innervates the m. rectus lateralis, which abducts the eye.

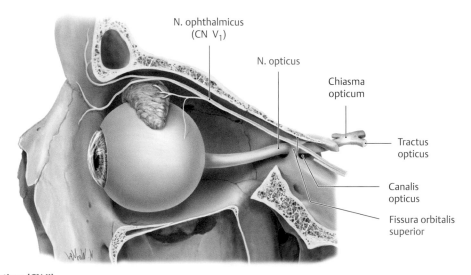

N. ophthalmicus (CN V₁)

N. opticus

Chiasma opticum

Tractus opticus

Canalis opticus

Fissura orbitalis superior

Fig. 26.21 Nervus opticus (CN II)
N. opticus in the left orbita, left lateral view. (From Schuenke M, Schulte E, Schumacher U. THIEME Atlas of Anatomy, Vol 3. Illustrations by Voll M and Wesker K. 3rd ed. New York: Thieme Publishers; 2020.)

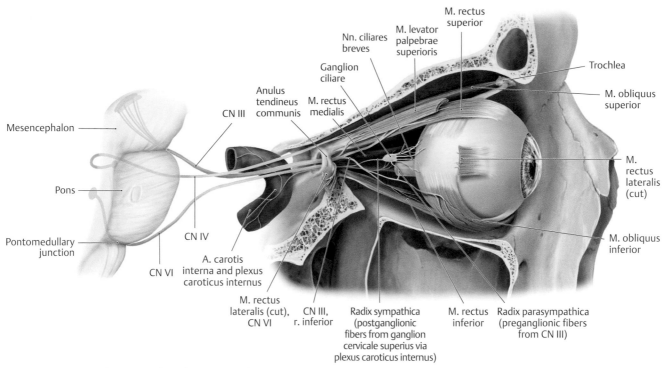

Fig. 26.22 Nervus oculomotorius (CN III), nervus trochlearis (IV), and nervus abducens (VI)
Course of the nerves innervating the mm. externi bulbi oculi, right orbita, lateral view. ((From Gilroy AM et al. Atlas of Anatomy. 4th ed. 2020. Based on: Schuenke M, Schulte E, Schumacher U. THIEME Atlas of Anatomy. Head, Neck, and Neuroanatomy. Illustrations by Voll M and Wesker K. 3rd ed. New York: Thieme Medical Publishers; 2020.)

CN V, the **n. trigeminus,** is the primary sensory nerve of the face (**Figs. 26.23** and **26.24**). Its small motor component innervates the muscles of mastication.

- The general somatic sensory neurons, which form the sensory root, synapse in sensory nuclei that are distributed along the truncus encephali and down into the pars cervicalis medullae spinalis.
- A small motor root in the n. mandibularis (CN V$_3$) contains branchial motor fibers.
- Branches of the n. trigeminus are spatially associated with the parasympathetic ganglia of the head and distribute post-ganglionic parasympathetic fibers to their target organs.

- The n. trigeminus has three divisions:
  1. The **ophthalmic division (CN V$_1$)** (see Section 28.1)
     - contains only somatic sensory fibers;
     - passes through the wall of the sinus cavernosus and fissura orbitalis superior into the orbita;
     - is associated with the **ganglion ciliare** (see Section 24.4);
     - distributes visceral motor fibers from the facial nerve (CN VII) to the gl. lacrimalis via the n. lacrimalis;
     - innervates the orbita, the cornea, and the skin on the top of the nose, forehead, and scalp;
     - functions as the sensory component of the corneal reflex via the **n. nasociliaris**; and
     - has **n. lacrimalis, n. frontalis,** and **n. nasociliaris** branches

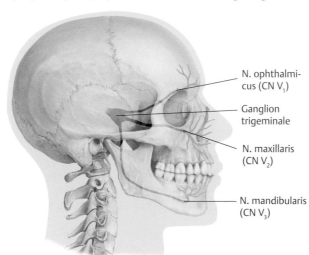

Fig. 26.23 Divisions of the nervus trigeminus
Right lateral view. (From Schuenke M, Schulte E, Schumacher U. THIEME Atlas of Anatomy, Vol 3. Illustrations by Voll M and Wesker K. 3rd ed. New York: Thieme Publishers; 2020.)

BOX 26.6: CLINICAL CORRELATION

TRIGEMINAL NEURALGIA
Trigeminal neuralgia, a pathology of the sensory root of the n. trigeminus (CN V), most commonly affects the n. maxillaris (CN V$_2$) and least frequently affects the n. ophthalmicus (CN V$_1$). The disorder is characterized by unilateral electric shock-like pain in the area supplied by the nerve. It usually lasts several seconds to several minutes. As the condition progresses, the pain may last longer, and there may be a shorter period between attacks. The pain may be initiated by touching a trigger point in the face by eating, talking, brushing teeth, or shaving. It is believed that trigeminal neuralgia is caused by the loss of myelin on the sensory root due to the pressure from an abnormal blood vessel. Surgery to destroy the nerve root or ganglion may be effective but may lead to permanent facial numbness.

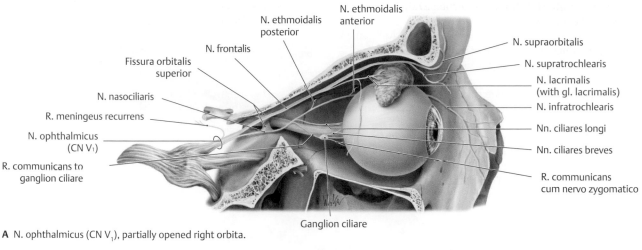

A N. ophthalmicus (CN V₁), partially opened right orbita.

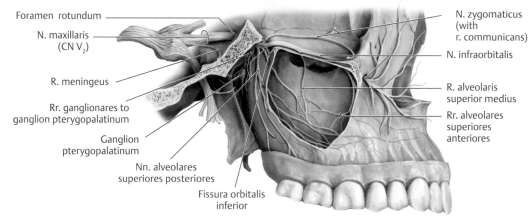

B N. maxillaris (CN V₂), partially opened right sinus maxillaris with the arcus zygomaticus removed.

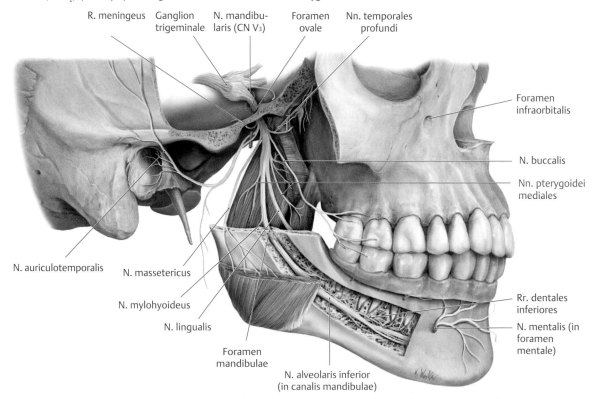

C N. mandibularis (CN V₃), partially opened mandibula with the arcus zygomaticus removed. *Note*: The n. mylohyoideus branches from the n. alveolaris inferior just before the foramen mandibulae.

Fig. 26.24 Nervus trigeminus (CN V)
Course of the n. trigeminus divisions. (From Schuenke M, Schulte E, Schumacher U. THIEME Atlas of Anatomy, Vol 3. Illustrations by Voll M and Wesker K. 3rd ed. New York: Thieme Publishers; 2020.)

2. The **n. maxillaris (CN V₂)** (see Section 27.6)
   - contains only somatic sensory fibers;
   - travels through the sinus cavernosus and the foramen rotundum to enter the **fossa pterygopalatina**;
   - is associated with the **ganglion pterygopalatinum** (see Section 26.4);
   - distributes visceral motor fibers to the gll. palatinae and gll. nasales via the n. nasopalatinus and n. palatinus major and n. palatinus minor;
   - distributes visceral motor fibers to the gl. lacrimalis via the n. zygomaticus which joins the n. lacrimalis of CN V1;
   - innervates the skin of the midface (from the lower eyelid to the upper lip) and structures associated with the maxilla, such as the sinus maxillaris, palatum, cavitas nasi, and dentes maxillares; and
   - has **n. infraorbitalis, n. zygomaticus, n. palatinus major** and **minor, n. alveolaris superior,** and **n. nasopalatinus** branches.
3. The **n. mandibularis (CN V₃)** (see Sections 27.4 and 27.5)
   - contains somatic sensory and branchial motor fibers;
   - passes through the foramen ovale into the **fossa infratemporalis**;
   - is associated with the **ganglion oticum** and **ganglion submandibulare** (see Section 26.4);

- distributes visceral motor fibers of the n. facialis (CN VII) to the gll. submandibulares and gll. sublinguales via the n. lingualis;
- distributes visceral motor fibers of the n. glossopharyngeus (CN IX) to the gl. parotidea via the n. auriculotemporalis;
- has a sensory component that innervates skin over the lower jaw and lateral face and structures associated with the mandibula, such as the lower teeth, **art. temporomandibularis**, floor of the mouth, and anterior tongue;
- has a motor component that innervates the **m. digastricus** (venter anterior), **m. mylohyoideus, m. tensor veli palatini,** and **m. tensor tympani**, as well as the **musculi masticatorii** (see Sections 27.2 and 27.8); and
- has **n. meningea, n. buccalis, n. auriculotemporalis, n. lingualis, n. alveolaris inferior,** and **rr. musculares** (to muscles noted above).

CN VII, the **n. facialis,** is the primary motor nerve of the face but also has sensory and visceral components (**Figs. 26.25, 26.26, 26.27**). It contains a motor root that innervates the muscles of facial expression, and an intermediate nerve that carries special sensory (for taste) and visceral motor fibers (parasympathetic) and somatic sensory fibers. Both the motor root and the intermediate nerve

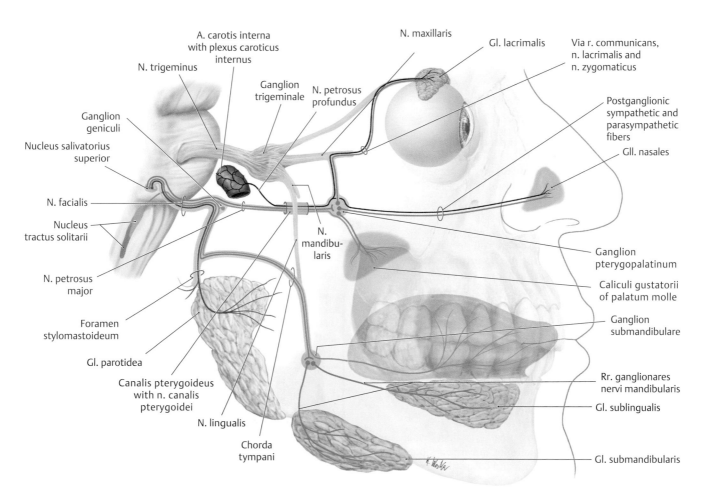

Fig. 26.25 Course of the nervus facialis
Visceral motor (parasympathetic) and special visceral sensory (taste) fibers shown in blue and green respectively. Postganglionic sympathetic fibers are shown in black, right lateral view. (From Gilroy AM et al. Atlas of Anatomy. 4th ed. 2020. Based on: Schuenke M, Schulte E, Schumacher U. THIEME Atlas of Anatomy. Head, Neck, and Neuroanatomy. Illustrations by Voll M and Wesker K. 3rd ed. New York: Thieme Medical Publishers; 2020.)

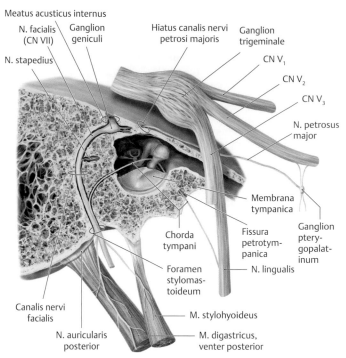

A N. facialis in the os temporale. (From Gilroy AM et al. Atlas of Anatomy. 4th ed. 2020. Based on: Schuenke M, Schulte E, Schumacher U. THIEME Atlas of Anatomy. Head, Neck, and Neuroanatomy. Illustrations by Voll M and Wesker K. 3rd ed. New York: Thieme Medical Publishers; 2020.)

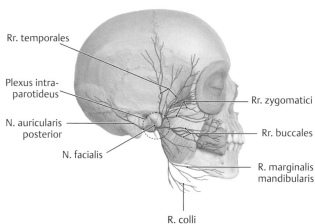

B Plexus intraparotideus. (From Schuenke M, Schulte E, Schumacher U. THIEME Atlas of Anatomy, Vol 3. Illustrations by Voll M and Wesker K. 3rd ed. New York: Thieme Publishers; 2020.)

Fig. 26.26 Nervus facialis (CN VII)
Branches of the n. facialis, right lateral view.

pass through the meatus acusticus internus into the **canalis facialis** of the os temporale,

— The motor root (radix motoria)
  • exits the skull through the foramen stylomastoideum
  • contains branchiomotor fibers, which
    ○ innervate the **m. stylohyoideus**, **m. stapedius**, and **m. digastricus** (venter posterior) (see **Figs. 27.28** and **27.29**);
    ○ form most of the n. auricularis posterior, which innervates the m. auricularis posterior and the m. occipitofrontalis, venter posterior; and
    ○ form the nerves of the **plexus intraparotideus** within the gl. parotideus, which innervates the muscles of facial expression (see Section 27.1). Branches of the parotid plexus include the **rr. temporales**, **rr. zygomatici**, **rr. buccales**, **rr. marginalis mandibularis**, and **rr. colli**.

— The three branches of the intermediate nerve (**nervus intermedius**) arise within the canalis facialis, including
  • the **n. petrosus major** (parasympathetic), which passes through the fossa cranii media and combines with the **deep petrosal nerve** (sympathetic) to form the **n. canalis pterygoidei** (see Section 27.6). The visceral motor (parasympathetic) fibers synapse in the ganglion pterygopalatinum and are distributed to glands of the nasal mucosa and palate and to the gl. lacrimalis.
  • the **chorda tympani,** which passes through the cavitas auris media, exits through the foramen stylomastoideum

to the fossa infratemporalis and travels with the n. lingualis of CN V$_3$. It carries
  ○ visceral motor fibers that synapse in the ganglion submandibulare and supply the gl. submandibularis and gl. sublingualis, and
  ○ special visceral sensory fibers for taste from the anterior part of the tongue and palate.
  • general somatic sensory fibers carried by the n. auricularis posterior, which transmit sensations from the auris externa to the **ganglion geniculi**, the sensory ganglion of the n. facialis, located in the os temporale.

BOX 26.7: CLINICAL CORRELATION

BELL'S PALSY

Bell's palsy is paralysis of the facial muscles due to a lesion of the n. facialis (CN VII). Symptoms usually begin suddenly and affect one side of the face only. They include drooping of the corner of the mouth, eyebrow, and lower eyelid, and the inability to smile, whistle, blow out cheeks, wrinkle the forehead, blink, or close the eyes forcefully. Taste is impaired on the anterior two thirds of the tongue (due to involvement of the chorda tympani), decreased tear production leads to dry eyes (due to involvement of the n. petrosus major), sensitivity to sounds is increased (due to paralysis of the m. stapedius), and the lower jaw and tongue deviate to the opposite side (due to paralysis of the venter posterior of m. digastricus).

BOX 26.8: CLINICAL CORRELATION

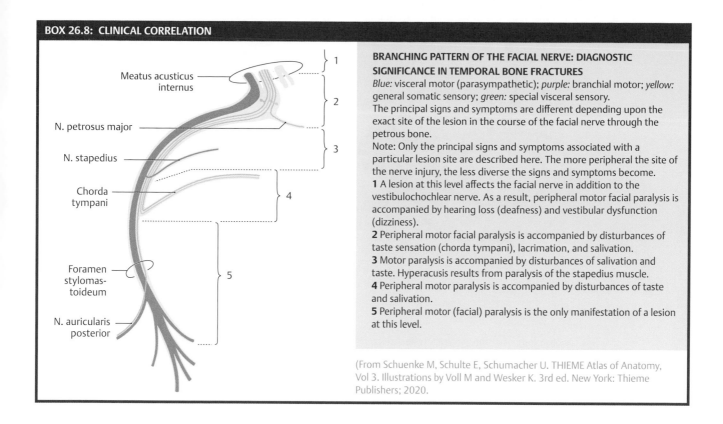

BRANCHING PATTERN OF THE FACIAL NERVE: DIAGNOSTIC SIGNIFICANCE IN TEMPORAL BONE FRACTURES

Blue: visceral motor (parasympathetic); *purple:* branchial motor; *yellow:* general somatic sensory; *green:* special visceral sensory.

The principal signs and symptoms are different depending upon the exact site of the lesion in the course of the facial nerve through the petrous bone.

Note: Only the principal signs and symptoms associated with a particular lesion site are described here. The more peripheral the site of the nerve injury, the less diverse the signs and symptoms become.

1 A lesion at this level affects the facial nerve in addition to the vestibulochochlear nerve. As a result, peripheral motor facial paralysis is accompanied by hearing loss (deafness) and vestibular dysfunction (dizziness).

2 Peripheral motor facial paralysis is accompanied by disturbances of taste sensation (chorda tympani), lacrimation, and salivation.

3 Motor paralysis is accompanied by disturbances of salivation and taste. Hyperacusis results from paralysis of the stapedius muscle.

4 Peripheral motor paralysis is accompanied by disturbances of taste and salivation.

5 Peripheral motor (facial) paralysis is the only manifestation of a lesion at this level.

(From Schuenke M, Schulte E, Schumacher U. THIEME Atlas of Anatomy, Vol 3. Illustrations by Voll M and Wesker K. 3rd ed. New York: Thieme Publishers; 2020.

CN VIII, the **n. vestibulocochlearis**, is the sensory nerve of hearing and balance. The nerve enters the os temporale with the n. facialis through the meatus acusticus internus.

— The two branches of the n. vestibulocochlearis carry special sensory fibers (**Fig. 26.27;** see Section 28.2):

- The **n. cochlearis** supplies the **cochlea** and its **spiral organ,** the organ of hearing.
- The **n vestibularis**, which contains the **ganglion vestibulare**, supplies the **utriculus**, **sacculus**, and **canales semicirculares**, the organs of balance.

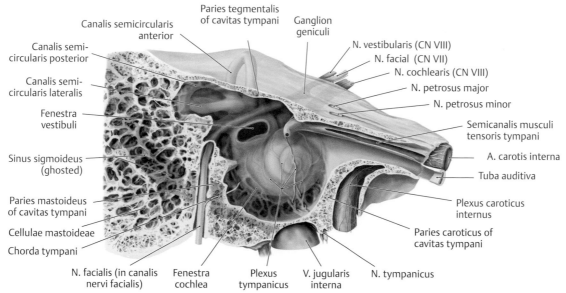

A N. vestibulocochlearis in the os temporale, paries labyrinthicus of the cavitas tympani. (From Gilroy AM et al. Atlas of Anatomy. 4th ed. 2020. Based on: Schuenke M, Schulte E, Schumacher U. THIEME Atlas of Anatomy. Head, Neck, and Neuroanatomy. Illustrations by Voll M and Wesker K. 3rd ed. New York: Thieme Medical Publishers; 2020.)

Fig. 26.27 **Nervus vestibulocochlearis (CN VIII)**

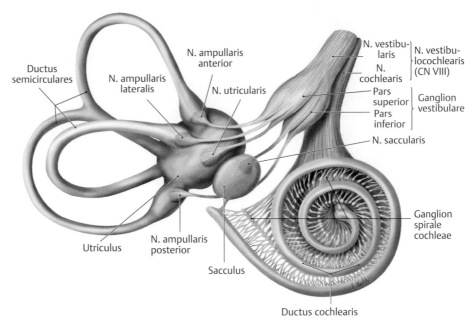

B Ganglion vestibulare and ganglion spirale cochleae. (From Schuenke M, Schulte E, Schumacher U. THIEME Atlas of Anatomy, Vol 3. Illustrations by Voll M and Wesker K. 3rd ed. New York: Thieme Publishers; 2020.)

Fig. 26.27 *(continued)* **Nervus vestibulocochlearis (CN VIII)**

CN IX, the **n. glossopharyngeus**, leaves the skull through the foramen jugulare and contains special sensory (taste), visceral sensory, somatic motor, and visceral motor components (**Figs. 26.28** and **26.29; Table 26.5**).

— Somatic motor fibers innervate the **m. stylopharyngeus**.
— Visceral motor fibers arise with the **n. tympanicus**, a branch of the n. glossopharyngeus. Carrying sensory and visceral motor fibers, it runs through the **cavitas tympani** of the **auris media** (see Section 28.2), where it contributes to the **plexus tympanicus**. It gives rise to the n. petrosus minor.
  ◦ The **n. petrosus minor** passes through the fossa cranii media and foramen ovale carrying visceral motor

(preganglionic parasympathetic) fibers that synapse in the ganglion oticum. Postganglionic fibers travel with the n. auriculotemporalis (CN V_3) to innervate the gl. parotidea.
  ◦ Sensory fibers of the plexus tympanicus supply the cavitas tympani and **tuba auditiva.**
— Special sensory fibers transmit taste from the posterior third of the tongue.
— Visceral sensory fibers transmit information from the **tonsils, soft palate,** posterior third of the tongue, **pharynx,** and, via the **branch to the sinus caroticus,** from receptors in the carotid body and sinus caroticus at the bifurcation of the a. carotis communis.

BOX 26.9: ANATOMIC NOTES

PETROSAL NERVES OF THE HEAD
Three nn. petrosi are associated with autonomic innervation of the head. Two nerves carry *preganglionic parasympathetic nerves:*
— The n. petrosus major, a branch of CN VII, forms the parasympathetic part of the n. canalis pterygoidei, which synapses in the ganglion pterygopalatinum. Postganglionic fibers travel via the n. zygomaticus (CN V_2) to the n. lacrimalis (CN V_1) in the orbita where they innervate the gl. lacrimalis. They also innervate glands in the cavitas nasi via branches of the n. maxillaris (CN V_2).

— The n. petrosus minor, a branch of CN IX, arises from the plexus tympanicus in the auris media and synapses in the ganglion oticum. Postganglionic fibers travel briefly with the n. auriculotemporalis (CN V_3) before innervating the gl. parotidea.
One nerve carries *postganglionic sympathetic fibers:*
— The n. petrosus profundus arises from the plexus caroticus internus and forms the sympathetic component of the n. canalis pterygoidei. These fibers pass through the fossa pterygopalatina without synapsing in the ganglion, and are distributed to the gl. lacrimalis and gll. nasales along the same routes as the n. petrosus major.

Table 26.5 Branches of Nervus Glossopharyngeus

①	N. tympanicus
②	R. sinus carotici
③	R. musculi stylopharyngei
④	Rr. tonsillares
⑤	Rr. linguales
⑥	Rr. pharyngei

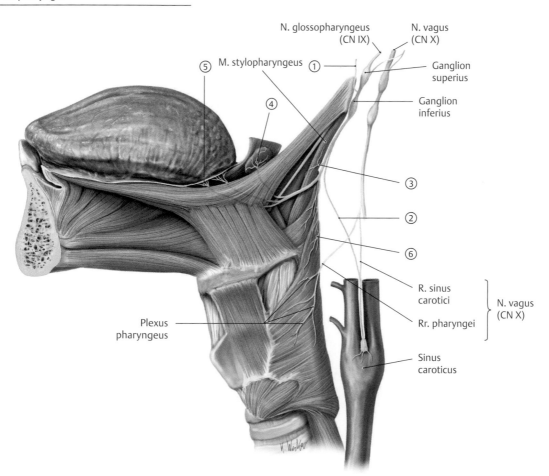

Fig. 26.28 Nervus glossopharyngeus (CN IX)
Course of the n. glossopharyngeus, left lateral view. The numbers are explained in **Table 26.5**. (From Schuenke M, Schulte E, Schumacher U. THIEME Atlas of Anatomy, Vol 3. Illustrations by Voll M and Wesker K. 3rd ed. New York: Thieme Publishers; 2020.)

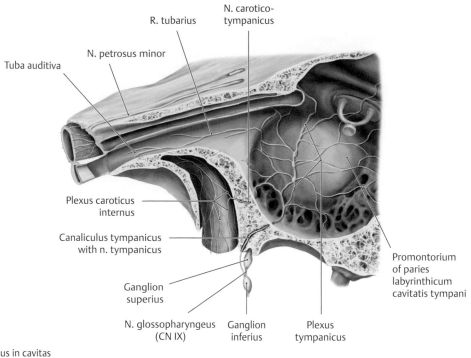

A N. glossopharyngeus in cavitas tympani, left anterolateral view.

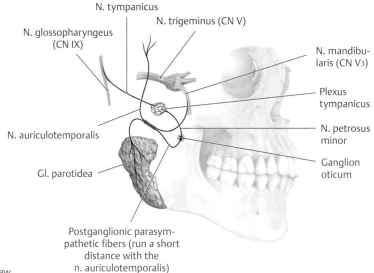

B Visceral motor fibers of the n. glossopharyngeus, right lateral view.

Fig. 26.29 Branches of the nervus glossopharyngeus
(From Schuenke M, Schulte E, Schumacher U. THIEME Atlas of Anatomy, Vol 3. Illustrations by Voll M and Wesker K. 3rd ed. New York: Thieme Publishers; 2020.)

CN X, the **n. vagus**, has the most extensive distribution of the nn. craniales (**Fig. 26.30; Table 26.6**).
— Branchial motor fibers innervate the muscles of the soft palate (except m. tensor veli palatini), pharynx (except m. stylopharyngeus), and larynx, and the m. palatoglossus of the tongue.
— Visceral motor fibers innervate smooth muscle and glands of the pharynx, larynx, thoracic organs, and abdominal praeenteron and mesenteron.
— General somatic sensory fibers transmit sensation from the dura in the fossa cranii posterior, the skin of auris externa, and the meatus acusticus externus.

— Visceral sensory fibers transmit sensation from mucosa of the lower pharynx, the larynx, lungs and airway, the heart, the abdominal praeenteron and mesenteron, and the chemoreceptors of the aortic body and baroreceptors of the arcus aortae.
— Special sensory fibers carry taste from the epiglottis.
— The n. vagus has cervical, thoracic, and abdominal segments.
  • In the neck
    ◦ each n. vagus leaves the skull through the foramen jugulare and descends within the vagina carotica of the neck, and
    ◦ its branches are **rr. pharyngeales**, **the n. laryngeus superior**, **rr. cardiaci cervicales**, (parasympathetic)

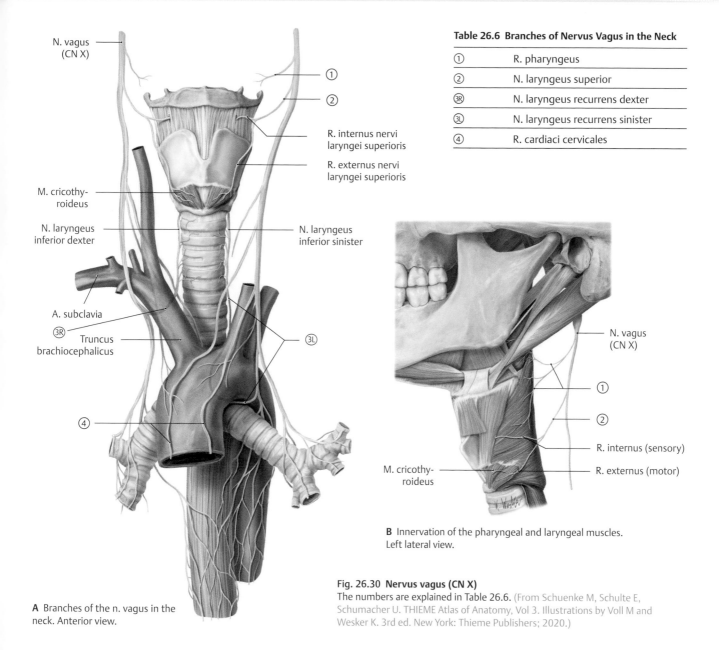

Table 26.6 Branches of Nervus Vagus in the Neck

①	R. pharyngeus
②	N. laryngeus superior
③R	N. laryngeus recurrens dexter
③L	N. laryngeus recurrens sinister
④	R. cardiaci cervicales

B Innervation of the pharyngeal and laryngeal muscles. Left lateral view.

Fig. 26.30 Nervus vagus (CN X)
The numbers are explained in Table 26.6. (From Schuenke M, Schulte E, Schumacher U. THIEME Atlas of Anatomy, Vol 3. Illustrations by Voll M and Wesker K. 3rd ed. New York: Thieme Publishers; 2020.)

A Branches of the n. vagus in the neck. Anterior view.

and the **n. laryngeus recurrens dexter** (which arises from the n. vagus dexter and recurs around the a. subclavia dextra).

- In the thorax
  ○ the n. vagus dexter and n. vagus sinister enter the thorax posterior to the art. sternoclavicularis and merge on the surface of the oesophagus oesophagus as the plexus oesophagus (see Section 5.2), and
  ○ their branches are the n. laryngeus recurrens sinister (which arises from the n. vagus sinister and recurs

around the arcus aortae, where it becomes known as the **n. laryngeus inferior**) and the rr. cardiaci thoracici and rr. bronchiales (parasympathetic).

- In the abdomen
  ○ truncus vagalis dexter and truncus vagalis sinister arise from the plexus oesophagus and pass through the hiatus oesophageus of the diaphragma as the truncus vagalis anterior and truncus vagalis posterior; and
  ○ their parasympathetic branches are distributed to organs of the praeenteron, mesenteron, and retroperitoneum.

CN XI, the **n. accessorius**, contains general somatic motor fibers, which originate in a nucleus of the upper segments of the medulla spinalis (**Fig. 26.31**).

— The nerve emerges with the upper five or six cervical spinal nerves and ascends within the canalis vertebralis. It enters the skull through the foramen magnum and exits through the foramen jugulare with the n. vagus and n. glossopharyngeus (CN IX).

— It innervates the m. sternocleidomastoideus and then crosses the lateral region of the neck to innervate the m. trapezius.

— Traditionally this nerve was believed to have a spinal root, as described above, and a cranial root, arising from the nucleus ambiguous in the medulla. The two roots travel together through the foramen jugulare before the cranial root splits off to join the n. vagus. Current thinking distinguishes the cranial root as part of the n. vagus; the spinal root is now considered to be the n. accessorius (CN XI).

CN XII, the **n. hypoglossus**, contains only general somatic motor fibers (**Fig. 26.32**).

— The n. hypoglossus leaves the skull through the canalis hypoglossi and runs forward, medial to the angulus mandibulae, to enter the cavitas oris.

— It innervates all of the muscles of the tongue except the m. palatoglossus.

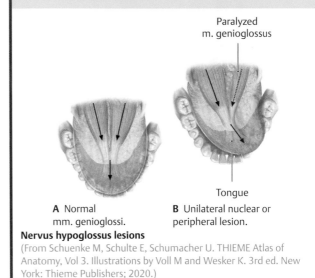

BOX 26.10: CLINICAL CORRELATION

INJURY TO THE NERVUS HYPOGLOSSUS

Injury to the n. hypoglossus causes ipsilateral paralysis of half of the tongue. When the tongue is protruded, the tip deviates toward the paralyzed side because the action of the m. genioglossus on the unaffected side is unopposed. Symptoms mainly manifest as slurring of speech. Over time, the tongue becomes weak and atrophies.

Paralyzed
m. genioglossus

Tongue

A Normal
mm. genioglossi.

B Unilateral nuclear or
peripheral lesion.

Nervus hypoglossus lesions
(From Schuenke M, Schulte E, Schumacher U. THIEME Atlas of Anatomy, Vol 3. Illustrations by Voll M and Wesker K. 3rd ed. New York: Thieme Publishers; 2020.)

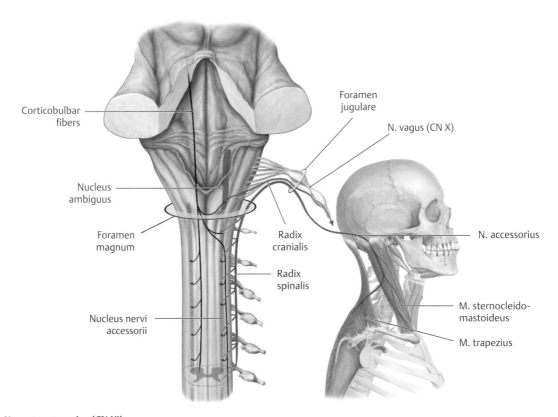

Fig. 26.31 Nervus accessorius (CN XI)
Truncus encephali with the cerebellum removed, posterior view. (From Schuenke M, Schulte E, Schumacher U. THIEME Atlas of Anatomy, Vol 3. Illustrations by Voll M and Wesker K. 3rd ed. New York: Thieme Publishers; 2020.)

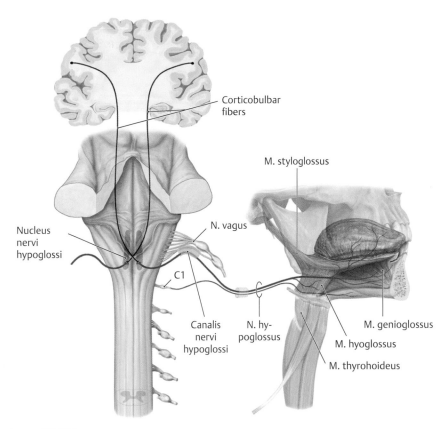

Fig. 26.32 Nervus hypoglossus (CN XII)
Truncus encephali with the cerebellum removed, posterior view. *Note*: C1, which innervates m. thyrohyoideus and m. geniohyoideus, runs briefly with the n. hypoglossus. (From Schuenke M, Schulte E, Schumacher U. THIEME Atlas of Anatomy, Vol 3. Illustrations by Voll M and Wesker K. 3rd ed. New York: Thieme Publishers; 2020.)

26.4 Autonomic Nerves of the Head

— Sympathetic nerves of the head arise as postganglionic fibers from the ganglion cervicale superius (**Fig. 26.33; Table 26.7;** see Section 25.4).

- The **plexus caroticus internus** of sympathetic fibers surrounds the a. carotis interna and its branches within the skull. A similar **plexus caroticus externus** follows the branches of the a. carotis externa on the face.
- Sympathetic fibers often travel with the parasympathetic nerves, but they do not synapse in the parasympathetic ganglia.

— The cranial portion of the parasympathetic (visceral motor) system is associated with the n. oculomotorius (CN III), n. facialis (CN VII), n. glossopharyngeus (CN IX), and n. vagus (CN X) (**Fig. 26.34; Table 26.8**).

- Preganglionic parasympathetic fibers traveling with the n. oculomotorius (CN III), n. facialis (CN VII), and n. glosso-pharyngeus (CN IX) synapse in the four parasympathetic ganglia of the head: the ganglion ciliare, ganglion pterygo-palatinum, ganglion submandibulare, and ganglion oticum.
- Parasympathetic nerves traveling with the n. vagus (CN X) extend into the thorax and abdomen and synapse in ganglia of plexus nervosum in those regions.
- Parasympathetic ganglia of the head are usually attached to, or in close association with, a branch of the n. trigeminus (CN V). The postganglionic parasympathetic fibers travel to their target organ by "piggybacking" on these trigeminal branches.

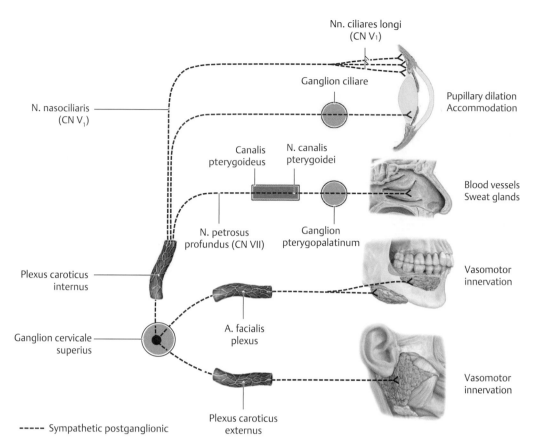

Fig. 26.33 Sympathetic innervation of the head
Sympathetic preganglionic fibers of the head originate in the cornu laterale of the medulla spinalis (T!–T3). They exit into the truncus sympathicus and ascend to synapse in the ganglion cervicale superius. Postganglionic fibers then travel with arterial plexuses (a. carotis interna, a. facialis, and a. carotis externa). Although these fibers often travel with parasympathetic fibers through the parasympathetic ganglia, they do not synapse in these ganglia. Similar to parasympathetic fibers, sympathetic nerves may "piggyback" on branches of the n. trigeminus (CN V) to reach their target organ. (From Schuenke M, Schulte E, Schumacher U. THIEME Atlas of Anatomy, Vol 3. Illustrations by Voll M and Wesker K. 3rd ed. New York: Thieme Publishers; 2020.)

Table 26.7 Sympathetic Fibers in the Head

Nucleus	Path of Presynaptic Fibers	Ganglion	Postsynaptic Fibers	Target Organs
Cornu laterale of medulla spinalis (T1–L2)	Enter truncus sympathicus and ascend to ganglion cervicale superius	Ganglion cervicale superius	Plexus caroticus internus → n. nasociliaris (CN V1) → nn. ciliares longi (CN V1)	M. dilatator pupillae (mydriasis)
			Postganglionic fibers → ganglion ciliare* → nn. ciliares breves (limited number of fibers)	M. ciliaris (sparse sympathetic fibers contributing to accommodation)
			Plexus caroticus internus → n. petrosus profundus → n. canalis pterygoidei → ganglion pterygopalatinum* → branches of n. maxillaris (CN V2)	Glands of cavitas nasi Sweat glands Blood vessels
			A. facialis plexus → ganglion submandibulare*	Gl. submandibularis Gl. sublingualis
			Plexus caroticus externus	Gl. parotidea

*Passes through without synapsing.
→, is continuous with.

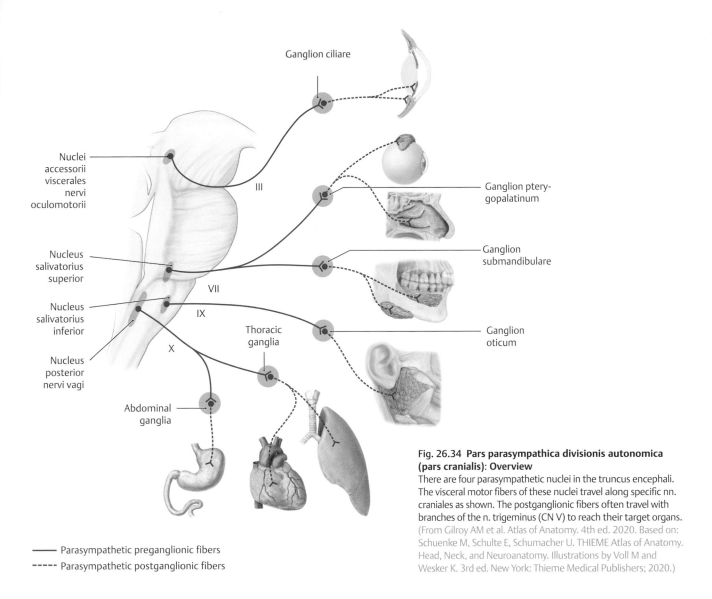

Ganglion ciliare

Nuclei accessorii viscerales nervi oculomotorii

Nucleus salivatorius superior

Nucleus salivatorius inferior

Nucleus posterior nervi vagi

III

VII

IX

X

Thoracic ganglia

Abdominal ganglia

Ganglion ptery-gopalatinum

Ganglion submandibulare

Ganglion oticum

Fig. 26.34 Pars parasympathica divisionis autonomica (pars cranialis): Overview
There are four parasympathetic nuclei in the truncus encephali. The visceral motor fibers of these nuclei travel along specific nn. craniales as shown. The postganglionic fibers often travel with branches of the n. trigeminus (CN V) to reach their target organs. (From Gilroy AM et al. Atlas of Anatomy. 4th ed. 2020. Based on: Schuenke M, Schulte E, Schumacher U. THIEME Atlas of Anatomy. Head, Neck, and Neuroanatomy. Illustrations by Voll M and Wesker K. 3rd ed. New York: Thieme Medical Publishers; 2020.)

——— Parasympathetic preganglionic fibers
----- Parasympathetic postganglionic fibers

Table 26.8 Parasympathetic Ganglia in the Head

Nucleus	Path of Presynaptic Fibers	Ganglion	Postsynaptic Fibers	Target Organs
Nuclei accessorii viscerales nervi oculomotorii	N. oculomotorius (CN III)	Ganglion ciliare	Nn. ciliares breves (CN V$_1$)	M. ciliaris (accommodation) M. sphincter pupillae (miosis)
Nucleus salivatorius superior	N. intermedius (CN VII root) → n. petrosus major → n. canalis pterygoidei	Ganglion pterygopalatinum	N. maxillaris (CN V$_2$) → n. zygomaticus → anastomosis → n. lacrimalis (CN V$_1$) • Rr. orbitales • Rr. nasales posteriores superiores • N. nasopalatinus • Nn. palatini majores and minores	• Gl. lacrimalis • Glands of cavitas nasi and sinus paranasales • Glands of gingiva • Glands of palata durum and molle • Gll. pharyngeales
	N. intermedius (CN VII root) → chorda tympani → n. lingualis (CN V$_3$)	Ganglion submandibulare	Glandular branches	Gl. submandibularis Gl. sublingualis
Nucleus salivatorius inferior	N. glossopharyngeus (CN IX) → n. tympanicus → n. petrosus minor	Ganglion oticum	N. auriculotemporalis (CN V$_3$)	Gl. parotidea
Nucleus posterior nervi vagi	N. vagus (X)	Ganglia near organs	Fine fibers in organs, not individually named	Thoracic and abdominal viscera

→, is continuous with.

27 Anterior, Lateral, and Deep Regions of the Head

The anatomy of the head can be divided into smaller regions that lie anterior and lateral to the neurocranium and form the superficial and deep structures of the face. They include the scalp; the regio parotidomasseterica; the fossa temporalis, fossa infratemporalis, and fossa pterygopalatina; and the cavitas nasi and cavitas oris.

27.1 The Scalp and Face

The **scalp** covers the neurocranium and extends from the linea nuchalis superior of the os occipitale, which mark the superior limit of the neck, to the arcus superciliaris of the os frontale. The face extends from the forehead to the chin and to the ears on either side.

— The scalp is composed of five layers **(Fig. 27.1)**:
  • Skin
  • Connective tissue containing the vessels of the scalp
  • Aponeurosis of the **m. occipitofrontalis**, **m. temporoparietalis**, and **m. auricularis superior** (galea aponeurotica)
  • Loose areolar tissue
  • Periosteum of the skull (pericranium)

Note that the first letter of each layer spells **"SCALP"**—a handy mnemonic.

— Muscles of facial expression (musculi faciei) lie in the loose connective tissue layer of the face and scalp. Their origin on bones of the face and insertion into the overlying skin allows them to create facial movements **(Fig. 27.2; Tables 27.1** and **27.2)**.
— Most arteries that supply the face and scalp are branches of the a. carotis externa (see **Fig. 24.21**) and include the following:
  • The a. labialis superior, a. labialis inferior, a. nasalis lateralis, and rr. angulares of a. facialis, which supply the face between the eye and lower lip
  • The r. mentalis of the a. alveolaris inferior, which supplies the chin
  • The a. temporalis superficialis, a. auricularis posterior, and a. occipitalis, which supply the lateral and posterior parts of the scalp
  • The a. supratrochlearis and a. supraorbitalis from the a. ophthalmicus (a branch of a. carotis interna), which supply the anterior scalp. These arteries anastomose with

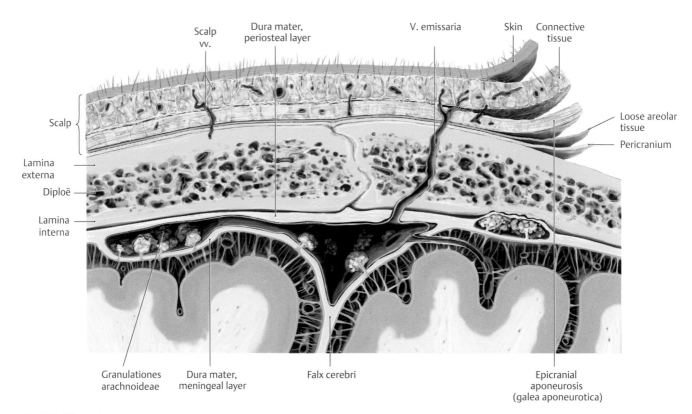

Fig. 27.1 The scalp
(From Schuenke M, Schulte E, Schumacher U. THIEME Atlas of Anatomy, Vol 3. Illustrations by Voll M and Wesker K. 3rd ed. New York: Thieme Publishers; 2020.)

the a. angularis on the face and form a connection between circulations arising from a. carotis interna and a. carotis externa (see **Box 24.5**).

— Superficial veins of the head drain the face and scalp. Most of these veins follow the arteries of similar name and territory but drain to the v. facialis and v. retromandibularis, which terminate in the v. jugularis interna and v. jugularis externa, respectively.

— Veins of the scalp have deep connections to
  • **vv. diploicae**, which run within the diploë layer of the skull, and
  • **vv. emissariae**, which drain through the skull from the sinus durae matris.

BOX 27.1: CLINICAL CORRELATION

SCALP INFECTIONS

Infections of the scalp spread easily over the calvaria through the loose connective tissue layer. Spread into the posterior neck is inhibited by the attachment of the m. occipitofrontalis to the os occipitale and os temporale. Laterally, spread is inhibited beyond the zygomatic arches by the attachment of the galea aponeurotica to the arcus zygomaticus via the fascia temporalis. Anteriorly, however, infections can spread to the eyelids and nose under the m. frontalis. Additionally, vv. emissariae may carry infections intracranially to the sinus durae matris and can result in meningitis.

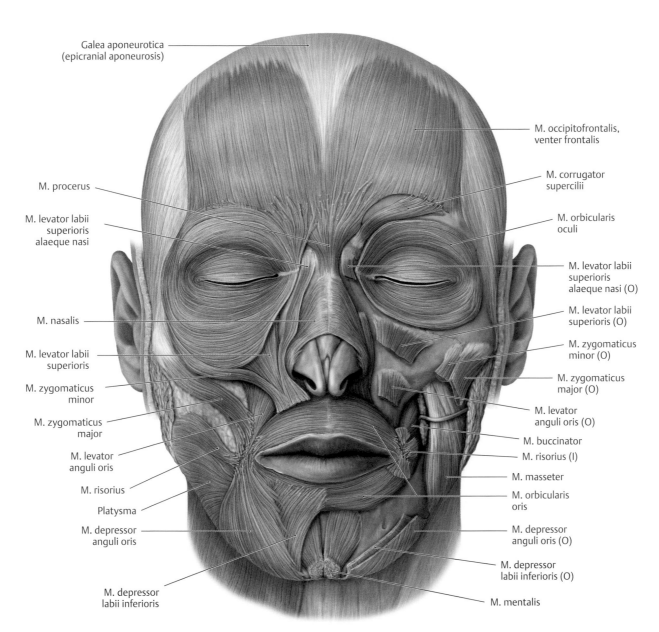

A Anterior view. Muscle origins (0) and insertion (I) indicated on left side of face.

Fig. 27.2 Muscles of facial expression (musculi faciei) (*continued on page 504*)

(*continued on page 504*)

(From Schuenke M, Schulte E, Schumacher U. THIEME Atlas of Anatomy, Vol 3. Illustrations by Voll M and Wesker K. 3rd ed. New York: Thieme Publishers; 2020.)

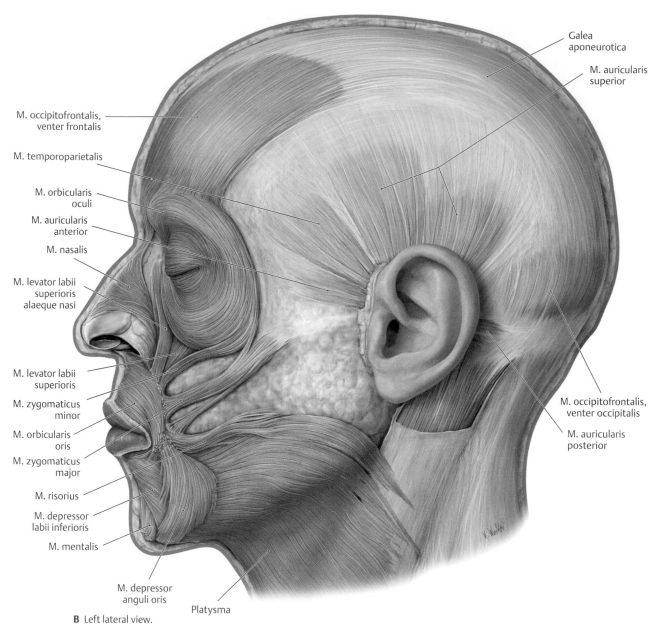

B Left lateral view.

Fig. 27.2 (*continued*) **Muscles of facial expression (musculi faciei)**

Table 27.1 **Muscles of Facial Expression (Musculi Faciei): Forehead, Nose, and Ear**

Muscle	Origin	Insertion*	Main Action(s)**
Calvaria			
M. occipitofrontalis (venter frontalis)	Galea aponeurotica	Skin and tela subcutanea of eyebrows and forehead	Elevates eyebrows, wrinkles skin of forehead
Rima palpebrarum and nose			
M. procerus	Os nasale, cartilago nasi lateralis (upper part)	Skin of lower forehead between eyebrows	Pulls medial angle of eyebrows inferiorly, producing transverse wrinkles over bridge of nose
M. orbicularis oculi	Margo medialis orbitae, lig. palpebrale mediale, os lacrimale	Skin around margin of orbita, tarsi superior and inferior	Acts as orbital sphincter (closes eyelids) • Pars palpebralis gently closes • Pars orbitalis tightly closes (as in winking)
M. nasalis	Maxilla (superior region of eminentia canina)	Cartilagines nasi	Flares nostrils by drawing ala (side) of nose toward septum nasi

Table 27.1 (*continued*) **Muscles of Facial Expression (Musculi Faciei): Forehead, Nose, and Ear**

Muscle	Origin	Insertion*	Main Action(s)**
M. levator labii superioris alaeque nasi	Proc. frontalis maxillae	Cartilago alaris of nose and upper lip	Elevates upper lip
Auris			
M. auricularis anterior	Fascia temporalis (anterior portion)	Helix of the ear	Pull ear superiorly and anteriorly
M. auricularis superior	Galea aponeurotica on side of head	Upper portion of auricula	Elevate ear
M. auricularis posterior	Proc. mastoideus	Convexity of concha auriculae	Pull ear superiorly and posteriorly

* There are no bony insertions for the muscles of facial expression.

** All muscles of facial expression are innervated by the n. facialis (CN VII) via rr. temporales, zygomatici, buccales, marginales mandibulares, or rr. cervicales (rr. colli) arising from the plexus intraparotideus.

Table 27.2 Muscles of Facial Expression (Musculi Faciei): Mouth and Neck

Muscle	Origin	Insertion*	Main Action(s)**
Mouth			
M. zygomaticus major	Facies lateralis ossis zygomatici (posterior part)	Skin at corner of the mouth	Pulls corner of mouth superiorly and laterally
M. zygomaticus minor		Upper lip just medial to corner of the mouth	Pulls upper lip superiorly
M. levator labii superioris alaeque nasi	Proc. frontalis maxillae	Cartilago alaris of nose and upper lip	Elevates upper lip
M. levator labii superioris	Proc. frontalis maxillae and regio infraorbitalis	Skin of upper lip, cartilago alaris of nose	Elevates upper lip, dilates nostril, raises angulus oris
M. depressor labii inferioris	Mandibula (anterior portion of linea obliqua)	Lower lip at midline; blends with muscle from opposite side	Pulls lower lip inferiorly and laterally
M. levator anguli oris	Maxilla (below foramen infraorbitale)	Skin at angulus oris	Raises angulus oris, helps form sulcus nasolabialis
M. depressor anguli oris	Mandibula (linea obliqua below dentes caninus, premolaris, and molaris primus)	Skin at angulus oris; blends with m. orbicularis oris	Pulls angulus oris inferiorly and laterally
M. buccinator	Mandibula, proc. alveolaris maxillae and pars alveolaris mandibulae, raphe pterygomandibularis	Angulus oris, m. orbicularis oris	Presses cheek against molar teeth, working with the tongue to keep food between occlusal surfaces and out of vestibulum oris; expels air from cavitas oris/resists distension when blowing. *Unilateral:* Draws mouth to one side
M. orbicularis oris	Deep surface of skin Superiorly: maxilla (planum medianum) Inferiorly: Mandibula	Mucous membrane of lips	Acts as oral sphincter • Compresses and protrudes lips (e.g., when whistling, sucking, and kissing) • Resists distension (when blowing)
M. risorius	Fascia over m. masseter	Skin of angulus oris	Retracts angulus oris as in grimacing
M. mentalis	Mandibula (incisive fossa)	Skin of chin	Elevates and protrudes lower lip
Neck			
Platysma	Skin over lower neck and upper lateral thorax	Mandibula (margo inferior), skin over lower face, angulus oris	Depresses and wrinkles skin of lower face and mouth; tenses skin of neck; aids in forced depression of the mandibula

* There are no bony insertions for the muscles of facial expression.

** All muscles of facial expression are innervated by the n. facialis (CN VII) via rr. temporales, zygomatici, buccales, marginales mandibulares, or rr. cervicales (rr. colli) arising from its plexus intraparotideus.

— Primary sensory nerves of the face and scalp (**Fig. 27.3**) include
  • the **n. supraorbitalis** and **n. supratrochlearis** (cranial nerve [CN] V₁);
  • the n. infraorbitalis and **n. zygomaticotemporalis** and **n. zygomaticofacialis** (V₂);
  • the n. auriculotemporalis, n. buccalis, and **n. mentalis** (a branch of the n. alveolaris inferior) nerves (V₃);
  • the **n. auricularis magnus** and **n. occipitalis minor**, which are rami anteriores of C2 and C3 via the plexus cervicalis; and
  • the **n. occipitalis major** and **n. occipitalis tertius**, which are rami posteriores of C2 and C3, respectively.

— Motor nerves of the face and scalp (**Fig. 27.4**) include
  • the rr. temporales, rr. zygomatici, rr. buccales, and r. marginalis mandibularis of the n. facialis (CN VII), which innervate muscles of the face;
  • the rr. temporales and n. auricularis posterior of the n. facialis, which innervate muscles of the scalp; and
  • the muscular branches of the n. mandibularis of the n. trigeminus (CN V₃), which innervate the muscles of mastication (musculi masticatorii).

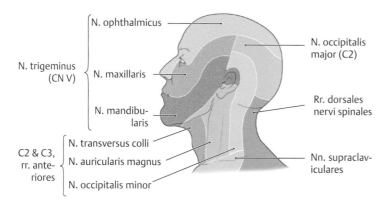

A Cutaneous innervation of the head and neck, left lateral view. The occiput and nuchal regions are supplied by the rr. dorsales *(blue)* of the nn. spinales (the n. occipitalis major is the r. dorsalis of C2).

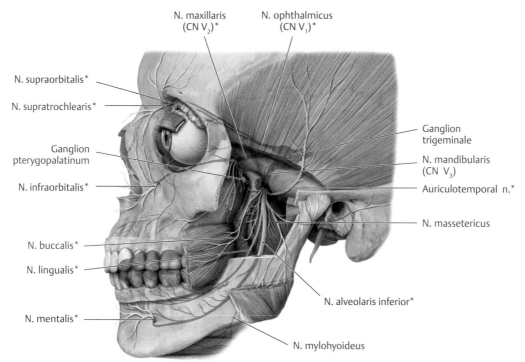

B Divisions of n. trigeminus, left lateral view. *Indicates sensory nn.

Fig. 27.3 Cutaneous innervation of the face
(From Gilroy AM et al. Atlas of Anatomy. 4th ed. 2020. Based on: Schuenke M, Schulte E, Schumacher U. THIEME Atlas of Anatomy. Head, Neck, and Neuroanatomy. Illustrations by Voll M and Wesker K. 3rd ed. New York: Thieme Medical Publishers; 2020.)

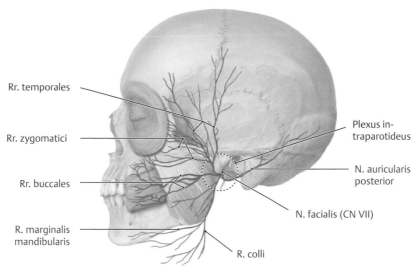

Rr. temporales

Rr. zygomatici

Rr. buccales

R. marginalis mandibularis

R. colli

Plexus in-traparotideus

N. auricularis posterior

N. facialis (CN VII)

A Motor innervation of the muscles of facial expression.

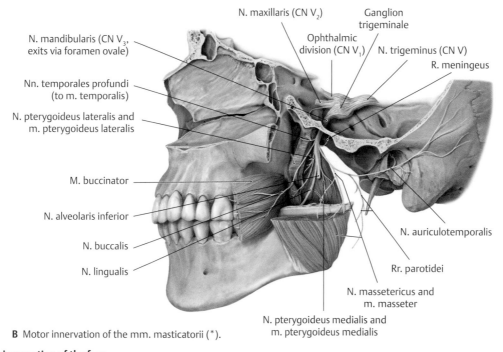

N. mandibularis (CN V₃, exits via foramen ovale)

Nn. temporales profundi (to m. temporalis)

N. pterygoideus lateralis and m. pterygoideus lateralis

M. buccinator

N. alveolaris inferior

N. buccalis

N. lingualis

N. maxillaris (CN V₂)

Ophthalmic division (CN V₁)

Ganglion trigeminale

N. trigeminus (CN V)

R. meningeus

N. auriculotemporalis

Rr. parotidei

N. massetericus and m. masseter

N. pterygoideus medialis and m. pterygoideus medialis

B Motor innervation of the mm. masticatorii (*).

Fig. 27.4 Motor innervation of the face
Left lateral view. (A) Five branches of the n. facialis (CN VII) provide motor innervation to the muscles of facial expression. (B) The n. mandibularis of the n. trigeminus (CN V₃) supplies motor innervation to the mm. masticatorii. (From Gilroy AM et al. Atlas of Anatomy. 4th ed. 2020. Based on: Schuenke M, Schulte E, Schumacher U. THIEME Atlas of Anatomy. Head, Neck, and Neuroanatomy. Illustrations by Voll M and Wesker K. 3rd ed. New York: Thieme Medical Publishers; 2020.)

27.2 The Articulatio Temporomandibularis and Muscles of Mastication

The **art. temporomandibularis** (TMJ), the articulation between the caput mandibulae and fossa mandibularis of the os temporale, is located within the fossa infratemporalis. The fossa mandibularis is a depression in the pars squamosa ossis temporalis; the tuberculum articulare lies anteriorly, and the meatus acusticus externus canal lies posteriorly (**Fig. 27.5**).

— The joint is enclosed by a fibrous joint capsule and stabilized externally by several ligaments: the **lig. laterale**, the strongest

of these, strengthens the capsula fibrosa that surrounds the joint. **Lig. sphenomandibulare** and **lig. stylomandibulare** support the joint during chewing (**Fig. 27.6**).

— Within the joint and attached to the joint capsule a fibrocartilaginous articular disk divides the joint space into an upper part for gliding movements and a lower part for hinge movements.

— Four muscles—**m. temporalis, m. masseter, m. pterygoideus lateralis**, and **m. pterygoideus medialis**—act at the art. temporomandibularis to move the mandibula during chewing (**Figs. 27.7, 27.8, 27.9, 27.10; Table 27.3**). They reside in the parotid

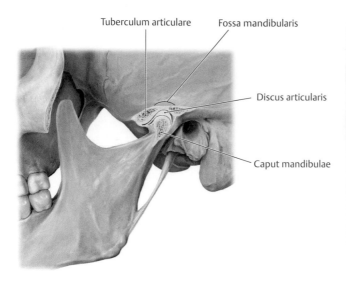

Fig. 27.5 Articulatio temporomandibularis
The caput mandibulae articulates with the fossa mandibularis in the art. temporomandibularis. Sagittal section, left lateral view. (From Gilroy AM et al. Atlas of Anatomy. 4th ed. 2020. Based on: Schuenke M, Schulte E, Schumacher U. THIEME Atlas of Anatomy. Head, Neck, and Neuroanatomy. Illustrations by Voll M and Wesker K. 3rd ed. New York: Thieme Medical Publishers; 2020.)

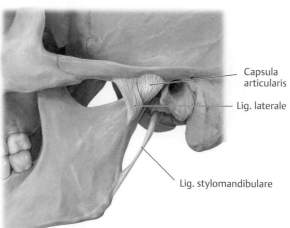

A Lateral view of the left art. temporomandibularis.

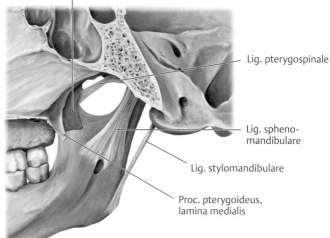

B Medial view of the right art. temporomandibularis.

Fig. 27.6 Ligaments of the articulatio temporomandibularis
(From Schuenke M, Schulte E, Schumacher U. THIEME Atlas of Anatomy, Vol 3. Illustrations by Voll M and Wesker K. 3rd ed. New York: Thieme Publishers; 2020.)

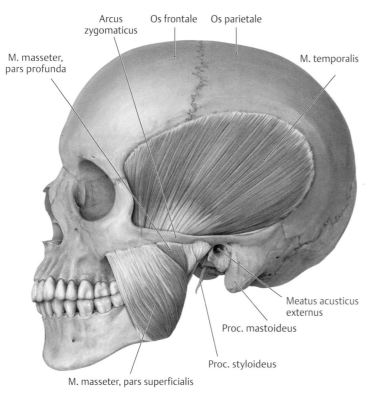

Fig. 27.7 Musculus masseter and musculus temporalis
Left lateral view. (From Schuenke M, Schulte E, Schumacher U. THIEME Atlas of Anatomy, Vol 3. Illustrations by Voll M and Wesker K. 3rd ed. New York: Thieme Publishers; 2020.)

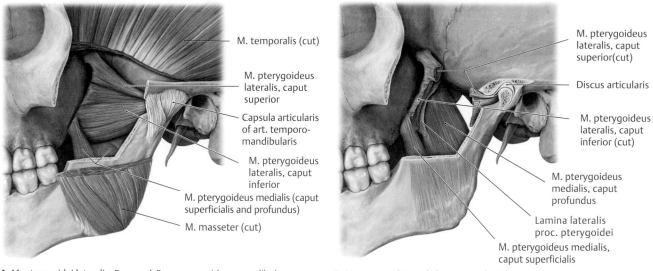

A M. pterygoidei lateralis. *Removed:* Proc. coronoideus mandibula.

B M. pterygoidei medialis. *Removed:* M. temporalis, m. masseter. *Cut:* M. pterygoidei lateralis.

Fig. 27.8 Musculi pterygoidei lateralis and medialis
Left lateral view. (From Schuenke M, Schulte E, Schumacher U. THIEME Atlas of Anatomy, Vol 3. Illustrations by Voll M and Wesker K. 3rd ed. New York: Thieme Publishers; 2020.)

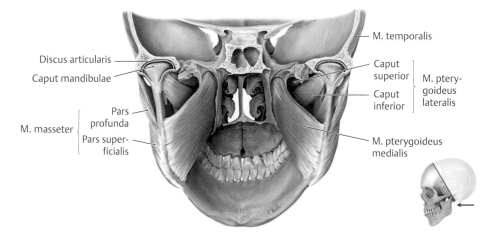

Fig. 27.9 Masticatory muscular sling
Oblique posterior view. *Revealed:* Muscular sling formed by the m. masseter and m. pterygoideus medialis that embed the mandibula. (From Schuenke M, Schulte E, Schumacher U. THIEME Atlas of Anatomy, Vol 3. Illustrations by Voll M and Wesker K. 3rd ed. New York: Thieme Publishers; 2020.)

Table 27.3 Muscles of Mastication

Muscle		Origin	Insertion	Innervation	Action
M. masseter		Pars superficialis: Arcus zygomaticus (anterior two thirds)	Angulus mandibulae (tuberositas masseterica)	N. mandibularis (CN V$_3$) via n. massetericus	Elevates (entire muscle) and protrudes (superficial fibers) mandibula
		Pars profunda: Arcus zygomaticus (posterior one third)			
M. temporalis		Fossa temporalis (linea temporalis inferior ossis parietalis)	Proc. coronoiodeus mandibulae (apex and medial surface)	N. mandibularis (CN V$_3$) via nn. temporales profundi	*Vertical fibers:* elevate mandibula *Horizontal fibers:* retract (retrude) mandibula *Unilateral:* lateral movement of mandibula (chewing)
M. pterygoideus lateralis	Caput superior	Ala major ossis sphenoidalis (crista infratemporalis)	Art. temporomandibularis (discus articularis)	N. mandibularis (CN V$_3$) via n. pterygoideus lateralis	*Bilateral:* protrudes mandibula (pulls discus articularis forward) *Unilateral:* lateral movements of mandibula (chewing)
	Caput inferior	Lamina lateralis processus pterygoidei (lateral surface)	Proc. condylaris mandibulae		
M. pterygoideus medialis	Caput superficiale	Tuber maxillae	Tuberositas pterygoidea on medial surface of the angulus mandibulae	N. mandibularis (CN V$_3$) via n. pterygoideus medialis	*Bilateral:* elevates mandibula with m. masseter; contributes to protrusion *Unilateral:* small grinding movements
	Caput profundum	Medial surface of lamina lateralis processus pterygoidei and fossa pterygoidea			

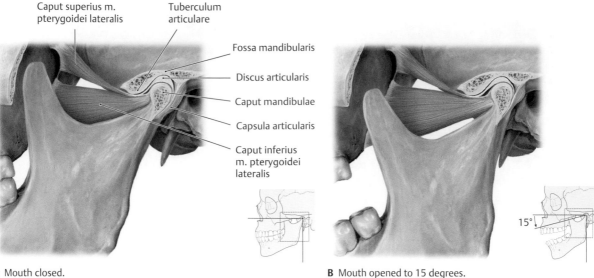

A Mouth closed.

B Mouth opened to 15 degrees.

C Mouth opened past 15 degrees.

Fig. 27.10 Movement of the articulatio temporomandibularis
Left lateral view. During the first 15 degrees of mandibular depression (opening of the mouth), the head of the mandibula remains in the fossa mandibularis. Past 15 degrees, the caput mandibulae glides forward onto the tuberculum articulare. (From Gilroy AM et al. Atlas of Anatomy. 4th ed. 2020. Based on: Schuenke M, Schulte E, Schumacher U. THIEME Atlas of Anatomy. Head, Neck, and Neuroanatomy. Illustrations by Voll M and Wesker K. 3rd ed. New York: Thieme Medical Publishers; 2020.)

BOX 27.2: CLINICAL CORRELATION

DISLOCATION OF THE ARTICULATIO TEMPOROMANDIBULARIS
During yawning (or other activities in which the mouth opens very widely), the caput mandibulae moves forward from the fossa mandibularis onto the tuberculum articulare. In some individuals this may cause the condylus mandibulae to slide in front of the tuberculum articulare, where it locks the mandibula in the protruded position. The ligamenta supporting the joint become stretched, which causes severe spasm (trismus) of the m. masseter, m. pterygoideus medialis, and m. temporalis.

region and in the fossa temporalis and fossa infratemporalis. All are innervated by CN V_3, the n. mandibularis of the n. trigeminus.

- The mm. masticatorii act primarily to close the jaw and move the upper teeth against the lower teeth in a grinding motion. The mouth is opened primarily by the mm. suprahyoidei with the assistance of the m. pterygoideus lateralis.
- The m. temporalis is the most powerful of these muscles and does approximately half of the work of mastication.
- The m. masseter, which has superficial and deep parts, raises the mandibula and closes the mouth.
- The m. pterygoideus lateralis initiates opening of the mouth, which is then continued by the mm. suprahyoidei. Because it's attached to the discus articularis, it guides the movement of the joint.
- The m. pterygoideus medialis runs almost perpendicular to the m. pterygoideus lateralis and contributes to the **masticatory muscular sling**.
- The m. masseter and m. pterygoideus medialis form a muscular sling that suspends the mandibula. By combining the actions of both muscles, the sling enables powerful closure of the jaws.

27.3 Parotid Region

The parotid region (regio parotideamasseterica) lies superficial to the ramus of the mandibulae and includes the gl. parotidea and its surrounding structures (**Figs. 27.11** and **27.12**).

- The **parotid gland (gl. parotidea)**, the largest of the three salivary glands, lies anterior to the ear on the lateral side of the face.
  - A superficial part of the gland lies on the m. masseter.
  - A deep part of the gland curves around the posterior edge of the ramus mandibulae.
  - A tough fascia parotidea derived from the deep cervical fascia encloses the gland.

- Secretomotor (parasympathetic) fibers to the gl. parotidea arise with the n. glossopharyngeus (CN IX) and synapse in the ganglion oticum. Postganglionic fibers hitchhike on the n. auriculotemporalis CN V$_3$.
- The **ductus parotideus** crosses the m. masseter superficially to pierce the m. buccinator and enter the mouth, where it opens into the oral vestibule opposite the second upper molar tooth.
- The plexus intraparotideus, formed by the n. facialis (CN VII), is embedded within the gl. parotidea and gives rise to five branches that supply muscles of the face: the rr. temporales, rr. zygomatici, rr. buccales, r. marginalis mandibularis, and r. cervicalis (r. colli) (see **Fig. 27.24**).

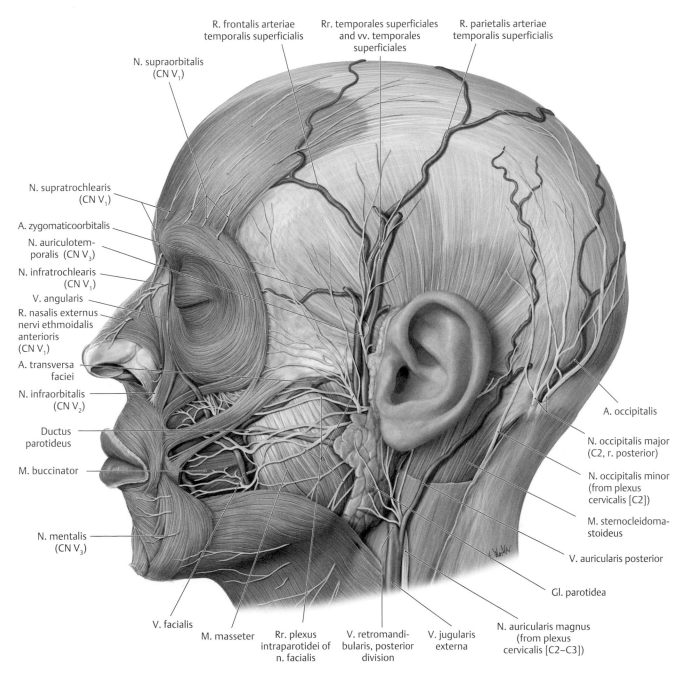

Fig. 27.11 Glandula parotidea
Left lateral view. *Note:* The ductus parotideus penetrates the m. buccinator to open opposite the second upper molar. (From Gilroy AM et al. Atlas of Anatomy. 4th ed. 2020. Based on: Schuenke M, Schulte E, Schumacher U. THIEME Atlas of Anatomy. Head, Neck, and Neuroanatomy. Illustrations by Voll M and Wesker K. 3rd ed. New York: Thieme Medical Publishers; 2020.)

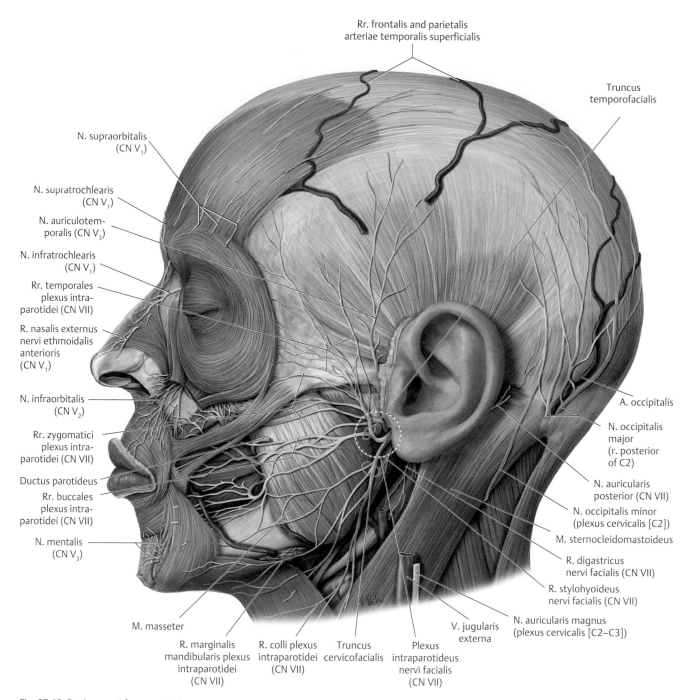

Rr. frontalis and parietalis
arteriae temporalis superficialis

Truncus
temporofacialis

N. supraorbitalis
(CN V₁)

N. supratrochlearis
(CN V₁)

N. auriculotem-
poralis (CN V₃)

N. infratrochlearis
(CN V₁)

Rr. temporales
plexus intra-
parotidei (CN VII)

R. nasalis externus
nervi ethmoidalis
anterioris
(CN V₁)

N. infraorbitalis
(CN V₂)

Rr. zygomatici
plexus intra-
parotidei (CN VII)

Ductus parotideus

Rr. buccales
plexus intra-
parotidei (CN VII)

N. mentalis
(CN V₃)

A. occipitalis

N. occipitalis
major
(r. posterior
of C2)

N. auricularis
posterior (CN VII)

N. occipitalis minor
(plexus cervicalis [C2])

M. sternocleidomastoideus

R. digastricus
nervi facialis (CN VII)

R. stylohyoideus
nervi facialis (CN VII)

N. auricularis magnus
(plexus cervicalis [C2–C3])

M. masseter

R. marginalis
mandibularis plexus
intraparotidei
(CN VII)

R. colli plexus
intraparotidei
(CN VII)

Truncus
cervicofacialis

Plexus
intraparotideus
nervi facialis
(CN VII)

V. jugularis
externa

Fig. 27.12 Regio parotideamasseterica
Left lateral view. *Removed:* Gl. parotidea, m. sternocleidomastoideus, and vv. capitis. (From Gilroy AM et al. Atlas of Anatomy. 4th ed. 2020. Based on: Schuenke M, Schulte E, Schumacher U. THIEME Atlas of Anatomy. Head, Neck, and Neuroanatomy. Illustrations by Voll M and Wesker K. 3rd ed. New York: Thieme Medical Publishers; 2020.)

— Structures traversing, or embedded within, the gl. parotidea include
  • the plexus intraparotideus of n. facialis (CN VII);
  • the v. retromandibularis, formed by the v. temporalis superficialis and v. maxillaris;
  • the a. carotis externa and the origin of its rami terminales, the a. temporalis superficialis and a. maxillaris; and
  • the nll. parotidei, which drain the gl. parotidea, the auris externa, the forehead, and the regio parotideamasseterica.

27.4   Fossa Temporalis

The fossa temporalis lies superior and medial to the regio parotideamasseterica and covers the lateral aspect of the head (**Figs. 27.13** and **27.14**).

— The boundaries of the fossa temporalis are
  • anteriorly, the proc. frontalis of the os zygomaticum and proc. zygomaticus of the os frontale;
  • laterally, the arcus zygomaticus;
  • medially, the os frontale, os parietale, ala major of os sphenoidale, and pars squamosa of os temporale; and
  • inferiorly, the fossa infratemporalis.

Fig. 27.13 Fossa temporalis

Left lateral view. The fossa temporalis lies on the lateral surface of the skull, medial and superior to the arcus zygomaticus. (From Gilroy AM et al. Atlas of Anatomy. 4th ed. 2020. Based on: Schuenke M, Schulte E, Schumacher U. THIEME Atlas of Anatomy. Head, Neck, and Neuroanatomy. Illustrations by Voll M and Wesker K. 3rd ed. New York: Thieme Medical Publishers; 2020.)

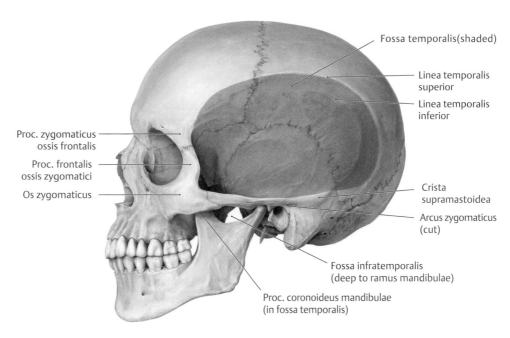

Fossa temporalis(shaded)

Linea temporalis superior

Linea temporalis inferior

Proc. zygomaticus ossis frontalis

Proc. frontalis ossis zygomatici

Os zygomaticus

Crista supramastoidea

Arcus zygomaticus (cut)

Fossa infratemporalis (deep to ramus mandibulae)

Proc. coronoideus mandibulae (in fossa temporalis)

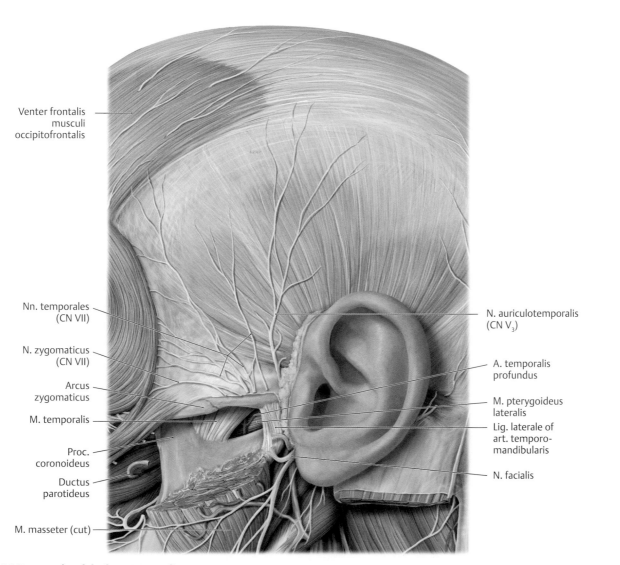

Venter frontalis musculi occipitofrontalis

Nn. temporales (CN VII)

N. zygomaticus (CN VII)

Arcus zygomaticus

M. temporalis

Proc. coronoideus

Ductus parotideus

M. masseter (cut)

N. auriculotemporalis (CN V₃)

A. temporalis profundus

M. pterygoideus lateralis

Lig. laterale of art. temporo-mandibularis

N. facialis

Fig. 27.14 Topography of the fossa temporalis

Left lateral view. *Cut:* M. masseter. *Revealed:* Fossa temporalis and art. temporomandibularis. (From Baker EW. Anatomy for Dental Medicine, 2nd ed. New York: Thieme; 2015)

— The fossa temporalis contains
  • the m. temporalis and **fascia temporalis**,
  • the a. temporalis superficialis and v. temporalis superficialis,
  • the **aa. temporales profundi** from the **a. maxillaris**, and
  • the **nn. temporales profundi** and **n. auriculotemporalis** of the **n. mandibularis** of the **n. trigeminus** (CN V₃).

27.5   Fossa Infratemporalis

The fossa infratemporalis lies deep to the ramus mandibulae and is continuous superiorly with the fossa temporalis (**Fig. 27.15**).
— The bony boundaries of the fossa infratemporalis are
  • anteriorly, the posterior wall of the maxilla;
  • posteriorly, the fossa mandibularis of the os temporale;
  • medially, the proc. pterygoideus lamina lateralis of os sphenoidale;
  • laterally the ramus mandibulae; and
  • superiorly, the os temporale and ala major of os sphenoidale.

— The fossa infratemporalis communicates with the orbita anteriorly, the fossa pterygopalatina medially, and the fossa cranii media superiorly.
— The contents of the fossa infratemporalis (**Figs. 27.16** and **27.17**) include
  • the art. temporomandibularis,
  • the m. pterygoideus medius and m. pterygoideus lateralis and the inferior part of m. temporalis,
  • the a. maxillaris and its branches (**Table 27.4**),
  • the plexus venosus pterygoideus,
  • the n. mandibularis of the n. trigeminus (CN V₃) and its branches,
  • the ganglion oticum, and
  • the chorda tympani of the n. facialis (CN VII).
— The n. mandibularis (CN V₃), the nerve of the fossa infratemporalis and the only division of the n. trigeminus that carries general sensory and somatic motor fibers, distributes postganglionic parasympathetic (visceral motor) fibers that arise from the ganglion oticum and ganglion submandibulare (**Fig. 27.18, Table 27.5**; see **Fig. 27.4**).

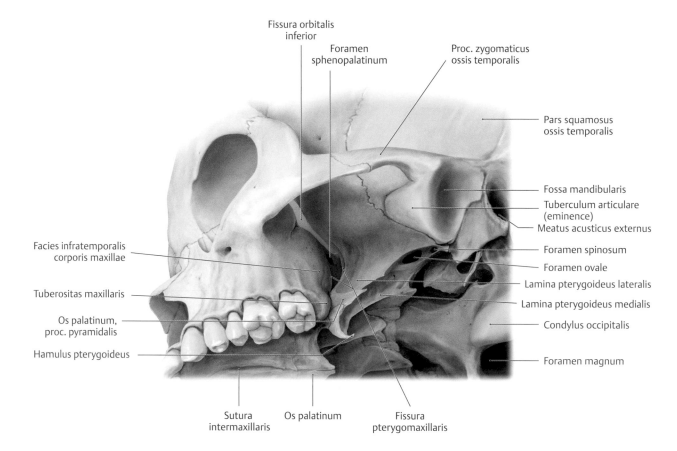

Fig. 27.15 Bony boundaries of the fossa infratemporalis
Oblique external view of the base of the skull. (From Gilroy AM et al. Atlas of Anatomy. 4th ed. 2020. Based on: Schuenke M, Schulte E, Schumacher U. THIEME Atlas of Anatomy. Head, Neck, and Neuroanatomy. Illustrations by Voll M and Wesker K. 3rd ed. New York: Thieme Medical Publishers; 2020.)

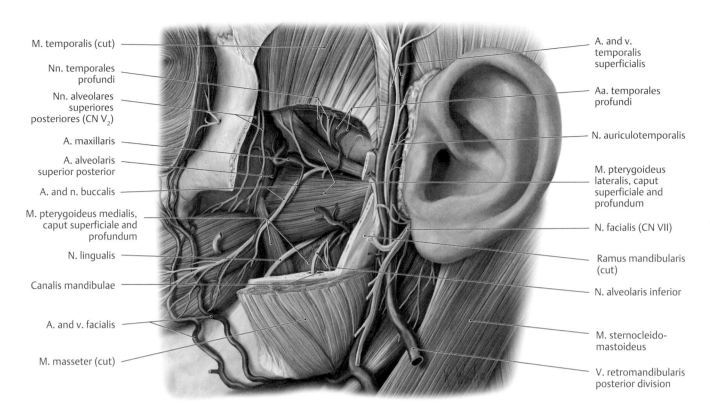

M. temporalis (cut)

Nn. temporales profundi

Nn. alveolares superiores posteriores (CN V₂)

A. maxillaris

A. alveolaris superior posterior

A. and n. buccalis

M. pterygoideus medialis, caput superficiale and profundum

N. lingualis

Canalis mandibulae

A. and v. facialis

M. masseter (cut)

A. and v. temporalis superficialis

Aa. temporales profundi

N. auriculotemporalis

M. pterygoideus lateralis, caput superficiale and profundum

N. facialis (CN VII)

Ramus mandibularis (cut)

N. alveolaris inferior

M. sternocleido-mastoideus

V. retromandibularis posterior division

Fig. 27.16 Fossa infratemporalis: Superficial layer
Left lateral view. *Removed:* Ramus mandibularis. (From Gilroy AM et al. Atlas of Anatomy. 4th ed. 2020. Based on: Schuenke M, Schulte E, Schumacher U. THIEME Atlas of Anatomy. Head, Neck, and Neuroanatomy. Illustrations by Voll M and Wesker K. 3rd ed. New York: Thieme Medical Publishers; 2020.)

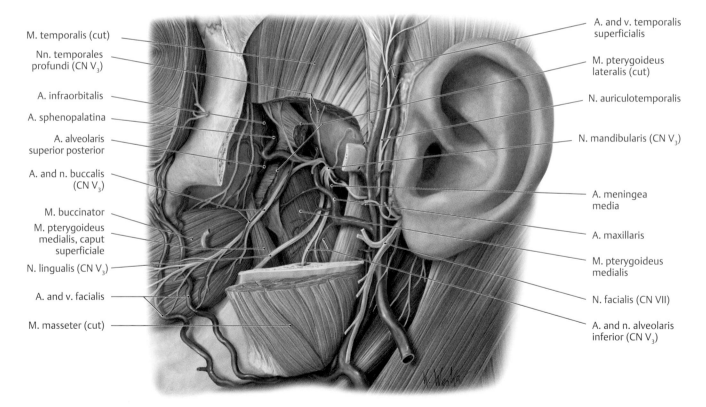

M. temporalis (cut)

Nn. temporales profundi (CN V₃)

A. infraorbitalis

A. sphenopalatina

A. alveolaris superior posterior

A. and n. buccalis (CN V₃)

M. buccinator

M. pterygoideus medialis, caput superficiale

N. lingualis (CN V₃)

A. and v. facialis

M. masseter (cut)

A. and v. temporalis superficialis

M. pterygoideus lateralis (cut)

N. auriculotemporalis

N. mandibularis (CN V₃)

A. meningea media

A. maxillaris

M. pterygoideus medialis

N. facialis (CN VII)

A. and n. alveolaris inferior (CN V₃)

Fig. 27.17 Fossa infratemporalis: Deep dissection
Left lateral view. *Removed:* M. pterygoideus lateralis (both heads).
Revealed: Deep fossa infratemporalis and n. mandibularis as it enters the canalis mandibulae via the foramen ovale in the roof of the fossa. (From Gilroy AM et al. Atlas of Anatomy. 4th ed. 2020. Based on: Schuenke M, Schulte E, Schumacher U. THIEME Atlas of Anatomy. Head, Neck, and Neuroanatomy. Illustrations by Voll M and Wesker K. 3rd ed. New York: Thieme Medical Publishers; 2020.)

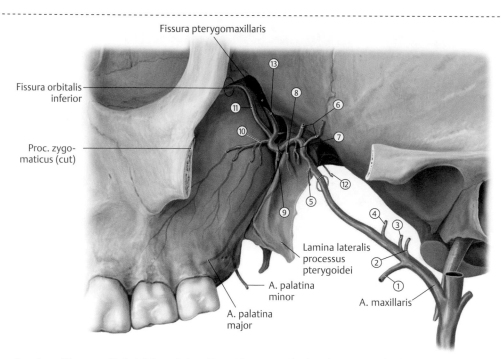

Branches of the a. maxillaris, left lateral view. (From Gilroy AM et al. Atlas of Anatomy. 4th ed. 2020. Based on: Schuenke M, Schulte E, Schumacher U. THIEME Atlas of Anatomy. Head, Neck, and Neuroanatomy. Illustrations by Voll M and Wesker K. 3rd ed. New York: Thieme Medical Publishers; 2020.)

Table 27.4 Branches of the Arteria Maxillaris

Part	Artery		Distribution
Pars mandibularis (between the origin and the first circle around artery)	① A. alveolaris inferior		Mandibula, dentes, gingiva
	② A. tympanica superior		Cavitas tympani
	③ A. auricularis profunda		Art. temporomandibularis, meatus acusticus externus
	④ A. meningea media		Calvaria, dura mater, fossa cranii anterior and media
Pars pterygoideus (between circles around the artery)	⑤ A. masseterica		M. masseter
	⑥ Aa. temporales profundae		M. temporalis
	⑦ Rr. pterygoidei		Mm. pterygoidei
	⑧ A. buccalis		Tunica mucosa buccae
Pars pterygopalatina (from second circle through the pterygomaxillary fissure)	⑨ A. palatina descendens	A. palatina major	Palatum durum
		A. palatina minor	Palatum molle, tonsilla palatina, pharyngeal wall
	⑩ A. alveolaris superior posterior		Dentes molares maxillares, sinus maxillaris, gingiva
	⑪ A. infraorbitalis		Alveoli dentales maxillae, maxillary incisors and canines, sinus maxillaris, and skin of the midface
	⑫ A. canalis pterygoidei		Upper nasopharynx, tuba auditiva, and sinus sphenoidalis
	⑬ A. sphenopalatina	Aa. nasales posteriores laterales	Lateral wall of cavitas nasi and choanae
		Rr. septales posteriores	Septum nasi

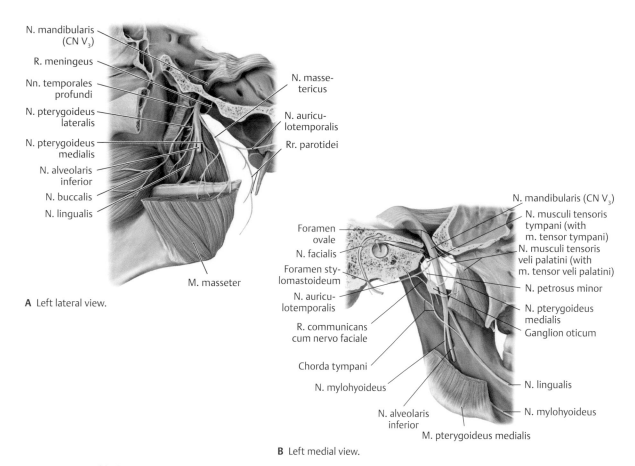

A Left lateral view.

B Left medial view.

Fig. 27.18 Nervus mandibularis (CN V₃) in the fossa infratemporalis
(From Gilroy AM et al. Atlas of Anatomy. 4th ed. 2020. Based on: Schuenke M, Schulte E, Schumacher U. THIEME Atlas of Anatomy. Head, Neck, and Neuroanatomy. Illustrations by Voll M and Wesker K. 3rd ed. New York: Thieme Medical Publishers; 2020.)

Table 27.5 Nerves of the Fossa Infratemporalis

Nerve	Nerve Fibers	Distribution
Muscular branches (CN V₃)	Branchial motor	Mm. masticatorii; m. mylohyoideus; m. tensor tympani; m. tensor veli palatini, anterior belly of m. digastricus
N. auriculotemporalis (CN V₃)	General sensory	Auriculus, regio temporalis. and art. temporomandibularis
	Visceral motor from n. glossopharyngealis (CN IX)	Gl. parotidea
N. alveolaris inferior (CN V₃)	General sensory	Dentes mandibulares; mental branch supplies skin of lower lip and chin
N. lingualis (CN V₃)	General sensory	Anterior two thirds of lingua, floor of mouth, and lingual mandibular gingiva
N. buccalis (CN V₃)	General sensory	Skin and mucous membrane of cheek
R. meningeus (CN V₃)	General sensory	Dura of fossa cranii media
Chorda tympani (CN VII)	Special sensory taste	Anterior two thirds of lingua
	Visceral motor	Gll. submandibulares and sublinguales via ganglion submandibulare and n. lingualis (CN V₃).

27.6   Fossa Pterygopalatina

The **fossa pterygopalatina**, a narrow space located medial to the fossa infratemporale, is an important distribution center for branches of the n. maxillaris of the n. trigeminus (CN V_2) and the accompanying branches of the a. maxillaris.

— The bony boundaries of the fossa pterygopalatina **(Fig. 27.19)** are
  • superiorly, the apex of the orbita;
  • anteriorly, the sinus maxillaris;
  • posteriorly, the os sphenoidale, proc. pterygoideus, lamina lateralis;
  • laterally, the **fissura pterygomaxillaris**; and
  • medially, the lamina perpendicularis ossis palatini.

— Contents of the fossa pterygopalatina include
  • the pars pterygopalatina of a. maxillaris, its branches, and its accompanying veins;
  • the n. canalis pterygoidei;
  • the ganglion pterygopalatinum; and
  • the n. maxillaris of the n. trigeminus (CN V_2) and its branches.

— The fossa pterygopalatina communicates anteriorly with the orbita, medially with the cavitas nasi and palate, and posteriorly with the fossa cranii media and basis cranii **(Table 27.6)**.

— The a. maxillaris passes from the fossa infratemporalis to the fossa pterygopalatina through the fissura pterygomaxillaris (see **Table 27.4**). Its branches accompany the branches of the n. maxillaris (CN V_2) to supply the nose, palate, and pharynx.

— The **n. canalis pterygoidei**, which enters the fossa pterygopalatina from the fossa cranii medius, is an autonomic nerve that carries
  • preganglionic parasympathetic fibers from the **n. petrosus major,** a branch of the **n. facialis** (CN VII); and
  • postganglionic sympathetic fibers from the **deep petrosal nerve,** which arises from the plexus caroticus internus.

— The ganglion pterygopalatinum receives general sensory fibers from the **n. pertrosus profundus** (CN V_2) and parasympathetic and sympathetic fibers from the n. canalis pterygoidei. Only the parasympathetic fibers synapse in the ganglion; general sensory and sympathetic fibers pass through the ganglion but do not synapse there **(Table 27.7)**.

— The n. maxillaris of the n. trigeminus (CN V_2)
  • passes from the fossa cranii media to the fossa pterygopalatina through the **foramen rotundum;**
  • suspends the ganglion pterygopalatinum by two small **rr. ganglionares,** which transmit general sensory fibers of the n. maxillaris;
  • distributes postganglionic parasympathetic (secretomotor) and sympathetic (vasoconstrictive) fibers to the gll. lacrimales, gll. nasales, gll. palatinae, and gll. pharyngeales; and
  • distributes general sensory fibers to the midface, sinus maxillaris, dentes maxillares, cavitas nasi, palate, and superior pharynx.

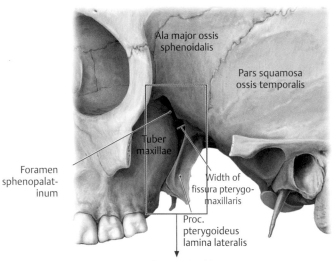

Ala major ossis sphenoidalis

Pars squamosa ossis temporalis

Tuber maxillae

Foramen sphenopalatinum

Width of fissura pterygomaxillaris

Proc. pterygoideus lamina lateralis

See detail in **B** and **Table 27.6**

A Left lateral view. The lateral approach through the fossa infratemporalis via the fissura pterygomaxillaris.

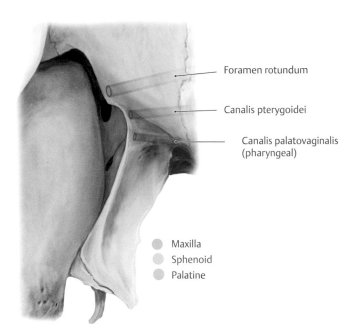

Foramen rotundum

Canalis pterygoidei

Canalis palatovaginalis (pharyngeal)

○ Maxilla
○ Sphenoid
○ Palatine

B Left lateral view. This color-coded version shows the location of the role of ossis palatini.

Fig. 27.19 Fossa pterygopalatina
(From Gilroy AM et al. Atlas of Anatomy. 4th ed. 2020. Based on: Schuenke M, Schulte E, Schumacher U. THIEME Atlas of Anatomy. Head, Neck, and Neuroanatomy. Illustrations by Voll M and Wesker K. 3rd ed. New York: Thieme Medical Publishers; 2020.)

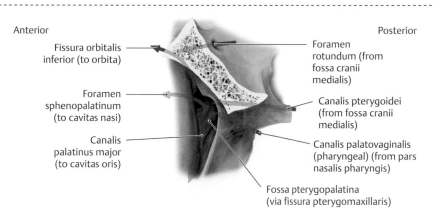

Anterior

Fissura orbitalis
inferior (to orbita)

Foramen
sphenopalatinum
(to cavitas nasi)

Canalis
palatinus major
(to cavitas oris)

Posterior

Foramen
rotundum (from
fossa cranii
medialis)

Canalis pterygoidei
(from fossa cranii
medialis)

Canalis palatovaginalis
(pharyngeal) (from pars
nasalis pharyngis)

Fossa pterygopalatina
(via fissura pterygomaxillaris)

(From Gilroy AM et al. Atlas of Anatomy. 4th ed. 2020. Based on: Schuenke M, Schulte E, Schumacher U. THIEME Atlas of Anatomy. Head, Neck, and Neuroanatomy. Illustrations by Voll M and Wesker K. 3rd ed. New York: Thieme Medical Publishers; 2020.)

Table 27.6 Communications of the Fossa Pterygopalatina

Communication	Direction	Via	Transmitted structures
Fossa cranii medialis	Posterosuperiorly	Foramen rotundum	• N. maxillaris (CN V$_2$)
Fossa cranii medialis	Posteriorly in anterior wall of foramen lacerum	Canalis pterygoidei	• N. canalis pterygoidei, formed from: 　◦ N. petrosus major (preganglionic parasympathetic fibers from CN VII) 　◦ N. petrosus profundus (postganglionic sympathetic fibers from plexus caroticus internus) • A. canalis pterygoidei • Vv. canalis pterygoidei
Orbita	Anterosuperiorly	Fissura orbitalis inferior	• Branches of n. maxillaris (CN V$_2$): 　◦ N. infraorbitalis 　◦ N. zygomaticus • A. infraorbitalis (and accompanying vv.) • Vv. communicantes between v. ophthalmica inferior and vv. plexus pterygoideus
Cavitas nasi	Medially	Foramen sphenopalatinum	• Rr. nasales posteriores superiores mediales and laterales and posteriores inferiores (from n. nasopalatinus, CN V$_2$) • A. sphenopalatina (with accompanying vv.)
Cavitas oris	Inferiorly	Canalis palatinus major (foramen)	• N. palatina descendens major (CN V$_2$) and a. palatina major • Branches that emerge through canalis palatinae minores: 　◦ Nn. palatinae minores (CN V$_2$) and aa. palatinae minores
Pars nasalis pharyngis	Inferoposteriorly	Canalis palatovaginalis (pharyngeal)	• Rr. pharyngeales of n. maxillaris (CN V$_2$), and a. pharyngealis
Fossa infratemporalis	Laterally	Fissura pterygomaxillaris	• Pars pterygopalatina a. maxillaris • N., a., and v. alveolaris posterior superior

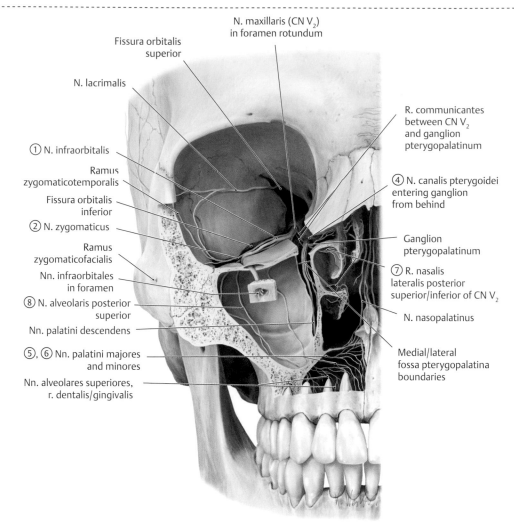

N. maxillaris (CN V₂)
in foramen rotundum

Fissura orbitalis
superior

N. lacrimalis

R. communicantes
between CN V₂
and ganglion
pterygopalatinum

① N. infraorbitalis

Ramus
zygomaticotemporalis

④ N. canalis pterygoidei
entering ganglion
from behind

Fissura orbitalis
inferior

② N. zygomaticus

Ganglion
pterygopalatinum

Ramus
zygomaticofacialis

⑦ R. nasalis
lateralis posterior
superior/inferior of CN V₂

Nn. infraorbitales
in foramen

⑧ N. alveolaris posterior
superior

N. nasopalatinus

Nn. palatini descendens

⑤, ⑥ Nn. palatini majores
and minores

Medial/lateral
fossa pterygopalatina
boundaries

Nn. alveolares superiores,
r. dentalis/gingivalis

Coronal view of the fossa pterygopalatina
(From Gilroy AM et al. Atlas of Anatomy. 4th ed. 2020. Based on: Schuenke M, Schulte E, Schumacher U.
THIEME Atlas of Anatomy. Head, Neck, and Neuroanatomy. Illustrations by Voll M and Wesker K. 3rd ed. New
York: Thieme Medical Publishers; 2020.)

Table 27.7 Nerves of the Fossa Pterygopalatina

Nerve	Motor Innervation	Sensory Distribution
① N. infraorbitalis (CN V₂)		Skin of the midface, sinus maxillaris, teeth, and gingiva
② N. zygomaticus (CN V₂)–communicating branch from n. zygomaticotemporalis		Skin of lateral cheek, temple
③ Rr. orbitales (CN V₂)		Orbita, sinus ethmoidalis, and sinus sphenoidalis
④ N. canalis pterygoidei (CN VII)	Visceral motor (preganglionic parasympathetic and postganglionic sympathetic) to glands of the nasal mucosa and palatum; gl. lacrimalis	
⑤ N. palatinus major (CN V₂)		Hard palate and palatal gingiva
⑥ N. palatinus minor (CN V₂)		Palatum molle, tonsilla palatina
⑦ Medial and lateral rr. nasales posteriores superiores and inferiores (CN V₂)		Septum nasi, upper lateral nasal wall, sinus ethmoidalis
⑧ Posterior superior alveolar n. (CN V₂)		Sinus maxillaris, cheeks, buccal gingiva, maxillary molars

27.7 Cavitas Nasi

The **cavitas nasi** is located in the middle of the face between the orbitae and sinus maxillaris and above the cavitas oris.

Structure of the Cavitas Nasi

The nose has an external portion and paired internal cavitates nasi that are separated by a septum nasi (**Figs. 27.20** and **27.21**).
— The external nose consists of
  • anteriorly, the **cartilago alaris** and **cartilagines nasi laterales**, which form the nasal **ala** and **crura** surrounding the nostrils and the **apex nasi**, or tip of the nose; and
  • posteriorly, the os frontale, maxilla, and os nasale, which form the **radix nasi**, or bridge, of the nose.
— The nasal cavities are pyramidally shaped spaces that communicate anteriorly with the outside through the **nares** (anterior nasal apertures) and posteriorly with the pars nasalis pharyngis through the **choanae.**
— The lateral walls of the cavitates nasi are formed by the concha nasalis superior and concha nasalis media of os ethmoidale; the conchae nasales inferiores; and the maxilla, os palatinum, os lacrimale, and os nasale.
  • The conchae nasales superior, media, and inferior are scrolllike bony processes that project into the cavitas nasi.
  • The **meatus nasi superior**, **meatus nasi medius**, and **meatus nasi inferior** are recesses below the respective conchae nasales.
— The septum nasi forms the medial wall of each cavitas nasi and consists of the vomer, the lamina perpendicularis of os ethmoidale, and the cartilago septi nasi.
— The **palatum durum**, consisting of the maxilla and os palatinum, forms the inferior surface of the cavitates nasi and separates them from the cavitas oris (see Section 27.8).
— **Sinus paranasales** are air-filled cavities within bones of the skull that communicate with the cavitates nasi (**Fig. 27.22; Table 27.8**).
  • Paired **sinus frontalis**, which are usually asymmetrical, lie above the radix nasi and drain into the meatus nasi medius through a **ductus frontonasalis** into the **hiatus semilunaris.**
  • **Sinus sphenoidalis**, which form within the body of the os sphenoidale, lie between the right and left sinus cavernosus and drain into the **recessus sphenoethmoidalis** in the posterosuperior part of the cavitates nasi above the concha superior.
  • **Cellulae ethmoidales** compose the medial wall of the orbita and are formed by numerous thin-walled ethmoid air cells. They lie between the orbitae above the cavitates nasi and drain into the meatus nasi superior and meatus nasi medius.
  • Paired **sinus maxillaris**, the largest of the sinus paranasales, lie on either side of the cavitates nasi, inferior to the orbitae, and drain into the meatus nasi medius.
— A **ductus nasolacrimalis** drains tears from the medial corner of each eye and empties into the meatus nasi inferior on each side.

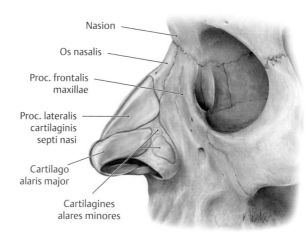

A Left lateral view.

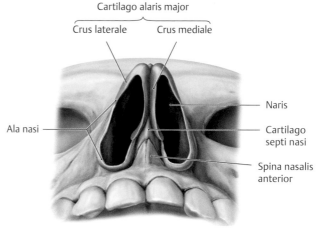

B Inferior view.

Fig. 27.20 Skeleton of the nose
The skeleton of the nose is composed of an upper bony portion and a lower cartilaginous portion. The proximal portions of the nostrils (alae) are composed of connective tissue with small embedded pieces of cartilage. (From Schuenke M, Schulte E, Schumacher U. THIEME Atlas of Anatomy, Vol 3. Illustrations by Voll M and Wesker K. 3rd ed. New York: Thieme Publishers; 2020.)

BOX 27.3: CLINICAL CORRELATION

INFECTION OF THE SINUS MAXILLARIS
Infections arising in the cavitas nasi may spread to any of the sinus paranasales, but the sinus maxillaris are the most commonly affected. Mucus builds up within the sinus maxillaris and is unable to drain because their ostia are located high on the superomedial walls. The ostia are also commonly obstructed by inflammation of the mucous membranes of the sinuses (maxillary sinusitis). Maxillary sinusitis usually follows the common cold or influenza virus but may also arise from the spread of infections from posterior dentes maxillares.

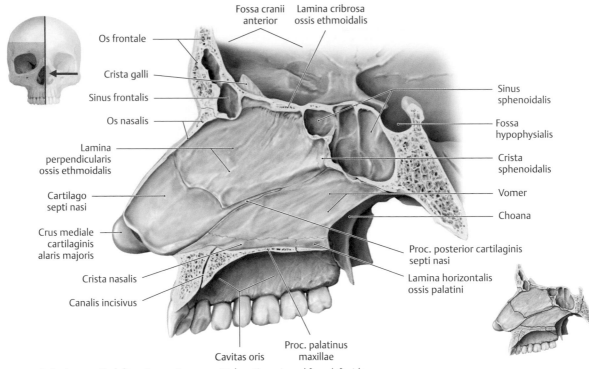

A Septum nasi in left cavitas nasi, parasagittal section, viewed from left side.

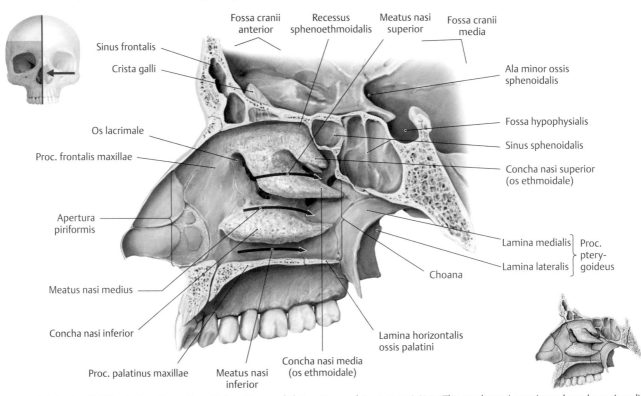

B Lateral wall of the right cavitas nasi, sagittal section, medial view. *Removed:* Septum nasi. *Note:* The concha nasi superior and concha nasi media are parts of the os ethmoidale, whereas the concha nasi inferior is a separate bone. *Arrows* indicate the direction of airflow through the concha nasi.

Fig. 27.21 Bones of the cavitas nasi

The left and right cavitates nasi are flanked by lateral walls and separated by the septum nasi. Air enters the cavitas nasi through the apertura piriformis and travels through three passages: the meatus nasi superior, medius, and inferior (**B**, *arrows*). These passages are separated by the concha nasi superior, media, and inferior. Air leaves the nose through the choanae, entering the nasopharynx. (From Schuenke M, Schulte E, Schumacher U. THIEME Atlas of Anatomy, Vol 3. Illustrations by Voll M and Wesker K. 3rd ed. New York: Thieme Publishers; 2020.)

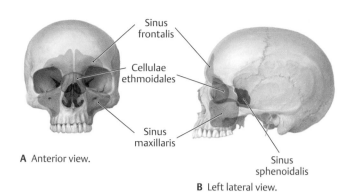

A Anterior view.

B Left lateral view.

Fig. 27.22 Location of the sinus paranasales
The sinus paranasales (sinus frontalis, maxillaris, and sphenoidalis and cellulae ethmoidales) are air-filled cavities that reduce the weight of the crabium. (From Schuenke M, Schulte E, Schumacher U. THIEME Atlas of Anatomy, Vol 3. Illustrations by Voll M and Wesker K. 3rd ed. New York: Thieme Publishers; 2020.)

Neurovasculature of the Cavitas Nasi

— The a. carotis externa, via its maxillary and facial branches, and the a. carotis interna, via its ophthalmic branch, supply the cavitas nasi. The area of overlap between the external and internal circulations is referred to as Kiesselbach's area **(Fig. 27.23)**.
  • Nasal branches of the a. maxillaris include
    ○ the aa. nasales posteriores laterales and rr. septales posteriores, branches of the a. sphenopalatina; and
    ○ the a. palatina major, a branch of the a. palatina descendens.
  • Branches of the a. facialis include the a. nasalis lateralis and a septal artery, a branch of the a. labialis superior.
  • Branches of the a. ophthalmicus include a. ethmoidalis anterior and a. ethmoidalis posterior.
— Veins that drain the cavitas nasi form a submucosal plexus venosus that drains into the v. ophthalmica, v. facialis, and v. sphenopalatina.
— The n. olfactorius (CN I) and the n. ophthalmicus (CN V₁) and n. maxillaris (CN V₂) divisions of the n. trigeminus innervate the nose **(Fig. 27.24)**.
  • Nn. olfactorii, which are responsible for smell, arise from the olfactory epithelium in the roof of the cavitas nasi. They pass through the lamina cribrosa and end in the bulbi olfactorii.
  • Rr. infratrochleares and rr. ethmoidales anteriores of CN V₁ and the r. infraorbitalis of CN V₂ innervate the external nose.
  • The rr. ethmoidales anteriores and posteriores of CN V₁ innervate the external nose and the mucosa of the anterosuperior cavitas nasi through internal, external, medial, and lateral nasal branches.
  • The posterior nasal branches of the n. nasopalatinus on the septum and nasal branches of the n. palatinus major on the lateral walls (both branches of CN V₂) innervate the mucosa of the posteroinferior cavitas nasi.

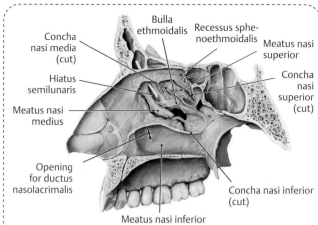

Openings of the sinus paranasales and ductus nasolacrimalis
Right nasal cavity, sagittal section, medial view. Mucosal secretions from the sinuses and ductus nasolacrimalis drain into the nose. (From Schuenke M, Schulte E, Schumacher U. THIEME Atlas of Anatomy, Vol 3. Illustrations by Voll M and Wesker K. 3rd ed. New York: Thieme Publishers; 2020.)

Table 27.8 Nasal Passages into which Sinuses Empty

Sinuses/duct		Nasal Passage	Via
Sinus sphenoidalis *(blue)*		Recessus sphenoethmoidalis	Direct
Cellulae ethmoidales *(green)*	Cellulae posteriores	Meatus nasi superior	Direct
	Cellulae anteriores and mediae	Meatus nasi medius	Bulla ethmoidalis
Sinus frontalis *(yellow)*		Meatus nasi medius	Ductus frontonasalis into hiatus semilunaris
Sinus maxillaris *(orange)*		Meatus nasi medius	Hiatus semilunaris
Ductus nasolacrimalis *(red)*		Meatus nasi inferior	Direct

BOX 27.4: CLINICAL CORRELATION

EPISTAXIS
Bleeding, or epistaxis, of the highly vascular nasal mucosa is a common consequence of nasal trauma, and even minor trauma can disrupt the veins in the vestibule. Most bleeding originates from the arteries of Kiesselbach's area, where branches of the a. carotis interna and a. carotis externa anastomose in the anterior third of the cavitas nasi. These include the a. sphenopalatina, a. palatina major, a. ethmoidalis anterior, and a. labialis superior.

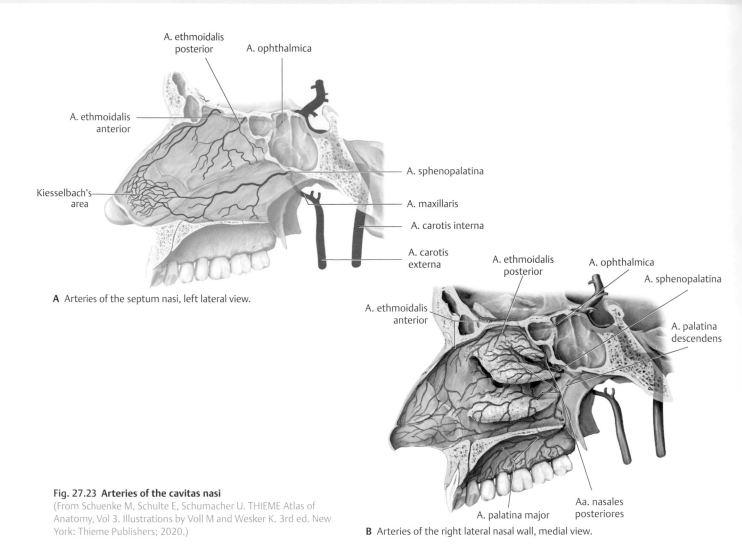

A   Arteries of the septum nasi, left lateral view.

Fig. 27.23 Arteries of the cavitas nasi
(From Schuenke M, Schulte E, Schumacher U. THIEME Atlas of Anatomy, Vol 3. Illustrations by Voll M and Wesker K. 3rd ed. New York: Thieme Publishers; 2020.)

B   Arteries of the right lateral nasal wall, medial view.

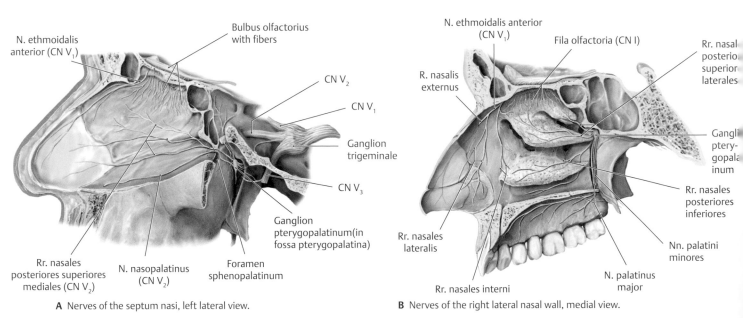

A   Nerves of the septum nasi, left lateral view.

B   Nerves of the right lateral nasal wall, medial view.

Fig. 27.24 Nerves of the cavitas nasi
(From Schuenke M, Schulte E, Schumacher U. THIEME Atlas of Anatomy, Vol 3. Illustrations by Voll M and Wesker K. 3rd ed. New York: Thieme Publishers; 2020.)

27.8 Oral Region

The cavitas oris, located below the cavitas nasi and anterior to the pharynx, is bounded superiorly by the palate, inferiorly by the tongue and muscular floor, anteriorly by the lips, posteriorly by the uvula, and laterally by the cheeks (**Fig. 27.25**).

Lips, Cheeks, Gingiva, Teeth, and Oral Cavity

— The **lips (labia oris)** frame the mouth and surround the **oral fissure (rima oris)**, the opening into the cavitas oris.
- The lips contain the sphincter-like m. obicularis oris and m. labialis superior and m. labialis inferior. Externally, they are covered by skin; internally, they are covered by the tunica mucosa of the cavitas oris.
- The **philtrum,** an external midline depression on the upper lip (labium superius), extends superiorly to the septum nasi.
- **Labial frenula** are midline folds of tunica mucosa that attach the inner surfaces of the upper and lower lips (labia superius and labia inferius) to the gums.

BOX 27.5: DEVELOPMENTAL CORRELATION

CLEFT LIP
Cleft lip is a congenital defect that occurs early in embryonic life when the prominentia maxillaris and the prominentia nasalis medialis fail to fuse. It is seen in ~ 1:1,000 live births and is more common in males than females. The cleft may be unilateral or bilateral and is described as complete when it extends into the nose and incomplete when it appears as a notch in the lip. Corrective surgery is usually performed when the infant is around 10 weeks old.

— The **cheeks (buccae)**, continuous with the lips, form the walls of the mouth and the **buccal region (regio buccalis)** of the face.
- The m. buccinator, innervated by the buccal branch of the n. facialis (CN VII), forms the movable wall of the cheek.

- Corpora adiposa buccae, encapsulated cushions of fat that lie superficial to the m. buccinator, are proportionately large in infants and reduced in adults.
- The os zygomaticum and arcus zygomaticus form the "cheek bone."

— Teeth are anchored in **alveoli** (sockets) of the **arcus dentalis maxillaris** and **arcus dentalis mandibularis** (**Figs. 27.26**).
- Children have 20 dentes decidui, which are replaced at predictable intervals between ages 7 and 25 years.
- Adult have 32 teeth, consisting of dentes incisivus, caninus, premolaris, and molaris. Teeth are numbered 1 to 16 from right to left along the maxillary arch, and 17 to 32 from left to right along the mandibular arch.

— The **gingivae,** or gums, made of fibrous tissue covered by the tunica mucosa of the cavitas oris, are firmly attached to the maxilla and mandible.

— The cavitas oris, or mouth, is divided into two regions: the **vestibulum oris** and the **cavitas oris propria** (**Fig. 27.27**).
- The vestibulum oris is the narrow space between the lips and cheeks and the arcus dentalis maxillaris and mandibularis.
- The cavitas oris propria is the space bounded anteriorly and laterally by the upper and lower arcus dentalis. Superiorly, the **palate (palatum)** forms the roof, and inferiorly, the tongue rests on a muscular floor.

— The cavitas oris connects posteriorly to the pharynx through a narrow space, the **isthmus faucium**.

— Muscles that form the floor of the mouth, the **mm. suprahyoidei**, are attached to the os hyoideum in the neck (**Fig. 27.28; Table 27.9**). They have a complex innervation with contributions from the n. trigeminus and n. facialis and the C1 n. spinalis via the n. hypoglossus. (**Fig. 27.29;** see also **Fig. 25.7**).

— The a. lingualis, a. facialis, and a. maxillaris branches of the a. carotis externa supply the lips, cheeks, floor of the mouth, and upper and lower teeth.

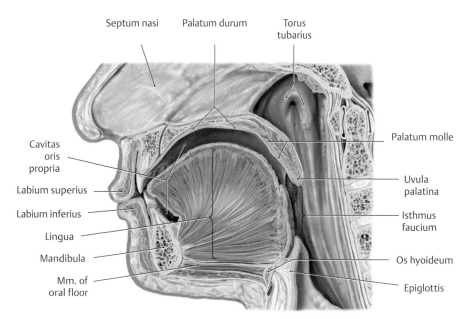

Septum nasi · Palatum durum · Torus tubarius · Palatum molle · Cavitas oris propria · Labium superius · Labium inferius · Lingua · Mandibula · Mm. of oral floor · Uvula palatina · Isthmus faucium · Os hyoideum · Epiglottis

Fig. 27.25 Organization and boundaries of the cavitas oris
Midsagittal section, left lateral view. (From Schuenke M, Schulte E, Schumacher U. THIEME Atlas of Anatomy, Vol 3. Illustrations by Voll M and Wesker K. 3rd ed. New York: Thieme Publishers; 2020.)

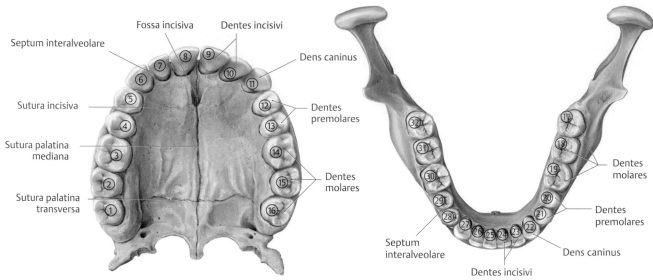

A Dentes maxillares. Inferior view of the maxilla.

B Dentes mandibulares. Superior view of the mandibula.

Fig. 27.26 Dentes permanentes
(From Gilroy AM et al. Atlas of Anatomy. 4th ed. 2020. Based on: Schuenke M, Schulte E, Schumacher U. THIEME Atlas of Anatomy. Head, Neck, and Neuroanatomy. Illustrations by Voll M and Wesker K. 3rd ed. New York: Thieme Medical Publishers; 2020.)

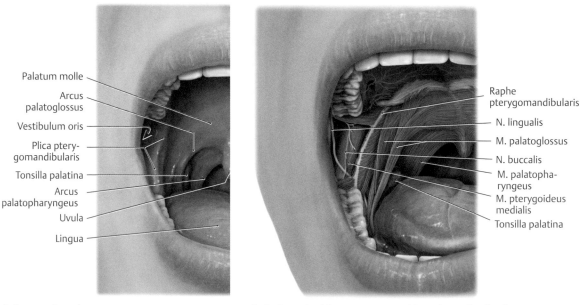

A Open cavitas oris.

B Cavitas oris with mucosa removed from the roof and walls.

Fig. 27.27 Cavitas oris topography
Right side, anterior view. (From Gilroy AM et al. Atlas of Anatomy. 4th ed. 2020. Based on: Schuenke M, Schulte E, Schumacher U. THIEME Atlas of Anatomy. Head, Neck, and Neuroanatomy. Illustrations by Voll M and Wesker K. 3rd ed. New York: Thieme Medical Publishers; 2020.)

— The n. trigeminus (CN V) transmits sensation from the mouth.
  • The n. alveolaris superior from the n. maxillaris (CN V$_2$) innervates the upper teeth.
  • N. alveolaris inferior, n. lingualis, and n. buccalis of the n. mandibularis (CN V$_3$) innervate the cheek, lower teeth, and floor of the mouth.
— Visceral motor fibers carried by the chorda tympani (CN VII) synapse in the submandibular ganglion in the floor of the mouth. Postganglionic fibers travel via the n. lingualis to innervate the gll. submandibulares and gll. sublinguales. (**Fig. 27.29**).

The Palate

The palate forms the roof of the cavitas oris and the floor of the cavitas nasi and separates the cavitas oris from the pharynx posteriorly.

— Nasal mucosa covers the superior surface, and oral mucosa, densely packed with mucus-secreting palatine glands, covers the inferior surface.
— The palate has anterior and posterior regions.
  • The **hard palate (palatum durum)**, formed by the proc. palatinus of the maxillae and the lamina horizontalis of the ossa palatina, makes up the anterior two thirds of the palate (**Fig. 27.30**).

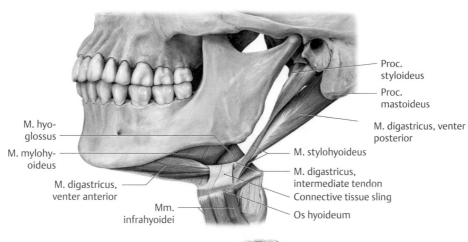

A Left lateral view.

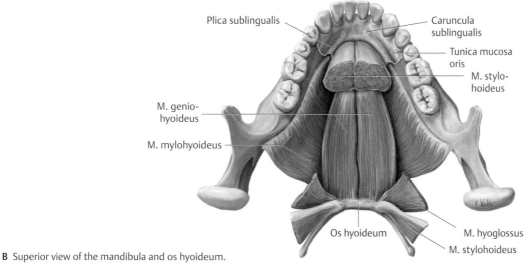

B Superior view of the mandibula and os hyoideum.

Fig. 27.28 Muscles of the oral floor: musculi suprahyoidei
(From Gilroy AM et al. Atlas of Anatomy. 4th ed. 2020. Based on: Schuenke M, Schulte E, Schumacher U. THIEME Atlas of Anatomy. Head, Neck, and Neuroanatomy. Illustrations by Voll M and Wesker K. 3rd ed. New York: Thieme Medical Publishers; 2020.)

Table 27.9 Musculi Suprahyoidei

Muscle		Origin	Insertion/Placement		Innervation	Action
M. digastricus	Venter anterior	Mandibula (fossa digastrica)	Corpus ossis hyoideum	Via an intermediate tendon with a fibrous loop	N. mylohyoideus (from CN V₃)	Elevates os hyoideum (during swallowing), assists in opening the mandibula
	Venter posterior	Os temporale (incisuramastoidea, medial to proc. mastoideus)			N. facialis (CN VII)	
M. stylohyoideus		Proc. stylohyoideus ossis temporalis		Via a split tendon		
M. mylohyoideus		Mandibula (linea mylohyoidea)		Via median tendon of insertion (mylohyoid raphe)	N. mylohyoideus (from CN V₃)	Tightens and elevates oral floor, draws os hyoideum forward (during swallowing), assists in opening mandibula and moving it side to side (mastication)
M. geniohyoideus		Mandibula (spina mentalis inferior)		Corpus hyoideum	R. anterior of C1 via n. hypoglossus (CN XII)	Draws os hyoideum forward (during swallowing), assists in opening mandibula
M. hyoglossus		Os hyoideum (superior border of cornu majus)	Sides of the tongue		N. hypoglossus (CN XII)	Depresses the tongue

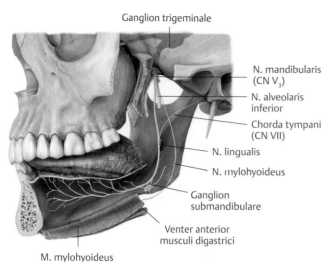

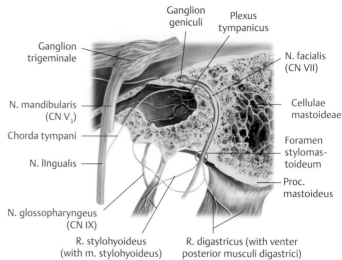

A N. mylohyoideus (CN V₃). Left lateral view with left half of the mandibula removed.

B N. facialis (CN VII). Sagittal section through the pars petrosa ossis temporalis at the level of the proc. mastoideus, lateral view.

Fig. 27.29 Nerves in the floor of the mouth
(From Schuenke M, Schulte E, Schumacher U. THIEME Atlas of Anatomy, Vol 3. Illustrations by Voll M and Wesker K. 3rd ed. New York: Thieme Publishers; 2020.)

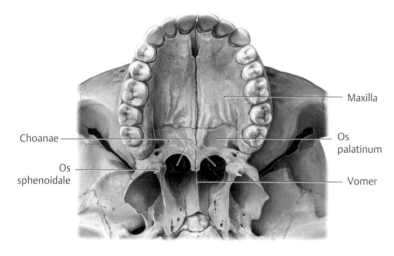

Fig. 27.30 Palatum durum
Inferior view. (From Schuenke M, Schulte E, Schumacher U. THIEME Atlas of Anatomy, Vol 3. Illustrations by Voll M and Wesker K. 3rd ed. New York: Thieme Publishers; 2020.)

BOX 27.6: DEVELOPMENTAL CORRELATION

CLEFT PALATE

Cleft palate is a congenital defect that occurs early in embryonic life when the lateral processi palatini fail to fuse with each other, with the septum nasi, and/or with the median processi palatini. It is seen in ~ 1:2,500 live births and is more common in females than males. The cleft (a fissure or opening) is described as complete when it involves the palatum molle and palatum durum and incomplete when it appears as a "hole" in the roof of the mouth (usually in the soft palate). In each case the uvula is usually also split. The cleft connects the cavitas oris directly to the cavitas nasi. Initial treatment involves the use of a prosthetic device called a palatal obturator to seal the cleft until corrective surgery is performed when the infant is between 6 and 12 months old.

- The **soft palate (palatum molle)**, the posterior third of the palate, has an anterior aponeurotic part that is attached to the palatum durum and a posterior muscular part with an unattached posterior margin that ends in a conical projection, the **uvula** (see **Fig. 27.25**).
- During swallowing, muscles of the palatum molle can tense and elevate it against the posterior pharyngeal wall to prevent food from passing into the cavitas nasi. They can also draw the palate downward against the tongue to prevent food from entering the pharynx. Muscles of the palatum molle include the **m. tensor veli palatini, m. levator veli palatini, m. uvulae, m. palatoglossus,** and **m. palatopharyngeus**. (**Fig. 27.31; Table 27.10**).
- The paired **arcus palatoglossus** and **arcus palatopharyngeus**, formed by the **m. palatoglossus** and **m. palatopharyngeus**, respectively, anchor the soft palate to the tongue and pharynx (see **Fig. 27.27**).
- A. palatina major, a. palatina minor, and a. sphenopalatina of the a. maxillaris supply the palate (**Fig. 27.32;** see also **Fig. 27.23B**).
- The n. palatinus major, n. palatinus minor, and n. nasopalatinus branches of n. maxillaris (CN V₂) carry sensory innervation from the palate (see **Fig. 27.24B**).

Fig. 27.31 Muscles of the palatum molle

Inferior view. The palatum molle forms the posterior boundary of the cavitas oris, separating it from the pars oralis pharyngis. (From Gilroy AM et al. Atlas of Anatomy. 4th ed. 2020. Based on: Schuenke M, Schulte E, Schumacher U. THIEME Atlas of Anatomy. Head, Neck, and Neuroanatomy. Illustrations by Voll M and Wesker K. 3rd ed. New York: Thieme Medical Publishers; 2020.)

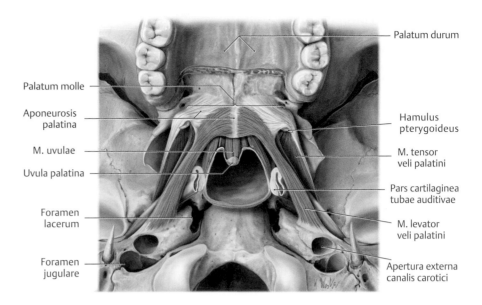

Palatum durum

Palatum molle

Aponeurosis palatina

M. uvulae

Uvula palatina

Foramen lacerum

Foramen jugulare

Hamulus pterygoideus

M. tensor veli palatini

Pars cartilaginea tubae auditivae

M. levator veli palatini

Apertura externa canalis carotici

Table 27.10 Muscles of the Palatum Molle

Muscle	Origin	Insertion	Innervation	Action
M. tensor veli palatini	Lamina medialis proc. pterygoidei (fossa scaphoidea); spina ossis sphenoidalis; cartilago tubae auditivae	Aponeurosis palatina	N. pterygoideus medialis (CN V₃)	Tightens palatum molle; opens ostium pharyngeum tubae auditivae (during swallowing, yawning)
M. levator veli palatini	Cartilago tubae auditivae; pars petrosa ossis temporalis		N. vagus via plexus pharyngeus	Raises palatum molle to horizontal position
M. uvulae	Uvula (mucosa)	Aponeurosis palatina; spina nasalis posterior		Shortens and raises uvula
M. palatoglossus	Lingua (side)	Aponeurosis palatina		Elevates the tongue (posterior portion); pulls palatum molle onto the tongue
M. palatopharyngeus				Tightens palatum molle; during swallowing pulls pharyngeal walls superiorly, anteriorly, and medially

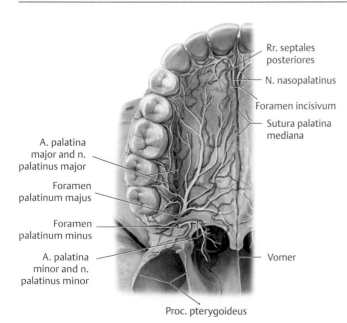

Rr. septales posteriores

N. nasopalatinus

Foramen incisivum

Sutura palatina mediana

A. palatina major and n. palatinus major

Foramen palatinum majus

Foramen palatinum minus

A. palatina minor and n. palatinus minor

Vomer

Proc. pterygoideus

Fig. 27.32 Neurovasculature of the palatum durum

Inferior view. The palatum durum receives sensory innervation primarily from terminal branches of the n. maxillaris of the n. trigeminus (CN V₂). The arteries of the palatum durum arise from the a. maxillaris. (From Schuenke M, Schulte E, Schumacher U. THIEME Atlas of Anatomy, Vol 3. Illustrations by Voll M and Wesker K. 3rd ed. New York: Thieme Publishers; 2020.)

The Tongue (Lingua)

The tongue (lingua) is a muscular organ that is involved in speech, taste, and manipulation of food during the initial phase of swallowing. Two thirds of the tongue lies in the cavitas oris; the remainder forms the anterior wall of the pars oralis pharyngis, the part of the pharynx posterior to the cavitas oris.

— The tongue has three parts **(Fig. 27.33)**:
  • the **root (radix)**, the attached posterior portion;
  • the **body (corpus)**, the largest portion, between the root and apex; and
  • the **apex,** the anterior tip.
— The **sulcus terminalis,** a groove on the dorsum of the tongue, divides the anterior two thirds of the tongue from the posterior third. A small pit at the center of the groove, the **foramen caecum**, marks the embryonic origin of the gl. thyroidea.
— Numerous papillae linguales, many containing taste buds, give the mucosa of the anterior two thirds of the tongue its rough texture.
  • **Papillae vallatae**, the largest of the papillae linguales, are arranged in a row directly anterior to the sulcus terminalis.
  • **Papillae foliatae** are found on the small lateral folds of the lingual mucosa and are not well developed.
  • **Papillae filiformes** contain afferent nerve endings that are sensitive to touch but not to taste. These are highly keratinized and facilitate rasplike licking activity.
  • **Papillae fungiformes** are most numerous at the apex and margins of the tongue.
— The **tonsilla lingualis** is a collection of noduli lymphoidei distributed over the mucosa of the posterior part of the tongue. Tonsillae linguales have crypts that are flushed by glands below them.
— The **frenulum of the tongue (frenulum linguae)**, a midline mucosal fold, attaches the inferior surface of the tongue to the floor of the cavitas oris and restricts its movement.
— Extrinsic muscles of the tongue, which originate outside the tongue and are responsible primarily for tongue movements, include the **m. genioglossus, m. hyoglossus**, and **m. styloglossus (Fig. 27.34; Table 27.11)**. The m. palatoglossus acts on the tongue but is actually a muscle of the palate and is innervated accordingly by the vagus nerve (CN X).
— Intrinsic muscles of the tongue have no bony attachments and are responsible for changing the shape of the tongue. They include the **m. longitudinalis superior** and **inferior** and the **m. transversus linguae** and **m. verticalis linguae.**

Table 27.11 Muscles of the Tongue*

Extrinsic muscles	Intrinsic muscles
• M. genioglossus	• M. longitudinalis superior
• M. hyoglossus	• M. longitudinalis inferior
• M. styloglossus	• M. transversus linguae
	• M. verticalis linguae

* All extrinsic and intrinsic muscles of the tongue are innervated by the n. hypoglossus (CN XII).

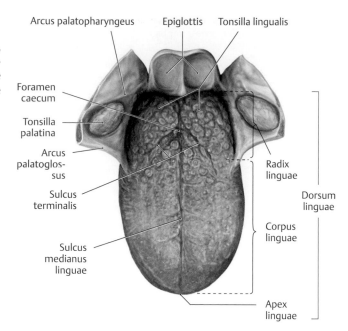

Fig. 27.33 Structure of the tongue
Superior view. The V-shaped sulcus terminalis divides the tongue into an anterior (oral, presulcal) and a posterior (pharyngeal, postsulcal) part. (From Schuenke M, Schulte E, Schumacher U. THIEME Atlas of Anatomy, Vol 3. Illustrations by Voll M and Wesker K. 3rd ed. New York: Thieme Publishers; 2020.)

— All extrinsic and intrinsic muscles of the tongue are innervated by the n. hypoglossus (CN XII).
— The aa. linguales, branches of the a. carotis externa, supply the tongue. The vv. linguales accompany the arteries and drain into the v. jugularis interna.
— Lymph from the tongue ultimately drains to deep cervical and jugular nodes in the neck, although the drainage from the various parts of the tongue follows four different pathways **(Fig. 27.35; Table 27.12)**. These drainage routes can be clinically important in the metastasis of lingual tumors.
— The five nn. craniales (n. trigeminus, n. facialis, n. glossopharyngeus, n. vagus, and n. hypoglossus) that innervate the tongue carry motor, general sensory, and special sensory fibers **(Fig. 27.36; Table 27.13)**.

Table 27.12 Lymphatic Drainage of the Tongue

Area of the Tongue	Drainage Pattern	Primary Nodes
Radix	Bilaterally	Nll. cervicales profundi superiores
Medial part of the corpus	Bilaterally	Nll. cervicales profundi inferiores
Lateral parts of the corpus	Ipsilaterally	Nll. submandibulares
Apex and frenulum	Midline—bilaterally Sides—ipsilaterally	Nll. submentales

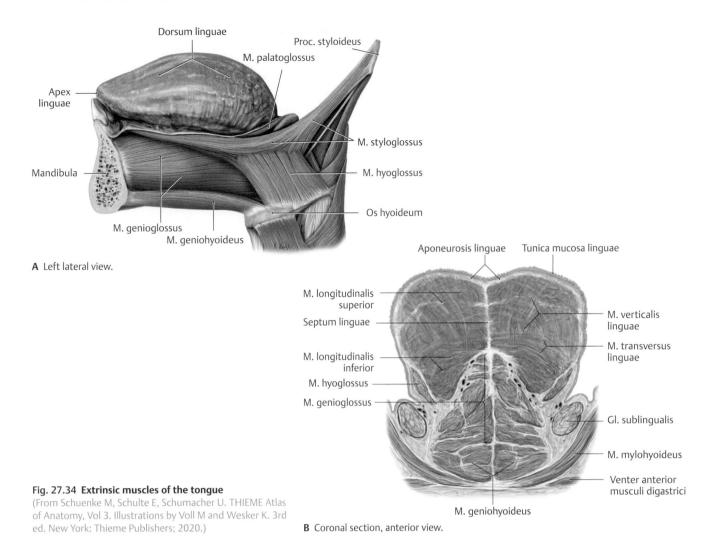

A Left lateral view.

Fig. 27.34 Extrinsic muscles of the tongue
(From Schuenke M, Schulte E, Schumacher U. THIEME Atlas of Anatomy, Vol 3. Illustrations by Voll M and Wesker K. 3rd ed. New York: Thieme Publishers; 2020.)

B Coronal section, anterior view.

A Left lateral view.

B Anterior view.

Fig. 27.35 Lymphatic drainage of the tongue and oral floor
Lymph flows to the nll. submentales and submandibulares of the tongue and oral floor, which ultimately drain into the jugular lymph nodes along the v. jugularis interna. Because the lymph nodes receive drainage from both the ipsilateral and contralateral sides **(B)**, tumor cells may become widely disseminated in this region (e.g., metastatic squamous cell carcinoma, especially on the lateral border of the tongue, frequently metastasizes to the opposite side). (From Schuenke M, Schulte E, Schumacher U. THIEME Atlas of Anatomy, Vol 3. Illustrations by Voll M and Wesker K. 3rd ed. New York: Thieme Publishers; 2020.)

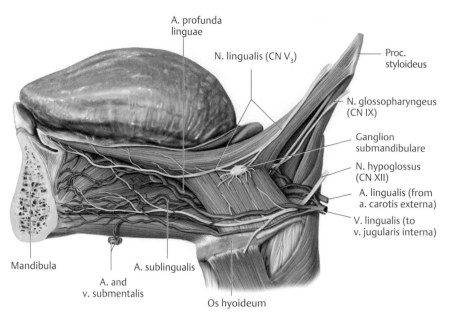

Fig. 27.36 Neurovasculature of the tongue
Left lateral view. (From Schuenke M, Schulte E, Schumacher U. THIEME Atlas of Anatomy, Vol 3. Illustrations by Voll M and Wesker K. 3rd ed. New York: Thieme Publishers; 2020.)

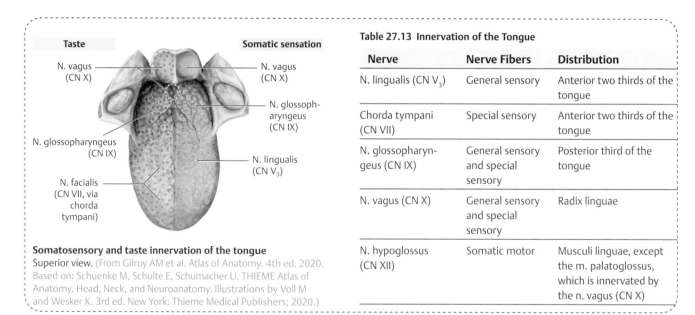

Somatosensory and taste innervation of the tongue
Superior view. (From Gilroy AM et al. Atlas of Anatomy. 4th ed. 2020. Based on: Schuenke M, Schulte E, Schumacher U. THIEME Atlas of Anatomy. Head, Neck, and Neuroanatomy. Illustrations by Voll M and Wesker K. 3rd ed. New York: Thieme Medical Publishers; 2020.)

Table 27.13 Innervation of the Tongue

Nerve	Nerve Fibers	Distribution
N. lingualis (CN V₃)	General sensory	Anterior two thirds of the tongue
Chorda tympani (CN VII)	Special sensory	Anterior two thirds of the tongue
N. glossopharyngeus (CN IX)	General sensory and special sensory	Posterior third of the tongue
N. vagus (CN X)	General sensory and special sensory	Radix linguae
N. hypoglossus (CN XII)	Somatic motor	Musculi linguae, except the m. palatoglossus, which is innervated by the n. vagus (CN X)

Salivary Glands (Glandulae Salivariae)

Three pairs of salivary glands (glandulae salivariae), the gll. parotideae, gll. submandibulares, and gll. sublinguales, produce and secrete saliva into the mouth (**Fig. 27.37**).

— The **gl. sublingualis**, the smallest of the three glands, lies deep to the mucosa of the floor of the mouth, forming the **plicae sublinguales**, onto which it secretes saliva through numerous small ducts.

— The **gl. submandibularis** has a superficial part located in the neck and a deep part located in the floor of the mouth, which connect around the posterior border of the m. mylohyoideus. The **ductus submandibularis (Wharton's)** opens via the **sublingual papilla** at the base of the lingual frenulum.

— The gl. parotidea, the largest of the three glands, is located in the regio parotideamasseterica on the lateral side of the head, anterior to the ear. The ductus parotideus opens into the vestibulum oris at the parotid papilla located opposite to the second dens molaris (see Section 27.3).

— The a. facialis, a. lingualis, a. maxillaris, and a. temporalis superficialis supply the gll. salivariae. Veins of similar names accompany the arteries and drain into the v. retromandibularis.

— The gll. submandibularis and gll. sublingualis receive parasympathetic secretomotor fibers via the chorda tympani (a branch of CN VII) and ganglion submandibulare.

— The gl. parotidea receives secretomotor (parasympathetic) fibers of the n. glossopharyngeus (CN IX) that synapse in the ganglion oticum.

— Sympathetic innervation to the glands arises as postganglionic fibers from the ganglion cervicale superius and follows the branches of the a. carotis externa.

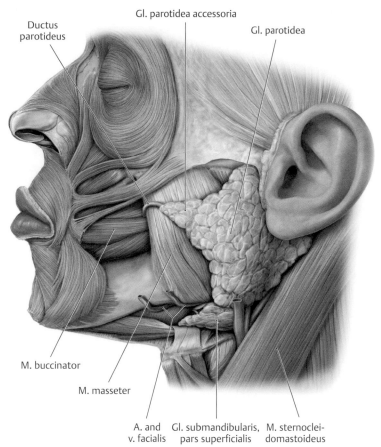

Ductus parotideus

Gl. parotidea accessoria

Gl. parotidea

M. buccinator

M. masseter

A. and v. facialis

Gl. submandibularis, pars superficialis

M. sternocleidomastoideus

A Gl. parotidea, left lateral view.

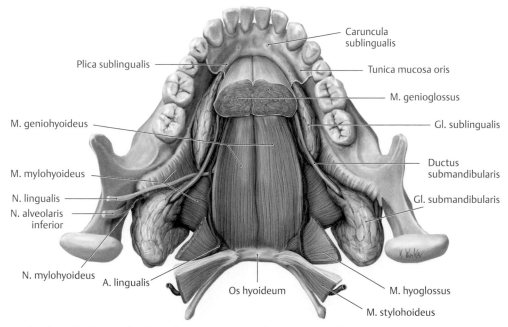

Plica sublingualis

Caruncula sublingualis

Tunica mucosa oris

M. genioglossus

M. geniohyoideus

Gl. sublingualis

M. mylohyoideus

Ductus submandibularis

N. lingualis

N. alveolaris inferior

Gl. submandibularis

N. mylohyoideus

A. lingualis

Os hyoideum

M. hyoglossus

M. stylohoideus

B Gll. submandibulares and sublinguales, superior view with tongue removed.

Fig. 27.37 Glandulae salivariae

(From Schuenke M, Schulte E, Schumacher U. THIEME Atlas of Anatomy, Vol 3. Illustrations by Voll M and Wesker K. 3rd ed. New York: Thieme Publishers; 2020.)

27.9   Pharynx and Tonsils

The **pharynx,** a fibromuscular tube that forms part of the upper airway and the upper digestive tract, transmits air from the cavitas nasi to the trachea and food from the cavitas oris to the oesophagus.

Regions of the Pharynx

The pharynx, which extends from the basis cranii to the inferior aspect of the larynx (cartilago cricoidea), is divided into three regions (**Figs. 27.38** and **27.39**): the nasopharynx, the oropharynx, and the laryngopharynx.

— The **nasopharynx (pars nasalis pharyngis)**, the uppermost part of the pharynx, lies posterior to the cavitas nasi and above the palatum molle. The body of the sphenoid forms its roof. Anteriorly, the nasopharynx communicates with the cavitas nasi through the paired choanae.

  • The orifices (openings) of the tuba auditiva are located on the lateral pharyngeal wall. Above the orifice, the pars cartilaginea of the tube protrudes into the pharynx to form a bulge, the **torus tubarius.**

  • A **plica salpingopharyngea**, formed by the **m. salpingopharyngeus** deep to the mucosa, extends inferiorly from the torus tubarius.

— The **oropharynx (pars oralis pharyngis)**, which lies posterior to the cavitas oris, extends superiorly to the palatum molle and inferiorly to the top of the larynx. The posterior tongue forms the anterior boundary.

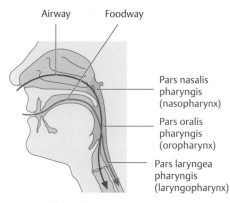

Fig. 27.38 **Regions of the pharynx**
Midsagittal section, left lateral view. The *blue arrow* indicates flow of air and the *red arrow*, passage of food. (From Schuenke M, Schulte E, Schumacher U. THIEME Atlas of Anatomy, Vol 3. Illustrations by Voll M and Wesker K. 3rd ed. New York: Thieme Publishers; 2020.)

  • Two arches, the anterior arcus palatoglossus (fold) and the posterior posterior arcus palatopharyngeus, (fold), formed by the palatoglossus and m. palatopharyngeus, respectively, separate the oropharynx from the cavitas oris. Both muscles are innervated by the n. vagus (CN X).

  • The tonsilla palatina lies between these arches in the tonsillar fossa.

  • A median fold of mucosa divides the space between the base of the tongue and the epiglottis. The spaces on either side of the fold are called **valleculae.**

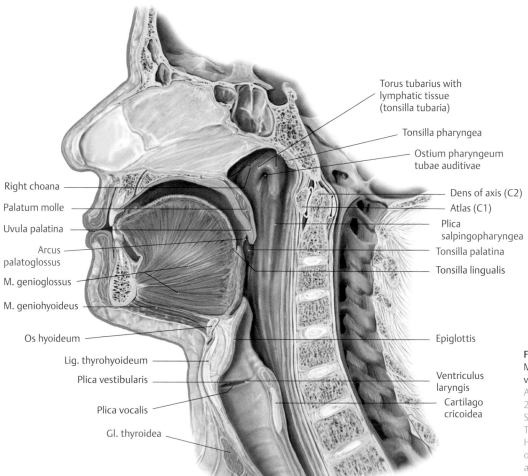

Fig. 27.39 **Pharynx**
Midsagittal section, left lateral view. (From Gilroy AM et al. Atlas of Anatomy. 4th ed. 2020. Based on: Schuenke M, Schulte E, Schumacher U. THIEME Atlas of Anatomy. Head, Neck, and Neuroanatomy. Illustrations by Voll M and Wesker K. 3rd ed. New York: Thieme Medical Publishers; 2020.)

— The **laryngopharynx (pars laryngea pharyngis)**, which lies posterior to the larynx, extends from the epiglottis to the inferior border of the cartilago cricoidea, where it narrows and is continuous with the oesophagus.
  - The laryngopharynx communicates with the larynx through the **aditus laryngis.**
  - **Aryepiglottic folds** separate the aditus laryngis from mucosal-lined fossae on the lateral walls of the pharynx called **recessus piriformis**.

BOX 27.7: CLINICAL CORRELATION

RECESSUS PIRIFORMIS

The recessus piriformis are small fossae that lie on either side of the aditus laryngis. Occasionally small foreign objects that are swallowed or inhaled or bits of food (such as a peanut) can become lodged in these spaces. In such cases, the internal laryngeal and inferior laryngeal nerves, which lie deep to the mucosa in this area, can be vulnerable to injury.

Muscles of the Pharynx

An outer circular layer and inner longitudinal layer of skeletal muscles form the walls of the pharynx (**Figs. 27.40** and **27.41; Tables 27.14** and **27.15**). Pharyngeal muscles coordinate with muscles of the floor of the mouth and soft palate during swallowing (**Fig. 27.42**).

— Circular **m. constrictor pharyngis superior**, **m. constrictor pharyngis medius**, and **m. constrictor pharyngis inferior** propel a bolus of food downward through the oropharynx and laryngopharynx; all are innervated by the n. vagus (CN X).
— Longitudinal muscles, the **m. salpingopharyngeus** and **m. palatopharyngeus** innervated by the n. vagus (CN X) and plexus pharyngeus, and the **m. stylopharyngeus** innervated by the n. glossopharyngeus (CN IX), elevate the pharynx to prevent food from entering the nasopharynx.

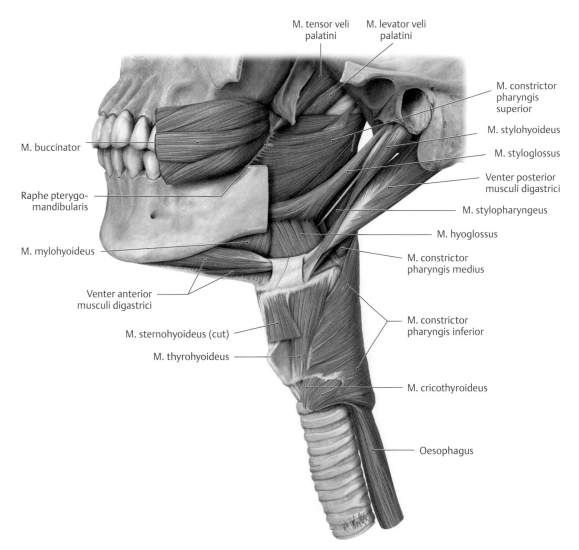

Fig. 27.40 Musculi pharyngis
Left lateral view. (From Gilroy AM et al. Atlas of Anatomy. 4th ed. 2020. Based on: Schuenke M, Schulte E, Schumacher U. THIEME Atlas of Anatomy. Head, Neck, and Neuroanatomy. Illustrations by Voll M and Wesker K. 3rd ed. New York: Thieme Medical Publishers; 2020.)

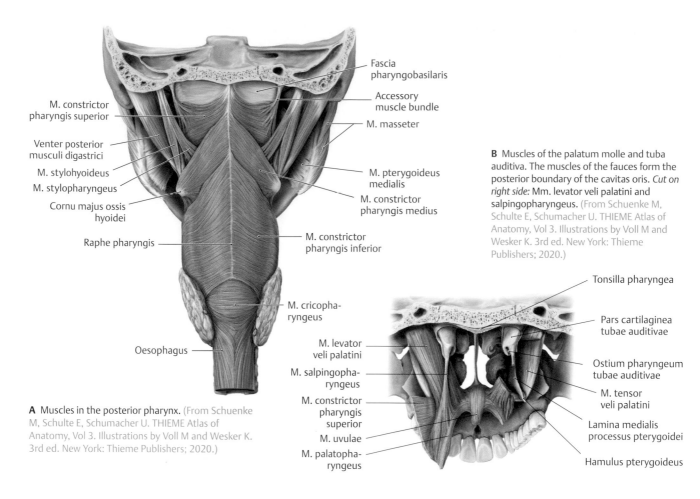

M. constrictor pharyngis superior

Venter posterior musculi digastrici

M. stylohyoideus

M. stylopharyngeus

Cornu majus ossis hyoidei

Raphe pharyngis

Oesophagus

M. cricopharyngeus

Fascia pharyngobasilaris

Accessory muscle bundle

M. masseter

M. pterygoideus medialis

M. constrictor pharyngis medius

M. constrictor pharyngis inferior

A Muscles in the posterior pharynx. (From Schuenke M, Schulte E, Schumacher U. THIEME Atlas of Anatomy, Vol 3. Illustrations by Voll M and Wesker K. 3rd ed. New York: Thieme Publishers; 2020.)

B Muscles of the palatum molle and tuba auditiva. The muscles of the fauces form the posterior boundary of the cavitas oris. *Cut on right side:* Mm. levator veli palatini and salpingopharyngeus. (From Schuenke M, Schulte E, Schumacher U. THIEME Atlas of Anatomy, Vol 3. Illustrations by Voll M and Wesker K. 3rd ed. New York: Thieme Publishers; 2020.)

Tonsilla pharyngea

Pars cartilaginea tubae auditivae

Ostium pharyngeum tubae auditivae

M. tensor veli palatini

Lamina medialis processus pterygoidei

Hamulus pterygoideus

M. levator veli palatini

M. salpingopharyngeus

M. constrictor pharyngis superior

M. uvulae

M. palatopharyngeus

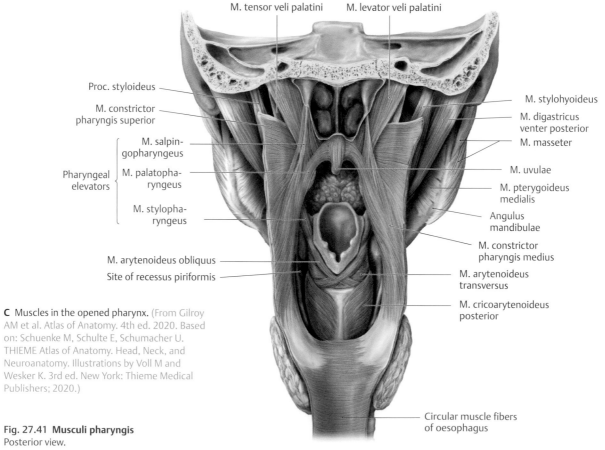

M. tensor veli palatini

M. levator veli palatini

Proc. styloideus

M. constrictor pharyngis superior

Pharyngeal elevators

M. salpingopharyngeus

M. palatopharyngeus

M. stylopharyngeus

M. arytenoideus obliquus

Site of recessus piriformis

M. stylohyoideus

M. digastricus venter posterior

M. masseter

M. uvulae

M. pterygoideus medialis

Angulus mandibulae

M. constrictor pharyngis medius

M. arytenoideus transversus

M. cricoarytenoideus posterior

Circular muscle fibers of oesophagus

C Muscles in the opened pharynx. (From Gilroy AM et al. Atlas of Anatomy. 4th ed. 2020. Based on: Schuenke M, Schulte E, Schumacher U. THIEME Atlas of Anatomy. Head, Neck, and Neuroanatomy. Illustrations by Voll M and Wesker K. 3rd ed. New York: Thieme Medical Publishers; 2020.)

Fig. 27.41 Musculi pharyngis
Posterior view.

Table 27.14 Muscles of the Pharynx: Pharyngeal Constrictors

Muscle	Origin	Insertion	Innervation	Action
M. constrictor pharyngis superior	Pterygoid hamulus, pterygomandibular raphe, mylohyoid line of mandible, lateral lingua	Tuberculum pharyngeum of os occipitale via raphe pharyngis medius	N. vagus (CN X) via plexus pharyngeus	Constricts the upper pharynx
M. constrictor pharyngis medius	Cornu majus and minus ossis hyoidei, lig. stylohyoideus	Raphe pharyngis		Constricts the middle pharynx
M. constrictor pharyngis inferior	Thyroid lamina, cornu minus ossis hyoidei, cartilago cricoidea	Raphe pharyngis; m. cricopharyngeus encircles pharynge-al-esophageal junction	N. vagus via plexus pharyngeus, nn. laryngei recurrens and externus (CN X)	Constricts lower pharynx; m. cricopharyngeus: sphincter between pars laryngea pharyngis and oesophagus

Table 27.15 Muscles of the Pharynx: Pharyngeal Elevators

Muscle	Origin	Insertion	Innervation	Action
M. palatopharyngeus (arcus palatopharyngeus)	Aponeurosis palatina (superior surface) and posterior border of os palatinum	Cartilago thyroidea (posterior border) or lateral pharynx	N. vagus (CN X) via plexus pharyngeus	*Bilaterally:* Elevates the pharynx anteromedially.
M. salpingopharyngeus	Pars cartilaginea tubae auditivae (inferior surface)	Along plica salpingopharyngea to m. palatopharyngeus		*Bilaterally:* Elevates the pharynx; may also open tuba auditiva.
M. stylopharyngeus	Proc. styloideus (medial surface of base)	Lateral pharynx, mixing with pharyngeal constrictors, m. palatopharyngeus, and cartilago thyroidea (posterior border)	N. glossopharyn-geus (CN IX)	*Bilaterally:* Elevates the pharynx and larynx.

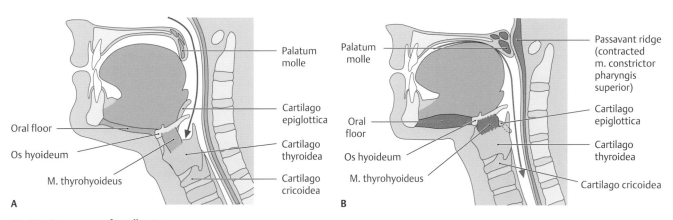

Fig. 27.42 Anatomy of swallowing

As part of the airway, the larynx in the adult is located at the inlet to the digestive tract **(A)**. During swallowing, therefore, the airway must be briefly occluded to keep food from entering the trachea. During the reflexive phase of swallowing, muscles on the floor of the mouth and the mm. thyrohyoideus elevate the larynx while the epiglottis covers the aditus laryngis, sealing off the lower airway. In addition, the palatum molle tightens, elevates, and opposes the posterior pharyngeal wall, sealing off the upper airway **(B)**. (From Schuenke M, Schulte E, Schumacher U. THIEME Atlas of Anatomy, Vol 3. Illustrations by Voll M and Wesker K. 3rd ed. New York: Thieme Publishers; 2020.)

Tonsils

— **Tonsils (tonsillae)**, masses of lymphoid tissue found in the mucosal lining of the pharynx, form an incomplete circular ring called the **anulus lymphoideus pharyngis** (Waldeyer's ring) around the superior part of the pharynx **(Fig. 27.43)**. They include
  • one **tonsillae pharyngeae** (also known as adenoid) in the mucous membrane of the roof and posterior wall of the pharynx;
  • paired **tonsillae tubariae**, extensions of the pharyngeal tonsil, near the orifices of the pharyngotympanic tube;
  • paired **tonsillae palatinae** in the fossae between the palatoglossal and palatopharyngeal arches;
  • **tonsillae linguales** on the posterior one third of the dorsum of the tongue; and
  • pairs of **lateral bands** that lie along the salpingopharyngeal folds.
— Tonsillae are supplied by branches of the a. facialis, a. palatina ascendens, a. lingualis, a. palatina descendens, and a. pharyngea ascendens.

— Tonsillar lymphatic vessels drain to the nl. jugulodigastricus near the angulus mandibulae before draining to the deep nll. cervicales profundi.
— A tonsillar nerve plexus is formed by the n. glossopharyngeus (CN IX) and n. vagus (CN X).

BOX 27.8: CLINICAL CORRELATION

TONSILLECTOMY

During a tonsillectomy, the tonsillae palatinae are removed from the tonsillar bed along with their accompanying fascia. The n. glossopharyngeus, which lies on the lateral wall of the pharynx, is vulnerable to injury during the procedure and may result in loss of sensation and taste from the posterior one third of the tongue. Bleeding may occur from the large v. palatina externa or from the tonsillar branches of the a. facialis, a. pharyngea ascendens, a. maxillaris, and a. lingualis. The a. carotis interna may also be vulnerable because it runs just lateral to the tonsilla.

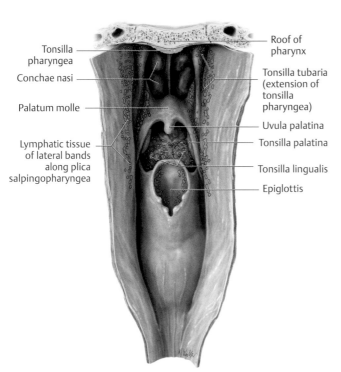

Tonsilla pharyngea
Conchae nasi
Palatum molle
Lymphatic tissue of lateral bands along plica salpingopharyngea

Roof of pharynx
Tonsilla tubaria (extension of tonsilla pharyngea)
Uvula palatina
Tonsilla palatina
Tonsilla lingualis
Epiglottis

Fig. 27.43 Tonsillae: Anulus lymphoideus pharyngis (Waldeyer's ring) Posterior view of the opened pharynx. (From Schuenke M, Schulte E, Schumacher U. THIEME Atlas of Anatomy, Vol 3. Illustrations by Voll M and Wesker K. 3rd ed. New York: Thieme Publishers; 2020.)

Neurovasculature of the Pharynx

— Direct and indirect branches of the a. carotis externa supply the pharynx. These include the a. facialis, a. lingualis, a. palatina ascendens, a. palatina descendens, and a. pharyngea acendens (see **Fig. 24.21**).
— Venous drainage of the pharynx passes through the pharyngeal plexus venosus to the v. jugularis interna (see **Fig. 24.26**).
— Sensory innervation of the pharyngeal mucosa varies by region **(Fig. 27.44)**.
  • The n. maxillaris (CN V_2) innervates the upper part of the nasopharynx.
  • The n. glossopharyngeus (CN IX) primarily innervates the oropharynx, although its territory extends into both the nasopharynx and laryngopharynx.
  • The n. vagus (CN X) via its n. laryngeus internus innervates the laryngopharynx.

BOX 27.9: CLINICAL CORRELATION

GAG REFLEX

The gag reflex is a reflexive contraction of the mm. pharyngis that protects the airway by preventing accidental ingestion and aspiration. It is elicited by touching the palatum molle or back of the tongue. The n. glossopharyngeus (CN IX) is the afferent limb, and the n. vagus (CN X) serves as the efferent limb of the reflex.

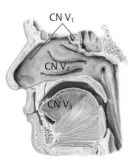
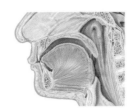
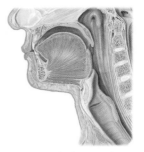

CN V₁
CN V₂
CN V₃

A N. maxillaris in the nasopharynx.   **B** N. glossopharyngeus in the oropharynx.   **C** N. vagus in the laryngopharynx.

Fig. 27.44 Sensory innervation of the pharynx
(From Schuenke M, Schulte E, Schumacher U. THIEME Atlas of Anatomy, Vol 3. Illustrations by Voll M and Wesker K. 3rd ed. New York: Thieme Publishers; 2020.)

BOX 27.10: CLINICAL CORRELATION

FASCIA AND POTENTIAL TISSUE SPACES IN THE HEAD
Fascial boundaries are the key to outlining pathways for the spread of infection. Potential spaces in the head, shown on this figure, become true spaces when they are infiltrated by products of infection. These spaces are defined by bones, muscles and fascia and initially confine an infection but eventually allow it to spread through communications between spaces.

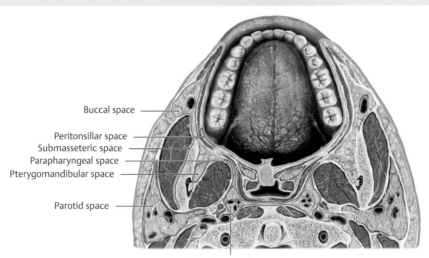

Buccal space

Peritonsillar space
Submasseteric space
Parapharyngeal space
Pterygomandibular space

Parotid space

Retropharyngeal space

Transverse section at the level of the fossa tonsillaris, superior view. (From Gilroy AM et al. Atlas of Anatomy. 4th ed. 2020. Based on: Schuenke M, Schulte E, Schumacher U. THIEME Atlas of Anatomy. Head, Neck, and Neuroanatomy. Illustrations by Voll M and Wesker K. 3rd ed. New York: Thieme Medical Publishers; 2020.)

28 The Eye and Ear

The eye (oculus), the organ of vision, and the ear (auris), which contains the organs for hearing and balance, are anatomically the most complex of the sense organs. The eyes, enclosed within the bony orbita, are prominent features of the face. The ears have superficial and deep components that are related to the os temporale on the sides of the head.

28.1 The Eye (Oculus)

The anatomy of the eye includes the bony orbita, the eyelids (palpebrae) and lacrimal apparatus (apparatus lacrimalis), the eyeball (bulbus oculi), and six extraocular muscles.

The Bony Orbita

The paired **orbitae** lie on either side of the superior part of the cavitas nasi, above the sinus maxillaris and below the fossa cranii anterior (see **Fig. 24.15**). These cavities are shaped like quadrangular pyramids with the apex directed posteriorly and the base opening onto the face (**Fig. 28.1**).

— Seven bones of the skull form the bony orbita:
   1. the os frontale which forms the paries superior,
   2. the maxilla, which forms the paries inferior,
   3. the os ethmoidale,

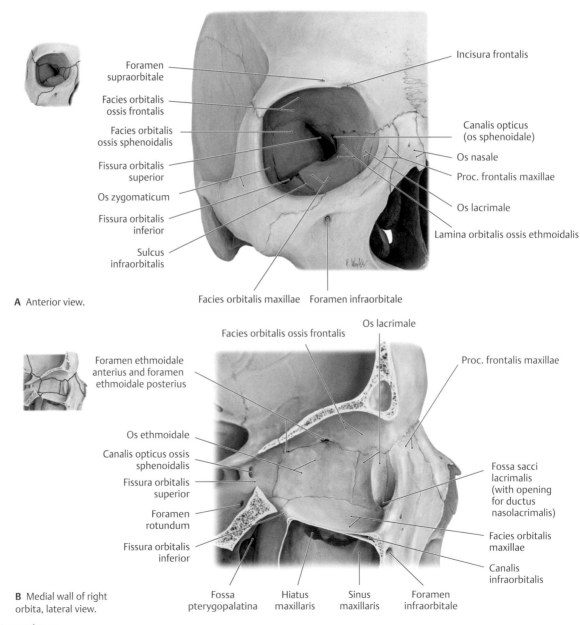

A Anterior view.

B Medial wall of right orbita, lateral view.

Fig. 28.1 **Ossa orbitae**
(From Schuenke M, Schulte E, Schumacher U. THIEME Atlas of Anatomy, Vol 3. Illustrations by Voll M and Wesker K. 3rd ed. New York: Thieme Publishers; 2020.)

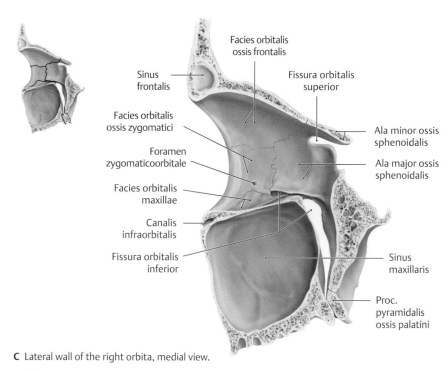

C Lateral wall of the right orbita, medial view.

Fig. 28.1 (*continued*) **Ossa orbitae**

4. os lacrimale,
5. os palatinum, and
6. os sphenoidale, which form the paries medialis. and
7. the os zygomaticum which, along with the os sphenoidale forms the paries lateralis.

— The bulbus oculi occupies the anterior part of the orbita, accompanied by six extraocular muscles, ophthalmic vessels, and six nn. craniales (n. opticus [CN II], n. oculomotorius [CN III], n. trochlearis [CN IV], n. trigeminus [CN V], n. abducens [CN VI], and n. facialis [CN VII]) (**Fig. 28.2**). Periorbital fat supports and surrounds these structures.

— Three openings at the apex of the orbit allow passage of nerves and vessels between the fossa cranii media and the orbita: the **canalis opticus**, **fissura orbitalis superior**, and **fissura orbitalis inferior** (**Table 28.1**).

— Several other openings transmit nerves and vessels onto the face—**foramen supraorbitale and foramen infraorbitale, incisura frontalis, and foramen zygomatico-orbitale**—and into the cavitas nasi—**foramen ethmoidale anterius** and **foramen ethmoidale posterius**. The **canalis nasolacrimalis**, a passageway between the orbit and nasal cavity, transmits the **ductus nasolacrimalis**.

Table 28.1 Openings in the Orbita for Neurovascular Structures

Opening*	Nerves	Vessels
Canalis opticus	N. opticus (CN II)	A. ophthalmica
Fissura orbitalis superior	N. oculomotorius (CN III) N. trochlearis (CN IV) N. abducens (CN VI) N. trigeminus, n. ophthalmicus division (CN V$_1$) • N. lacrimalis • N. frontalis • N. nasociliaris	V. ophthalmica superior
Fissura orbitalis inferior	N. infraorbitalis (CN V$_2$), n. zygomaticus (CN V$_2$)	A. and v. infraorbitalis, v. ophthalmica inferior
Canalis infraorbitalis	N. infraorbitalis (CN V$_2$)	A. and v. infraorbitalis
Foramen supraorbitale	R. lateralis nervi supraorbitalis	A. supraorbitalis
Incisura frontalis	R. medialis nervi supraorbitalis	A. supratrochlearis
Foramen ethmoidale anterius	N. ethmoidalis anterior	A. and v. ethmoidalis anterior
Foramen ethmoidale posterius	N. ethmoidalis posterior	A. and v. ethmoidalis posterior

* The canalis nasolacrimalis transmits the ductus nasolacrimalis.

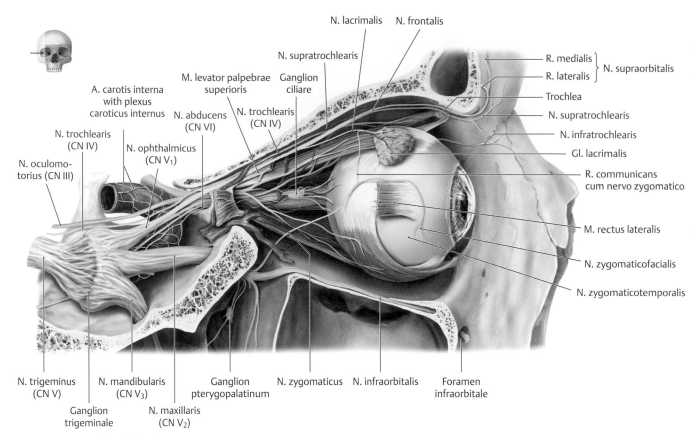

Fig. 28.2 Topography of the orbita
Right orbita, lateral view. (From Schuenke M, Schulte E, Schumacher U. THIEME Atlas of Anatomy, Vol 3. Illustrations by Voll M and Wesker K. 3rd ed. New York: Thieme Publishers; 2020.)

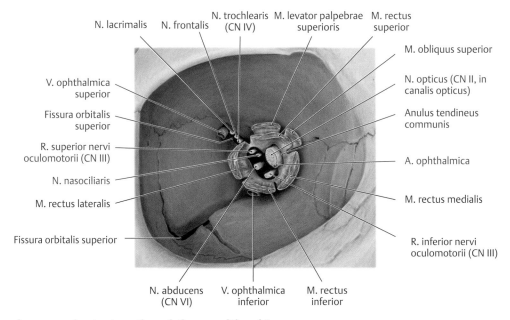

Fig. 28.3 Passage of neurovascular structures through the apex of the orbita
Anterior view. (From Gilroy AM et al. Atlas of Anatomy. 4th ed. 2020. Based on: Schuenke M, Schulte E, Schumacher U. THIEME Atlas of Anatomy. Head, Neck, and Neuroanatomy. Illustrations by Voll M and Wesker K. 3rd ed. New York: Thieme Medical Publishers; 2020.)

— An **anulus tendineus communis** at the apex of the orbita surrounds the canalis opticus and part of the fissura orbitalis superior and serves as the origin for four of the extraocular muscles (**Fig. 28.3**). The n. opticus (CN II) and a. ophthalmica enter the orbita through the canalis opticus and thus pass through the anulus tendineus. Other structures entering through part of the fissura orbitalis superior enclosed by the ring include the **superior** and **inferior branches** of the n. oculomotorius (CN III), the **n. nasociliaris** of the n. ophthalmicus (CN V₁), and the n. abducens (CN VI).

Orbital Region, Eyelids, and Lacrimal Apparatus

The upper and lower **eyelids (palpebrae)** are movable folds of skin that protect the bulbus oculi from injury, irritation, and light. They are separated from each other by the **palpebral fissure (rima palpebraum)** (**Fig. 28.4**).
— The eyelids are covered externally by skin and internally by the **tunica conjunctiva palpebrarum**. This thin inner membrane reflects at the **superior** and **inferior fornices** onto the anterior bulbus oculi as the **tunica conjunctiva bulbi**. When the eyes are closed, the tunica conjunctiva palpebrarum and tunica conjunctiva bulbi form the **saccus conjunctivalis**.
— **Tarsal plates** or **tarsus**, bands of dense connective tissue that provide support for both the upper and lower eyelids, are attached to **lig. palpebrale laterale** and **lig. palpebrale mediale**, which connect to the margo lateralis and margo

medialis of the orbita, respectively. Gll. tarsales within the tarsal plates lubricate the edges of the eyelids to prevent them from sticking together.
— The **m. orbicularis oculi** (see **Fig. 27.2**), innervated by the n. facialis (n. cranialis [CN] VII), closes the eye in a sphincter-like fashion. The **m. levator palpebrae superioris**, innervated by the n. oculomotorius (CN III) and attached to the superior tarsal plate, opens the eye by lifting the upper eyelid.
— The **septum orbitale**, a thin membranous sheet, extends from the orbital rim, where it's continuous with the periosteum, into the tarsal plates of the eyelids. On the upper eyelid it also blends with the tendon of the m. levator palpebrae superioris. The septum holds the orbital fat within the orbita and helps limit the spread of infection to and from the orbita.

The **lacrimal apparatus (apparatus lacrimalis)** produces and drains tears that cleanse and lubricate the outer surface of the eye (**Fig. 28.5**).
— The **gl. lacrimalis**, which produces and secretes tears, resides in the fossa lacrimalis in the supralateral aspect of the orbita. Secretomotor parasympathetic fibers from the n. facialis (CN VII) stimulate the gland (see **Fig. 26.25**).
— Blinking of the eye sweeps the tears across the eye toward the medial angle, where they drain via **superior** and **inferior puncta** (openings) into **canaliculi lacrimalis** and the **saccus lacrimalis**, the dilated superior part of the ductus nasolacrimalis.

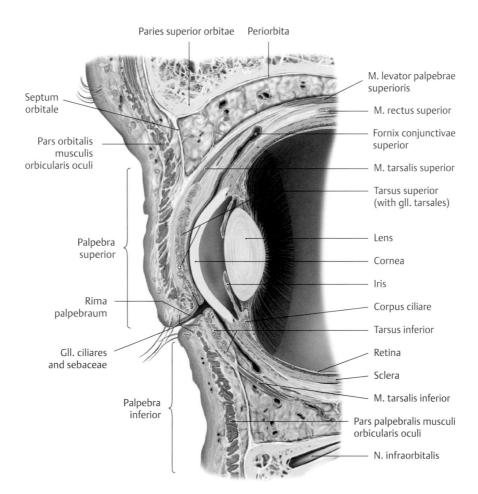

Fig. 28.4 Palpebrae and tunica conjunctiva
Sagittal section through the anterior cavitas orbitalis.
(From Gilroy AM et al. Atlas of Anatomy. 4th ed. 2020. Based on: Schuenke M, Schulte E, Schumacher U. THIEME Atlas of Anatomy. Head, Neck, and Neuroanatomy. Illustrations by Voll M and Wesker K. 3rd ed. New York: Thieme Medical Publishers; 2020.)

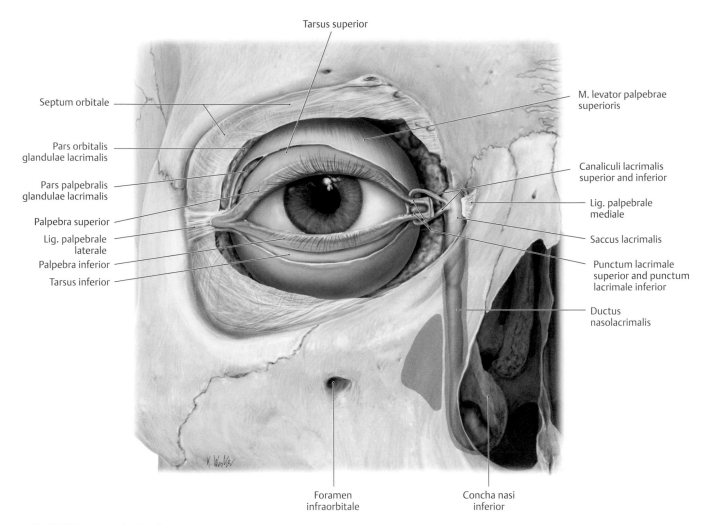

Tarsus superior

Septum orbitale

Pars orbitalis glandulae lacrimalis

Pars palpebralis glandulae lacrimalis

Palpebra superior

Lig. palpebrale laterale

Palpebra inferior

Tarsus inferior

M. levator palpebrae superioris

Canaliculi lacrimalis superior and inferior

Lig. palpebrale mediale

Saccus lacrimalis

Punctum lacrimale superior and punctum lacrimale inferior

Ductus nasolacrimalis

Foramen infraorbitale

Concha nasi inferior

Fig. 28.5 Apparatus lacrimalis
Right eye, anterior view.
Removed: Septum orbitale (partial). *Divided:* M. levator palpebrae superioris (tendon of insertion). (From Schuenke M, Schulte E, Schumacher U. THIEME Atlas of Anatomy, Vol 3. Illustrations by Voll M and Wesker K. 3rd ed. New York: Thieme Publishers; 2020.)

— The **ductus nasolacrimalis** is a membranous structure that begins in the medial angle of the eye and terminates in the inferior meatus of the cavitas nasi. Tears drain into the cavitas nasi via this duct.

The Eyeball (Bulbus Oculi)

The eyeball (bulbus oculi), the organ of vision, has three concentric layers that form its outer walls: the sclera, the choroidea, and the retina (**Fig. 28.6**).

— The **sclera**, the white part of the eye, forms the posterior five sixths of the outer tunica fibrosa bulbi; the **cornea**, the transparent part of the sclera, forms the anterior sixth. This outer layer is largely avascular but provides structure to the bulbus oculi.

— The **choroidea**, the middle vascular layer, provides oxygen and nutrients to the underlying retina (**Fig. 28.7**).

• The **corpus ciliare** connects the choroidea with the circumference of the iris. Short, smooth muscle fibers, **fibrae zonularis**, which attach the corpus ciliare to the lens, control the thickness and refractive power of the lens and therefore the focus of the eye.

• The **iris**, an adjustable muscular diaphragm, surrounds a central aperture, the **pupilla** (**Fig. 28.8**).
  ○ The **m. sphincter pupillae** of the iris responds to parasympathetic stimulation to constrict the pupilla.
  ○ The **m. dilatator pupillae** of the iris responds to sympathetic stimulation to dilate the pupilla.

— The **retina**, the inner sensory layer, has a posterior **pars optica** that is sensitive to light and a **pars caeca** that continues anteriorly over the corpus ciliare and iris.
  • The **discus nervi optici**, a point on the retina where the nervus opticus exits the bulbus oculi, lacks photoreceptors and therefore is insensitive to light and is known as the **blind spot**.
  • The **macula lutea** of the retina, a spot lateral to the discus nervi opitici, is an area of intense visual acuity.
  • The **fovea centrali3s**, a depression in the macula lutea, is the area of greatest visual acuity.

— Light passes through four refractive media before focusing on the retina of the eye:
  1. The cornea, the primary refractive medium for light entering the eye

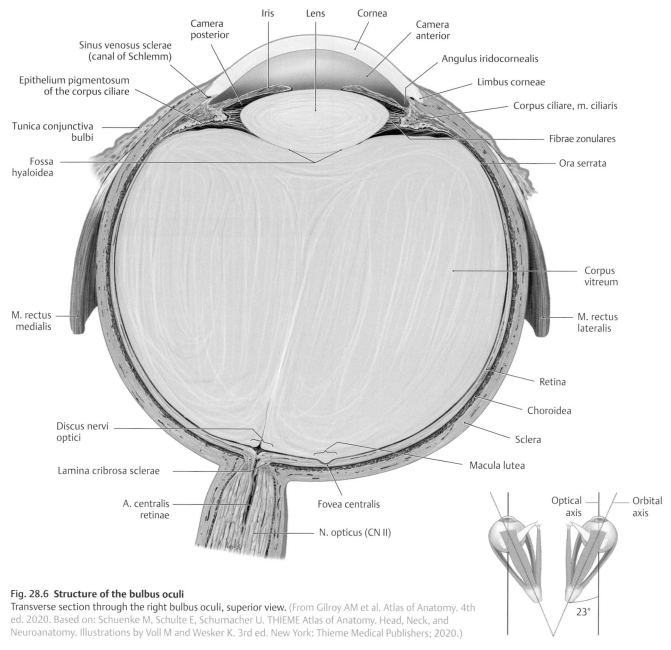

Fig. 28.6 Structure of the bulbus oculi
Transverse section through the right bulbus oculi, superior view. (From Gilroy AM et al. Atlas of Anatomy. 4th ed. 2020. Based on: Schuenke M, Schulte E, Schumacher U. THIEME Atlas of Anatomy. Head, Neck, and Neuroanatomy. Illustrations by Voll M and Wesker K. 3rd ed. New York: Thieme Medical Publishers; 2020.)

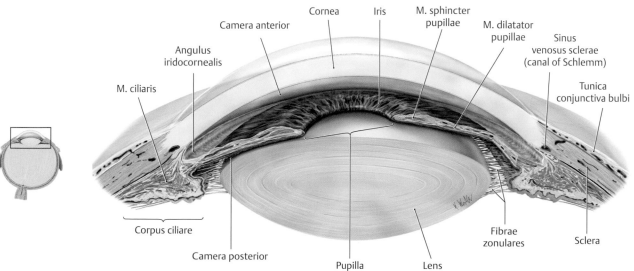

Fig. 28.7 Cornea, iris, and lens
Transverse section through the anterior segment of the eye, anterosuperior view. (From Gilroy AM et al. Atlas of Anatomy. 4th ed. 2020. Based on: Schuenke M, Schulte E, Schumacher U. THIEME Atlas of Anatomy. Head, Neck, and Neuroanatomy. Illustrations by Voll M and Wesker K. 3rd ed. New York: Thieme Medical Publishers; 2020.)

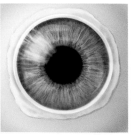
A Normal pupilla size.

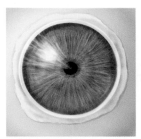
B Maximum constriction (miosis).

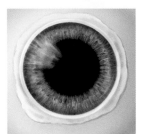
C Maximum dilation (mydriasis).

Fig. 28.8 Pupilla
Pupilla size is regulated by two intraocular muscles of the iris: the m. sphincter pupillae, which narrows the pupilla (parasympathetic innervation), and the m. dilatator pupillae, which enlarges it (sympathetic innervation). (From Schuenke M, Schulte E, Schumacher U. THIEME Atlas of Anatomy, Vol 3. Illustrations by Voll M and Wesker K. 3rd ed. New York: Thieme Publishers; 2020.)

BOX 28.1: CLINICAL CORRELATION

PRESBYOPIA AND CATARACTS
The lens of the eye undergoes age-related changes that affect vision in the older patient. The loss of elasticity of the lens, and the subsequent loss of accommodation, diminishes a patient's ability to focus on near objects, a condition known as presbyopia. Opacities of the lens or its capsule, known as cataracts, reduce the amount of light that reaches the retina, resulting in blurred, cloudy vision. Treatment involves surgical removal of the affected lens and replacement with a plastic lens implant.

BOX 28.2: CLINICAL CORRELATION

GLAUCOMA
Glaucoma refers to a group of eye diseases that involve increased intraocular pressure and atrophy of the n. opticus. In primary open-angle glaucoma, the most common form, venous channels in the angle between the cornea and the iris that allow drainage of the humor aquosus from the anterior and posterior chambers are blocked. The subsequent buildup of humor aquosus results in raised intraocular pressure and eventual damage to the n. opticus. This leads to a gradual loss of peripheral vision that progresses to tunnel vision. Pressure on the retina can lead to blindness.

---

2. The **humor aquosus**, a watery solution that fills the **camera anterior** and **camera posterior** of the eye that lie anterior to the lens and corpus ciliare. The balance between its production and drainage determines the intraocular pressure.

3. The **lens**, a transparent biconcave disk that focuses objects on the retina by changing its thickness. In the process of **accommodation**, which is mediated by parasympathetic stimulation, the m. ciliaris contracts, causing the lens to thicken and bring near objects into focus. When the m. ciliaris relaxes, the lens flattens, allowing the eye to focus on far objects (**Fig. 28.9**).

4. The **humor vitreus**, a jelly-like substance that fills the chamber of the eye posterior to the lens.

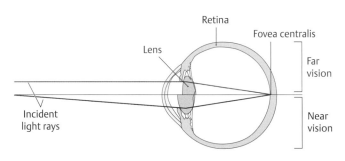

A Normal dynamic of the lens.

B Abnormal lens dynamic.

Fig. 28.9 Light refraction by the lens
Transverse section, superior view.
In the normal (emmetropic) eye, light rays are refracted by the lens (and cornea) to a focal point on the retinal surface (fovea centralis). Tensing of the fibrae zonulares, with relaxation of the m. ciliaris, flattens the lens in response to parallel rays arriving from a distant source (far vision). Contraction of the m. ciliaris, with relaxation of fibrae zonulares, causes the lens to assume a more rounded shape (near vision). (From Gilroy AM et al. Atlas of Anatomy. 4th ed. 2020. Based on: Schuenke M, Schulte E, Schumacher U. THIEME Atlas of Anatomy. Head, Neck, and Neuroanatomy. Illustrations by Voll M and Wesker K. 3rd ed. New York: Thieme Medical Publishers; 2020.)

Extraocular Muscles (Musculi Externi Bulbi Oculi)

— The six extraocular muscles (musculi externi bulbi oculi) that control the movement of the bulbus oculi (**Fig. 28.10**; **Table 28.2**) include
  • four mm. rectus, the **m. rectus superior**, **m. rectus medialis**, **m. rectus inferior**, and **m. rectus lateralis**, that originate from a **anulus tendineus communis** at the apex of the orbita; and
  • two mm. obliquus, the **m. obliquus superior** that arises near the apex and reflects back via the trochlea to attach to the bulbus oculi, and the **m. obliquus inferior** that arises from the medial aspect of the orbital floor.
— The muscles allow six cardinal directions of gaze, which are the normal movements of the bulbus oculi tested during clinical evaluation of ocular mobility.

Neurovasculature of the Orbita

The orbital region is an area of arterial and venous anastomoses (**Fig. 28.11**; see Sections 24.3 and 24.4).
  • Branches of the a. carotis externa, the a. infraorbitalis (a branch of the a. maxillaris), and a. facialis, anastomose with the a. supraorbital of the a. carotis interna. This potential anastomosis can serve an important function if the a. maxillaris is ligated (such as for severe nosebleeds).
  • The anastomosis between the extracranial v. angularis and intracranial v. ophthalmica superior can serve as a conduit for bacterial infections of the face passing into intracranial venous pathways.
— The a. ophthalmica supplies most structures of the orbit (**Fig. 28.12**). One of its branches, the **a. centralis retinae**, runs within the n. opticus and is the sole arterial supply to the retina through its terminal branches.
  • The a. ophthalmica anastomoses with the a. facialis through its r. supratrochlearis and with the a. maxillaris through a. ethmoidalis anterior and a. ethmoidalis posterior and a. meningea media.
— The **v. ophthalmica superior** and **v. ophthalmica inferior**, which drain structures in the orbita, primarily drain into the sinus cavernosus but also communicate with the v. facialis and plexus venosus pterygoideus (**Fig. 28.13**).

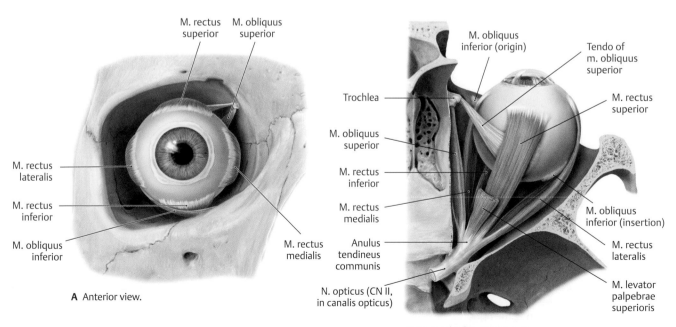

A Anterior view.

B Opened orbit, superior view.

Fig. 28.10 Musculi externi bulbi oculi
Right eye. (From Schuenke M, Schulte E, Schumacher U. THIEME Atlas of Anatomy, Vol 3. Illustrations by Voll M and Wesker K. 3rd ed. New York: Thieme Publishers; 2020.)

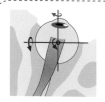 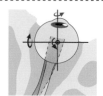 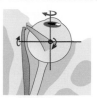 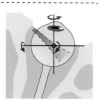

A M. rectus superior. **B** M. rectus medialis. **C** M. rectus inferior. **D** M. rectus lateralis. **E** M. obliquus superior. **F** M. obliquus inferior.

(From Schuenke M, Schulte E, Schumacher U. THIEME Atlas of Anatomy, Vol 3. Illustrations by Voll M and Wesker K. 3rd ed. New York: Thieme Publishers; 2020.)

Table 28.2 Actions of the Musculi Externi Bulbi Oculi

Muscle	Origin	Insertion	Action* Vertical Axis (red)	Action* Horizontal Axis (black)	Action* Anteroposterior Axis (blue)	Innervation
M. rectus superior	Anulus tendineus communis (common annular tendon)	Sclera oculi	Elevates	Adducts	Rotates medially	R. superior nervi oculomotorii (CN III)
M. rectus medialis			–	Adducts	–	R. inferior nervi oculomotorii (CN III)
M. rectus inferior			Depresses	Adducts	Rotates laterally	
M. rectus lateralis			–	Abducts	–	N. abducens (CN VI)
M. obliquus superior	Os sphenoidale+		Depresses	Abducts	Rotates medially	N. trochlearis (CN IV)
M. obliquus inferior	Margo orbitalis medialis		Elevates	Abducts	Rotates laterally	R. inferior nervi oculomotorii (CN III)

*Starting from gaze directed anteriorly.
+The tendon of insertion of the m. obliquus superior passes through a tendinous loop (trochlea) attached to the superomedial margo orbitalis.

BOX 28.5: CLINICAL CORRELATION

OCULOMOTOR NERVE INJURY

The n. oculomotorius innervates most of the extraocular muscles. With paralysis of these muscles, the eye is directed downward and outward because of the unopposed action of the m. rectus lateralis (innervated by the n. abducens) and m. obliquus superior (innervated by the n. trochlearis) (A). The m. dilatator pupillae is also unopposed, so the pupilla remains fully dilated. Paralysis of the m. levator palpebrae superioris causes the palpebra superior to droop (B).

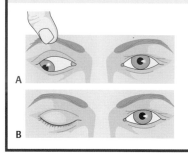

(From Schuenke M, Schulte E, Schumacher U. THIEME Atlas of Anatomy, Vol 3. Illustrations by Voll M and Wesker K. 3rd ed. New York: Thieme Publishers; 2020.)

— Six nn. craniales (n. opticus, n. oculomotorius, n. trochlearis, n. trigeminus, n. abducens, and n. facialis) innervate structures in the orbita. All of these nerves pass through the sinus cavernosus before entering the orbita at its apex (**Table 28.3**; **Figs. 28.14** and **28.15**).
  • The n. opticus (CN I) transmits images from the retina.
  • The n. oculomotorius (CN III), n. trochlearis (CN IV), and n. abducens (CN VI) innervate the extraocular muscles.

• The n. ophthalmicus of the n. trigeminus (CN V₁) carries general sensory fibers from structures in the orbit and distributes postganglionic autonomic fibers to target organs of the orbita and face.
• The n. facialis (CN VII) provides secretomotor (parasympathetic) innervation to the gl. lacrimalis.
— Autonomic innervation of structures in the orbita includes the following:
  • Sympathetic fibers from the plexus caroticus innervate the corpus ciliare and m. dilatator pupillae (responsible for pupillary dilation).
  • Parasympathetic fibers from the n. oculomotorius (CN III) synapse in the ganglion ciliare and travel via the nn. ciliares breves to innervate the corpus ciliare and m. sphincter pupillae (responsible for pupil constriction).
  • Parasympathetic fibers from the n. facialis (CN VII) synapse in the ganglion pterygopalatinum and travel via the n. zygomaticus (CN V₂) to innervate the gl. lacrimalis (responsible for tear secretion).

BOX 28.6: CLINICAL CORRELATION

HORNER'S SYNDROME

Horner's syndrome is a kaleidoscope of symptoms resulting from disruption of the truncus sympathicus cervicalis in the neck. The absence of sympathetic innervation is manifested on the affected side of the face as pupillary constriction (miosis), a sunken eye (enophthalmos), drooping of the palpebra superior (ptosis), loss of sweating (anhidrosis), and vasodilation.

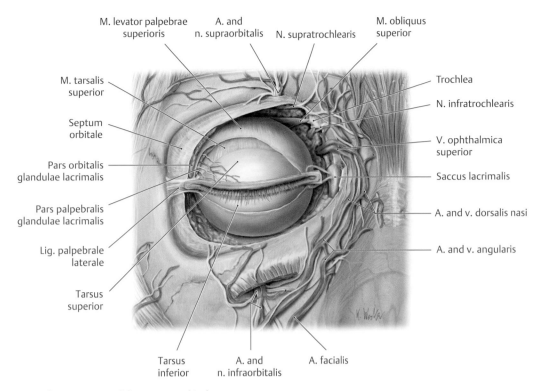

M. levator palpebrae superioris
A. and n. supraorbitalis
N. supratrochlearis
M. obliquus superior
M. tarsalis superior
Trochlea
N. infratrochlearis
Septum orbitale
V. ophthalmica superior
Pars orbitalis glandulae lacrimalis
Saccus lacrimalis
Pars palpebralis glandulae lacrimalis
A. and v. dorsalis nasi
Lig. palpebrale laterale
A. and v. angularis
Tarsus superior
Tarsus inferior
A. and n. infraorbitalis
A. facialis

Fig. 28.11 Neurovascular structures of the septum orbitale
Anterior orbital structures have been exposed by partial removal of the septum orbitale. (From Schuenke M, Schulte E, Schumacher U. THIEME Atlas of Anatomy, Vol 3. Illustrations by Voll M and Wesker K. 3rd ed. New York: Thieme Publishers; 2020.)

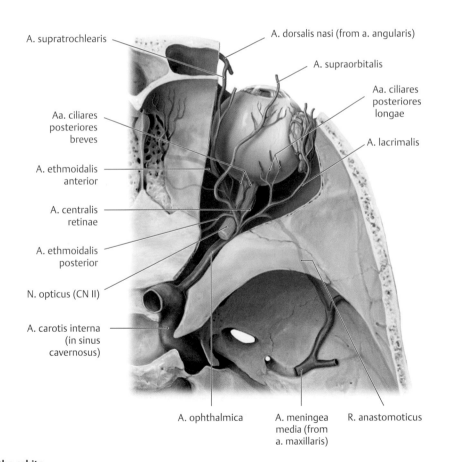

A. supratrochlearis
A. dorsalis nasi (from a. angularis)
A. supraorbitalis
Aa. ciliares posteriores longae
Aa. ciliares posteriores breves
A. lacrimalis
A. ethmoidalis anterior
A. centralis retinae
A. ethmoidalis posterior
N. opticus (CN II)
A. carotis interna (in sinus cavernosus)
A. ophthalmica
A. meningea media (from a. maxillaris)
R. anastomoticus

Fig. 28.12 Arteries of the orbita
Right orbita, superior view. *Opened:* Canalis opticus and paries superior orbitae. (From Schuenke M, Schulte E, Schumacher U. THIEME Atlas of Anatomy, Vol 3. Illustrations by Voll M and Wesker K. 3rd ed. New York: Thieme Publishers; 2020.)

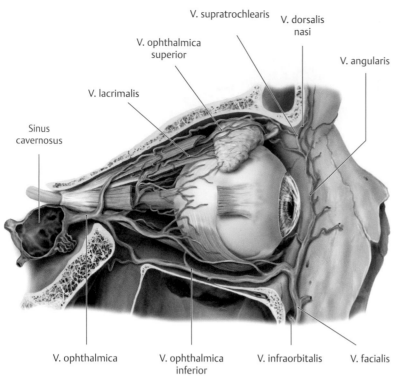

V. supratrochlearis   V. dorsalis nasi

V. ophthalmica superior

V. lacrimalis

V. angularis

Sinus cavernosus

Fig. 28.13 Veins of the orbita
Right orbita, lateral view. *Removed:* Paries lateralis orbitae. *Opened:* Sinus maxillaris. (From Schuenke M, Schulte E, Schumacher U. THIEME Atlas of Anatomy, Vol 3. Illustrations by Voll M and Wesker K. 3rd ed. New York: Thieme Publishers; 2020.)

V. ophthalmica   V. ophthalmica inferior   V. infraorbitalis   V. facialis

Table 28.3 Nerves of the Orbita

Nerve	Nerve Fibers	Distribution
N. opticus (CN II)	Special sensory for vision	Retina
N. oculomotorius (CN III)	Somatic motor	Muscles of the orbita, except the m. rectus lateralis and m. obliquus superior
	Parasympathetic: synapse in ganglion ciliare; postsynaptic fibers travel with n. nasociliaris (CN V$_1$)	M. sphincter pupillae and corpus ciliare
N. trochlearis (CN IV)	Somatic motor	M. obliquus superior
N. ophthalmicus (CN V$_1$)		
N. lacrimalis	General sensory	Gl. lacrimalis, upper lateral bulbus oculi
N. frontalis		
- N. supratrochlearis	General sensory	Anterior scalp
- N. supraorbitalis	General sensory	Anterior scalp
Nn. ciliares breves	General sensory Parasympathetic (CN III) and sympathetic	Corpus ciliare and iris
N. nasociliaris		
- N. ethmoidalis anterior and posterior	General sensory	Cavitas nasi, sinus ethmoidalis and sinus sphenoidalis
- N. infratrochlearis	General sensory	Nasus externus, conjunctiva, saccus lacrimalis
- Nn. ciliares longi	General sensory Sympathetic (plexus caroticus)	Iris and cornea M. dilatator pupillae
N. abducens (CN VI)	Somatic motor	M. rectus lateralis
N. facialis (CN VII)	Parasympathetic: synapse in ganglion pterygopalatinum; postsynaptic fibers travel with n. zygomaticus (CN V$_2$)	Gl. lacrimalis

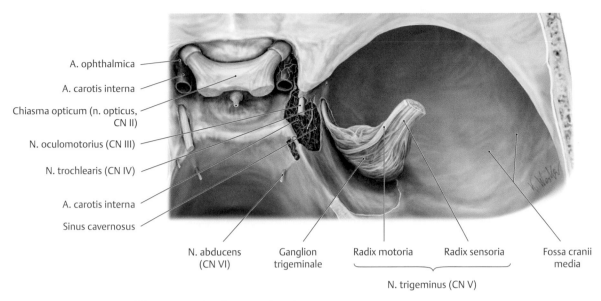

A. ophthalmica

A. carotis interna

Chiasma opticum (n. opticus, CN II)

N. oculomotorius (CN III)

N. trochlearis (CN IV)

A. carotis interna

Sinus cavernosus

N. abducens (CN VI)

Ganglion trigeminale

Radix motoria

Radix sensoria

Fossa cranii media

N. trigeminus (CN V)

Fig. 28.14 Intracavernous course of the nn. craniales that enter the orbita
Superior view of the sella turcica and fossa cranii media, right side. The lateral and superior walls of the sinus cavernosus have been opened and the ganglion trigeminale has been retracted laterally. The three nn. craniales that supply the ocular muscles (CN III, CN IV, and CN VI) pass through the sinus cavernosus with CN V$_1$ and CN V$_2$ and the a. carotis interna. All of the nerves course along the lateral wall of the sinus except CN VI, which runs directly through the sinus in close proximity to the artery. Because of this relationship, the CN VI may be damaged as a result of a sinus thrombosis or an intracavernous aneurysm of the a. carotis interna. (From Gilroy AM et al. Atlas of Anatomy. 4th ed. 2020. Based on: Schuenke M, Schulte E, Schumacher U. THIEME Atlas of Anatomy. Head, Neck, and Neuroanatomy. Illustrations by Voll M and Wesker K. 3rd ed. New York: Thieme Medical Publishers; 2020.)

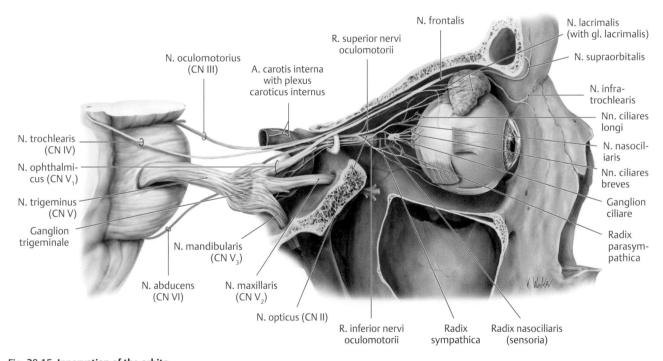

N. frontalis

N. lacrimalis (with gl. lacrimalis)

R. superior nervi oculomotorii

N. supraorbitalis

N. oculomotorius (CN III)

A. carotis interna with plexus caroticus internus

N. infra-trochlearis

Nn. ciliares longi

N. trochlearis (CN IV)

N. ophthalmi-cus (CN V$_1$)

N. nasoci-liaris

N. trigeminus (CN V)

Nn. ciliares breves

Ganglion trigeminale

Ganglion ciliare

N. mandibularis (CN V$_3$)

Radix parasym-pathica

N. abducens (CN VI)

N. maxillaris (CN V$_2$)

N. opticus (CN II)

R. inferior nervi oculomotorii

Radix sympathica

Radix nasociliaris (sensoria)

Fig. 28.15 Innervation of the orbita
Right orbita, lateral view. *Removed:* Temporal bony wall. (From Schuenke M, Schulte E, Schumacher U. THIEME Atlas of Anatomy, Vol 3. Illustrations by Voll M and Wesker K. 3rd ed. New York: Thieme Publishers; 2020.)

28.2   The Ear (Auris)

The ear (auris), which contains the organs for hearing and equilibrium, is divided into auris externa, auris media, and auris interna (**Fig. 28.16**).

The External Ear (Auris Externa)

The external ear (auris externa) collects and conducts sound.
— The auricula, the visible external part of the ear, is composed mostly of a skeleton of elastic cartilage that is covered by skin (**Fig. 28.17**).
  • Inferiorly is the soft (non-cartilaginous) **lobule**.
  • Anteriorly, the small part projecting posteriorly over the opening of the auditory canal is the **tragus**, which is separated from the **antitragus** by a small notch.
  • The posterior margin of the auricle is defined by the **helix**, which curves around the **scapha** and ends at the **concha**, a depression at the entrance to the auditory canal.
  • The rim of the **antihelix** begins at the antitragus and curves superiorly, forming the **cymba concha**. Superiorly its crura diverge to form the **fossa triangularis**.
— The **meatus acusticus externus** (external auditory canal), a canal that extends 2 to 3 cm from the auricula to the tympanic membrane, conducts sound waves toward the auris media. The outer third of the canal is cartilaginous, and the inner two thirds are formed by the os temporale. Gll. ceruminosae and gll. sebaceae in the subcutaneous tissue lining the cartilaginous part secrete earwax.

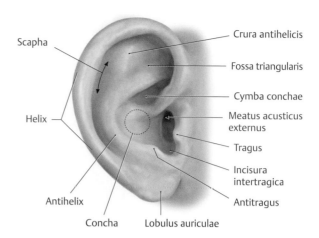

Fig. 28.17 Structure of the auricula
Right auricula, lateral view. (From Gilroy AM et al. Atlas of Anatomy. 4th ed. 2020. Based on: Schuenke M, Schulte E, Schumacher U. THIEME Atlas of Anatomy. Head, Neck, and Neuroanatomy. Illustrations by Voll M and Wesker K. 3rd ed. New York: Thieme Medical Publishers; 2020.)

— The **membrana tympanica**, a thin, transparent membrane, separates the auris externa and auris media.
  • Skin covers the membrana tympanica externally, and a mucous membrane lines it internally.
  • The concave outer surface of the membrane has a central conelike depression, the **umbo**.
  • A thin, superior portion of the membrane, the **flaccid part** (pars flaccida), is distinct from the rest of the membrane, the **tense part** (pars tensa).

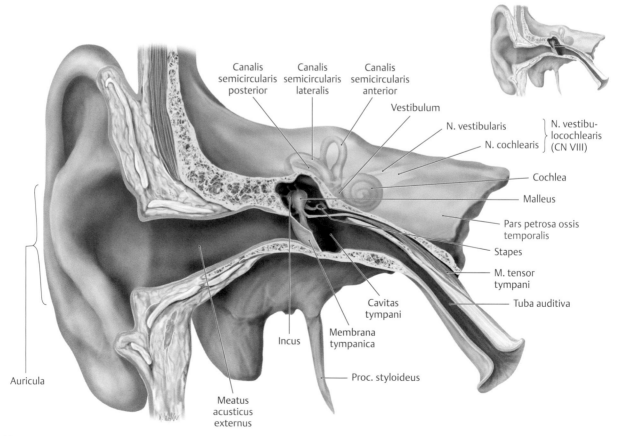

Fig. 28.16 Ear
Coronal section through the right ear, anterior view. (From Schuenke M, Schulte E, Schumacher U. THIEME Atlas of Anatomy, Vol 3. Illustrations by Voll M and Wesker K. 3rd ed. New York: Thieme Publishers; 2020.)

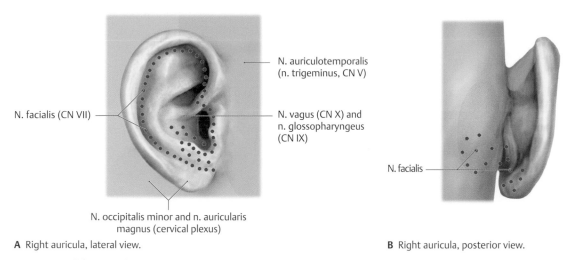

N. auriculotemporalis
(n. trigeminus, CN V)

N. facialis (CN VII)

N. vagus (CN X) and
n. glossopharyngeus
(CN IX)

N. occipitalis minor and n. auricularis
magnus (cervical plexus)

A Right auricula, lateral view.

N. facialis

B Right auricula, posterior view.

Fig. 28.18 Innervation of the auricula
(From Schuenke M, Schulte E, Schumacher U. THIEME Atlas of Anatomy, Vol 3. Illustrations by Voll M and Wesker K. 3rd ed. New York: Thieme Publishers; 2020.)

— A. auricularis posterior and a. auricularis anterior, branches of the a. temporalis superficialis, supply the auris externa.
— Sensation from the auris externa is transmitted by the cervical plexus and three cranial nerves **(Fig. 28.18)**:
  • the n. auricularis magnus (cervical plexus) from the auricula;
  • the n. auriculotemporalis, a branch of CN V_3, from the auricula and external surface of the membrana tympanica;
  • the n. auricularis of the n. vagus (CN X) from the external surface of the membrana tympanica; and
  • the n. glossopharyngeus (CN IX) from the internal surface of the membrana tympanica.

The Middle Ear (Auris Media)

— The middle ear (auris media), also known as the **cavitas tympani**, is an air-filled chamber housed in the pars petrosa of the os temporale **(Figs. 28.19, 28.20, 28.21)**.
  • Anteriorly, a **tuba auditiva**, which connects the cavitas tympani to the nasopharynx, helps equalize pressure in the auris media.
  • Posteriorly, the **aditus** (inlet) to the **mastoid antrum** (a cavity in the proc. mastoideus of os temporale) connects the cavitas tympani to the bony meshwork of **cellulae mastoideae**.

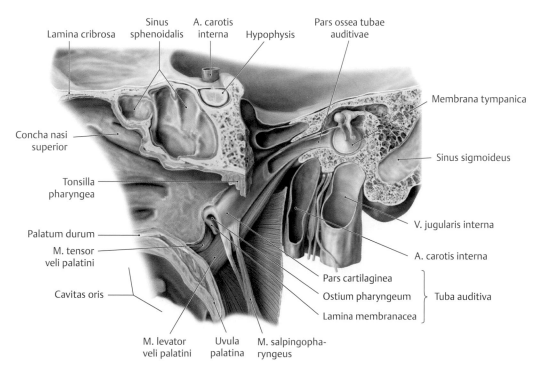

Lamina cribrosa

Sinus sphenoidalis

A. carotis interna

Hypophysis

Pars ossea tubae auditivae

Membrana tympanica

Concha nasi superior

Sinus sigmoideus

Tonsilla pharyngea

Palatum durum

M. tensor veli palatini

V. jugularis interna

A. carotis interna

Cavitas oris

Pars cartilaginea
Ostium pharyngeum   } Tuba auditiva
Lamina membranacea

M. levator veli palatini

Uvula palatina

M. salpingopharyngeus

Fig. 28.19 Cavitas tympani and tuba auditiva
Medial view of opened cavitas tympani. (From Gilroy AM et al. Atlas of Anatomy. 4th ed. 2020. Based on: Schuenke M, Schulte E, Schumacher U. THIEME Atlas of Anatomy. Head, Neck, and Neuroanatomy. Illustrations by Voll M and Wesker K. 3rd ed. New York: Thieme Medical Publishers; 2020.)

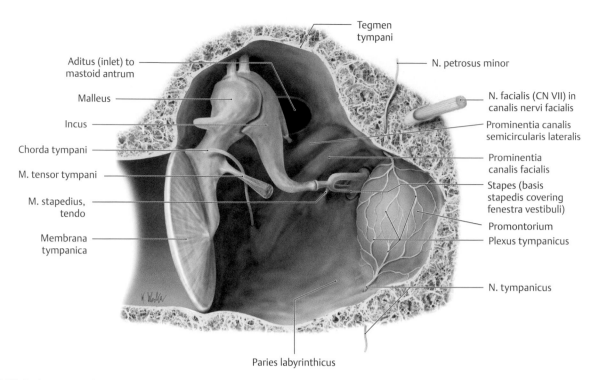

Fig. 28.20 Cavitas tympani
Right cavitas tympani, anterior view. *Removed:* Anterior wall. (From Gilroy AM et al. Atlas of Anatomy. 4th ed. 2020. Based on: Schuenke M, Schulte E, Schumacher U. THIEME Atlas of Anatomy. Head, Neck, and Neuroanatomy. Illustrations by Voll M and Wesker K. 3rd ed. New York: Thieme Medical Publishers; 2020.)

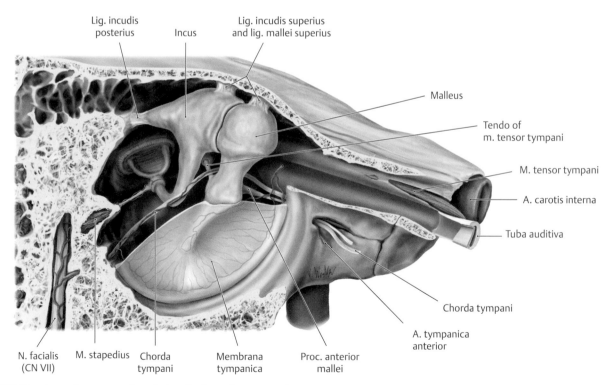

Fig. 28.21 Muscles and neurovascular relations in the cavitas tympani
Right auris media, lateral view. (From Schuenke M, Schulte E, Schumacher U. THIEME Atlas of Anatomy, Vol 3. Illustrations by Voll M and Wesker K. 3rd ed. New York: Thieme Publishers; 2020.)

- A thin bony plate, the **tegmen tympani**, forms the roof of the cavitas tympani and separates it from the fossa cranii media.
- The medial wall, which separates the cavitas tympani from the auris interna, has a **promontorium**, covered by the plexus tympanicus, and two openings, the **fenestra vestibuli** and **fenestra cochleae** (see Fig. 28.20).
- The **ossicula auditus**, the **malleus**, **incus**, and **stapes** bones of the auris media, articulate with each other through synovial joints and form a bony chain between the membrana tympanica and the fenestra vestibuli of the auris interna.
  - The manubrium mallei is embedded in the membrana tympanica, and its head articulates with the incus.
  - The **incus** articulates with the malleus and stapes.
  - The **caput stapedis** articulates with the incus, and its base fits into the fenestra vestibuli of the labyrinthus osseus of the auris interna.
- Muscles of the auris media dampen the movements of the ossicula auditus, thereby lessening the sound transmitted from the auris externa.
  - The **m. tensor tympani**, which is innervated by a branch of the n. mandibularis (CN V₃), lessens the damage from loud sounds by tensing the membrana tympanica.
  - The **m. stapedius**, which is innervated by a branch of the n. facialis (CN VII), dampens the vibrations of the stapes on the fenestra vestibuli.
- The aa. pharyngea ascendens, a. maxillaris, and a. auricularis posterior from the a. carotis externa and a small branch of the a. carotis interna supply the auris media.
- The chorda tympani, a branch of the n. facialis (CN VII), has no branches in the auris media but passes between the malleus and incus to exit the cavity through a small opening in the os temporale.
- The n. glossopharyngeus (CN IX) transmits sensation from the cavitas tympani and tuba auditiva. Preganglionic parasympathetic fibers carried in the n. tympanicus (a branch of the n. glossopharyngeus) synapse in the ganglion oticum. The postganglionic fibers join with sympathetic fibers of the plexus carotis internus to form the plexus tympanicus (see **Fig. 26.29**).

BOX 28.7: CLINICAL CORRELATION

OTITIS MEDIA

Otitis media is an infection of the auris media that occurs commonly in children often following an upper respiratory tract infection. Fluid that accumulates in the auris media can temporarily diminish hearing, and inflammation of the lining of the cavitas tympani can block the tuba auditiva.

BOX 28.8: CLINICAL CORRELATION

HYPERACUSIS

The m. stapedius protects the delicate auris interna by modifying the vibrations of very loud sounds as they are transmitted through the auris media to the stapes. Paralysis of the muscle resulting from a lesion of the n. facialis causes an extreme sensitivity to sound, a condition known as hyperacusis.

The Internal Ear (Auris Interna)

- The internal ear (auris interna), which contains the organ for hearing, the auditory apparatus, and the organ for balance, the vestibular apparatus, is encased within the pars petrosa of os temporale (**Figs. 28.22** and **28.23**) and consists of the following:
  - A bony **otic capsule**, which forms the walls of the labyrinthus osseus

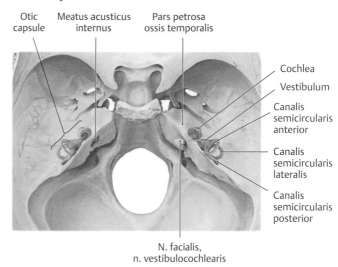

Fig. 28.22 Projection of the otic capsule of the inner ear onto the skull
Pars petrosa ossis temporalis, superior view. (From Schuenke M, Schulte E, Schumacher U. THIEME Atlas of Anatomy, Vol 3. Illustrations by Voll M and Wesker K. 3rd ed. New York: Thieme Publishers; 2020.)

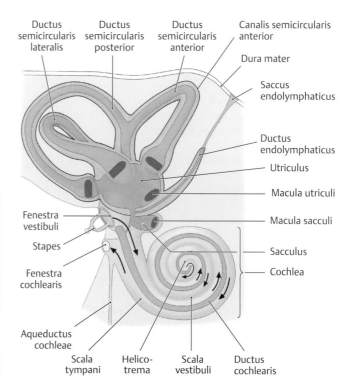

Fig. 28.23 Schematic of the auris interna
Right lateral view. The auris interna is embedded within the pars petrosa ossis temporalis. It is composed of a labyrinthus membranaceus filled with endolympha floating within a similarly shaped labyrinthus osseus filled with perilympha. (From Schuenke M, Schulte E, Schumacher U. THIEME Atlas of Anatomy, Vol 3. Illustrations by Voll M and Wesker K. 3rd ed. New York: Thieme Publishers; 2020.)

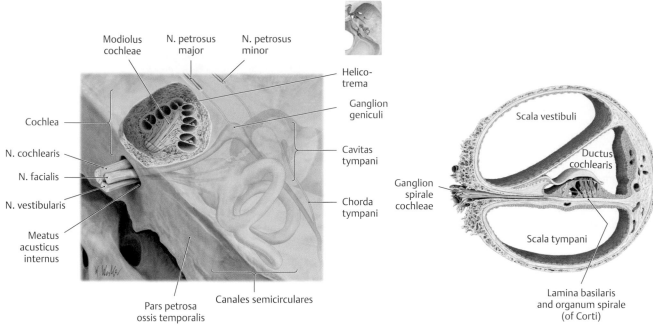

A Location of the cochlea. Superior view of the pars petrosa ossis temporalis with the cochlea sectioned transversely.

B Compartments of the canalis spiralis cochleae, cross section.

Fig. 28.24 Auditory apparatus
(From Schuenke M, Schulte E, Schumacher U. THIEME Atlas of Anatomy, Vol 3. Illustrations by Voll M and Wesker K. 3rd ed. New York: Thieme Publishers; 2020.)

- A **labyrinthus osseus**, a series of chambers and canals within the otic capsule containing the fluid **perilympha**. It includes the **cochlea**, the **vestibulum**, and the **canales semicirculares**.
- A **labyrinthus membranaceus**, a series of sacs and ducts suspended within the labyrinthus osseus, and filled with a fluid, **endolympha**. The labyrinthus membranaceus is made up of
  - the **ductus cochlearis** contained within the cochlea,
  - the **utriculus** and **sacculus** contained within the vestibulum, and
  - the **ductus semicirculares** contained within the canales semicirculares.
- The auditory apparatus consists of the following:
  - The **cochlea**, a space within the labyrinthus osseus that includes the bony **canalis spiralis cochleae**, which makes 2.5 turns around its axis, the **modiolus (Fig. 28.24)**. The basal turn of the cochlea forms the promontory on the medial wall of the auris media and contains the fenestra cochleae, which is closed by a membrane.
  - The **ductus cochlearis**, part of the labyrinthus membranaceus, which is a blind-ended duct filled with endolympha and suspended within the canalis cochleae **(Fig. 28.24)**:
    - The ductus cochlearis divides the canalis cochleae into two channels, the **scala vestibuli** and **scala tympani**, which are continuous with each other at the helicotrema, a space at the apex of the canal.
    - At the base of the cochlea, the scala vestibuli lies against the fenestra vestibuli, and the scala tympani lies against the fenestra cochleae.
  - The **organum spirale** (of Corti), which contains the sensory receptors for hearing, and is embedded in the **basement membrane** on the floor of the ductus cochlearis

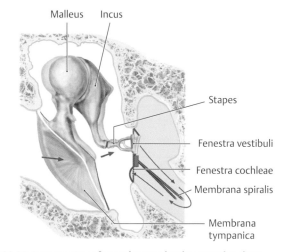

Fig. 28.25 Propagation of sound waves by the ossicular chain
(From Schuenke M, Schulte E, Schumacher U. THIEME Atlas of Anatomy, Vol 3. Illustrations by Voll M and Wesker K. 3rd ed. New York: Thieme Publishers; 2020.)

- The sequence of sound transmission through the ear involves **(Fig. 28.25)** the following:
  1. Transmission of sound waves from the auris externa and meatus acusticus externus to the membrana tympanica of the auris media. The waves vibrate the ossicula auditus and, in turn, the fenestra vestibuli that is attached to the basis stapedis.
  2. Transmission of vibrations of the fenestra vestibuli to the perilympha of the scala vestibuli, which creates pressure waves that displace the basement membrane and organum

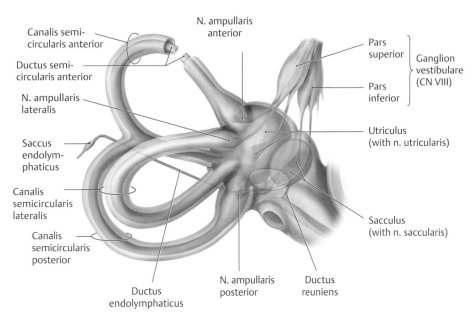

Fig. 28.26 Structure of the vestibular apparatus
(From Gilroy AM et al. Atlas of Anatomy. 4th ed. 2020. Based on: Schuenke M, Schulte E, Schumacher U. THIEME Atlas of Anatomy. Head, Neck, and Neuroanatomy. Illustrations by Voll M and Wesker K. 3rd ed. New York: Thieme Medical Publishers; 2020.)

spirale of the ductus cochlearis. Nerve endings in the organum spirale transmit impulses to the brain along the n. cochlearis.

3. Transmission of the pressure waves of the perilympha from the scala vestibuli along the scala tympani to the fenestra cochleae, with dissipation into the tympanic cavity.

— The vestibular apparatus consists of the following (**Fig. 28.26**):
  • The vestibulum of the labyrinthus osseus that communicates with the cochlea and canales semicirculares
    ◦ A small extension, the **aqueductus vestibuli**, communicates with the fossa cranii posterior and contains the **saccus endolymphaticus**, a membranous storage space for excess endolympha.
  • The utriculus and sacculus, part of the labyrinthus membranaceus, which lie within the vestibule
    ◦ The utriculus communicates with the ductus semicirculares; the saccule communicates with the ductus cochlearis.
    ◦ Both the utriculus and sacculus contain specialized sensory fields called **maculae**, which occupy different positions in space and are sensitive to movement of the endolympha in the horizontal and vertical planes.
  • Three canales semicirculares of the labyrinthus osseus, which are arranged perpendicular to one another and communicate with the vestibulum. Each canal has a swelling at one end, the **ampulla ossea**.
  • Three ductus semicirculares, parts of the labyrinthus membranaceus contained within the canales semicirculares, that communicate with the utricle
    ◦ An **ampulla** at one end of each ductus semicircularis contains the **crista ampullaris**, an area of sensory epithelium. The cristae ampullares respond to motion of the endolympha within the ducts caused by rotation of the head.
— The labyrinthus membranaceus receives its blood supply from the a. labyrinthi, a branch of the a. basilaris via its a. inferior anterior cerebelli.

— The **n. vestibularis** and **n. cochlearis** within the meatus acusticus internus form the n. vestibulocochlearis (CN VIII) (see **Fig. 26.27**).
  • The n. vestibularis innervates organs of the vestibular apparatus: the macula utriculi and macula sacculi and the cristae ampullares of the canales semicirculares. Neuron cell bodies lie within the ganglion vestibulare in the meatus acusticus internus.
  • The n. cochlearis innervates the organum spirale (of Corti) in the cochlea. Neuron cell bodies lie in the ganglion spirale of the cochlea at the modiolus cochleae.

BOX 28.9: CLINICAL CORRELATION

MENIERE'S DISEASE
Meniere's disease is an inner ear disorder resulting from blockage of the ductus cochlearis. Recurring episodes are characterized by tinnitus (ringing or buzzing in the ear), vertigo (the illusion of movement), and hearing loss. The hearing loss may fluctuate in intensity and from ear to ear but eventually becomes permanent.

BOX 28.10: CLINICAL CORRELATION

VERTIGO, TINNITUS, AND HEARING LOSS
Trauma to the ear can cause three types of symptoms: vertigo, tinnitus, and hearing loss. Vertigo refers to the illusion of movement, or dizziness, and results from injury to the canales semicirculares. Tinnitus refers to a ringing in the ears and is a disorder involving the ductus cochlearis. Causes of hearing loss can be either peripheral or centrally located. Conductive hearing loss occurs when there is impaired transmission of sound waves through the auditory canal to the ossicula auditus. Sensorineural hearing loss occurs when there is damage to the pathway between the cochlea and the brain.

29 Clinical Imaging Basics of the Head and Neck

Ultrasound provides excellent high-resolution detail of superficial structures of the neck (such as the thyroid (**Fig. 29.1**) and neck blood vessels) quickly, inexpensively, and safely—that is, without radiation exposure. Evaluation of deeper and intracranial structures requires computed tomography (CT) or magnetic resonance imaging (MRI). CT is fast, and best for emergent situations, such as trauma or other acute clinical scenarios (**Fig. 29.2**). CT is also superior in evaluation of the bones of the skull and skull base. MRI, however, is the workhorse for nonemergent imaging of the head and neck. MRI's superior soft tissue contrast makes it highly suitable for the brain, and for evaluating tumors of the head and neck (**Table 29.1**).

Vascular structures are an important focus in the radiology of the head and neck anatomy. Vessels can be imaged by ultrasound (**Fig. 29.3**), CT angiogram, MRI angiogram, or fluoroscopic catheter-based angiogram (**Fig. 29.4**). For evaluating the bone and air-filled spaces of the skull, CT provides the clearest detail (**Fig. 29.5**) but the soft tissues of the brain are seen best with MRI (**Figs. 29.6 and 29.7**).

X-rays of the skull have a limited clinical role but can be useful as a screening evaluation for developmental or acquired abnormalities of the cranium (such as abnormal skull shape or size) in children (**Fig. 29.8**).

Table 29.1 Suitability of Imaging Modalities for the Head and Neck

Modality	Clinical Uses
Radiographs (x-rays)	Used primarily for evaluation of the skull, and the soft tissues of the neck in children. Also used with angiographic studies (fluoroscopy) of the neck and intracranial vessels
CT (computed tomography)	Excellent for high detail evaluation of the skull and skull base, sinuses, cervical spine, and for evaluation of the deeper spaces of the neck
MRI (magnetic resonance imaging)	Excellent for evaluation of the soft tissues of the neck, orbitae, nn. craniales, and brain
Ultrasound	Used primarily for the thyroid and neck vessels. Also used for evaluation of other abnormalities in the more peripheral soft tissue structures of the neck especially in children (e.g., lymph nodes, branchial cleft cysts, thyroglossal duct cysts).

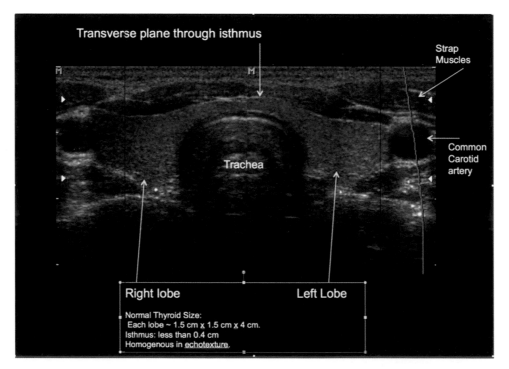

Fig. 29.1 Ultrasound of the glandula thyroidea
Transverse (axial) plane.
The gl. thyroidea is perfectly suited for ultrasound because of its position deep to the skin and subcutaneous tissues of the neck. This allows the use of a high-frequency linear transducer probe, which gives the highest resolution possible with ultrasound. The gl. thyroidea is homogeneously echoic, slightly more echogenic (whiter) than muscle. Note how the echogenic fascial planes delineate the strap muscles. The a. carotis communis appears black because of the fluid (blood) it contains. Ultrasound waves do not travel well through air, so the trachea is seen as a curved line anteriorly where the sound waves bounce off the air-filled structure. (Courtesy of Joseph Makris, MD, Baystate Medical Center.)

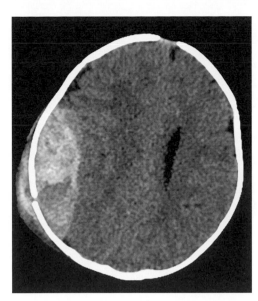

Fig. 29.2 CT of the head showing large epidural hematoma
This is a single axial image from a CT scan of the head in an unconscious patient after a severe motor vehicle accident. There is a large right-sided epidural hematoma (*white* = acute blood in the brain) compressing and displacing the brain. This patient requires immediate surgical evacuation of the hematoma. (Courtesy of Joseph Makris, MD, Baystate Medical Center.)

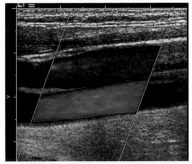

A Color Doppler is used to assess motion, more specifically, flow within a blood vessel. The trapezoid-shaped box within the image is the color Doppler "window." Outside of this window is simply gray scale ultrasound. Notice that in gray scale, blood vessels are *black*. The *red* and *blue* color scales indicate direction of flow and give an estimate of velocity. (From Schmidt G. Clinical Companions Ultrasound, Stuttgart: Thieme Publishers; 2007.)

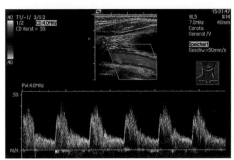

B Spectral ultrasound is used to give a graphical representation of the flow velocity vs. time. In this image, the spectral window is the small parallel lines placed within the deeper vessel. The waveform shown is arterial. Note the systolic peak and diastolic plateau. This deeper vessel is the a. carotis communis. (From Schmidt G. Clinical Companions Ultrasound. Stuttgart: Thieme Publishers; 2007.)

Fig. 29.3 Ultrasound of the a. carotis communis and v. jugularis
The skin surface is at the top of the image.

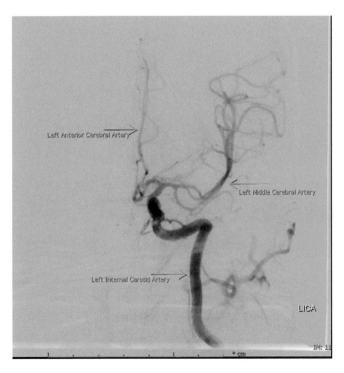

Fig. 29.4 Angiogram of the a. carotis interna sinistra
Anteroposterior view.
In this fluoroscopic study, bones are digitally subtracted in order to isolate the vessels. The image is a photo negative of the x-ray in which contrast in the vessels appears black. The catheter, inserted into the patient's groin and threaded through the aorta, enters the a. carotis interna sinistra. Contrast material is then injected directly into the artery, and fluoroscopic x-rays are taken of the area during the injection. Note that in the normal condition, blood vessels are smooth and without focal or diffuse dilation and the caliber of the vessels is uniform, tapering slightly as they progress distally, without narrowing or ending abruptly. (Courtesy of Joseph Makris, MD, Baystate Medical Center.)

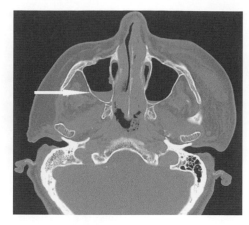

Fig. 29.5 CT of the head through the cavitas nasi and sinus maxillaris
Transverse (axial) plane, inferior view.
CT is superior for imaging the sinus paranasales because the high contrast readily differentiates air and bone from other structures. The air-filled sinuses are sharply contrasted against the soft tissues and even more so against the white bones. This feature also makes CT optimal for skull base imaging. Note in this patient there is some fluid in the right sinus maxillaris producing an air-fluid level (patient is supine, so the fluid settles in the posterior aspect of the sinus) and the mastoid air cells on the right are filled with fluid instead of air. Compare the normal left side with the abnormal right side. This patient has right maxillary sinusitis and mastoiditis. (Courtesy of Joseph Makris, MD, Baystate Medical Center.)

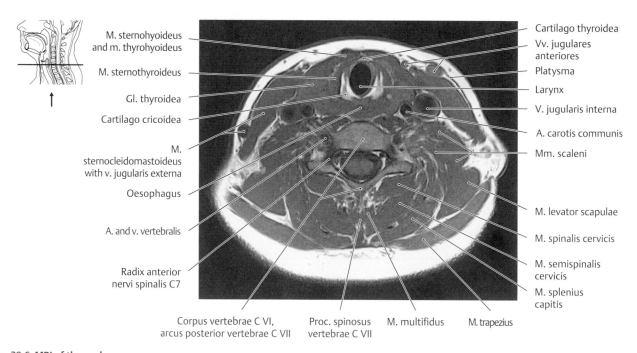

Fig. 29.6 MRI of the neck
Transverse (axial) plane, inferior view.
In this MRI sequence, fat is bright and muscles are *gray*. The fat planes between muscles allow differentiation of the adjacent muscles and identification of the spaces of the neck. (From Moeller TB, Reif E. Pocket Atlas of Sectional Anatomy, Vol 1, 4th ed. New York: Thieme Publishers; 2013.)

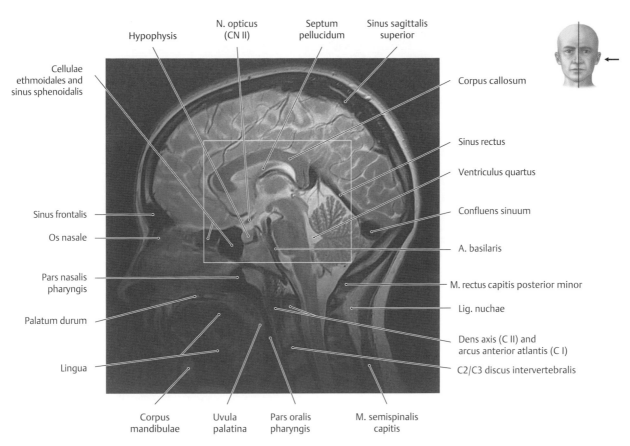

Fig. 29.7 MRI of the head

Midsagittal section.

In this MRI sequence, fluid is bright (note the bright CSF in the 4th ventricle) and soft tissues are shades of *gray*. However, note the subtle differences in gray scale that allow differentiation of the various soft tissues. This feature makes MRI superior to CT for use in imaging the brain. The brainstem structures and corpus callosum are sharply defined. The small amount of fluid interdigitating between the sulci of the cerebrum highlights the gross architecture of the brain. The layers of the scalp and skull are also well differentiated. (From Moeller TB, Reif E. Pocket Atlas of Sectional Anatomy, Vol 1, 4th ed. New York: Thieme Publishers; 2013.)

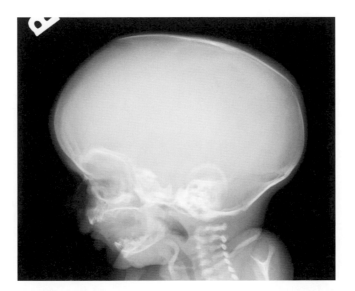

Fig. 29.8 Skull x-ray in infant

This infant was imaged for "abnormal head shape." Note the elongated appearance of the skull (scaphocephaly) in this child with sagittal suture craniosynostosis—premature fusion of the sagittal suture. The sutures of the skull normally remain open during childhood to allow for brain and head growth. Premature fusion of the sagittal suture limits transverse growth of the skull. To compensate, the skull grows abnormally long. These infants require surgical correction by re-opening the affected fused suture. (Courtesy of Joseph Makris, MD, Baystate Medical Center.)

Unit VIII   Review Questions: Head and Neck

1. Which bone of the skull contains the optic foramen, foramen ovale, and foramen spinosum?
   A. Os frontale
   B. Os temporale
   C. Os sphenoidale
   D. Os ethmoidale
   E. Os occipitale

2. The v. jugularis interna
   A. is located within the vagina carotica
   B. receives venous drainage from the brain
   C. is a tributary of the v. brachiocephalica
   D. receives blood from the v. facialis
   E. All of the above

3. The following structure runs within the falx cerebri.
   A. Sinus sagittalis inferior
   B. Sinus transversus
   C. Sinus sigmoideus
   D. Sinus cavernosus
   E. Ventriculus tertius

4. The a. vertebralis
   A. ascends through the foramina transversarium vertebrae cervicales
   B. arises from the first part of the a. axillaris
   C. terminates by joining with the a. cerebri posterior
   D. supplies branches to the gl. thyroidea
   E. supplies the posterior cerebral circulation

5. A man is taken to the emergency department after his wife noticed something wrong with the left side of his face during breakfast. He is found to have a problem with the nerve exiting the foramen stylomastoideum, a disorder called Bell's palsy. Which of the following problems is this patient likely to have?
   A. He is unable to open his left eye.
   B. He is unable to raise his eyebrow on the left side.
   C. He is unable to protrude his tongue to the right.
   D. He is unable to chew.
   E. He is unable to feel pressure on his left cheek.

6. A patient came to the emergency department with a broken mandibula resulting from an over-swung baseball bat. Which nerve is most likely affected by this injury?
   A. N. lingualis
   B. N. hypoglossus
   C. Rr. zygomatici of n. facialis
   D. N. alveolaris inferior
   E. Chorda tympani

7. The muscle of mastication that inserts into the proc. condylaris of the mandibula and its discus articularis and the capsula articularis of the art. temporomandibularis (TMJ) is the
   A. m. pterygoideus medialis
   B. m. pterygoideus lateralis
   C. m. temporalis
   D. m. masseter
   E. m. buccinator

8. A man develops acromegaly secondary to a tumor in his gl. pituitaria secreting growth hormone. A transsphenoidal resection of the tumor is scheduled. During this process, part of the inferior and posterior nasal septum is removed. Which bone forms this part of the septum nasi?
   A. Vomer
   B. Os ethmoidale
   C. Os palatinum
   D. Os temporale
   E. Os sphenoidale

9. The gl. lacrimalis is innervated by
   A. the n. facialis (VII)
   B. the postganglionic neurons with the cell bodies in the ganglion pterygopalatinum
   C. the parasympathetic neurons
   D. the n. lacrimalis
   E. All of the above

10. A 2-year-old boy seen by his pediatrician was noticeably irritable and tugging at his ear. When his mother asked him in a normal tone to sit quietly, he covered his ears screaming in pain and asked her not to shout at him. On exam he was found to have a fever, and his membrana tympanica was red and bulging. He was diagnosed with otitis media and started on antibiotics. The child's extreme sensitivity to sound (hyperacusis) suggests that the infection affected the m. stapedius. The nerve that innervates this muscle is a branch of what nerve?
    A. N. maxillaris
    B. N. mandibularis
    C. N. facialis
    D. N. glossopharyngeus
    E. N. vagus

11. The innervation for the m. sternothyroideus is the
    A. ansa cervicalis
    B. n. facialis
    C. n. hypoglossus
    D. n. accessorius
    E. n. laryngeus recurrens

12. A man was having an animated discussion with his friends when he started coughing after swallowing a piece of chicken at a fast-food restaurant. He soon became unable to speak or cough. Two paramedics who were taking a break at a nearby table quickly came to his help, and one stood behind the man and performed forceful abdominal thrusts (Heimlich maneuver). After several unsuccessful attempts to dislodge the aspirated food, the paramedics decide to perform an emergency airway procedure. What is the most superior site to perform this procedure so that the airway is secured below the plicae vocales?
    A. Superior to the os hyoideum
    B. Between the os hyoideum and the cartilago thyroidea
    C. Between the cartilago thyroidea and the cartilago cricoidea
    D. Between the cartilago thyroidea and the cartilago arytenoidea
    E. Superior to the manubrium in the fossa jugularis

13. A man is found to have a nodule in his neck. His calcitonin level is elevated, and a biopsy reveals medullary carcinoma of the gl. thyroidea. A thyroidectomy is performed. After surgery the patient's voice is found to be hoarse. What nerve was most likely injured during surgery?

   A. N. glossopharyyngeus
   B. N. hypoglossus
   C. Ansa cervicalis
   D. N. laryngeus recurrens
   E. N. phrenicus

14. A boy who has been vomiting is diagnosed with an obstruction in his gastrointestinal tract. He becomes severely dehydrated, and a sunken fonticulus anterior is felt. What is the youngest age at which this sign no longer would appear in a dehydrated child?

   A. 1 month
   B. 3 months
   C. 6 months
   D. 12 months
   E. 24 months

15. The nll. jugulodigastrici nodes that lie near the v. facialis and v. jugularis interna are also known as

   A. nll. parotidei
   B. nll. cervicales profundi superiores
   C. nll. cervicales profundi inferiores
   D. nll. retroauriculares
   E. nll. cervicales laterales

16. A patient develops severely elevated intracranial pressure due to a brain tumor obstructing the flow of cerebrospinal fluid (liquor cerebrospinalis, CSF). A shunt is placed to relieve this pressure because the CSF is blocked from being returned to the venous system. Where would this resorption normally take place?

   A. At the plexus choroideus
   B. At the foramen interventriculare
   C. At the aqueductus cerebri
   D. At the apertura lateralis
   E. At the granulationes arachnoideae

17. The n. vagus (CN X)

   A. leaves the skull through the carotid foramen
   B. innervates the sinus caroticus
   C. is transmitted through the fissura orbitalis superior
   D. innervates all of the muscles of the palatum molle
   E. None of the above

18. A 40-year-old obese woman has frequent headaches. At an eye exam, she is found to have papilledema (swelling of the discus opticus). It is suspected that she has elevated intracranial pressure. CT scan is negative for any strokes or tumors. She is diagnosed with idiopathic intracranial hypertension (pseudotumor cerebri). One complication of this disorder is downward displacement of the truncus encephali, which leads to stretching of the n. abducens. How would you diagnose if this complication occurred in this patient?

   A. She would be unable to move her eyes laterally.
   B. She would be unable to move her eyes medially.
   C. She would be unable to move her eyes superiorly.
   D. She would be unable to move her eyes inferiorly.
   E. She would be unable to rotate her eyes internally.

19. A 61-year-old firefighter was trapped for 12 hours in a collapsed building following an earthquake. Although he suffered a fractured tibia, the emergency department physician was also concerned about a deep scalp laceration that extended across the top of the patient's head. Infection from this laceration could spread

   A. to sinus durae matris through vv. emissariae
   B. into the neck in the loose areolar tissue
   C. laterally beyond the arcus zygomaticus
   D. to the spatium epidurale
   E. All of the above

20. A dentist who specializes in relief of facial pain is experimenting with a procedure to inject anesthetic into the fossa pterygopalatina through a lateral approach. The needle passes through the incisura mandibularis of the mandibula, traverses the fossa infratemporalis, and enters the fissura pterygomaxillaris. Which of the following structures would be at risk during the procedure?

   A. A. maxillaris
   B. N. mandibularis
   C. Plexus venosus pterygoideus
   D. Ganglion oticum
   E. All of the above

21. Which of the following drains into the meatus nasi inferior?

   A. Ductus nasolacrimalis
   B. Sinus frontalis
   C. Sinus ethmoidalis
   D. Sinus sphenoidalis
   E. Sinus maxillaris

22. Which of the following vessels accompanies the n. opticus through the canalis opticus?

   A. A. supratrochlearis
   B. A. supraorbitalis
   C. A. ophthalmicus
   D. V. ophthalmicus
   E. N. ophthalmicus

23. The nerve that innervates the musculus in the auris media that changes the shape of the membrana tympanica is the

   A. N. opticus
   B. N. oculomotorius
   C. N. trochlearis
   D. N. trigeminalis
   E. N. facialis

24. The branches of the plexus cervicalis

   A. originate from the anterior rami of C1 through C4
   B. innervate the m. sternocleidomastoideus
   C. carry preganglionic fibers that synapse in parasympathetic ganglia of the head
   D. include only nn. cutanei
   E. include the n. occipitalis major

25. Intubation is necessary during surgery because, due to muscle relaxants and other drugs administered during the procedure, patients are unable to fully relax the plicae vocales. Paralysis of which muscle prevents the relaxation of the plicae vocales?

   A. Mm. thyroarytenoidei
   B. Mm. cricoarytenoidei posteriores
   C. Mm. cricothyroidei
   D. Mm. arytenoidei transversi
   E. Mm. arytenoidei laterales

26. All of the innervation of the larynx, both sensory and motor, is supplied by
   A. the n. vagus
   B. the n. glossopharyngeus
   C. the n. laryngeus recurrens
   D. the n. laryngeus superior
   E. None of the above

27. Which is the only cartilago laryngis to completely encircle the airway?
   A. Cartilago thyroidea
   B. Cartilago cricoidea
   C. Cartilago epiglottica
   D. Cartilago arytenoidea
   E. Cartilago corniculata

28. A man is in a knife fight and receives a stab wound between the m. sternocleidomastoideus and the venter superior of the m. omohyoideus. Profuse bleeding ensues due to penetration of the a. carotis communis. Which structure within the same fascial sheath may also have been injured?
   A. V. jugularis externa
   B. N. phrenicus
   C. V. jugularis interna
   D. A. thyroidea superior
   E. Truncus sympathicus

29. A man with a long history of tobacco use goes to the dentist for a cleaning. The dentist notices a lesion on the lateral part of the body of the tongue and refers the patient to an otolaryngologist (ENT), who biopsies the lesion and determines that the patient has squamous cell carcinoma of the tongue. A CT of the patient's head and neck demonstrates metastasis to the nodi lymphoidei. The primary group of nodi lymphoidei for the drainage of this patient's cancer is
   A. Nll. cervicales profundi superiores
   B. Nll. cervicales profundi inferiores
   C. Nll. cervicales anteriores superficiales
   D. Nll. submandibulares
   E. Nll. submentales

30. All of the following bones form a part of the nasal walls or floor except
   A. Os frontale
   B. Os ethmoidale
   C. Maxilla
   D. Vomer
   E. Os palatinum

31. The action of the m. pterygoideus medius is to
   A. elevate the mandibula
   B. tense the palatum molle
   C. elevate the palatum molle
   D. elevate the os hyoideum
   E. retract the mandible

32. A 63-year-old man complains of difficulty speaking, chewing, and swallowing. On physical exam, you note that the patient's tongue is atrophied, and when asked to stick out his tongue and say "ahh," the patient's tongue deviates to the left. In obtaining a medical history, you learn that the patient underwent recent surgery on his a. carotis communis. Damage to which nerve has most likely caused the observed deficits?

   A. N. glossopharyngeus dexter
   B. N. hypoglossus dexter
   C. N. hypoglossus sinister
   D. N. lingualis dexter
   E. N. lingualis sinister

33. The n. mandibularis of the n. trigeminus (V$_3$) passes through the foramen ovale into the
   A. fossa infratemporalis
   B. fossa pterygopalatina
   C. orbita
   D. cavitas nasi
   E. cavitas oris

34. A man with hypertension and a long history of smoking suffers a series of transient ischemic attacks (TIAs). In the evaluation, a carotid bruit is heard. Further testing reveals severe stenosis of his a. carotis interna due to atherosclerosis. The TIAs were due to embolism of the atherosclerotic plaque. Which of the following is the first branch of the a. carotis interna likely to be affected by an embolism?
   A. A. thyroidea superior
   B. A. lingualis
   C. A. facialis
   D. A. maxillaris
   E. A. ophthalmica

35. A patient has thrombophlebitis of the right cavernous sinus due to a facial skin infection. The infection traveled via the v. angularis to the v. ophthalmica superior and into the sinus cavernosus. Which of the following is an additional symptom that this patient might exhibit?
   A. Jugular venous distension on the right
   B. Inability to smile
   C. Inability to chew on the right
   D. Loss of vision in the right eye
   E. Loss of sensation to the right cheek

36. Which of the following arteries is a branch of the a. carotis interna?
   A. A. cerebri posterior
   B. A. occipitalis
   C. A. labyrinthi
   D. A. ophthalmicus
   E. A. meningea media

37. A patient undergoes an ultrasound of the blood vessels in the neck. How can the sonographer quickly distinguish a normal v. jugularis from the a. carotis?
   A. The vein is blue on color doppler.
   B. The vein is easily collapsed by gentle pressure.
   C. The vein is black on grayscale ultrasound.
   D. The normal vein is echogenic.

38. A patient with hearing loss after trauma is suspected of having a fracture of the skull base and possible injury of the middle ear ossicles. Which imaging modality would be best to evaluate this?
   A. Ultrasound
   B. MRI
   C. X-ray
   D. Angiography
   E. CT

Answers and Explanations

1. **C.** The os sphenoidale forms the posterior orbita and the floor of the fossa cranii media between the os frontale and os temporale. Foramina of the os sphenoidale include the foramen opticum, foramen ovale, foramen rotundum, foramen spinosum, and fissura orbitalis superior (Section 24.1).

   A. The os frontale forms the forehead, the paries superior and margo supraorbitalis of the orbita, and the paries inferior of the fossa cranii anterior.

   B. The os temporale forms part of the fossa cranii media and fossa cranii posterior. Its foramina include the meatus acusticus internus and meatus acusticus externus, canalis caroticus, and foramen stylomastoideum.

   D. The os ethmoidale forms part of the fossa cranii anterior, paries medialis of the orbita, and parts of the septum nasi and paries lateralis nasi.

   E. The os occipitale forms most of the fossa cranii posterior. Its foramina include the foramen magnum, canalis condylaris, and foramen jugulare.

2. **E.** The v. jugularis interna is located within the vagina carotica (A), contains venous drainage from the brain (B), is a tributary of the v. brachiocephalica (C), and receives blood from the v. facialis (D) (Section 24.4).

   A. The v. jugularis interna runs within the vagina carotica with the a. carotis communis and n. vagus. B, C, and D are also correct (E).

   B. Cerebral venous drainage flow primarily to the vv. jugulares internae. A, C, and D are also correct (E).

   C. The vv. jugulares internae join the vv. subclaviae to form the vv. brachiocephalicae. A, B, and D are also correct (E).

   D. The v. facialis is a tributary of the v. jugularis interna. A through C are also correct (E).

3. **A.** The sinus sagittalis inferior runs in the inferior edge of the falx cerebri and ends as the sinus rectus (Section 26.1).

   B. The sinus transversus runs along the margo posterolateralis of the tentorium cerebelli.

   C. The sinus sigmoideus run in grooves of the os occipitale and os temporale.

   D. The sinus cavernosus lie lateral to the sella turcica between the meningeal and periosteal dura.

   E. The ventriculus tertius lies between the right and left thalami of the diencephalon.

4. **E.** The a. vertebralis dextra and sinistra join to form the a. basilaris. Together these arteries supply the posterior circulation of the brain (Section 26.2).

   A. The a. vertebralis ascends through the foramina transversarium vertebrae cervicales of C1–C6.

   B. The a. vertebralis is a branch of the a. subclavia.

   C. The a. vertebralis terminates by joining with the contralateral a. vertebralis to form the a. basilaris.

   D. The a. vertebralis does not supply branches to the gl. thyroidea.

5. **B.** CN VII, the n. facialis, exits the foramen stylomastoideum and is responsible for the muscles of facial expression, including the m. occipitofrontalis, which elevates the eyebrows (Section 26.3).

   A. The m. levator palpebrae superioris muscle elevates the eyelid and is innervated by CN III, the n. oculomotorius. In addition to the m. levator palpebrae superioris, the m. occipitofrontalis assists in raising the eyebrow, but because CN III is not affected the patient is able to open his eye. He is not, however, able to close his eye completely due to the paralysis of the m. orbicularis oculi.

   C. CN XII, the n. hypoglossus, innervates most of the tongue musculature. A left-sided hypoglossal injury would lead to the inability to protrude his tongue to the right.

   D. The mm. masticatori are innervated by the n. mandibularis division of CN V, the n. trigeminus. Although his ability to chew is unaffected, the patient does have some trouble eating because of paralysis to the m. buccinator, which assists in positioning food in the cavitas oris.

   E. Sensation to the cheek is conveyed through the n. maxillaris of the n. trigeminus.

6. **D.** The n. alveolaris inferior courses within the canalis mandibulae of the mandibula and would be injured in this patient (Section 26.3).

   A. The n. lingualis courses through the fossa infratemporalis and into the floor of the mouth.

   B. The n. hypoglossus courses anteriorly below the angulus mandibulae before entering the mouth at the margo posterior of the m. mylohyoideus.

   C. Rr. zygomatici of the n. facialis pass lateral to the m. masseter as they cross the cheek.

   E. The chorda tympani travels with the n. lingualis in the fossa infratemporalis and floor of the mouth.

7. **B.** The m. pterygoideus lateralis inserts into the proc. condylaris mandibulae and its discus articularis and the capsula articularis of the art. temporomandibularis (TMJ) (Section 27.2).

   A. The m. pterygoideus medialis inserts into the tuberositas pterygoidea on the medial surface of the angulus mandibulae.

   C. The m. temporalis inserts into the apex and medial surface of the proc. coronoideus mandibulae.

   D. The m. masseter inserts into the tuberositas masseterica at the angulus mandibulae.

   E. The m. buccinator inserts into the angulus oris and m. orbicularis oris.

8. **A.** The vomer makes up the inferior and posterior parts of the septum nasi (Section 27.7).

   B. The os ethmoidale, through its lamina perpendicularis, makes up the superior and posterior parts of the septum nasi.

   C. The os palatinum forms the posterior palate and does not contribute to the septum nasi.

   D. The os temporale forms the base and lateral side of the skull and does not contribute to the septum nasi.

   E. Although some of the os sphenoidale will be removed as a part of the procedure, it does not contribute to the septum nasi.

9. **E.** The gl. lacrimalis is innervated by visceral motor fibers (preganglionic parasympathetic [C]) of the n. petrosus major from the n. facialis (A). The postganglionic neuron is the n. zygomaticus of the n. maxillaris (V_2), which has its cell body in the ganglion pterygopalatinum (B) and is then distributed to the gl. lacrimalis. The n. lacrimalis

(D) provides sensory innervation to the lacrimal gland, conjunctiva, and upper eyelids (Section 26.3).

   A. The gl. lacrimalis is innervated by visceral motor fibers (preganglionic parasympathetic of the n. petrosus major of the n. facialis). B through D are also correct (E).

   B. The n. zygomaticus of the n. facialis carries postganglionic parasympathetic fibers from the ganglion pterygopalatinum to the gl. lacrimalis. A, C, and D are also correct (E).

   C. Parasympathetic fibers of the n. zygomaticus innervate the gl. lacrimalis. A, B, and D are also correct (E).

   D. The n. lacrimalis provides sensory innervation to the gl. lacrimalis, conjunctiva, and palpebrae superior. A through C are also correct (E).

10. **C.** The n. stapedius arises from the n. facialis in the canalis facialis to innervate the m. stapedius, which dampens sound waves transmitted through the auris media (Section 28.2).

   A. The n. maxillaris is distributed to the orbita, cavitas nasi, and cavitas oris, but it has no branches in the auris media.

   B. The n. mandibularis innervates the m. tensor tympani, which tenses the membrana tympanica.

   D. The n. glossopharyngeus transmits sensation from the cavitas tympani and tuba auditiva and joins with sympathetic fibers of the plexus caroticus and plexus caroticus internus to form the plexus tympanicus.

   E. The n. vagus transmits sensation from the external surface of the membrana tympanica.

11. **A.** The ansa cervicalis innervates all of the mm. infrahyoidei except the m. thyrohyoideus (Section 25.3 and **Table 21.4**).

   B. The r. cervicalis of n. facialis innervates the platysma.

   C. The n. hypoglossus innervates only the muscles of the tongue, including the m. genioglossus, m. hyoglossus, and intrinsic muscles of the tongue.

   D. The n. accessorius innervates the m. trapezius and the m. sternocleidomastoideus and contributes to the pharyngeal plexus that helps to control the m. pharyngis.

   E. The n. laryngeus recurrens, a branch of the n. vagus, innervates the intrinsic muscles of the larynx.

12. **C.** An emergency tracheotomy (or cricothyrotomy) is performed to secure an airway in a patient with respiratory failure who does not have time to have a procedure performed in the operating room. The quickest access to secure an airway is by incising the membrana cricothyroidea (Section 25.6).

   A. Superior to the hyoid bone is superior to the plicae vocales and is also a difficult access site given the presence of the mm. mylohyoidei.

   B. The membrana thyrohyoidea is between the os hyoideum and the cartilago thyroidea and is superior to the plicae vocales.

   D. Between the cartilago thyroidea and cartilago arytenoidea is too posterior to access the airway and is also at the level of the plicae vocales.

   E. Superior to the manubrium sterni in the fossa jugularis is a potential site for an airway (tracheostomy) but is more inferior to the membrane cricothyroidea. Also,

incising the tracheal cartilage or trying to access the airway between the cartilagines tracheales is too difficult without the benefit of being in the operating room. Another benefit of a cricothyrotomy versus a tracheostomy is that there are fewer structures at risk for injury such as blood vessels, the n. laryngeus recurrens, the gl. thyroidea, and the oesophagus.

13. **D.** The n. laryngeus recurrens is a branch of the n. vagus, which travels in the tracheoesophageal groove, lateral and posterior to the gl. thyroidea. Injury to this nerve causes hoarseness, among other complications (Sections 25.6 and 26.3).

   A., B., C., and **E.** The n. glossopharyngeus, n. hypoglossus, nerves of the ansa cervicalis, and the n. phrenicus do not travel close enough to the gl. thyroidea to be at risk during careful thyroid surgery.

14. **E.** The fonticulus anterior is the fibrous area at the junction of the os frontale and os parietale. It closes at 18 to 24 months of age (Section 24.1).

   A., B., C., D. The fonticulus anterior remains open until 18 to 24 months of age.

15. **B.** The nll. cervicales profundi superior lie between the v. jugularis and v. facialis and the venter posterior of m. digastricus (Section 24.5).

   A. The nll. parotidei are superficial nodes that overlie the gl. parotidea on the side of the face.

   C. The nll. cervicales profundi inferior lie in the neck near the inferior part of the v. jugularis interna.

   D. The nll. retroauriculares are superficial nodes that lie along the margo posterior of the auricula.

   E. The nll. cervicales laterales are superficial nodes that lie along the v. jugularis externa in the neck.

16. **E.** The CSF is reabsorbed into the venous system by the granulationes arachnoideae, which protrude into the sinus sagittalis superior (Section 26.2).

   A. The plexus choroideus is the site of CSF production in each of the four ventricles (the first and second [or lateral], the third, and the fourth).

   B. The foramen interventriculare is the communication between the ventriculi laterales.

   C. The aqueductus cerebri is the communication between the ventriculus tertius and ventriculus quartus.

   D. The aperturae laterales are the communication between the ventriculus quartus and the spatium subarachnoideum.

17. **E.** None of the answers above describes the n. vagus correctly (Section 26.3).

   A. The n. vagus leaves the skull through the foramen jugulare with the n. glossopharyngeus and n. accessorius.

   B. The sinus caroticus is innervated by the n. glossopharyngeus.

   C. The n. oculomotorius (III), n. trochlearis (IV), n. abducens (VI), n. ophthalmicus (V$_1$), and v. ophthalmica are transmitted through the fissura orbitalis superior.

   D. The n. vagus innervates all of the muscles of the palatum molle except the m. tensor veli palatini, which is supplied by the n. mandibularis of the n. trigeminus.

18. **A.** The n. abducens innervate the m. rectus lateralis, which move the eyes laterally (Section 26.3).

B. Medial movement of the eyes is controlled by the n. oculomotorius via the m. rectus medialis.

C. Superior movement of the eyes is controlled by the n. oculomotorius and n. trochlearis via the m. rectus superior and m. obliquus inferior.

D. Inferior movement of the eyes is controlled by the n. oculomotorius via the m. rectus inferior and m. obliquus superior.

E. Internal rotation of the eyes, also called intorsion or rotation along the long axis of the eye, is controlled by the n. trochlearis via the m. obliquus superior. This movement is normally prevented by the action of the m. obliquus inferior.

19. **A.** Vv. emissariae communicate with veins of the scalp and can carry infections intracranially to the sinus durae matris (Section 27.1).

B. The attachment of the m. occipitofrontalis to the skull prevents infections of the scalp from spreading into the neck.

C. The attachment of the aponeurosis epicranialis to the arci zygomatici prevents further lateral spread of infection.

D. Spread of infection intracranially occurs through the vv. emissariae, which communicate with the sinus durae matris, not with the spatium epidurale.

E. Not applicable.

20. **E.** The fossa infratemporale contains the a. maxillaris and many of its branches, n. mandibularis, the plexus pterygoideus, and the ganglion oticum, as well as the m. pterygoideus medialis and m. pterygoideus lateralis (Section 27.5).

A. The fossa infratemporale contains the a. maxillaris, but choices B, C, and D are also correct (E).

B. The fossa infratemporale contains the n. mandibularis, but choices A, C, and D are also correct (E).

C. The fossa infratemporale contains the plexus pterygoideus, but choices A, B, and D are also correct (E).

D. The fossa infratemporale contains the ganglion oticum, but choices A, B, and C are also correct (E).

21. **A.** The ductus nasolacrimalis drains tears from the medial corner of each eye into the meatus nasi inferior (Sections 27.7 and 28.1).

B. The sinus frontalis drains into the meatus nasi medius through a ductus frontonasalis.

C. The sinus ethmoidalis drains into the meatus nasi superior and meatus nasi medius.

D. The sinus sphenoidalis drains into the recessus sphenoethmoidalis in the posterosuperior part of the cavitas nasi.

E. The sinus maxillaris drains into the meatus nasi medius.

22. **C.** Only the a. ophthalmica and n. opticus enter the orbita through the canalis opticus (Sections 24.1 and 28.1).

A. The a. supratrochlearis is a branch of the a. ophthalmica in the orbita that supplies the scalp.

B. The a. supraorbitalis is a branch of the a. ophthalmica in the orbita that supplies the scalp.

D. The v. ophthalmicus enters the orbit through the fissura orbitalis superior.

E. The n. ophthalmicus (CN V$_1$) enters the orbita through the fissura orbitalis superior.

23. **D.** The n. mandibularis division of the n. trigeminus innervates the m. tensor tympani, which lessens damage from loud sounds by tensing the membrana tympanica (Section 28.2).

A. The n. opticus carries sensory innervation from the neural retina to the lateral geniculate nucleus.

B. The n. oculomotorius innervates most of the extraocular muscles of the eye and the intrinsic muscles of the eye.

C. The n. trochlearis innervates the m. obliquus superior of the eye.

E. The n. facialis innervates the m. stapedius, which dampens the vibrations of the stapes on the fenestra vestibuli.

24. **A.** The plexus cervicalis originates from the rami anteriores of C1–C4 (Section 25.4).

B. The n. accessorius (CN XI) innervates the m. sternocleidomastoideus.

C. Only the n. oculomotorius, n. facialis, and n. glossopharyngeus carry preganglionic parasympathetic nerves that synapse in the head.

D. The plexus cervicalis has both sensory and motor components. The sensory nerves of the plexus, the n. occipitalis minor, n. auricularis magnus, n. transversus cervicalis, and n. supraclavicularis innervate the skin of the anterior and lateral neck and lateral scalp. The ansa cervicalis, the motor part of the plexus, innervates most of the mm. infrahyoidei.

E. The n. occipitalis magnus is supplied by the rami posteriores of nn. spinales C1–C3 and is therefore not a branch of the plexus cervicalis.

25. **B.** The only muscles that relax the plicae vocales are the mm. cricoarytenoidei posteriores. Note that there are other results of anesthesia that also necessitate intubation (Section 25.6).

A. The m. thyroarytenoideus closes the plicae vocales.

C. The mm. cricothyroidei tighten the plicae vocales.

D. The mm. arytenoidei transversi close the plicae vocales.

E. The mm. arytenoidei laterales close the plicae vocales.

26. **A.** All of the innervation of the larynx, both sensory and motor, is supplied by the n. laryngeus superior and n. laryngeus recurrens from the n. vagus (CN X) (Section 25.6).

B. The n. glossopharyngeus (IX) innervates the cavitas tympani and tuba auditiva; the pharynx (sensory and motor), the tonsillae, palatum, posterior one third of the tongue (sensory and taste), and the m. stylopharyngeus. It also innervates the glomus caroticum and sinus caroticus.

C. The n. laryngeus recurrens is a branch of the n. vagus that innervates all of the muscles of the larynx except the m. cricothyroideus and carries sensation from the lower half of the larynx (from the vocal cords downward).

D. The n. laryngeus superior innervates the m. cricothyroideus, which helps to tense the plicae vocales, and provides sensation to the upper half of the larynx (above the vocal cords).

E. Not applicable.

27. **B.** The only cartilago laryngis to completely encircle the airway is the cartilago cricoidea (Section 25.6).

A. The U-shaped cartilago thyroidea has two laminae that join in the anterior midline to form a prominentia laryngea.

C. The cartilago epiglottica, a single leaf-shaped cartilage, forms the anterior wall of the aditus laryngis at the root of the tongue.

D. Paired arytenoid cartilages articulate with the superior borders of the laminae cartilagines cricoideae. Their proc. vocalis attach to the cartilago thyroidea through the ligg. vocales.

E. Cartilagenes corniculata appear as small tubercles within the plica aryepiglottica.

28. **C.** The a. carotis communis, v. jugularis interna, and n. vagus are contained within the vagina carotica (Section 25.2).

A. The v. jugularis externa is not within the vagina carotica.

B. The n. phrenicus lies on the m. scalenus anterior behind the vagina carotica.

D. The a. thyroidea superior is a branch of the a. carotis externa and does not travel in the vagina carotica.

E. The truncus sympathicus lies behind the vagina carotica.

29. **D.** The nll. submandibulares are the primary nodes of the lateral part of the body of the tongue (Section 27.8).

A. The nll. cervicales superiores profundi are the primary nodes of the root of the tongue.

B. The nll. cervicales inferiores profundi are the primary nodes of the medial parts of the body of the tongue.

C. The nll. cervicales anteriores superficiales are the primary nodes of the skin anterior muscles of the neck and are not the primary nodi lymphoidei of any part of the tongue.

E. The nll. submentales are the primary nodes of the apex linguae and frenulum linguae.

30. **A.** The os ethmoidale, maxilla, vomer, os palatinum, os lacrimale, os nasale, and conchae nasi inferiores form the bony skeleton of the cavitas nasi (Section 27.7).

B. The os ethmoidale forms the lamina cribrosa at the paries superior of the cavitas nasi, the concha nasi superior and concha nasi media of the lateral walls, and part of the septum nasi.

C. The maxilla forms the pars anterior of the palatum on the paries inferior of the cavitas nasi.

D. The vomer forms part of the septum nasi.

E. The os palatinum forms the pars posterior of the palatum on the paries inferior of the cavitas nasi.

31. **A.** The m. pterygoideus medialis forms a sling with the masseter muscle to elevate the mandibula (Section 27.2 and **Table 27.3**).

B. The m. tensor veli palatini tenses the palatum molle.

C. The m. levator veli palatini elevates the palatum molle.

D. The mm. suprahyoidei, including m. digastricus, m. geniohyoideus, m. stylohyoideus, and m. mylohyoideus, elevate the os hyoideum. The m. pterygoideus medialis can only elevate the os hyoideum secondarily by first elevating the mandibula.

E. The posterior part of the m. temporalis retracts the mandibula.

32. **C.** The n. hypoglossus (CN XII) innervates all muscles of the tongue except for the m. palatoglossus. When damaged, muscles on the affected side atrophy and fail to contribute to protrusion of the tongue. This causes the tongue to deviate to the side of the lesion (left side in this patient).

The nerve is at risk during surgery on the a. carotis communis because of its proximity to the bifurcatio carotidis (Section 26.3).

A. The m. stylopharyngeus is the only muscle innervated by the n. glossopharyngeus.

B. Damage to the n. hypoglossus dexter would cause atrophy of the right side of the tongue and deviation to the right side with protrusion.

D. The n. lingualis, a branch of n. mandibularis division of the n. trigeminus, transmits sensation from the anterior tongue. It also carries parasympathetic fibers via the chorda tympani to the gl. submandibularis and gl. sublingualis and taste from the anterior tongue.

E. The n. lingualis, a branch of n. mandibularis, transmits sensation from the anterior tongue. It also carries parasympathetic fibers via the chorda tympani to the gl. submandibularis and gl. sublingualis and taste from the anterior tongue.

33. **A.** The n. mandibularis enters the fossa infratemporale where it sends motor branches to mm. masticatori and sensory branches to the tongue, dentes mandibulares, cavitas oris, and skin of the lower and lateral face (Section 26.3).

B. The n. maxillaris division of the n. trigeminus nerve passes through the foramen rotundum to the fossa pterygopalatina.

C. The n. ophthalmicus branch of the n. trigeminus passes through the fissura orbitalis superior to the orbita.

D. The n. maxillaris of the n. trigeminus innervates the cavitas nasi.

E. The n. lingualis passes from the fossa infratemporale into the cavitas oris.

34. **E.** The aa. carotis internae do not have branches in the neck. The aa. ophthalmicae are the first major branches of the aa. carotis internae (Section 26.2).

A. The a. thyroidea superior is a branch of the a. carotis externa.

B. The a. lingualis is a branch of the a. carotis externa.

C. The a. facialis is a branch of the a. carotis externa.

D. The a. maxillaris is a branch of the a. carotis externa.

35. **E.** The sinus cavernosus contains the n. oculomotorius, n. trochlearis, n. abducens, n. ophthalmicus, and n. maxillaris divisions of the n. trigeminus. The n. maxillaris division of the n. trigeminus supplies sensation to the cheek (Section 26.1).

A. Jugular venous distension is caused by a decrease of venous return to the heart.

B. The inability to smile is caused by a lesion to the n. facialis.

C. The inability to chew is caused by a lesion to the n. mandibularis of the n. trigeminus.

D. Loss of vision is caused by a lesion to the n. opticus, which does not travel through the sinus cavernosus. Note that there are additional causes of loss of vision, none of which are related to the sinus cavernosus.

36. **D.** The a. ophthalmica is the first major branch of the a. carotis interna in the fossa cranii anterior (Section 24.3).

A. The a. cerebri posterior is the terminal branch of the a. basilaris.

B. The a. occipitalis is a branch of the a. carotis externa.

C. The a. labyrinthi is a branch of the a. basilaris.

E. The a. meningea media is a branch of the a. maxillaris, which is a branch of the a. carotis externa.

37. **B.** Ultrasound is a dynamic modality in which the structures are seen in real time as the sonographer manipulates the probe. Veins and arteries can be quickly and easily distinguished from each other by the application of gentle pressure on the probe. This will cause the veins with lower internal pressure to collapse temporarily, but the higher pressure arteries remain distended (Chapter 21).

A. The blue and red colors only indicate direction of blood flow relative to the transducer (red toward the transducer).

C. Although a normal vein is black (anechoic), a normal artery is black as well. Fluid, including un-clotted normal blood is black on grayscale ultrasound.

D. A normal vein is not echogenic. This would indicate a blood clot or other abnormality.

38. **E.** CT has excellent spatial resolution and is optimal for evaluating the bones of the skull base and assessing the anatomy/integrity of the tiny middle ear ossicles (Chapter 21).

A. Ultrasound would be a poor choice for bony evaluation and for deep structures.

B. Although MRI would be sensitive to the edema seen with skull base injuries, it has lower specificity for fractures and decreased spatial resolution compared with CT.

C. X-rays would not show the skull base or ossicles well, due to the overlapping cranium.

D. Angiography may be used to assess vascular integrity after trauma, but would not be helpful in this case.

Index

Note: Italicized page numbers represent clinical or developmental correlations and anatomic notes. Figures and tables are indicated by *f* and *t,* respectively, immediately following the page number.